Research Protocols for Ophthalmic Disease Mechanisms and Therapeutics: Glaucoma - Ocular Hypertension

Edited By

Najam A. Sharif

Vice President and Head of Research & Development
Nanoscope Therapeutics Inc. 2777 N. Stemmons Fwy,
Suite 1102, Dallas
TX-75207, USA

&

Sunny E. Ohia

Department of Pharmaceutical Sciences
College of Pharmacy and Health Sciences
Texas Southern University
Houston, Texas, USA

Research Protocols for Ophthalmic Disease Mechanisms and Therapeutics: Glaucoma - Ocular Hypertension

Editors: Najam A. Sharif & Sunny E. Ohia

ISBN (Online): 978-981-5324-33-4

ISBN (Print): 978-981-5324-34-1

ISBN (Paperback): 978-981-5324-35-8

First published in 2025.

Bentham Science Publishers Pte. Ltd.
No. 9 Raffles Place
Office No. 26-01
Singapore 048619
Singapore
Email: subscriptions@benthamscience.net

BENTHAM SCIENCE

CONTENTS

DEDICATION

This book is dedicated to God, my father (may his soul rest in peace, Amen), my mother, my siblings, my wife and children with whose blessings and support everything in my life has been rendered possible. *Najam A. Sharif*

Dedicated to my wife, Dr. Ekanem Ohia, and my children, Dr. Odochi Nwoko and Uchechukwu Ohia, Esq. *Sunny E. Ohia*

PREFACE

We are grateful for the opportunity to compile and edit this book, composed of two volumes, on materials and methods for conducting experiments to study the many aspects of the disease, ocular hypertension (OHT) and glaucoma, a constellation of potentially blinding diseases that afflict millions of patients worldwide. Additionally, it was important to guide readers about the drug / device discovery process and the basic aspects of drug development to treat the afore-mentioned eye diseases. Thus, salient features of Investigational New Drug (IND)-enabling studies for new compounds and devices are presented to underscore the ultimate purpose of the ocular research that is conducted in academia and industry, namely, to unearth mechanisms of ocular hypertensive disease and then find treatment options to mitigate and retard the disease process(es).

We have been conducting and supervising basic and applied ocular research for advancing knowledge about the pathogenesis of eye diseases, and drug discovery and development for more than three decades. Working in the pharmaceutical and academic arenas, respectively, and frequently guiding and mentoring junior staff, we realized there was a deficiency of a single source of key methods utilized for performing ocular pharmacology, disease mechanisms and therapeutics discovery research. To capture existing procedures and rapidly emerging techniques and technologies, we decided to develop this book. This project would not have been possible without the kind and generous help and support of our family members, Bentham Science Publishers and our many colleagues who have contributed to this endeavor. We have deliberately focused on OHT, which develops from elevated intraocular pressure (IOP) in the anterior chamber of the eye (ANCe) as a case study, since lowering and controlling IOP by pharmaceuticals, aqueous humor drainage devices and ocular surgery are the only currently approved medical treatments for OHT and for many forms of glaucoma. The topic of glaucomatous optic neuropathy (GON), which has several risk factors of which OHT is one, and that encompasses the many factors and events occurring at the optic nerve head, retina, optic nerve and the brain leading to potential blindness, will be covered in a follow-up book.

Protocols described in the various sections and chapters in the current two volumes cover a wide range of techniques that are currently being used in studying the anatomy, morphology, pathology, biochemistry, physiology, pharmacology, and molecular biology of the cells/tissues within the anterior chamber of the eye (ANCe). In Volume 1, Section 1, beginning with a brief review of the basic anatomy and physiology of the eye (Chapter 1), a treatise on research and development of drugs, their sources and screening paradigms *in vitro* and *in vivo* are described in Chapters 2 and 3. Since the majority of drugs used to treat elevated IOP engage with membranous and /or cytoplasmic receptors and/or enzymes, it is important to determine whether the tissues/cells contain the requisite drug targets. This is accomplished using specific protocols and a range of techniques (reverse transcriptase polymerase chain reaction [RT-PCR]; receptor binding; autoradiography and immunohistochemistry) that are described in Section 2 (Chapters 4-7). Once cellular binding site for target receptor/enzyme verification has been accomplished, it is necessary to demonstrate the functional activity associated with the target protein through drug-receptor engagement using well characterized reference compounds in suitable cell-based assays. Additional relevant cell types are also needed to potentially define off-target effects of test compounds and/or to find ocular cells that may contain the drug receptor/enzyme/transporter protein(s). This necessitates isolation, propagation and utility of cells from appropriate ANCe uveal tissues (*e.g.* cells from the ciliary muscle, ciliary processes, trabecular meshwork, Schlemm's canal) and other cells derived from the sclera, corneal and conjunctival tissues.

Suitable protocols needed for such endeavors are described in Section 3 (Chapters 8-13).

Cell- and tissue-based assays to permit interrogation of receptor/enzyme activity for compounds of interest are crucial in the quest to find new drugs for treating elevated IOP, and these are described in Section 4 (Chapters 14-24). Drug discovery screening, whether conducted manually or using automated high-through-screening platforms, requires the use of a broad range of biochemical and pharmacological techniques and technologies. Agonist or antagonist activity of reference and test compounds can be determined in isolated cells or tissues using a variety of functional parameters such as quantifying second messengers, cell impedance, cell volume changes, tissue contraction/relaxation, release of transmitters, cellular ionic changes, etc. The concentration-response data, including receptor/enzyme affinity, compound potency and intrinsic activity, can then help rank order compounds and find suitable hits for further optimization by the medicinal chemists. Once all the *in vitro* studies have been completed and suitable compounds selected to progress for testing in normal animals for ocular safety and tolerability, and then for efficacy, the more labor-intensive and expensive portion of drug/device discovery and development begins.

Although the *in vitro* pharmacological characterization of drug targets and test compounds is important, ultimately appropriate response(s) in animal models of disease dictates the final selection of a suitable lead compound, and back-ups, that can be further characterized via additional IND-enabling studies. These aspects are the subject matter covered in Volume 2 of this book. In the case of glaucoma/OHT, compounds should be safe (not causing eye irritation or other systemic/ central nervous system adverse effects) and be able to significantly lower and control IOP. Thus, Volume 2, Section 5 (Chapters 25-36) provides numerous protocols for such *in vivo* studies in various mammalian species (rodent, rabbit, dog, monkey) using induced methods to raise IOP in various animals. Since the aim of the IOP-reducing drugs for treating OHT/glaucoma is to promote AQH outflow from the ANCe and/or to reduce AQH production, a specific protocol dealing with AQH drainage devices (Chapter 36) is also provided. In the modern age the use of genetic medicine has come to fruition. Along the way, the discovery of naturally occurring mouse models of glaucoma and development of new animal models of OHT using genetic engineering has also been accomplished, and these are described in Section 6 (Chapters 37-39).

Once compound ocular safety and tolerability has been established, and some relative efficacy in a few models of OHT demonstrated, the lead compound and any back-up compounds can now be progressed to a stage where an ultimate formulation is selected for all remaining studies. Typically, a safe and comfortable drug formulation suitable for topical ocular dosing is developed and appropriate pharmacokinetic, pharmacodynamic and toxicological studies performed on the lead compound. Such investigations can be performed using protocols described in Section 7 (Chapters 40-42). The results from the *in vitro* and *in vivo* studies performed for the IND-ready compound(s) or device(s) using validated protocols and standard operating procedures (SOPs) using Good Laboratory Practices (GLP) and/or Good Manufacturing Practices (GMP) can then be assembled into dossiers for submission to the regulatory authority under an IND application. These and other key regulatory considerations need to be addressed through appropriate communications and interactions with the health agency and are out of scope for the current book.

Finally, we surmised that in this technologically advanced age we should provide the modern researchers in ocular physiology and pharmacology new methods to help advance basic and applied eye research and thus help discover new drugs and treatments for OHT/glaucoma. To that end, Section 8 (Chapters 43-48) provides some new information on modern techniques and technologies addressing some novel avenues of eye research delving into gene and cell therapies and studying cell-to-cell communication via nanotubes and study of metabolomics of cells in the ANCe.

In conclusion, both clinical and basic science ocular researchers, graduate students, postdoctoral fellows, optometrists, and ophthalmologists should find this book to be a comprehensive and one-stop-resource for methodologies needed to study ocular structure and function of cells and tissues of the ANCe. The preservation of our most precious sense, eyesight, and its potential restoration in patients afflicted with blinding eye diseases such as OHT/glaucoma is a goal worthy of pursuit. We hope that this collection of protocols helps eye scientists achieve such audacious goals. We extend our thanks and gratitude to all the authors and the publisher for making this book a reality.

Najam A. Sharif
Vice President and Head of Research & Development
Nanoscope Therapeutics Inc. 2777 N. Stemmons Fwy
Suite 1102, Dallas
TX-75207, USA

&

Sunny E. Ohia
Department of Pharmaceutical Sciences
College of Pharmacy and Health Sciences
Texas Southern University
Houston, Texas, USA

List of Contributors

Anthonia Okolie	Department of Pharmaceutical Sciences, College of Pharmacy and Health Sciences, Texas Southern University, Houston, Texas, USA
Amy Chen	Department of Ophthalmology, Novartis Institute of Biomedical Research, 22 Windsor St. Cambridge, MA-02452, USA
Andrea M. Unser	Colleges of Nanoscale Science and Engineering, SUNY Polytechnic Institute, 257 Fuller Road, Albany 12203, New York, USA
Aparna Rao	Hyderabad Eye Research Foundation, , , , LV Prasad Eye Institute, Patia, Bhubaneswar, MTC Campus, Bhubaneswar, Odisha, India
Alyssa Hostert	Department of Pharmacy Sciences, School of Pharmacy and Health Professions, Creighton University, Omaha, Nebraska, USA
Anna Van Koeverden	Department of Optometry & Vision, 202 Berkeley St, Parkville, The University of Melbourne, Victoria 3010, Australia
Abdelrahman Anter	Bascom Palmer Eye Institute, University of Miami Miller School of Medicine, Miami, FL 33136, USA
Adnan Dibas	Nanoscope Technologies, 1312 Brown Trail, Bedford, TX 76022, USA
Alex Leung	UCL Institute of Ophthalmology, University College London, London, United Kingdom
Anna Mueller	Bascom Palmer Eye Institute, University of Miami Miller School of Medicine, Miami, FL 33136, USA
Brianna Caroline Afiat	Department of Optometry & Vision, 202 Berkeley St, Parkville, The University of Melbourne, Victoria 3010, Australia
Bang Viet Bui	Department of Optometry & Vision, 202 Berkeley St, Parkville, The University of Melbourne, Victoria 3010, Australia
Betsy Benitez	Miami Integrative Metabolomics Research Center, Miami, FL 33136, USA
Catherine A. Opere	Department of Pharmacy Sciences, School of Pharmacy and Health Professions, Creighton University, Omaha, Nebraska, USA
Christopher W. Wilson	Department of Ophthalmology, Novartis Institute of Biomedical Research, 22 Windsor St. Cambridge, MA-02452, USA
Christine Tram Oanh Nguyen	Department of Optometry & Vision, 202 Berkeley St, Parkville, The University of Melbourne, Victoria 3010, Australia
Carol B. Toris	Havener Eye Institute, Department of Ophthalmology and Visual Sciences, The Ohio State University Wexner Medical Center, 915 Olentangy River Rd, Suite 3010B, Columbus, OH 43212, USA
Charles E. Amankwa	Department of Pharmacology and Neuroscience and The North Texas Eye Research Institute, University of North Texas Health Science Center, Fort Worth, TX 76107, USA
Dorette Z. Ellis	Department of Pharmaceutical Sciences, University of North Texas System College of Pharmacy, North Texas Eye Research Institute, University of North Texas Health Science Center, Fort Worth, Texas, USA

Da Zhao	Department of Optometry & Vision, 202 Berkeley St, Parkville, The University of Melbourne, Victoria 3010, Australia
Dharmalingam Kuppamuthu	Department of Biotechnology, Aravind Medical Research Foundation - Affiliated to Alagappa University, Karaikudi, Tamil Nadu, India Department of Proteomics, Aravind Medical Research Foundation, Madurai, Tamil Nadu, India
Fatima Muili	Department of Pharmaceutical Sciences, College of Pharmacy and Health Sciences, Texas Southern University, Houston, Texas, USA
Fatima Shirazee	Department of Pathology and Molecular Medicine, McMaster University, Hamilton, Canada
Ganesh Prasanna	Department of Ophthalmology, Novartis Institute of Biomedical Research, 22 Windsor St. Cambridge, MA-02452, USA
Gowri Priya Chidambaranathan	Department of Immunology and Stem Cell Biology, Aravind Medical Research Foundation, Madurai, Tamil Nadu, India Department of Biotechnology, Aravind Medical Research Foundation - Affiliated to Alagappa University, Karaikudi, Tamil Nadu, India
Gulab Zode	Department of Pharmacology and Neuroscience and The North Texas Eye Research Institute, University of North Texas Health Science Center, Fort Worth, TX 76107, USA
Hanna Rao	Department of Arts and Science, McMaster University, Hamilton, Ontario, Canada
Iswarya Radhakrishnan	Department of Immunology and Stem Cell Biology, Aravind Medical Research Foundation, Madurai, Tamil Nadu, India Department of Biotechnology, Aravind Medical Research Foundation - Affiliated to Alagappa University, Karaikudi, Tamil Nadu, India
Isabella Moceri	Miami Integrative Metabolomics Research Center, Miami, FL, 33136, USA
J. Cameron Millar	North Texas Eye Research Institute (NTERI), Department of Pharmacology & Neuroscience, University of North Texas Health Science Center (UNTHSC), 3500 Camp Bowie Boulevard, Room IREB-511, Fort Worth, TX 76107, USA
Judith West-Mays	Department of Pathology and Molecular Medicine, McMaster University, Hamilton, Canada
James E. Chastain	Novartis Institutes for BioMedical Research (Retired), The Woodlands, 26 Dawning Flower Dr., The Woodlands, TX 77375, USA
Jack Hopkins	UCL Institute of Ophthalmology, University College London, London, United Kingdom
Karen Y. Torrejon	Colleges of Nanoscale Science and Engineering, SUNY Polytechnic Institute, 257 Fuller Road, Albany 12203, New York, USA
Kalu K. Ngele	Department of Pharmaceutical Sciences, College of Pharmacy and Health Sciences, Texas Southern University, Houston, Texas, USA
Krishnadas Subbaiah	Glaucoma Services, Aravind Eye Hospital and Post Graduate Institute of Ophthalmology, Madurai, Tamil Nadu, India

Len Pinchuk	Research & Development, InnFocus Inc. (A Santen Co.), 12415 S.W. 136 Ave., Unit 3, Miami, FL 33186, USA
Mary J. Kelley	Department of Ophthalmology, Casey Eye Institute Oregon Health & Science University Portland, Oregon, USA
Mohammad Shahidullah	Department of Physiology and Department of Ophthalmology & Vision Science, College of Medicine, University of Arizona, 1501 N Campbell Avenue, Tucson, AZ 85724, USA
Munmun Chakraborthy	Hyderabad Eye Research Foundation, , , , LV Prasad Eye Institute, Patia, Bhubaneswar, MTC Campus, Bhubaneswar, Odisha, India
Muthukkaruppan Veerappan	Department of Immunology and Stem Cell Biology, Aravind Medical Research Foundation, Madurai, Tamil Nadu, India
Najam A. Sharif	Vice President and Head of Research & Development Nanoscope Therapeutics Inc., 2777 N. Stemmons Fwy, Suite 1102, Dallas, TX-75207, USA
Nozhat Choudry	Santen Inc., 6401 Hollis Street, Suite 125, Emeryville, CA-94608, USA
Nicholas Delamere	Department of Physiology and Department of Ophthalmology & Vision Science, College of Medicine, University of Arizona, 1501 N Campbell Avenue, Tucson, AZ 85724, USA
Onkar N. Singh	CMC/Manufacturing/Technical Operations, Alentia Therapeutics Inc., Fort Worth, 2648 Gosling Way, Fort Worth, TX-76118, USA
Peter G. Klimko	Novartis Pharmaceuticals Corporation, Fort Worth, TX 76107, USA
Pujhitha Ramesh	Colleges of Nanoscale Science and Engineering, SUNY Polytechnic Institute, 257 Fuller Road, Albany 12203, New York, USA
Pratik Bhankele	Department of Pharmacy Sciences, School of Pharmacy and Health Professions, Creighton University, Omaha, Nebraska, USA
Pei Ying Lee	Department of Optometry & Vision, 202 Berkeley St, Parkville, The University of Melbourne, Victoria 3010, Australia
Rachel N. Andrews	Therapeutic Area Lead for Ophthalmology, Safety Assessment – Toxicology, Genentech Research and Development, A Member of the Roche Group, 1 DNA Way, MS# 441A, South San Francisco, CA 94080, USA
Raj Patil	OKYO Pharma Ltd, 420 Lexington Ave, Suite 1402, New York, NY-10170, USA
Sunny E. Ohia	Department of Pharmaceutical Sciences, College of Pharmacy and Health Sciences, Texas Southern University, Houston, Texas, USA
Saima Chaudhry	Univ N. Texas at Arlington, 701 S Nedderman Dr, Arlington, TX-76019, USA
Suchismita Acharya	AyuVis Research Inc., 3500 Camp Bowie Blvd, EAD #116J, Fort Worth, TX 76107, USA Department of Pharmacology & Neuroscience, North Texas Eye Research Institute, Fort Worth, TX 76107, USA
Shan Fan	Department of Ophthalmology and Visual Sciences, University of Nebraska Medical Center, Omaha, Nebraska, USA

Sanjoy K. Bhattacharya	University of Miami Miller School of Medicine, 1638 NW 10th Avenue, Suite 707Am Miami, FL 33136, USA
Shahid Husain	Department of Ophthalmology, Storm Eye Institute, Medical University of South Carolina, 167 Ashley Ave, Charleston, SC-29425, USA
Samarendra Mohanty	Nanoscope Technologies, 1312 Brown Trail, Bedford, TX 76022, USA
Schuichi Koizumi	Department of Neuropharmacology, Interdisciplinary Graduate School of Medicine & GLIA Center, University of Yamanashi, Yamanashi, Japan
Sam Yacoub	Department of Pharmacology and Neuroscience and The North Texas Eye Research Institute, University of North Texas Health Science Center, Fort Worth, TX 76107, USA
Shin-ichi Ohnuma	UCL Institute of Ophthalmology, University College London, London, United Kingdom
Ted S. Acott	Department of Ophthalmology, Casey Eye Institute Oregon Health & Science University Portland, Oregon, USA
Thomas R. Vollmer	Department of Ophthalmology, Novartis Institute of Biomedical Research, 22 Windsor St. Cambridge, MA-02452, USA
Ursula Schlötzer-Schrehardt	Department of Ophthalmology, Friedrich-Alexander University Erlangen-Nürnberg, Schwabachanlage 6, 91054 Erlangen, Germany
Veluchamy A. Barathi	Translational Pre-Clinical Model Platform, Singapore Eye Research Institute, ACP in Ophthalmology & Visual Sciences, DUKE-NUS Graduate Medical School, Department of Ophthalmology, Yong Loo Lin School of Medicine, National University of Singapore, Singapore 119077, Singapore
VijayKrishna Raghunathan	Department of Ophthalmology, Novartis Institutes for BioMedical Research, 22 Windsor St, Cambridge, MA 02139, USA
Vickie Hoi Ying Wong	Department of Optometry & Vision, 202 Berkeley St, Parkville, The University of Melbourne, Victoria 3010, Australia
Vladimir Bantseev	Therapeutic Area Lead for Ophthalmology, Safety Assessment – Toxicology, Genentech Research and Development, A Member of the Roche Group, 1 DNA Way, MS# 441A, South San Francisco, CA 94080, USA
Wei Zhang	North Texas Eye Research Institute (NTERI), Department of Pharmacology & Neuroscience, University of North Texas Health Science Center (UNTHSC), 3500 Camp Bowie Boulevard, Room IREB-511, Fort Worth, TX 76107, USA
Ya Fatou Njie-Mbye	Department of Pharmaceutical Sciences, College of Pharmacy and Health Sciences, Texas Southern University, Houston, Texas, USA
Yasushi Kato	Research & Development, InnFocus Inc. (A Santen Co.), 12415 S.W. 136 Ave., Unit 3, Miami, FL 33186, USA
Youichi Shinozaki	Department of Neuropharmacology, Interdisciplinary Graduate School of Medicine & GLIA Center, University of Yamanashi, Yamanashi, Japan Visual Research Project, Tokyo Metropolitan Institute of Medical Science, Tokyo, Japan

Zheng He Department of Optometry & Vision, 202 Berkeley St, Parkville, The University of Melbourne, Victoria 3010, Australia

OCULAR HYPERTENSION (OHT) AND GLAUCOMA AND REASONS FOR STUDYING THEM

CHAPTER 1

Basic Anatomy and Physiology of the Human Eye

Fatima Muili[1], **Anthonia Okolie**[1], **Catherine A. Opere**[2], **Ya Fatou Njie-Mbye**[1] and **Sunny E. Ohia**[1,*]

[1] *Department of Pharmaceutical Sciences, College of Pharmacy and Health Sciences, Texas Southern University, Houston, Texas, USA*

[2] *Department of Pharmacy Sciences, School of Pharmacy and Health Professions, Creighton University, Omaha, Nebraska, USA*

Abstract: The eye is an exquisitely designed sensory organ adapted to respond to ambient white light. It is composed of many specialized structures and cell types that have defined functions. Good vision is important for us to perceive our environment and to conduct our daily life activities. In simple terms, the eyes detect light and convert it into electrochemical impulses, which the brain decodes into the final images we perceive. Thus, in higher organisms, the eye is a complex optical system that collects light from the surrounding environment, regulates its intensity through the pupil, and focuses it *via* the lens to form an image at the back of the eye. This image is then converted into a set of electrical impulse signals transmitted *via* the retinal ganglion cells (neurons) and their axons (bundled into the optic nerve) to the thalamic and suprachiasmatic nuclei and, ultimately, to the visual cortex. Visual perception in these higher brain systems, therefore, is reliant on proper and optimal functioning of all components of the retina-optic nerve-brain structure system. Defects along this visual axis result in many types of eye diseases of which glaucoma (made up of many disorders) is one of the major leading causes of worldwide visual impairment that can lead to blindness. The eye structure and function at a high level are described in this chapter.

Keywords: Anatomy, Glaucoma, Light, Ocular diseases, Ocular hypertension, Physiology, Vision.

INTRODUCTION

As the key sensory organ involved in vision, the photoreceptors in the retina of the eye respond to the environmental light, and the optic nerve from retinal ganglion cells transmits this information to the brain's visual centers for processing. Due to its unique location and functions, the eye is isolated and some-

* **Corresponding author Sunny E. Ohia:** Department of Pharmaceutical Sciences, College of Pharmacy and Health Sciences, Texas and Southern University, Houston, Texas, USA; E-mail: sunny.ohia@TSU.edu

Najam A. Sharif and Sunny E. Ohia (Eds.)

what protected from the blood-vitreous, blood-retinal, and blood-aqueous compartments. Due to the latter features, the eye has distinctly unique pharmacodynamic and pharmacokinetic characteristics (Goodman and Gilman, 2023).

The eye globe comprises and is surrounded by three tissue layers named sclera, choroid, and retina, and the globe can be split into the anterior and the posterior segments. Within the anterior segment are the following tissues: cornea, lens, iris, trabecular meshwork, canal of Schlemm, and the ciliary body. Conversely, the posterior segment houses and/or is connected to the vitreous humor, retina, choroid, and optic nerve (Fig. **1**). Tissues that are involved in focusing the incoming light onto the retina include the cornea, iris, and lens. However, it is the multi-layered retina that converts the photons of light into chemical-electric signals, which are relayed to the brain thalamic and visual centers for image generation and visual perception. Meanwhile, physiological balance, appropriate intraocular pressure maintenance, and nourishment of ocular tissues are provided by the choroid, aqueous humor, vitreous humor, and the lacrimal gland system.

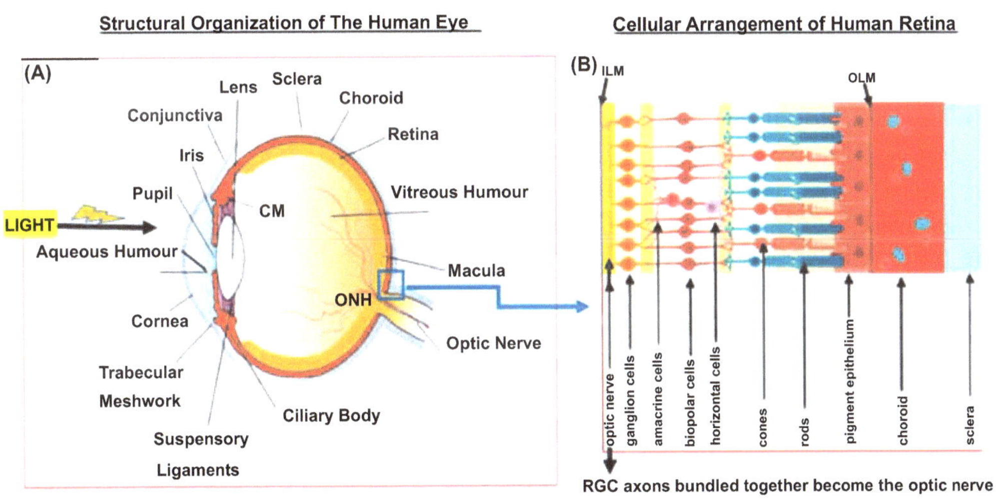

Fig. (1). Key structural elements of the human eye: anterior segment (**A**) and Posterior Segment (**P**).

EXTRAOCULAR STRUCTURES

Eye Lids

This specialized thin layer of skin is responsible for protecting the eye, with the inner portion lined with the palpebral portion of the conjunctiva, which keeps the eyes moist *via* the blink response. The eyelids also protect the eyeball from airborne pollutants, chemicals, and potential mechanical injuries. The cornea and conjunctiva are highly innervated with sensory nerves, and they initiate the blink response. The oily film produced by the meibomian glands and the aqueous lacrimal secretion from the eyelids keep the cornea and conjunctiva moist and prevent excessive tear evaporation.

Lacrimal System

Secretory glands and excretory (nasolacrimal) ducts are part of the lacrimal system. This system includes lacrimal glands located in the temporal outer portion of the orbit innervated by the autonomic nerves and accessory glands located in the conjunctiva (Krause and Wolfring glands). The meibomian glands are located on the posterior and inferior surface to the eyelashes, whereas orifices of the glands are positioned posterior to the eyelashes and secrete oils that slow down tear evaporation. Capillary action and blinking permits the tears to flow through the lacrimal drainage system and out to the nasal cavities.

Orbit

The bony cavity of the skull that houses and protects the eyeball is the orbit. This structure has multiple fissures and foramina that house the nerves, muscles, and blood vessels. Connective tissue, adipose tissue, and six extraocular muscles align and support the eyes within the orbit to permit binocular vision. The retrobulbar region is immediately behind the eye.

OCULAR STRUCTURES (ANTERIOR SEGMENT)

Cornea

The cornea is composed of five layers (epithelium, bowman's membrane, stroma, Descemet's membrane, and endothelium) and is a transparent and avascular tissue. Six cell layers form the hydrophobic epithelial layer, which is fundamentally interconnected with the tear film. An average adult cornea is approximately 11.5 – 12.0 mm in diameter and 0.5 mm thick (Rüfer *et al.*, 2005). The corneal limbus area receives the blood supply, and the tears and aqueous humor support the metabolic processes of the cornea. The cornea and the tear film are important in providing some of the important optical power of the eyes (Donaldson *et al.*, 2017).

Limbus

The transitional zone between the cornea and the sclera, consisting of conjunctival epithelium, Schlemm's canal, and the trabecular meshwork, is the limbus. The conjunctival epithelium contains the corneal epithelium stem cells, tenons capsule, episcleral, corneoscleral stroma, canal of Schlemm, and trabecular meshwork. The tears and limbal blood vessels provide important nutrients and immunological defense mechanisms for the cornea and adjoining conjunctival tissue.

Anterior Chamber

While the iris forms the base of the anterior chamber, the cornea forms the roof of the latter chamber. The anterior chamber contains ~250 μL of aqueous humor, which is produced by the ciliary body. Normally, the production and drainage of the aqueous humor are equal, and thus, the intraocular pressure and shape of the eyeball are maintained. The flow of the aqueous humor occurs through the pupil into the anterior chamber from where it drains through the trabecular meshwork into the canal Schlemm and then back into the systemic circulation. This is the conventional outflow pathway accounting for about 80% of the total drainage. The alternate outflow pathway is the uveal scleral pathway, which drains from the ciliary across muscle through uveal tissues into the sclera and can account for up to 20% of the total outflow of aqueous humor (Fig. **2**). The aqueous humor provides nourishment to the tissues within the anterior chamber and contributes to the optical system of the eye by functioning as a refractive medium. The aqueous humor also removes the metabolic waste in the anterior chamber and helps maintain a "normal" intraocular pressure of 14-21 mmHg.

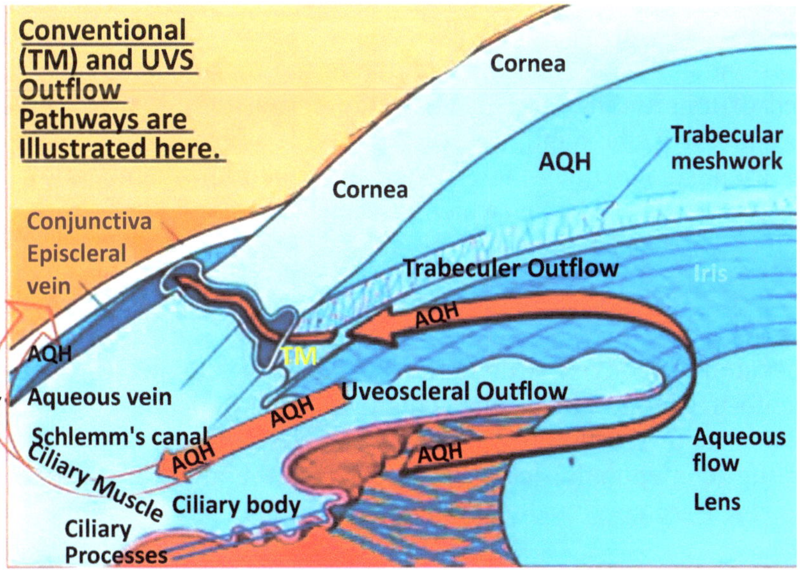

(Adapted from Sharif NA, 2021)

Fig. (2). Aqueous humor outflow pathways in the human eye anterior segment.

Posterior Chambers

While the anterior surface of the lens and the ciliary processes form the base, the posterior surface of the iris forms the roof of the posterior chamber, which can contain about 50 μL of aqueous humor.

Trabecular Meshwork

This tissue is a sieve-like structure through which the aqueous humor drains from the anterior chamber. It connects to the Schlemm's canal, which is connected to the aqueous veins in the sclera. As mentioned above, 80- 90% of aqueous humor drains from the anterior chamber *via* the trabecular meshwork, which can get blocked by cell debris and aberrantly accumulated matrix materials and thereby raise the intraocular pressure (Ou Y *et al.*, 2021).

Canal of Schlemm

Within the posterior part of the corneoscleral junction is located the circular Schlemm's canal. This canal permits the drainage of aqueous humor from the trabecular meshwork into the episcleral venous plexus and then into the systemic circulation. Along with the trabecular meshwork, the Schlemm's canal is responsible for maintaining fluid homeostasis in the eye (Karpinich *et al.*, 2014).

Iris

The iris provides the color of the eye due to the melanocytes present in it. It is composed of longitudinal and circular smooth muscles, which help control the diameter and size of the pupil, thus regulating the amount of light passing into the eye. The iris also separates the anterior and posterior chambers of the eye. Its anterior surface is the stroma, which contains parasympathetic and sympathetic nerves, blood vessels, smooth muscles, and melanocytes.

Lens

The transparent, biconvex structure, suspended by zonules, that focuses visual images onto the retina is the lens. This tissue anatomically originates from the ciliary body and is about 10mm in diameter and enclosed in a capsule. Proliferating lens epithelial cells located under the anterior portion of the lens capsule, which are continually produced throughout life, form the fibers of the lens.

Zonule

The circumferential suspensory ligaments that connect the lens to the ciliary body and assist in focusing visual images onto the retina are referred to as the zonules. These are composed of fibers that span the gap between the lens and the adjacent non-pigmented ciliary epithelium (Shi Y *et al.*, 2013).

Ciliary Body

Ciliary muscles and ciliary processes comprise the ciliary body. While non-pigmented ciliary epithelial cells within the ciliary processes form the aqueous humor, it is the ciliary muscles that change the shape of the lens (accommodation) when the eye focuses on an object. The ciliary smooth muscle consists of the outer longitudinal, middle radial, and inner circular layers. The ciliary processes are located at the anterior-innermost point of the ciliary body and they form the aqueous humor to fill the anterior chamber of the eye (Glasser, 2006).

OCULAR STRUCTURES (POSTERIOR SEGMENT)

Vitreous Humor

The posterior segment of the eye contains a transparent gelatinous medium that accounts for about 80% of the volume of the eye and is made primarily of water (80-90%) and various proteins. Together with the aqueous humor, the vitreous humor helps maintain the shape of the eyeball, and its transparency aids light to reach the retina. The vitreous humor (~ 3ml) acts as a diffusion barrier between the anterior and posterior segments of the eye.

Retina

The retina forms the light-sensitive innermost layer of tissue in the posterior segment of the eye for vision perception. It is a thin, transparent, highly specialized, and organized structure comprising millions of neurons, blood vessels (choroid), and light-sensitive photoreceptors (rods and cones). While the rods mediate peripheral and dim light vision, the cones are dense in the center of the retina (fovea) and are responsible for color vision. The retinal pigment epithelium adjoining the choroid on the one side and photoreceptors on the other side is responsible for vitamin A metabolism to create the light-sensitive chromophore, phagocytosis of the rod outer segments, and various transport processes.

Choroid

The choroid is a highly vascularized middle layer of the retina that supplies nutrients to interior structures of the retina, maintains the ocular temperature, modulates the volume of the eye, and removes retinal metabolic waste. Choroidal vasculature is derived from the ophthalmic artery and the anterior ciliary artery, and blood flow through this structure comprises about 85% of the total blood circulation of the eye.

Sclera

The sclera is the white fibrous tissue that covers the outermost layer of the eye, extending from the cornea to the optic nerve, which helps maintain the shape of the eyeball and offers protection to the more delicate inner tissues of the eye. Scleral thickness ranges from about 0.3 to 1.35mm and is comprised of sclera fibrocytes and a rich supply of nerve endings. Several blood vessels connect to the sclera through an emissary vein to provide blood flow and drain the iris, ciliary body, choroid, and optic nerve.

Optic Nerve

The optic nerve is a myelinated nerve that conducts the electrical activity generated by the retinal ganglion cells, the most high-order neurons, to the brain's thalamic relay centers, amongst other nuclei. The thalamic and suprachiasmatic nuclei, in turn, process and integrate this information and send it on to the visual cortical centers for final processing, integration, and creation of images the person perceives. The suprachiasmatic nucleus is also involved in regulating the sleep-wake cycle of mammals.

CONCLUSION

The specialization and the unique structural and functional domains of the eye are indeed complex and require attention to understand. Nevertheless, the specific anatomy and physiology of the eye provide the basis for our vision and need to be appreciated and cherished. Understanding the described basic anatomy, physiology, and pathology of the eye is important for a reader who plans to embark on research studies using the protocols described in this book. Disorders of the eye include diseases such as glaucoma, cataracts, dry eye disease, age-related macular degeneration, and diabetic retinopathy. It is hoped that the information provided in this chapter will be foundational and useful to the ocular researchers, the uninitiated, and those who already work in this field.

REFERENCES

Donaldson, PJ, Grey, AC, Maceo Heilman, B, Lim, JC & Vaghefi, E (2017) The physiological optics of the lens. *Prog Retin Eye Res,* 56, e1-e24.
[http://dx.doi.org/10.1016/j.preteyeres.2016.09.002] [PMID: 27639549]

Goodman and Gilman's. *The Pharmacological Basis of Therapeutics. Surgical Neurology International, 14*, 91

[http://dx.doi.org/10.25259/SNI_184_2023]

Glasser, A (2006) Restoration of accommodation. *Curr Opin Ophthalmol,* 17, 12-8.
[http://dx.doi.org/10.1097/01.icu.0000193069.32369.e1] [PMID: 16436919]

Karpinich, NO & Caron, KM (2014) Schlemm's canal: more than meets the eye, lymphatics in disguise. *J Clin Invest,* 124, 3701-3.
[http://dx.doi.org/10.1172/JCI77507] [PMID: 25061871]

Ou. Y & Ou Y (2021). Glaucoma and the Importance of the Eye's Drainage System, Bright Focus Foundation, Available from: https://www.brightfocus.org/glaucoma/article/glaucoma-and-importance-e-es-drainage- system

Rüfer, F, Schröder, A & Erb, C (2005) White-to-white corneal diameter: normal values in healthy humans obtained with the Orbscan II topography system. *Cornea,* 24, 259-61.
[http://dx.doi.org/10.1097/01.ico.0000148312.01805.53] [PMID: 15778595]

Sharif, NA (2021) Therapeutic Drugs and Devices for Tackling Ocular Hypertension and Glaucoma, and Need for Neuroprotection and Cytoprotective Therapies. *Front Pharmacol,* 12, 729249.
[http://dx.doi.org/10.3389/fphar.2021.729249] [PMID: 34603044]

Shi, Y, Tu, Y, De Maria, A, Mecham, RP & Bassnett, S (2013) Development, composition, and structural arrangements of the ciliary zonule of the mouse. *Invest Ophthalmol Vis Sci,* 54, 2504-15.
[http://dx.doi.org/10.1167/iovs.13-11619] [PMID: 23493297]

CHAPTER 2

Introduction to Ocular Hypertension and Glaucoma and an Overview of Drug Screening Funnels for Discovering and Characterizing New Intraocular Pressure-Reducing Compounds

Najam A. Sharif[1,*] and **Saima Chaudhry**[2]

[1] *Vice President and Head of Research & Development Nanoscope Therapeutics Inc., 2777 N. Stemmons Fwy, Suite 1102, Dallas, TX-75207, USA*

[2] *Univ N. Texas at Arlington, 701 S Nedderman Dr, Arlington, TX-76019, USA*

Abstract: Many forms of glaucoma prevail in our aging population. However, all forms cause a characteristic optic nerve and retinal ganglion cell (RGC) degeneration, which results in visual impairment and can ultimately cause blindness. The most common types of glaucoma are open-angle glaucoma (OAG) and angle-closure glaucoma (ACG), which afflict over 75 million individuals worldwide. Both these types of glaucoma involve an abnormal accumulation of aqueous humor (AQH) in the anterior chamber of the eye. This raises the intraocular pressure (IOP) which radiates out to cause mechanical damage to tissues at the back of the eye. Whilst no cure is available, the elevated IOP (ocular hypertension; OHT) is treatable with topical ocularly instilled drugs that either slow down the production of AQH or open up the congested AQH outflow pathway, which involves digestion of accumulated extracellular matrix in and around the trabecular meshwork and/or the ciliary muscle bundles. Furthermore, surgery and/or implantation of AQH microshunts in the anterior chamber can alleviate the OHT. Due to its chronic nature, medicated eyedrops are usually the first-line treatments involving the use of prostaglandin/prostanoid FP- and/or EP2-receptor agonists. Combination products are used if one drug fails to lower and control the elevated IOP. Drug discovery of new receptor- or enzyme-targeted molecules for OHT/glaucoma treatment is still warranted since existing drugs have several deficiencies and produce ocular and/or systemic side effects. This chapter addresses various elements of ocular hypotensive drug discovery and development.

Keywords: Drug discovery, Glaucoma, Intraocular pressure, Ocular hypertension, Trabecular meshwork, Vision.

* **Corresponding author Najam A. Sharif:** Vice President and Head of Research & Development Nanoscope Therapeutics Inc., 2777 N. Stemmons Fwy, Suite 1102, Dallas, TX-75207, USA; Tel: +1(817)-565-7686; E-mail: nsharif@nanostherapeutics.com

Najam A. Sharif and Sunny E. Ohia (Eds.)

INTRODUCTION

Eyesight is our most precious sense that is vital for our daily activities, learning, socializing, and ultimate survival. Unfortunately, millions to over a billion individuals worldwide suffer from various preventable visual impairments and eye diseases (WHO, 2019). One of the leading causes of vision loss is a constellation of neurodegenerative disorders of the eye called glaucoma, of which the four major classes are open-angle glaucoma (OAG), angle-closure glaucoma (ACG), secondary glaucomas (SGs) and normotensive glaucoma (NTG) (Tham *et al.*, 2014; Weinreb *et al.*, 2014; Sharif, 2017, 2018, 2021). Globally, there are currently more than 75 million patients who suffer from OAG and ACG (Tham *et al.*, 2014). Whilst all types of glaucoma damage the optic nerve, retina, and visual centers in the brain, the underlying pathogenic culprit causing OAG, ACG, and SGs involves defects in the aqueous humor (AQH) drainage system (trabecular meshwork [TM] and Schlemm's canal [SC]) located in the anterior chamber of the eye (ANCe) (Grierson and Howes, 1987; Sacca *et al.*, 2005; Izotti *et al.*, 2011; Buffault *et al.*, 2020; Fig. **1**). At a highly simplified level, the aging process and pathological accumulation of extracellular proteins and cellular debris (De Groef *et al.*, 2016) within the TM and in the juxtacanalicular area slow down the egress of AQH, which raises the intraocular pressure (IOP). Since the AQH is constantly being produced by the ciliary epithelium (Civan and Macknight, 2004) and its drainage is reduced (Acott *et al.*, 2020), the IOP continues to slowly increase. Over time, the elevated IOP's mechanical force is exerted on all tissues of the eye. The stretching and distorting pressure adversely affects the most vulnerable tissues at the back of the eye, where the retinal ganglion cell axons coalesce before exiting the eye to form the optic nerve. Over time, the effects of this abnormally raised pressure at the optic nerve head and lamina cribosa initiate local inflammation (Hernandez *et al.*, 1989; Burgoyne *et al.*, 2005; McElnea *et al.*, 2011) (Fig. **2**). The secreted cytokines and proteases injure/kill the RGC axons and the cell bodies causing a loss of connectivity to the brain centers, which culminates in visual impairment (Gupta *et al.*, 2007; Fig. **2**). In OAG and ACG, over decades of asymptomatic destruction of RGCs due to the imperceptibly increased IOP, the patient's eyesight continues to deteriorate (Gazzard *et al.*, 2003). When over 600k RGCs are lost, the patient begins to notice the loss of visual contrast, reduced color vision, and patchy blind spots in the visual field (Crab *et al.*, 2016). It is now critical to lower and control the IOP, the only modifiable and treatable biomarker for OAG, ACG, and SGs, in order to preserve the remaining eyesight (Heill *et al.*, 2002; Kass *et al.*, 2002). Many drugs, surgical techniques, and AQH drainage microshunts are available to reduce the IOP, but they all have various shortcomings (Newman-Casey *et al.*, 2015; Sharif *et al.*, 2023) that limit their clinical utility (Weinreb *et al.*, 2014; Sharif, 2017, 2018, 2021; Sadruddin *et al.*, 2019; Sharif *et al.*, 2023). Therefore, there continues to be an unmet medical need to find new treatment modalities for all types of glaucoma, not just IOP-lowering therapeutics but neuroprotective agents as well (Sharif, 2018, 2021).

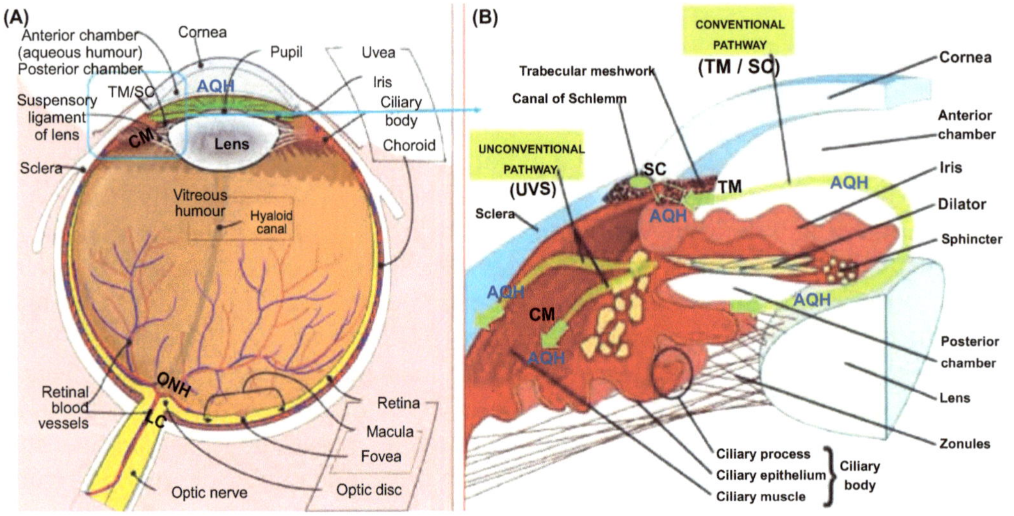

Fig. (1). The anatomy of the human eye (**A**) and the anterior chamber of the eye (**B**).

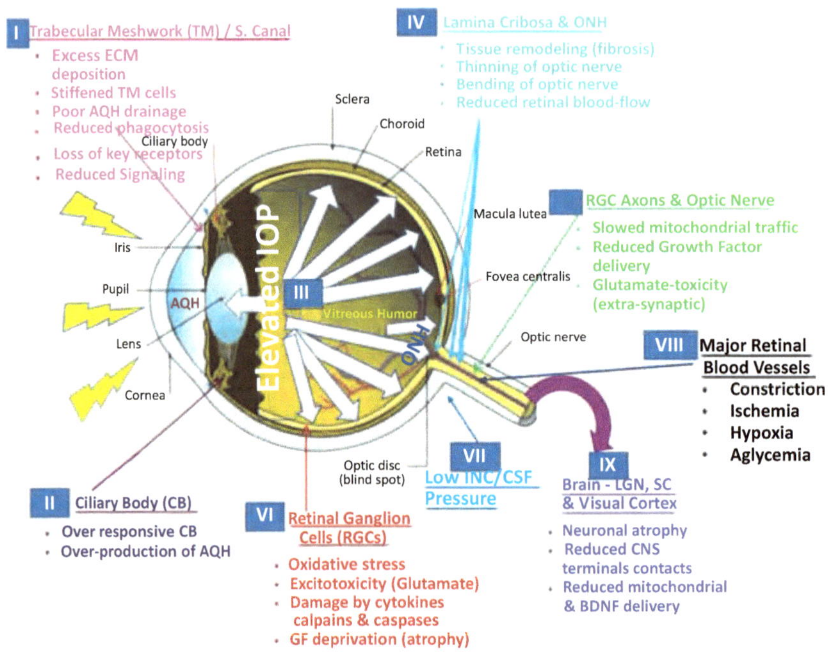

Fig. (2). The effects of chronically elevated IOP on ocular structures and functions that contribute to visual impairment.

As an exquisitely designed and important sensory organ, the eye is relatively inaccessible to systemic circulation due to blood-aqueous, blood-vitreous, and blood-retinal barriers. This arrangement is a protective mechanism. Consequently, most of the existing therapeutic drugs to treat OHT/glaucoma are administered *via* the topical ocular route. Such drugs need to penetrate the five-layered cornea and/or gain entry through the conjunctival tissue in order to reach the ANCe and the AQH (Fig. **1**). Here, they interact with and either stimulate or inhibit their cognate receptors/enzymes/ion channels located on target cells of the ciliary processes or ciliary muscle and/or TM and SC to impart their ocular hypotensive activity (Fig. **3**). Drug formulation and delivery of the therapeutic agent to the AQH is therefore challenging and is determined by many factors including physicochemical properties of the molecules and their pharmacokinetics. The pharmacodynamic aspects of drug efficacy are then dictated by the ambient drug concentration achieved at the active site, the full or partial engagement with the cellular target(s) within the ANCe, and the activation or inhibition of the signal transduction pathway that ultimately leads to IOP reduction (Fig. **3**).

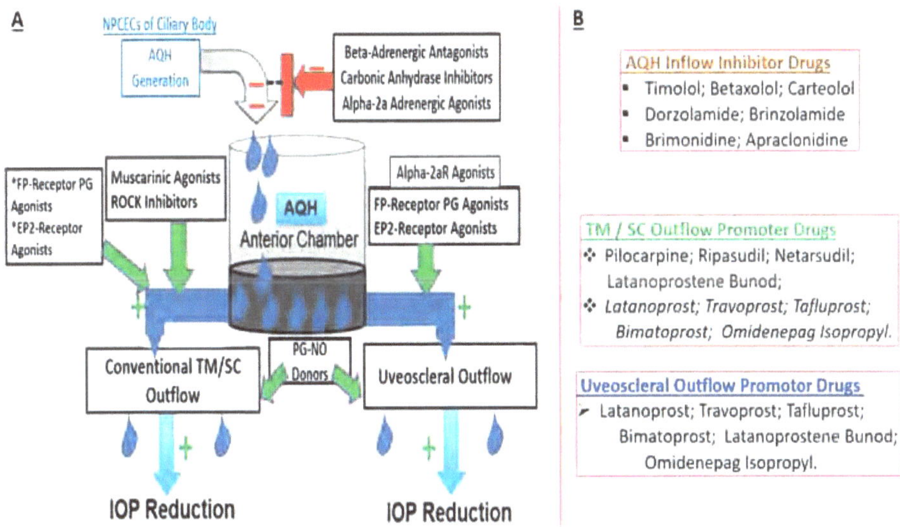

Fig. (3). The pictogram illustrates the production source and drainage routes of AQH from the anterior chamber of the eye and the effects of various drugs that lower IOP (**A**) by promoting AQH efflux or by inhibiting the generation of AQH (**B**). Under normal conditions, the major outflow pathway for AQH drainage is the TM/SC route. Outflow-stimulating drugs can either open up the conventional TM/SC route and/or the uveoscleral outflow pathway to help reduce IOP.

SCREENING FUNNELS- AN OVERVIEW

Drug discovery research is a long, torturous, and expensive endeavor. To shorten this process, compound screening funnels (Fig. **4**) have been developed that exploit known knowledge (*e.g.*, genetics, cellular, and tissue localization) (Davis and Sharif, 1999; Sharif *et al.*, 2005) about the target protein (receptor/enzyme/ion-channel/transporter), its functional coupling mechanism(s) (*e.g.*, induction of second messenger production, tissue relaxation, and transmitter release) (Ohia *et al.*,2018; Ohia and Jumblatt, 1990; Harris *et al.*, 2001), and linkage to the disease (*e.g.*, ocular hypertension). Additional known details about the potential therapeutic product profile help to define and refine the stage-gat--passing-criteria (*e.g.*, affinity or potency equilibrium constant of < 100 nM; Full or partial agonist) to help accept or reject compounds being tested. Compounds that pass the *in vitro* testing stage can then be tested in appropriate animal models for ocular safety (*e.g.*, ocular irritation, redness, inflammation, tearing, discharge), general safety (*e.g.*, gross behavioral changes), and efficacy (*e.g.*, ability to lower and control intraocular pressure) (Quigley, 2018; Sharif, 2017, 2018). *Via* such iterative screening processes, medicinal chemists can then make changes to the compound structure to enhance the affinity, potency, selectivity, and eventually *in vivo* efficacy of the compound or the compound series, hopefully with reduced side effect potential. The types of therapeutic targets, passing criteria, and end-points of typical screening funnels for *in vitro* assays and animal models are shown in Fig. (**4**). The types of screening techniques and technologies available and the functional readouts indicating target engagement are shown in Figs. (**3-6**).

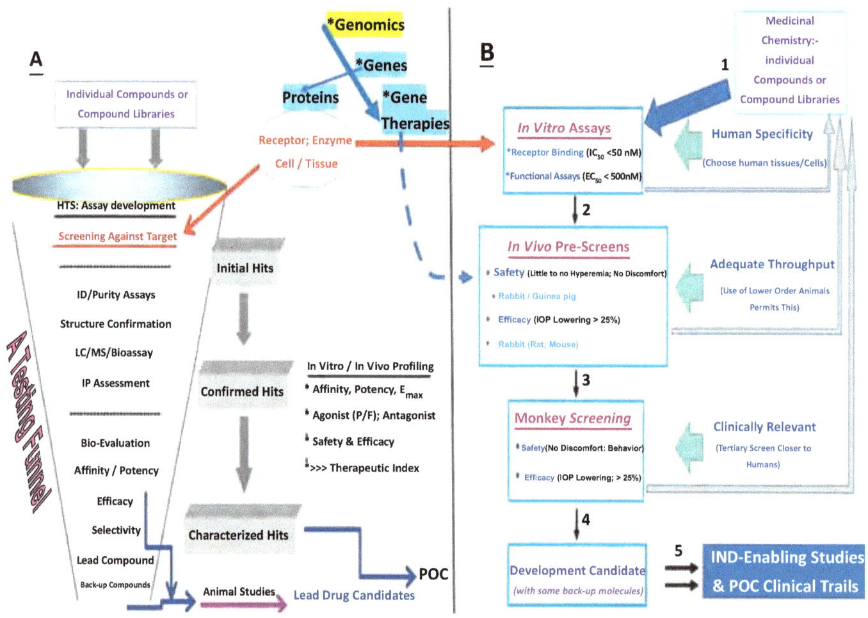

Fig. (4). A high-level view of screening funnels for compound sources and their physiochemical properties determination (**A**) followed by their testing in various *in vitro* assays and animal models (**B**).

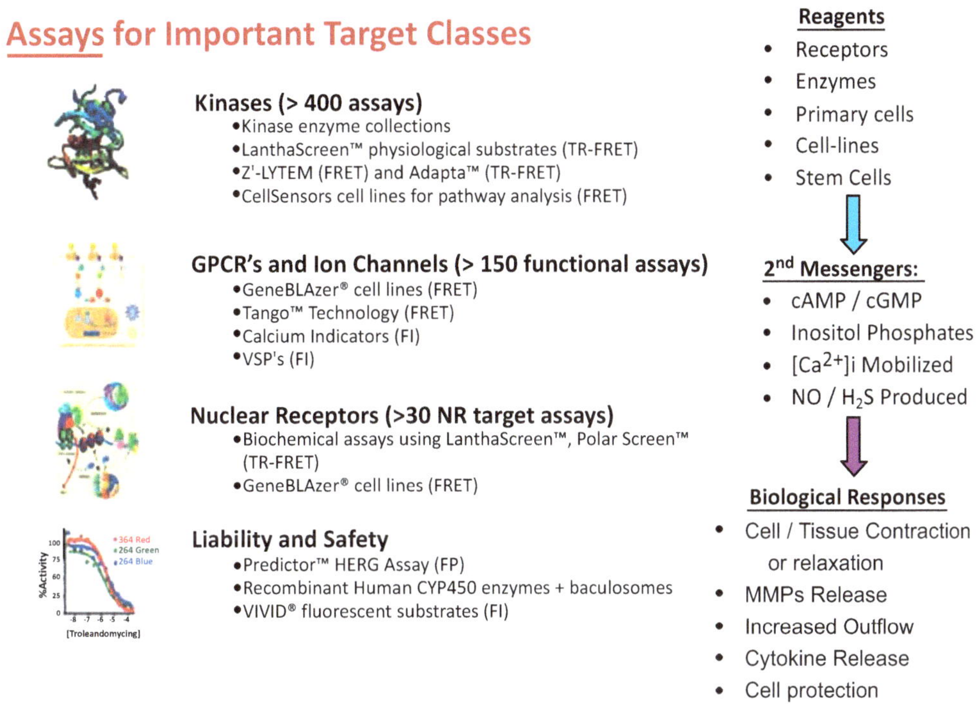

Fig. (5). various target classes, reagents, assays, and functional readouts/biomarkers induced during target engagement are depicted. These parameters help characterize the potential drug candidates, leading to their rank ordering and selection for additional studies, especially *in vivo* investigations.

Cell Analysis Applications	Cell Analysis Instrument Platforms	Cell Analysis Products
Cell Culture	Flow Cytometers	Antibodies
Cell Imaging	Fluorescence Microscopy	Antibody & Protein Labeling Kits
Cell Isolation & Expansion	Microplate Readers	Streptavidin Conjugates
Cell Signaling Pathways	Fluorescence Microplate Assays	Targeted Fluorescent Proteins
Cell Structure	Cell Counter	Cell Proliferation Kits
Cell Tracing & Tracking	Luminex Bead Detection System	Magnetic Cell Separation Kit
Cell Function Assays	Chemiluminescence Detection	ELISA Kits & Luminex Assays
Exosomes	Laser Capture Microdissection	Quantum Dots & Microspheres
Flow Cytometry	Small Animal In Vivo Imaging	Fluorophores
Labeling Chemistry	Super-Resolution Microscopy (SRM)	Chamber Slide & Chambered Coverglass
Microbiology		
Neuroscience		
Single Cell Analysis		
Stem Cell Research		

Fig. (6). Examples of some currently available cell analysis applications, instrument platforms, and cell analysis products.

While the investigative new drug (IND)-enabling studies covering the safety, toxicology, metabolism, and pharmacokinetics are beyond the scope of this chapter and book, the information gathered from the screening funnels is critically important to reach specific goals in the drug discovery process and help select the most promising drug candidate(s) for more detailed studies. The pharmacological characteristics of the final selected compound and potential back-up compounds are defined by such investigations. They can then form the basis of regulatory filings and are necessary for transitioning the compound to full development status and eventual IND/clinical trials. The protocols described in this book are, therefore, immensely important to permit the performance of appropriate discovery and refinement experiments of test compounds of interest. Although certain gene-directed therapies (Figs. **7** and **8**) for OHT and glaucoma offer novel approaches to treat the latter diseases, they can even be assessed in appropriately designed screening funnels. Overall, it is hoped that this book will fulfill our aims and expectations to serve the needs of the readers and researchers working in the OHT/glaucoma field and especially focused on the ANCe. Future studies will cover the protocols needed for conducting assays and using specific animal models of disease directed to the retina, optic nerve, and the associated brain visual centers and the topics of neurodegeneration, neuroprotection, and neuro-regeneration since the OHT and glaucomatous optic neuropathy impacts the back of the eye structures and function.

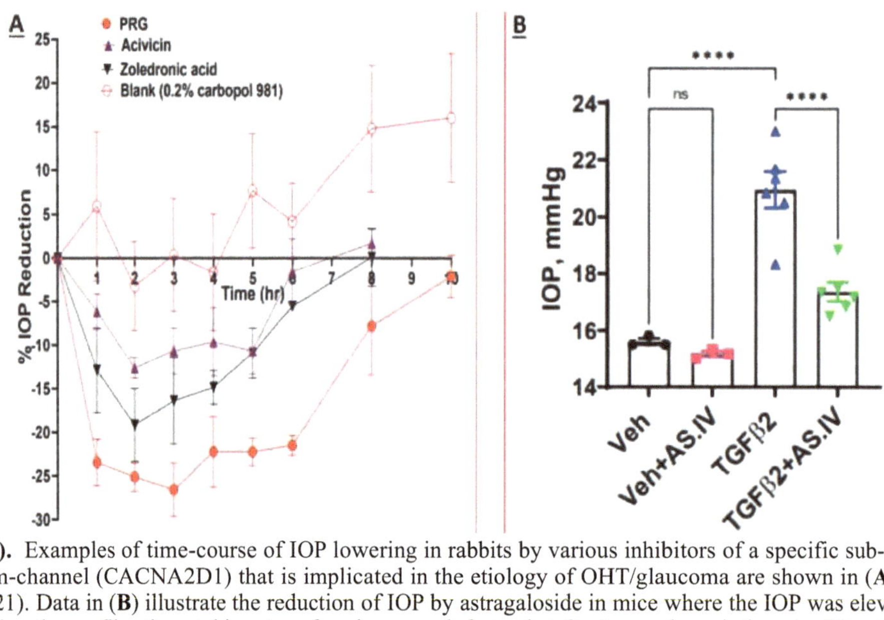

Fig. (7). Examples of time-course of IOP lowering in rabbits by various inhibitors of a specific sub-class of calcium-channel (CACNA2D1) that is implicated in the etiology of OHT/glaucoma are shown in (**A**) (Li *et al.*, 2021). Data in (**B**) illustrate the reduction of IOP by astragaloside in mice where the IOP was elevated by delivering the profibrotic cytokine, transforming growth factor-beta2, *via* an adenoviral vector (Kasetti *et al.*, 2021).

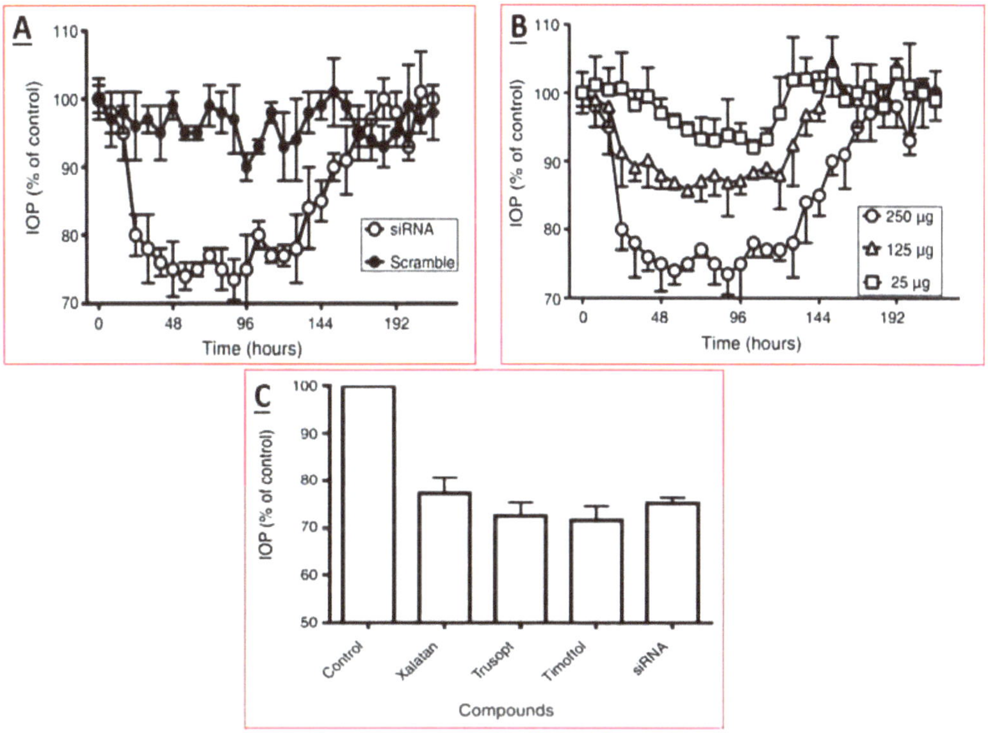

Fig. (8). The IOP-lowering effects of a short interfering RNA (siRNA) directed to the beta2-adrenergic receptor in rabbits are shown in (**A**), with the effect being dose-related (**B**). Comparative IOP-lowering efficacy of the siRNA to the beta2-receptor and various ocular hypotensive drugs in rabbits is depicted in (**C**) (Loma *et al.*, 2018).

CONCLUSION

OHT/glaucoma treatment requires novel modalities that can help the patients tackle the symptoms of their disease, which slowly increases their visual impairment over time. Reduction of raised IOP in a durable manner is the goal, and new drugs need to be more efficacious, with multiple mechanisms of action and fewer side effects than the existing approved medicines. The screening funnels and strategies described in the current chapter provide relatively robust and effective ways to test new compounds and progress them toward IND-enabling studies and, ultimately, to proof-of-concept clinical trials.

REFERENCES

Acott, TS, Vranka, JA, Keller, KE, Raghunathan, V & Kelley, MJ (2021) Normal and glaucomatous outflow regulation. *Prog Retin Eye Res,* 82, 100897.
[http://dx.doi.org/10.1016/j.preteyeres.2020.100897] [PMID: 32795516]

Buffault, J, Labbé, A, Hamard, P, Brignole-Baudouin, F & Baudouin, C (2020) The trabecular meshwork: Structure, function and clinical implications. A review of the literature. *J Fr Ophtalmol,* 43, e217-30.

[http://dx.doi.org/10.1016/j.jfo.2020.05.002] [PMID: 32561029]

Burgoyne, CF, Crawford Downs, J, Bellezza, AJ, Francis Suh, J-K & Hart, RT (2005) The optic nerve head as a biomechanical structure: a new paradigm for understanding the role of IOP-related stress and strain in the pathophysiology of glaucomatous optic nerve head damage. *Prog Retin Eye Res,* 24, 39-73.
[http://dx.doi.org/10.1016/j.preteyeres.2004.06.001] [PMID: 15555526]

Civan, MM & Macknight, ADC (2004) The ins and outs of aqueous humour secretion. *Exp Eye Res,* 78, 625-31.
[http://dx.doi.org/10.1016/j.exer.2003.09.021] [PMID: 15106942]

Crabb, DP (2016) A view on glaucoma—are we seeing it clearly? *Eye (Lond),* 30, 304-13.
[http://dx.doi.org/10.1038/eye.2015.244] [PMID: 26611846]

Davis, TL & Sharif, NA (1999) Quantitative autoradiographic visualization and pharmacology of FP-prostaglandin receptors in human eyes using the novel phosphor-imaging technology. *J Ocul Pharmacol Ther,* 15, 323-36.
[http://dx.doi.org/10.1089/jop.1999.15.323] [PMID: 10463871]

De Groef, L, Andries, L, Siwakoti, A, Geeraerts, E, Bollaerts, I, Noterdaeme, L, Etienne, I, Papageorgiou, AP, Stalmans, I, Billen, J, West-Mays, JA & Moons, L (2016) Aberrant collagen composition of the trabecular meshwork results in reduced aqueous humor drainage and elevated IOP in MMP-9 Null Mice. *Invest Ophthalmol Vis Sci,* 57, 5984-95.
[http://dx.doi.org/10.1167/iovs.16-19734] [PMID: 27820954]

Gazzard, G, Foster, PJ, Devereux, JG, Oen, F, Chew, P, Khaw, PT & Seah, S (2003) Intraocular pressure and visual field loss in primary angle closure and primary open angle glaucomas. *Br J Ophthalmol,* 87, 720-5.
[http://dx.doi.org/10.1136/bjo.87.6.720] [PMID: 12770969]

Grierson, I & Howes, RC (1987) Age-related depletion of the cell population in the human trabecular meshwork. *Eye (Lond),* 1, 204-10.
[http://dx.doi.org/10.1038/eye.1987.38] [PMID: 3653434]

Gupta, N, Ly, T, Zhang, Q, Kaufman, PL, Weinreb, RN & Yücel, YH (2007) Chronic ocular hypertension induces dendrite pathology in the lateral geniculate nucleus of the brain. *Exp Eye Res,* 84, 176-84.
[http://dx.doi.org/10.1016/j.exer.2006.09.013] [PMID: 17094963]

Harada, C, Kimura, A, Guo, X, Namekata, K & Harada, T (2019) Recent advances in genetically modified animal models of glaucoma and their roles in drug repositioning. *Br J Ophthalmol,* 103, 161-6.
[http://dx.doi.org/10.1136/bjophthalmol-2018-312724] [PMID: 30366949]

Harris, LC, Awe, SO, Opere, CA, LeDay, AM, Ohia, SE & Sharif, NA (2001) [(^{3})H]-serotonin release from bovine iris-ciliary body: pharmacology of prejunctional serotonin (5-HT(7)) autoreceptors. *Exp Eye Res,* 73, 59-67.
[http://dx.doi.org/10.1006/exer.2001.1012] [PMID: 11428863]

Heijl, A, Leske, MC, Bengtsson, B, Hyman, L, Bengtsson, B & Hussein, M (2002) Reduction of intraocular pressure and glaucoma progression: results from the Early Manifest Glaucoma Trial. *Arch Ophthalmol,* 120, 1268-79.
[http://dx.doi.org/10.1001/archopht.120.10.1268] [PMID: 12365904]

Hernandez, MR, Luo, XX, Andrzejewska, W & Neufeld, AH (1989) Age-related changes in the extracellular matrix of the human optic nerve head. *Am J Ophthalmol,* 107, 476-84.
[http://dx.doi.org/10.1016/0002-9394(89)90491-1] [PMID: 2653045]

Izzotti, A, Longobardi, M, Cartiglia, C & Saccà, SC (2011) Mitochondrial damage in the trabecular meshwork occurs only in primary open-angle glaucoma and in pseudoexfoliative glaucoma. *PLoS One,* 6, e14567.
[http://dx.doi.org/10.1371/journal.pone.0014567] [PMID: 21283745]

Jain, A, Zode, G & Kasetti, RB (2017) CRISPR-Cas9-based treatment of myocilin associated glaucoma. *Proc Natl Acad Sci (USA),* 114, 1199-11204.

Kass, MA, Heuer, DK, Higginbotham, EJ, Johnson, CA, Keltner, JL, Miller, JP, Parrish, RK, II, Wilson, MR & Gordon, MO (2002) The Ocular Hypertension Treatment Study: a randomized trial determines that topical ocular hypotensive medication delays or prevents the onset of primary open-angle glaucoma. *Arch Ophthalmol,* 120, 701-13.
[http://dx.doi.org/10.1001/archopht.120.6.701] [PMID: 12049574]

Kasetti, RB, Maddineni, P, Millar, JC, Clark, AF & Zode, GS (2017) Increased synthesis and deposition of extracellular matrix proteins leads to endoplasmic reticulum stress in the trabecular meshwork. *Sci Rep,* 7, 14951.
[http://dx.doi.org/10.1038/s41598-017-14938-0] [PMID: 29097767]

Kasetti, RB, Maddineni, P, Kodati, B, Nagarajan, B & Yacoub, S (2021) Astragaloside IV Attenuates Ocular Hypertension in a Mouse Model of TGFβ2 Induced Primary Open Angle Glaucoma. *Int J Mol Sci,* 22, 12508.
[http://dx.doi.org/10.3390/ijms222212508] [PMID: 34830390]

Li, H, Ibrahim, MM, Chen, H, Li, W & Jablonski, MM (2021) In Silico Screening and *In Vivo* Evaluation of Potential CACNA2D1 Antagonists as Intraocular Pressure-Reducing Agents in Glaucoma Therapy. *Pharmaceuticals (Basel),* 14, 887.
[http://dx.doi.org/10.3390/ph14090887] [PMID: 34577587]

Loma, P, Guzman-Aranguez, A, de Lara, MJP & Pintor, J (2018) Beta2 adrenergic receptor silencing change intraocular pressure in New Zealand rabbits. *J Optomet,* 11.

McElnea, EM, Quill, B, Docherty, NG, Irnaten, M, Siah, WF, Clark, AF, O'Brien, CJ & Wallace, DM (2011) Oxidative stress, mitochondrial dysfunction and calcium overload in human lamina cribrosa cells from glaucoma donors. *Mol Vis,* 17, 1182-91.
[PMID: 21617752]

Newman-Casey, PA, Robin, AL, Blachley, T, Farris, K, Heisler, M, Resnicow, K & Lee, PP (2015) The most common barriers to glaucoma medication adherence. *Ophthalmology,* 122, 1308-16.
[http://dx.doi.org/10.1016/j.ophtha.2015.03.026] [PMID: 25912144]

Ohia, SE & Jumblatt, JE (1990) Prejunctional inhibitory effects of prostanoids on sympathetic neurotransmission in the rabbit iris-ciliary body. *J Pharmacol Exp Ther,* 255, 11-6.
[PMID: 2170622]

Ohia, SE, Njie-Mbye, YF, Robinson, J, Mitchell, L, Mckoy, M, Opere, CA & Sharif, NA (2018) Serotonin-2b/2c receptors mediate bovine ciliary muscle contraction: role in intraocular pressure regulation. *J Ocul Pharmacol Ther,* 34, 70-5.
[http://dx.doi.org/10.1089/jop.2017.0123] [PMID: 29364761]

Quigley, HA (2018) Use of animal models and techniques in glaucoma research: Introduction. *Methods Mol Biol,* 1695, 1-10.
[http://dx.doi.org/10.1007/978-1-4939-7407-8_1] [PMID: 29190013]

Saccà, SC, Pascotto, A, Camicione, P, Capris, P & Izzotti, A (2005) Oxidative DNA damage in the human trabecular meshwork: clinical correlation in patients with primary open-angle glaucoma. *Arch Ophthalmol,* 123, 458-63.
[http://dx.doi.org/10.1001/archopht.123.4.458] [PMID: 15824217]

Sadruddin, O, Pinchuk, L, Angeles, R & Palmberg, P (2019) Ab externo implantation of the MicroShunt, a poly (styrene-*block*-isobutylene-*block*-styrene) surgical device for the treatment of primary open-angle glaucoma: a review. *Eye Vis (Lond),* 6, 36.
[http://dx.doi.org/10.1186/s40662-019-0162-1] [PMID: 31807606]

Sharif, NA (2017) Ocular hypertension and glaucoma: a review and current perspectives. *Int. J Ophthalmol Vis Sci,* 2, 22-36.

Sharif, NA (2018) *i*Drugs and *i*Devices discovery and development - preclinical assays, techniques and animal model studies for ocular hypotensives and neuroprotectants. *J Ocul Pharmacol Ther,* 34, 7-39.
[http://dx.doi.org/10.1089/jop.2017.0125] [PMID: 29323613]

Sharif, NA (2021) Therapeutic drugs and devices for tackling ocular hypertension and glaucoma, and need for neuroprotection and cytoprotective therapies. *Front Pharmacol,* 12, 729249.
[http://dx.doi.org/10.3389/fphar.2021.729249] [PMID: 34603044]

Sharif, NA, Davis, TL & Williams, GW (2005) Ocular hypotensive DP-class prostaglandin receptor affinities determined by quantitative autoradiography on human eye sections. *J Ocul Pharmacol Ther,* 21, 121-32.
[http://dx.doi.org/10.1089/jop.2005.21.121] [PMID: 15857278]

Sharif, NA, Odani-Kawabata, N, Lu, F & Pinchuk, L (2023) FP and EP2 prostanoid receptor agonist drugs and aqueous humor outflow devices for treating ocular hypertension and glaucoma. *Exp Eye Res,* 229, 109415.
[http://dx.doi.org/10.1016/j.exer.2023.109415] [PMID: 36803996]

Tham, YC, Li, X, Wong, TY, Quigley, HA, Aung, T & Cheng, CY (2014) Global prevalence of glaucoma and projections of glaucoma burden through 2040: a systematic review and meta-analysis. *Ophthalmology,* 121, 2081-90.
[http://dx.doi.org/10.1016/j.ophtha.2014.05.013] [PMID: 24974815]

Weinreb, RN, Aung, T & Medeiros, FA (2014) The pathophysiology and treatment of glaucoma: a review. *JAMA,* 311, 1901-11.
[http://dx.doi.org/10.1001/jama.2014.3192] [PMID: 24825645]

WHO (2019). Blindness and vision impairment- https://www.who.int › News › Fact sheets. WHO Priority eye diseases. www.who.int/blindness/causes/priority/en/

CHAPTER 3

Protocols for Access to and Dose Selection of Selected IOP-Lowering Drugs

Suchismita Acharya[1,2,*] and **Peter G. Klimko**[3]

[1] *AyuVis Research Inc., 3500 Camp Bowie Blvd, EAD #116J, Fort Worth, TX 76107, USA*

[2] *Department of Pharmacology & Neuroscience, North Texas Eye Research Institute, Fort Worth, TX 76107, USA*

[3] *Novartis Pharmaceuticals Corporation, Fort Worth, TX 76107, USA*

Abstract: Described herein are high-level protocols to access selected small molecules with IOP-lowering properties when topically dosed as ophthalmic formulations, as well as dose selection for evaluation in appropriate animal models. Sources are provided for commercially available drugs, and high-level synthetic protocols are described for agents that are not commercially available. The agents described are approved for use in humans or have demonstrated robust pre-clinical activity. These are drawn from a diverse range of pharmacological classes, such as prostaglandin analogs, beta-adrenergic antagonists, carbonic anhydrase inhibitors, alpha-adrenergic agonists, and dual-activity prostaglandin-NO donors. Their physiological mechanisms of action have been characterized by the suppression of aqueous humor (AH) inflow, enhancement of AH conventional or uveoscleral outflow, and reduction of episcleral venous pressure.

Keywords: ATP-sensitive potassium channel openers, Adenosine receptor modulators, Alpha-adrenergic agonists, Antioxidant-NO donors, Beta-blockers, Carbonic anhydrase inhibitors, IOP lowering agents, Nitric oxide donors, Prostaglandins, Protein tyrosine phosphatase inhibitors, Rho kinase inhibitors.

INTRODUCTION

Given that the major glaucoma risk factor characterized to date is elevated intraocular pressure (IOP), frequently defined as sustained IOP values of ≥21mm Hg (Wijesinghe *et al.*, 2022), agents that lower IOP have been the mainstay of agents used to treat glaucoma. The preferred delivery method is usually *via* topical application of an ophthalmic formulation of a small molecule, which has the advantage of achieving a high tissue concentration while limiting systemic ex-

* **Corresponding author Suchismita Acharya:** AyuVis Research Inc., 3500 Camp Bowie Blvd, EAD #116J, Fort Worth, TX 76107, USA and Department of Pharmacology & Neuroscience, North Texas Eye Research Institute, Fort Worth, TX 76107, USA; Tel: 817-845-0304; E-mail: sacharya@ayuvis.com

Najam A. Sharif and Sunny E. Ohia (Eds.)

posure and subsequent side effects. Historic systemic administration of the carbonic anhydrase inhibitors acetazolamide and methazolamide are notable exceptions. Another is the investigative agent **FM-101**, an adenosine A3 receptor modulator which, unusually, is being studied as an oral formulation (see section 2 below).

IOP-lowering drugs can typically be classified based on three physiological mechanisms of action: decreasing aqueous humor flow through the ciliary body, increasing aqueous outflow facility through the trabecular meshwork (conventional outflow), or increasing aqueous humor outflow through the uveoscleral pathway (non-conventional outflow). The additional mechanism of lowering episcleral venous pressure has been reported for the Rho kinase inhibitor netarsudil (Sit *et al.*, 2021) and the ATP-sensitive potassium channel opener **QLS-101** (Chowdhury *et al.*, 2022). Note that some agents lower IOP *via* more than one physiological mechanism of action.

The purpose of this chapter is to provide a high-level description of methods to access leading IOP-lowering drugs and drug candidates to further pre-clinical investigations. A more comprehensive analysis of topics such as sustained-release drug delivery systems, alternative therapies, discussion of the mechanism of action, and clinical effects of these drugs is reported by Liu *et al.* (Liu *et al.*, 2022). In section 1, health authority-approved IOP-lowering agents that are commercially available, corresponding vendors, and the dosages reported to lower IOP in both rodent and large animal models are tabulated. Section 2 focuses on selected IOP-lowering agents that have not yet been approved by any health authority, with commercial access information provided or high-level synthetic protocols for those that are not commercially available.

Section 1: Access to Health Authority-Approved Iop-Lowering Agents

Table **1** is a list of drugs that health authorities have approved for lowering IOP in humans when they are applied as topical ophthalmic formulations. Prostaglandin FP receptor agonists are typically used as first-line agents (Klimko and Sharif, 2019), frequently with the addition of a beta-adrenergic antagonist (*e.g.*, timolol), an alpha-adrenergic agonist (*e.g.*, brimonidine), or a carbonic anhydrase inhibitor (*e.g.*, brinzolamide) if IOP control is insufficient. A fixed combination of 2 different classes (*e.g.*, fixed combination of brimonidine and brinzolamide; SIMBRINZA®) may be recommended as adjunctive therapy. The clinical impact of recently approved classes, such as dual-acting prostaglandin-nitric oxide donors and Rho kinase inhibitors, will be clarified over time.

Table 1A. Commercially available, regulatory-approved IOP-lowering compounds.

Name	Latanoprost (Xalatan)	Timolol	Netarsudil	Latanoprostene Bunod
Chemical structure	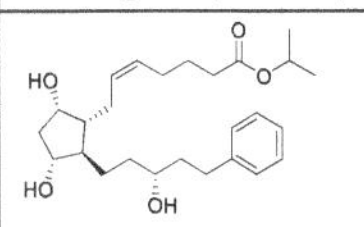	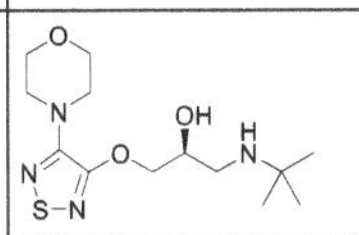	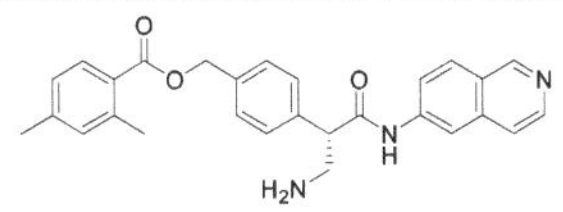	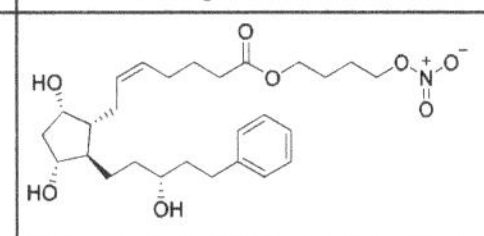
CAS #	130209-82-4	26921-17-5 (maleate salt)	1422144-42-0 (dimesylate salt)	860005-21-6
Therapeutic class	Prostaglandin FP receptor agonist	β-adrenergic blocker	Rho kinase inhibitor	Prostaglandin FP receptor agonist and nitric oxide donor
Mechanism of action	Increase in uveoscleral AH outflow	Decrease in AH formation	Increase in AH conventional outflow and reduction in episcleral venous pressure	Increase in AH uveoscleral and conventional outflow
Doses	-			
Rodent models	Mouse-0.01% (Aihara *et al.*, 2002) Rat- 50 ng (Husain *et al.*, 2006) Rabbit-unresponsive	Mouse (Dexamethasone induced OHT model): - 3 µL of a 5-mg/mL solution (Whitlock *et al.*, 2010); Rat (Hydrogel model)- 0.05% ;(Indian ink, laser coagulation) 0.5% (Yu *et al.*, 2020); (Seki *et al.*, 2005) Rabbit (Normotensive model): 0.5% (Lee *et al.*, 2022)	Rabbit (Normotensive model): 0.04% (Lin *et al.*, 2018)	Mouse (FP receptor knock-out mice: 0.006% (Saeki *et al.*, 2009) Rabbit (Saline induced OHT): 0.036% (Krauss *et al.*, 2011)
Large animal models	Dog-0.005% (Gelatt and MacKay, 2001) Monkey-0.005% (Serle *et al.*, 1998)	Dog (Natural glaucoma)-0.5% (Plummer *et al.*, 2006)	Dog (Normotensive model): 0.04% (Lin *et al.*, 2018)	Dog (Natural glaucoma): 0.036% (Krauss *et al.*, 2011) Monkey (Laser induced OHT): 0.036% (Krauss *et al.*, 2011)
Commercial source	Cayman Chemical (www.caymanchem.com); ThermoFisher (www.thermofisher.com); Key Organics (www.keyorganics.net)	For maleate salt: Sigma-Aldrich (www.sigmaaldrich.com), Cayman Chemical (www.caymanchem.com)	For dimesylate salt: Sigma-Aldrich (www.sigmaaldrich.com), Abovchem (www.abovchem.com); Combi-Blocks (www.combi-blocks.com)	Sigma-Aldrich (www.sigmaaldrich.com), Cayman Chemical (www.caymanchem.com),
Chemical structure	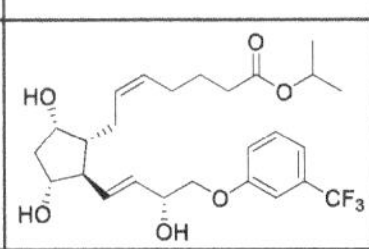	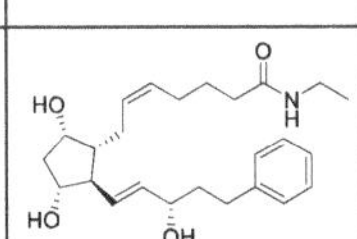	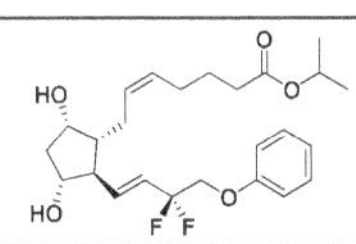	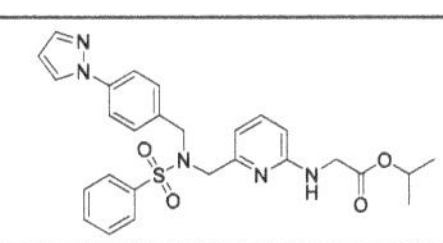
CAS #	157283-68-6	155206-00-1	209860-87-7	1187451-19-9
Therapeutic class	Prostaglandin FP receptor agonist	Prostaglandin FP receptor agonist	Prostaglandin FP receptor agonist	Prostaglandin EP_2 receptor agonist
Mechanism of action	Increase in AH uveoscleral outflow	Increase in AH uveoscleral outflow	Increase in AH uveoscleral outflow	Increase in AH conventional and uveoscleral outflow
Doses	-			

(Table 1A) cont.....

Name	Latanoprost (Xalatan)	Timolol	Netarsudil	Latanoprostene Bunod
Rodent models	-	Rat (Hydrogel model): 0.03% (Yu *et al.*, 2020)	Mouse (normotensive): 0.0015% (Ota *et al.*, 2007)	Rabbit (normotensive)-0.001--0.03%
Large animal models	Monkey (Laser induced OHT): 0.04% (Toris *et al.*, 2005)	Monkey laser-induced OHT: 0.03% (Woodward *et al.*, 2001)	Monkey laser-induced OHT: 0.0025% (Takagi *et al.*, 2004)	Dog, monkey (normotensive)-0.06% Monkey (laser-induced OHT)-0.01% (Kirihara *et al.*, 2015)
Commercial source	Sigma-Aldrich (www.sigmaaldrich.com), Cayman Chemical (www.caymanchem.com), Key Organics (www.keyorganics.com)	Sigma-Aldrich (www.sigmaaldrich.com), Cayman Chemical (www.caymanchem.com), Key Organics (www.keyorganics.com)	Cayman Chemical (www.caymanchem.com), MedChemExpress (www.medchemexpress.com), Key Organics (www.keyorganics.com)	MedChemExpress (www.medchemexpress.com), ChemScene (www.chemscene.com)

Table 1B. Commercially available, regulatory-approved IOP-lowering compounds.

Name	**Dorzolamide**	**Brinzolamide**	**Brimonidine**
Chemical structure	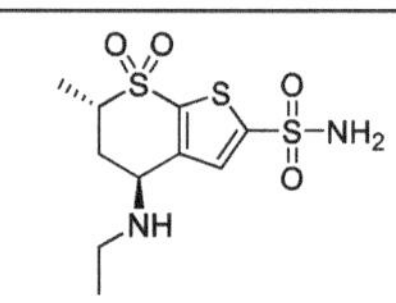	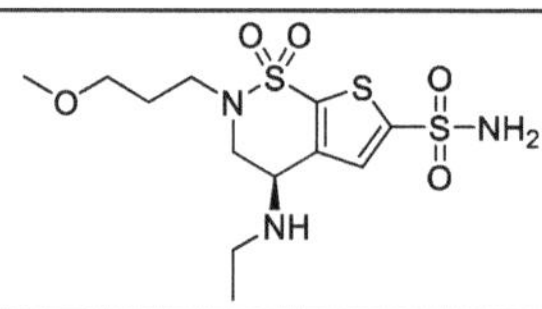	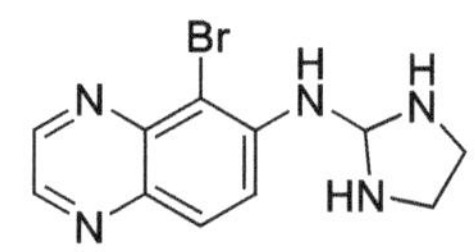
CAS #	130693-82-2 (HCl salt)	138890-62-7	59803-98-4
Therapeutic class	Carbonic anhydrase inhibitor	Carbonic anhydrase inhibitor	Alpha adrenergic agonist
Mechanism of action	Decrease in AH formation	Decrease in AH formation	Decrease in AH formation
Doses	-		
Rodent model	Mouse (DBA/2J): 2% (Chandra *et al.*, 2016) Rat (Indian ink injection and laser coagulation): 1% (Seki *et al.*, 2005) Rabbit (normotensive):2% (Reitsamer *et al.*, 2009)	Rabbit (normotensive):1% (Dong *et al.*, 2018)	Rabbit (normotensive): 0.1% (Burke and Schwartz, 1996)
Large animal models	-	Monkey (laser-induced) -1--2%	Dogs (natural glaucoma)-0.2%

(Table 1B) cont.....

Name	Dorzolamide	Brinzolamide	Brimonidine
Commercial source	Cayman Chemical (www.caymanchem.com), MedChemExpress (www.medchemexpress.com), Key Organics (www.keyorganics.com)	Cayman Chemical (www.caymanchem.com), MedChemExpress (www.medchemexpress.com), Key Organics (www.keyorganics.com)	Cayman Chemical (www.caymanchem.com), MedChemExpress (www.medchemexpress.com), Key Organics (www.keyorganics.com)

Abbreviations CAS: Chemical Abstracts Registry Number; NA: Not available.

Section 2. Access to Investigational Iop-Lowering Agents

Table **2** below lists selected investigational IOP-lowering agents that are commercially available. Taprenepag Isopropyl and **NCX-470** are members of pharmacological classes that already have health authority-approved members (prostaglandin EP2 receptor agonist Omenedipag Isopropyl and dual prostaglandin FP receptor agonist/ nitric oxide donor Latanoprostene Bunod, respectively).

Table 2. Commercially available investigational IOP-lowering compounds.

Name	Taprenepag Isopropyl (PF-04217329)	Razuprotafib (AKB 9778)	NCX-470
Chemical structure	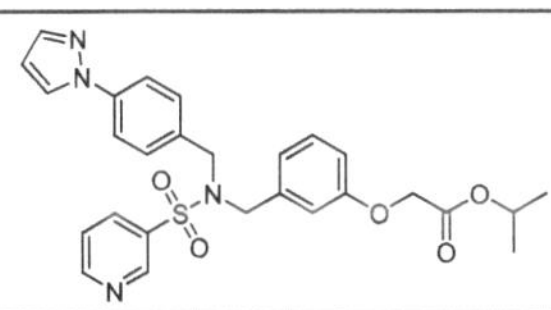	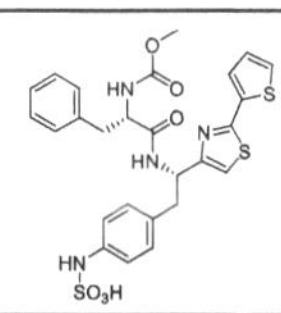	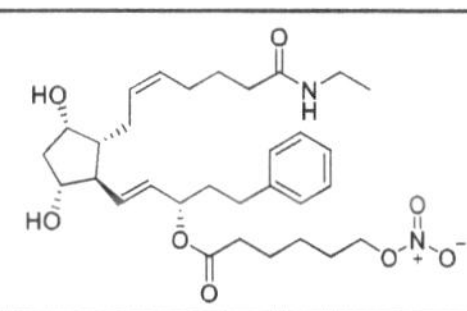
CAS #	1005549-94-9	1008510-37-9	1194396-71-8
Therapeutic class	Prostaglandin EP_2 agonist	Protein tyrosine phosphatase inhibitor	Prostaglandin FP receptor agonist and nitric oxide donor
Mechanism of action	Increase in AH conventional and uveoscleral outflow	Increase in AH conventional outflow	Increase in AH uveoscleral and conventional outflow
Doses	-		
Rodent models	Rabbit (normotensive): (0.2mg/mL-0.2mg/mL) (Prasanna *et al.*, 2011)	Mouse (WT, $Tie2^{+/-}$): 4% Rabbit (normotensive): 4% (Li *et al.*, 2020)	Rabbit (normotensive): 0.1% (Impagnatiello *et al.*, 2015a)

(Table 2) cont.....

Name	**Taprenepag Isopropyl (PF-04217329)**	**Razuprotafib (AKB 9778)**	**NCX-470**
Large animal models	Dogs (normotensive): 0.05 mg/mL-0.2 mg/mL (Prasanna *et al.*, 2011)	NA	Dog (normotensive)-0.04% Monkey (laser-induced OHT)-0.04% (Impagnatiello *et al.*, 2015b)
Commercial source	Sigma-Aldrich (www.sigmaaldrich.com), Medchem Express (www.medchemexpress.com), Aurora Fine Chemicals (www.aurorafinechemicals.com), BOC Sciences (www.bocsci.com)	Sigma-Aldrich (www.sigmaaldrich.com), MedChemExpress (www.medchemexpress.com), ChemScene (www.chemscene.com)	Cayman Chemical (www.caymanchem.com), AA Blocks LLC (www.aablocks.com)

Abbreviations CAS#: Chemical Abstracts Registry Number; NA: Not available.

Table **3** lists several investigative IOP-lowering agents that are not commercially available. These come from diverse pharmacological classes that have demonstrated IOP-lowering *via* several mechanisms, such as AH conventional or uveoscleral outflow enhancement and episcleral venous pressure reduction. Figs. (**1-4**) provide corresponding high-level descriptions of how to synthesize these compounds. Unusually, adenosine A3 receptor modulator **FM-101** is being evaluated in a phase 1/2a trial on subjects with ocular hypertension (entry number NCT04585100 at www.clinicaltrials.gov) for IOP-lowering *via* oral delivery instead of as a topical ophthalmic formulation.

Table 3. Investigational IOP-lowering agents that are not commercially available.

Name	**FM-101**	**Sepetaprost (ONO-9054)**	**QLS-101**	**SA-2**
Chemical structure	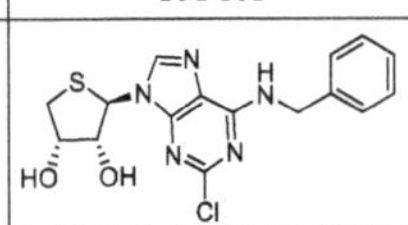	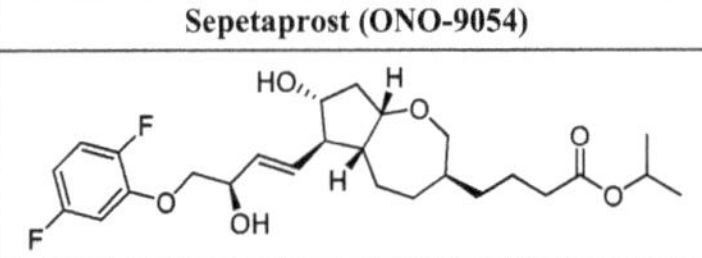	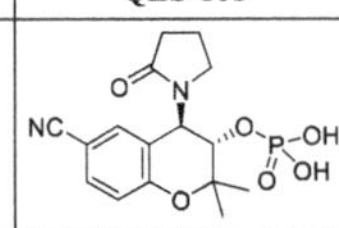	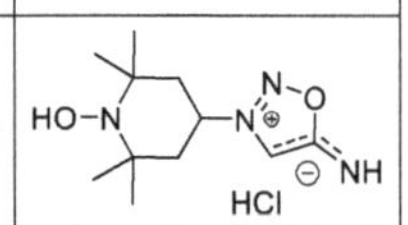
CAS #	945457-84-1	1262873-06-2	1802655-72-6	NA
Therapeutic class	Adenosine A3 receptor modulator	Prostaglandin FP and EP_3 receptor dual agonist	ATP-sensitive potassium channel opener	Nitric oxide donor-superoxide dismutase mimetic
Mechanism of action	Increase in AH conventional outflow and decrease in AH inflow	Increase in AH conventional and uveoscleral outflow	Decrease in episcleral venous pressure	Increase in AH conventional outflow and decrease episcleral venous pressure
Doses	-			
Rodent models	Mouse (glucocorticoid-induced OHT): 700 µM oral dose Rabbit (Normotensive): 500 µM, oral dose (Park *et al.*, 2020)	Mouse (normotensive): 0.003% (Yamagishi-Kimura *et al.*, 2022)	Mouse (normotensive): 0.2% (Pervan-Steel *et al.*, 2022)	Rat (Morrisons model)-2% Mouse (Ad5TGFβ induced OHT): 2% (Stankowska *et al.*, 2021)

(Table 3) cont.....

Name	FM-101	Sepetaprost (ONO-9054)	QLS-101	SA-2
Large animal models	NA	Monkey (Normotensive): 3 µg/mL-30 µg/mL (Yamane *et al.*, 2015)	NA	NA

Abbreviations CAS#: Chemical Abstracts Registry Number; NA: Not available.

The synthesis of **FM-101** is described in Yu *et al.* (2017) (as compound **3b**) and starts by protection of 4 of the hydroxy groups of D-mannose (Sigma-Aldrich Company; www.sigmaaldrich.com) with 2,2-dimethoxypropane under acidic conditions to provide the bis-acetonide tetrahydrofuranyl acetal **1**. Reduction with sodium borohydride affords diol **2**, which is converted to bis-mesylate **3** with mesyl chloride and base. Ring closure to tetrahydrothiophene **4** is affected by treatment with sodium sulfide. Selective mono-acetonide cleavage by treatment with acetic acid affords diol **5**, oxidative degradation of which with lead acetate provides thioacetal **6**. N-alkylation of 2,6-dichloropurine (Sigma-Aldrich Company; www.sigmaaldrich.com) with **6** followed by hydrochloric acid deprotection provides (2,6-chloropurin-7-yl)tetrahydrothiophene **7**. Selective displacement of the 6-chlorine with 3-chlorobenzylamine affords **FM-101** (CAS# 945457-84-1).

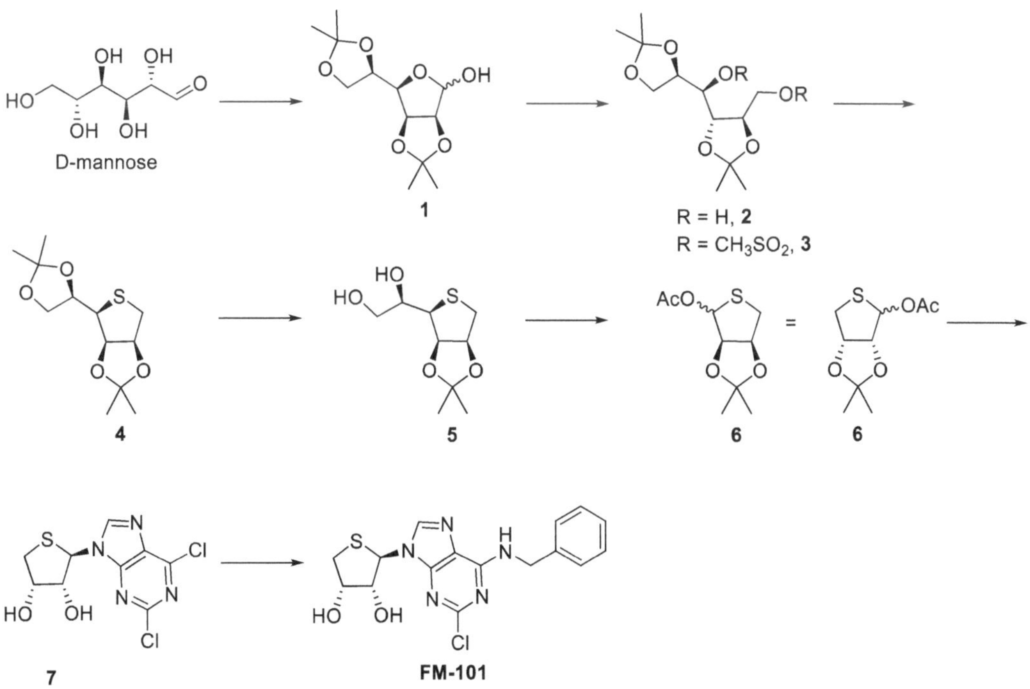

Fig. (1). Synthesis of FM-101, an adenosine A3 receptor modulator.

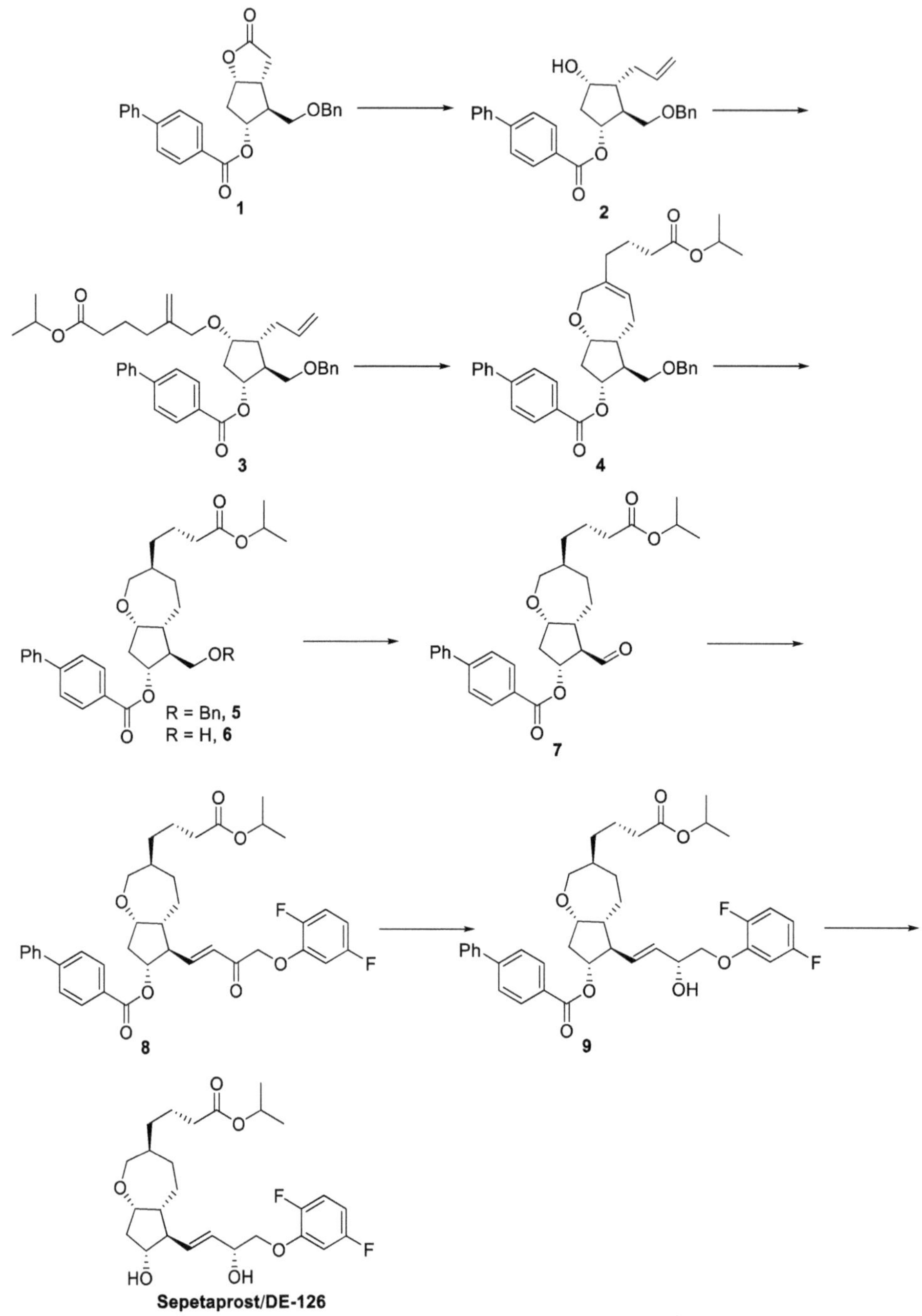

Fig. (2). Synthesis of Sepetaprost/DE-126, a dual prostaglandin FP/EP_3 receptor agonist.

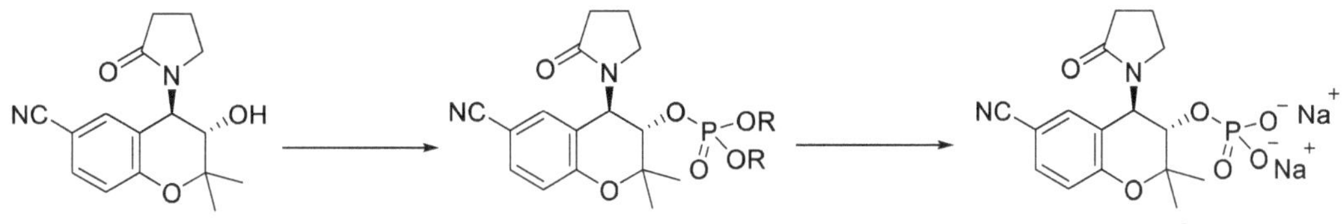

Levcromakalin R = Bn, (3*S*,4*R*)-**1** R = H, **QLS-101** (3*S*,4*R*)-**2** Chemical Abstracts Registry Number 1802655-71-5

Fig. (3). Synthesis of QLS-101, a phosphate ester prodrug of the ATP-sensitive potassium channel opener levcromakalin.

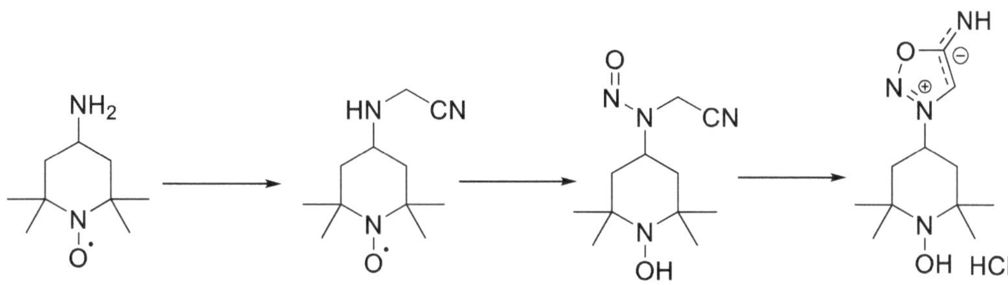

1 **2** **3** **SA-2**

Fig. (4). Synthesis of SA-2, a nitric oxide donor–antioxidant.

The synthesis of sepetaprost/**DE-126** is described in Moriguchi *et al.*'s study (2019) (example 13). Reduction of lactone **1** [commercially available from ASW MedChem, www.aswmedchem.com, 732-342-6911] with diisobutylaluminum hydride affords the corresponding lactol, which is treated with methyltripheny lphosphonium bromide and potassium *tert*-butoxide to provide allylcyclopentanol **2**. O-alkylation of **2** with isopropyl 5-(bromomethyl)-5-hexenoate [for preparation, see Moriguchi *et al.* (2019), example 3:2] under basic conditions provides allyl ether **3**, ruthenium carbene-catalyzed ring-closing metathesis of which affords hexahydro-oxepin **4**. Hydrogenation of **4** in the presence of a chiral catalyst gives 3*S*-octahydro-oxepin **5**, which is O-debenzylated by catalytic hydrogenation to give primary alcohol **6**. Oxidation of **6** under Moffat conditions is effected using dimethylsulfoxide, carbodiimide, and chloroacetic acid to provide aldehyde **7**, which undergoes Horner-Emmons olefination with dimethyl [3-(2,5-difluorophenoxy)-2-oxopropyl]phosphonate to yield *E* enone **8**. The ketone in **8** is reduced stereoselectively with (−)-B-chlorodiisopino campheylborane to give the *R* allyl alcohol **9**. Removal of the 4-phenylbenzoate group with lithium hydroxide affords sepetaprost/**DE-126**.

The synthesis of **QLS-101** and its disodium salt are described in Chowdhury *et al.* (2016); the structure of **QLS-101** has been disclosed in Pervan-Steel *et al.*'s study

(2022). Treatment of levcromakalin (Tocris Biosciences, www.tocris.com) with dibenzyl *N,N*-dimethylphosphoramidite gives the corresponding phosphite ester, which is oxidized with 30% hydrogen peroxide to provide phosphate ester (3*S*,4*R*)-**1**. Debenzylation with trimethylsilyl bromide affords **QLS-101**, which can be conveniently converted to the disodium salt using an ion exchange column to afford (3*S*, 4*R*)-**2**.

The synthesis of hybrid anti-oxidant-NO donor compound **SA-2** HCl was previously described (Acharya *et al.*, 2016) following the scheme shown in Fig. (**4**). Briefly, commercially available 4-amino TEMPO **1** (www.sigmaaldrich.com, Cat #163945) was treated with formaldehyde bisulfite in H_2O followed by heating with KCN at 50°C to produce the nitrile intermediate **2,** which was nitrosylated at 0°C using $NaNO_2$/HCl. Product formation was confirmed from LC/MS. The nitrosylated intermediate **3** is unstable and immediately converted to the 1,2,3-oxadiazole amine hydrochloride salt **SA-2** on treatment with excess methanolic HCl and overnight stirring.

For a more extensive listing and discussion of clinically useful and experimental IOP-lowering drugs, please consult some of the following references (Sharif, 2021; Liu *et al.*, 2022; Sharif *et al.*, 2023).

CONCLUSION

Reduction of IOP is still the main therapeutic strategy for preventing vision loss due to glaucoma. There are a number of compounds that, when applied as topical ocular formulations, have demonstrated IOP-lowering activity in the clinic and/or in experimental glaucoma models. Many of these agents are commercially available for further exploration of their biology, and those that are not commercially available can typically be synthesized by methods demonstrated in the peer-reviewed and patent literature.

REFERENCES

Acharya, S, Rogers, P, Krishnamoorthy, RR, Stankowska, DL, Dias, HVR & Yorio, T (2016) Design and synthesis of novel hybrid sydnonimine and prodrug useful for glaucomatous optic neuropathy. *Bioorg Med Chem Lett,* 26, 1490-4.
[http://dx.doi.org/10.1016/j.bmcl.2015.12.030] [PMID: 26832784]

Aihara, M, Lindsey, JD & Weinreb, RN (2002) Reduction of intraocular pressure in mouse eyes treated with latanoprost. *Invest Ophthalmol Vis Sci,* 43, 146-50.
[PMID: 11773025]

Burke, J & Schwartz, M (1996) Preclinical evaluation of brimonidine. *Surv Ophthalmol,* 41 (Suppl. 1), S9-S18.
[http://dx.doi.org/10.1016/S0039-6257(96)82027-3] [PMID: 8970245]

Chandra, S, Muir, ER, Deo, K, Kiel, JW & Duong, TQ (2016) Effects of Dorzolamide on Retinal and Choroidal Blood Flow in the DBA/2J Mouse Model of Glaucoma. *Invest Ophthalmol Vis Sci,* 57, 826-31.

[http://dx.doi.org/10.1167/iovs.15-18291] [PMID: 26934140]

Roy Chowdhury, U, Viker, KB, Stoltz, KL, Holman, BH, Fautsch, MP & Dosa, PI (2016) Analogs of the ATP-Sensitive Potassium (K_{ATP}) Channel Opener Cromakalim with *in vivo* Ocular Hypotensive Activity. *J Med Chem,* 59, 6221-31.
[http://dx.doi.org/10.1021/acs.jmedchem.6b00406] [PMID: 27367033]

Roy Chowdhury, U, Millar, JC, Holman, BH, Anderson, KJ, Dosa, PI, Roddy, GW & Fautsch, MP (2022) Effect of ATP-sensitive Potassium Channel Openers on Intraocular Pressure in Ocular Hypertensive Animal Models. *Invest Ophthalmol Vis Sci,* 63, 15.
[http://dx.doi.org/10.1167/iovs.63.2.15] [PMID: 35129587]

Dong, YR, Huang, SW, Cui, JZ & Yoshitomi, T (2018) Effects of brinzolamide on rabbit ocular blood flow *in vivo* and *ex vivo*. *Int J Ophthalmol,* 11, 719-25.
[http://dx.doi.org/10.18240/ijo.2018.05.03] [PMID: 29862168]

Gelatt, KN & MacKay, EO (2001) Effect of different dose schedules of latanoprost on intraocular pressure and pupil size in the glaucomatous Beagle. *Vet Ophthalmol,* 4, 283-8.
[http://dx.doi.org/10.1046/j.1463-5216.2001.00201.x] [PMID: 11906665]

Husain, S, Andy Whitlock, N, Rice, DS & Crosson, CE (2006) Effects of latanoprost on rodent intraocular pressure. *Exp Eye Res,* 83, 1453-8.
[http://dx.doi.org/10.1016/j.exer.2006.08.004] [PMID: 17027754]

Impagnatiello, F, Bastia, E, Toris, CB, Krauss, AH, Prasanna, G & Ongini, E (2015) NCX 470, a nitric oxide (NO)-donating bimatoprost lowers intraocular pressure in rabbits, dogs and non-human primate models of glaucoma. *Invest Ophthalmol Vis Sci,* 56, 5809.

Impagnatiello, F, Toris, CB, Batugo, M, Prasanna, G, Borghi, V, Bastia, E, Ongini, E & Krauss, AHP (2015) Intraocular Pressure–Lowering Activity of NCX 470, a Novel Nitric Oxide–Donating Bimatoprost in Preclinical Models. *Invest Ophthalmol Vis Sci,* 56, 6558-64.
[http://dx.doi.org/10.1167/iovs.15-17190] [PMID: 26457541]

Kirihara, T, Iwamura, R, Yoneda, K, Kawabata-Odani, N, Shimazaki, A & Kawazu, K (2015) DE-117, a selective EP2 agonist, lowered intraocular pressure in animal models. *Invest Ophthalmol Vis Sci,* 56, 5709-9.

Klimko, PG & Sharif, NA (2019) Discovery, characterization and clinical utility of prostaglandin agonists for the treatment of glaucoma. *Br J Pharmacol,* 176, 1051-8.
[http://dx.doi.org/10.1111/bph.14327] [PMID: 29665040]

Krauss, AHP, Impagnatiello, F, Toris, CB, Gale, DC, Prasanna, G, Borghi, V, Chiroli, V, Chong, WKM, Carreiro, ST & Ongini, E (2011) Ocular hypotensive activity of BOL-303259-X, a nitric oxide donating Prostaglandin F2α agonist, in preclinical models. *Exp Eye Res,* 93, 250-5.
[http://dx.doi.org/10.1016/j.exer.2011.03.001] [PMID: 21396362]

Lee, LY, Hsu, JH, Fu, HI, Chen, CC & Tung, KC (2022) Lowering the Intraocular Pressure in Rats and Rabbits by *Cordyceps cicadae* Extract and Its Active Compounds. *Molecules,* 27, 707.
[http://dx.doi.org/10.3390/molecules27030707] [PMID: 35163975]

Li, G, Nottebaum, AF, Brigell, M, Navarro, ID, Ipe, U, Mishra, S, Gomez-Caraballo, M, Schmitt, H, Soldo, B, Pakola, S, Withers, B, Peters, KG, Vestweber, D & Stamer, WD (2020) A Small Molecule Inhibitor of VE-PTP Activates Tie2 in Schlemm's Canal Increasing Outflow Facility and Reducing Intraocular Pressure. *Invest Ophthalmol Vis Sci,* 61, 12.
[http://dx.doi.org/10.1167/iovs.61.14.12] [PMID: 33315051]

Lin, CW, Sherman, B, Moore, LA, Laethem, CL, Lu, DW, Pattabiraman, PP, Rao, PV, deLong, MA & Kopczynski, CC (2018) Discovery and Preclinical Development of Netarsudil, a Novel Ocular Hypotensive Agent for the Treatment of Glaucoma. *J Ocul Pharmacol Ther,* 34, 40-51.
[http://dx.doi.org/10.1089/jop.2017.0023] [PMID: 28609185]

Liu, P, Wang, F, Song, Y, Wang, M & Zhang, X (2022) Current situation and progress of drugs for reducing intraocular pressure. *Ther Adv Chronic Dis,* 13, 20406223221140392.

[http://dx.doi.org/10.1177/20406223221140392] [PMID: 36479139]

Moriguchi, H., Tanaka, Y. Ino, T., Kame, T., Nishiyama, T., Tsujiyama, S., Ueda, O. (2019). Method for producing bicyclic compound. United States Patent Application Publication number US 2019/0315705 A1

Ota, T, Aihara, M, Saeki, T, Narumiya, S & Araie, M (2007) The IOP-lowering effects and mechanism of action of tafluprost in prostanoid receptor-deficient mice. *Br J Ophthalmol,* 91, 673-6. [http://dx.doi.org/10.1136/bjo.2006.105585] [PMID: 17124244]

Park, CW, Han, CT, Sakaguchi, Y, Lee, J & Youn, HY (2020) Safety evaluation of FM101, an A3 adenosine receptor modulator, in rat, for developing as therapeutics of glaucoma and hepatitis. *EXCLI J,* 19, 187-200. [http://dx.doi.org/10.17179/excli2019-2058] [PMID: 32256265]

Pervan-Steel, CL, Roy Chowdhury, U, Sookdeo, HK, Casale, RA, Dosa, PI, Htoo, TM, Fautsch, MP & Wirostko, BM (2022) Ocular Hypotensive Properties and Biochemical Profile of QLS-101, a Novel ATP-Sensitive Potassium (K_{ATP}) Channel Opening Prodrug. *Invest Ophthalmol Vis Sci,* 63, 26. [http://dx.doi.org/10.1167/iovs.63.4.26] [PMID: 35486069]

Plummer, CE, MacKay, EO & Gelatt, KN (2006) Comparison of the effects of topical administration of a fixed combination of dorzolamide–timolol to monotherapy with timolol or dorzolamide on IOP, pupil size, and heart rate in glaucomatous dogs. *Vet Ophthalmol,* 9, 245-9. [http://dx.doi.org/10.1111/j.1463-5224.2006.00469.x] [PMID: 16771760]

Prasanna, G, Carreiro, S, Anderson, S, Gukasyan, H, Sartnurak, S, Younis, H, Gale, D, Xiang, C, Wells, P, Dinh, D, Almaden, C, Fortner, J, Toris, C, Niesman, M, Lafontaine, J & Krauss, A (2011) Effect of PF-04217329 a prodrug of a selective prostaglandin EP2 agonist on intraocular pressure in preclinical models of glaucoma. *Exp Eye Res,* 93, 256-64. [http://dx.doi.org/10.1016/j.exer.2011.02.015] [PMID: 21376717]

Reitsamer, HA, Bogner, B, Tockner, B & Kiel, JW (2009) Effects of dorzolamide on choroidal blood flow, ciliary blood flow, and aqueous production in rabbits. *Invest Ophthalmol Vis Sci,* 50, 2301-7. [http://dx.doi.org/10.1167/iovs.08-2468] [PMID: 19182250]

Saeki, T, Tsuruga, H, Aihara, M, Araie, M & Rittenhouse, K (2009) Dose-Response Profile of PF-03187207 (PF-207) and Peak IOP Lowering Response Following Single Topical Administration to FP Receptor Knockout Mice vs. Wild Type Mice. *Invest Ophthalmol Vis Sci,* 50, 4064.

Seki, M, Tanaka, T, Matsuda, H, Togano, T, Hashimoto, K, Ueda, J, Fukuchi, T & Abe, H (2005) Topically administered timolol and dorzolamide reduce intraocular pressure and protect retinal ganglion cells in a rat experimental glaucoma model. *Br J Ophthalmol,* 89, 504-7. [http://dx.doi.org/10.1136/bjo.2004.052860] [PMID: 15774933]

Serle, J, Podos, SM, Kitazawa, Y & Wang, R-F (1998) A comparative study of latanoprost (Xalatan) and isopropyl unoprostone (Rescula) in normal and glaucomatous monkey eyes. *Jpn J Ophthalmol,* 42, 95-100. [http://dx.doi.org/10.1016/S0021-5155(97)00128-7] [PMID: 9587840]

Sharif, NA (2021) Therapeutic Drugs and Devices for Tackling Ocular Hypertension and Glaucoma, and Need for Neuroprotection and Cytoprotective Therapies. *Front Pharmacol,* 12, 729249. [http://dx.doi.org/10.3389/fphar.2021.729249] [PMID: 34603044]

Sharif N.A., Odani-Kawabata N., Lu F., Pinchuk L. (2023) FP and EP2 prostanoid receptor agonist drugs and aqueous humor outflow devices for treating ocular hypertension and glaucoma. Experimental Eye Research 299: 109415.

Sit, AJ, Gupta, D, Kazemi, A, McKee, H, Challa, P, Liu, KC, Lopez, J, Kopczynski, C & Heah, T (2021) Netarsudil Improves Trabecular Outflow Facility in Patients with Primary Open Angle Glaucoma or Ocular Hypertension: A Phase 2 Study. *Am J Ophthalmol,* 226, 262-9. [http://dx.doi.org/10.1016/j.ajo.2021.01.019] [PMID: 33524367]

Stankowska, DL, Millar, JC, Kodati, B, Behera, S, Chaphalkar, RM, Nguyen, T, Nguyen, KT, Krishnamoorthy, RR, Ellis, DZ & Acharya, S (2021) Nanoencapsulated hybrid compound SA-2 with long-lasting intraocular pressure-lowering activity in rodent eyes. *Mol Vis,* 27, 37-49.

[PMID: 33633438]

Takagi, Y, Nakajima, T, Shimazaki, A, Kageyama, M, Matsugi, T, Matsumura, Y, Gabelt, BAT, Kaufman, PL & Hara, H (2004) Pharmacological characteristics of AFP-168 (tafluprost), a new prostanoid FP receptor agonist, as an ocular hypotensive drug. *Exp Eye Res,* 78, 767-76.
[http://dx.doi.org/10.1016/j.exer.2003.12.007] [PMID: 15037111]

Toris, CB, Zhan, GL, Camras, CB & McLaughlin, MA (2005) Effects of travoprost on aqueous humor dynamics in monkeys. *J Glaucoma,* 14, 70-3.
[http://dx.doi.org/10.1097/01.ijg.0000146361.15163.ea] [PMID: 15650608]

Whitlock, NA, McKnight, B, Corcoran, KN, Rodriguez, LA & Rice, DS (2010) Increased intraocular pressure in mice treated with dexamethasone. *Invest Ophthalmol Vis Sci,* 51, 6496-503.
[http://dx.doi.org/10.1167/iovs.10-5430] [PMID: 20671272]

Wijesinghe, HK, Puthuran, GV, Ramulu, PY, Ponnat, AK, Reddy, MM, Mani, I, Krishnadas, SR & Gedde, SJ (2022) Intraocular Pressure Control Following Phacoemulsification in Eyes With Pre-existing Aurolab Aqueous Drainage Implant. *J Glaucoma,* 31, 456-61.
[http://dx.doi.org/10.1097/IJG.0000000000001946] [PMID: 34628424]

Woodward, DF, Krauss, AHP, Chen, J, Lai, RK, Spada, CS, Burk, RM, Andrews, SW, Shi, L, Liang, Y, Kedzie, KM, Chen, R, Gil, DW, Kharlamb, A, Archeampong, A, Ling, J, Madhu, C, Ni, J, Rix, P, Usansky, J, Usansky, H, Weber, A, Welty, D, Yang, W, Tang-Liu, DDS, Garst, ME, Brar, B, Wheeler, LA & Kaplan, LJ (2001) The pharmacology of bimatoprost (Lumigan). *Surv Ophthalmol,* 45 (Suppl. 4), S337-45.
[http://dx.doi.org/10.1016/S0039-6257(01)00224-7] [PMID: 11434936]

Yamagishi-Kimura, R, Honjo, M & Aihara, M (2022) The Roles Played by FP/EP3 Receptors During Pressure-lowering in Mouse Eyes Mediated by a Dual FP/EP3 Receptor Agonist. *Invest Ophthalmol Vis Sci,* 63, 24-4.
[http://dx.doi.org/10.1167/iovs.63.2.24] [PMID: 35147658]

Yamane, S, Karakawa, T, Nakayama, S, Nagai, K, Moriyuki, K, Neki, S, Suto, F, Kambe, T, Hirota, Y & Kawabata, K (2015) IOP-Lowering Effect of ONO-9054, A Novel Dual Agonist of Prostanoid EP3 and FP Receptors, in Monkeys. *Invest Ophthalmol Vis Sci,* 56, 2547-52.
[http://dx.doi.org/10.1167/iovs.14-16181] [PMID: 25788650]

Yu, J, Ahn, S, Kim, HJ, Lee, M, Ahn, S, Kim, J, Jin, SH, Lee, E, Kim, G, Cheong, JH, Jacobson, KA, Jeong, LS & Noh, M (2017) Polypharmacology of N^6 -(3-Iodobenzyl)adenosine-5′- *N* -methyluronamide (IB-MECA) and Related A $_3$ Adenosine Receptor Ligands: Peroxisome Proliferator Activated Receptor (PPAR) γ Partial Agonist and PPARδ Antagonist Activity Suggests Their Antidiabetic Potential. *J Med Chem,* 60, 7459-75.
[http://dx.doi.org/10.1021/acs.jmedchem.7b00805] [PMID: 28799755]

Yu, H, Zhong, H, Chen, J, Sun, J, Huang, P, Xu, X, Huang, S & Zhong, Y (2020) Efficacy, Drug Sensitivity, and Safety of a Chronic Ocular Hypertension Rat Model Established Using a Single Intracameral Injection of Hydrogel into the Anterior Chamber. *Med Sci Monit,* 26, e925852.
[http://dx.doi.org/10.12659/MSM.925852] [PMID: 32997651]

TARGET LOCALIZATION AND VERIFICATION STUDIES

CHAPTER 4

Protocols for Localizing Receptor mRNAs and Proteins by RT-PCR, *In Situ* Hybridization, and Autoradiography

Najam A. Sharif[1,*] and **Saima Chaudhry**[2]

[1] *Vice President and Head of Research & Development Nanoscope Therapeutics Inc., 2777 N. Stemmons Fwy, Suite 1102, Dallas, TX-75207, USA*

[2] *Univ N. Texas at Arlington, 701 S Nedderman Dr, Arlington, TX-76019, USA*

Abstract: Receptors, enzymes, transporters, and ion channels receive external signals and generate specific intracellular second messengers to mediate the biological response to the ligands that bind to the proteins on the cell membrane and/or to organelles inside the cells. In order to localize the potential target protein(s) that may be defective and/or those serving endogenous transmitter or drug activities in various tissues of the body, the use of reverse transcriptase-polymerase chain reaction and *in situ* hybridization coupled with quantitative receptor autoradiography are deployed. Such studies can be performed using isolated cells or postmortem tissues of animals and humans. Such techniques are powerful indicators of the presence or absence of the key receptors/enzymes and other protein targets that can help ensure target validation, localization, and engagement with exogenously delivered chemicals, drugs, antibodies, *etc.* These aspects are critical for drug discovery and can also indicate off-target side effects of drugs under study. These techniques will be described in this chapter.

Keywords: Transporters, Target `engagement, Drug interaction, Enzymes, Ion channels, Receptors, Signal transduction, Target localization.

INTRODUCTION

The drug discovery and development process is a lengthy and expensive endeavor regardless of the disease being targeted. Therefore, it is important to know if and where a drug molecule binds with target and off-target tissues and cells of the body. Consequently, a number of techniques have been developed, validated, and utilized in order to study the interaction and functional engagement of endogenous

* **Corresponding author Najam A. Sharif:** Vice President and Head of Research & Development Nanoscope Therapeutics Inc., 2777 N. Stemmons Fwy, Suite 1102, Dallas, TX-75207, USA; Tel: +1(817)-565-7686; E-mail: nsharif@nanostherapeutics.com

chemicals (*e.g.*, neurotransmitters) and potential drug candidates (small compounds, peptides, antibodies, *etc.*) with their target proteins (receptor, enzyme, transporter, or ion channel protein). This chapter describes protocols to perform reverse transcriptase-polymerase chain reaction (RT-PCR) and *in situ* hybridization (ISH) microscopy to obtain information about the presence/absence of the mRNAs of targeted proteins and their distribution. Autoradiography allows localization, visualization, and quantification of radioligand-protein complexes *in vitro* and *ex vivo*, depending on the study design and the expected outcome. These are important techniques to demonstrate the drug molecule-target protein interactions in cells and tissues of importance from an efficacy and potential safety perspective.

Prostaglandins (PGs) and serotonin (5-hydroxytryptamine; 5-HT) are endogenous transmitter substances that elicit their biological actions by interacting with specific cell membrane-bound receptors. Several sub-types of receptors for each class of transmitter have been identified and characterized using agonist and antagonist drugs. For instance, DP- (DP1-2), EP- (EP1-4), and FP-PG receptors exist, and receptor-selective drugs have been created that lower and control intraocular pressure (IOP) as treatments for many forms of glaucoma, a collection of neurodegenerative retinal/optic nerve/brain diseases (Weinreb *et al.*, 2014; Sharif, 2018-2022). Thus, the free acid forms of FP-receptor agonists (*e.g.*, latanoprost and travoprost) engage with their cognate receptors to stimulate phosphoinositide turnover in the cytoplasm, which produces inositol phosphates and diacylglycerol (Sharif *et al.*, 2023). These agents, in turn, liberate intracellular Ca^{2+} and lead to the phosphorylation of various enzymes and other proteins in the target cells. These activities culminate in the outflow of aqueous humor fluid (AQH) from both the unconventional uveoscleral outflow pathway (across the ciliary muscle and sclera) and, to some degree, from the conventional outflow pathway that involves trabecular meshwork/Schlemm's canal (TM/SC) and IOP reduction. Similarly, drugs that bind to EP2-receptors, for example, omidenepag (Sharif *et al.*, 2023), raise intracellular cAMP levels that induce a plethora of additional intracellular reactions to enhance relaxation of TM and digest extracellular matrix to promote AQH outflow from the anterior chamber of the eye *via* the unconventional and conventional outflow pathways to reduce IOP (Sharif *et al.*, 2023). A similar situation prevails for 5-HT2 receptors and subtypes. Hence, 5-HT2A-2C receptor-selective agonists exert strong ocular hypotensive actions when dosed topical ocularly in ocular hypertensive monkey eyes to suppress elevated IOP (Sharif et l., 2006; Sharif and Senchyna, 2006). Below are described some of the key methods to determine the presence/absence of the receptor mRNA and proteins for selected PGs and 5-HT, which serve as good examples for these ocular hypotensive activity mediators.

RT-PCR of Receptors in Eye Tissues of the Anterior Chamber

RT-PCR is a technique combining reverse transcription of RNA into DNA (in this context called complementary DNA or cDNA) and amplification of specific DNA targets using the polymerase chain reaction (PCR). It is primarily used to measure and quantify the amount of a specific RNA, which is accomplished by monitoring the amplifying reaction using fluorescence, a technique called real-time PCR, or, in other cases, quantitative PCR (qPCR). Combined RT-PCR and qPCR are utilized to assess gene expression and quantification of mRNAs. Some publications where receptor mRNAs were ascertained by RT-PCR include those by Ullmer *et al.* (1995), Senchyna *et al.* (2000), Kyveris *et al.* (2002), Sharif *et al.* (2002), Chidlow *et al.* (2004), and Sharif and Senchyna (2006). As examples, these publications provide the necessary procedures to determine mRNAs for FP- and TP- prostaglandin and serotonin receptors.

Isolation of Total RNA

- Aseptic isolation of total RNA from tissues isolated from the human cadaveric anterior chamber should be performed with the RNeasy Midi Kit (QIAGEN Inc., Mississauga, Ontario, Canada).
- Determination of the concentration and purity of total RNA should be performed by UV light absorption on a GeneQuant pro RNA/DNA calculator (Biochrom Ltd.; Cambridge, UK). If optical densities at 260 nm/280 nm are lower than 1.6, the preparations should be discarded.
- Use electrophoresis to determine the presence of intact RNA by loading it on 1% agarose-formaldehyde gels. RNA isolates can be accepted to be intact if the UV fluorescence of the 28S rRNA band is twice the intensity of the 18S rRNA band and if no UV fluorescence is found below the 18 rRNA band.

mRNA Detection by RT-PCR

- Synthesis of sense and antisense-specific primers ought to be based on an intron-exon boundary design in order to distinguish between the amplification of mRNA and genomic DNA and should be based on reported/published cDNA sequences. BLAST retrieval of human cDNA sequences (based on GenBank searches) should be used to design other primers.
- Procedures used to determine the RT-PCR-based detection of mRNAs for various 5-HT receptors in human ocular tissues will be illustrated (Fig. **1**).
- Total RNA (25 to 97 μg) should be isolated from the ocular tissue samples followed by conversion to cDNA in a 10 μl reverse transcription reaction solution containing 0.5 mg of total RNA of each sample, 1X first strand buffer (75 mM KCl; 50 mM Tris-HCl, pH 8.3; 3.0 mM $MgCl_2$), 1.7 mM $MgCl_2$, 1 mM each dNTP, 10 mM dTT, 2.5 mM oligo (dT)18, and 5 U/μl of SuperScript™ II

reverse transcriptase. Incubate reactants at 42 °C for 1 hr, heat at 95 °C for 5 minutes, and then cool at 4 °C for a minimum of 5 minutes and a maximum of 30 minutes.

- PCR should then be performed on 5 µl of the cDNA preparation (generated from 0.5 µg of total RNA), to which 44 µl of a PCR master mix containing 1X PCR buffer (55 mM KCl; 13 mM Tris-HCl, pH 8.3) 1 mM MgCl2, 10% dimethylsulphoxide (DMSO), 1.25 U/50 µl AmpilTaq Gold® with GeneAmp® DNA polymerase, and 0.2 µM sense and anti-sense primer in a total volume of 50 µl is added. The PCR is then carried out in a GeneAmp® PCR System 2400 thermocycler utilizing various parameters: an initial denaturing step of 10 minutes at 95 °C, denaturing at 94 °C for 30s, annealing at the optimal temperature for 30s, and extending at 72 °C for one minute. The final polymerization step is extended for an additional 7 minutes.
- PCR should be performed for 40 cycles, and appropriate precautions should be observed to prevent product contamination. For best results, the PCR process, amplification, and product processing should be performed on dedicated equipment and in separate isolated rooms. Additionally, several control reactions should be run in parallel during RT-PCR analyses. These include RT reactions conducted in the absence of the reverse transcriptase enzyme to confirm the absence of genomic DNA and/or cDNA contamination and RT reactions run without RNA to assess any reagent contamination.
- A negative control employs PCR amplification of 1.5 ng of human genomic DNA. Positive control RT-PCR reactions should be carried out using total human brain or lung RNA obtained commercially or harvested in the lab. Electrophoresis of 12 µl of PCR product on 1.5% agarose gels containing 1 µg/ml ethidium bromide and visualization by UV transillumination should be used to evaluate PCR amplification reactions. Using positive control and the molecular weight ladder can help identify the product and product identity can be confirmed by an endonuclease digestion procedure as described below.
- Each 5HT receptor mRNA is digested utilizing the appropriate restriction endonuclease enzyme in a final reaction volume of 25 µl. After digestion, the products should be resolved by electrophoresis (90 V; for 2.5 hrs) on a 2.0% agarose-TBE gel, which is stained with 1 µg/ml ethidium bromide. The gels should then be visualized and photographed using the GeneGenius and GeneSnap software, and the splice products must be identified using the positive control tissues and the molecular weight ladder. The other important internal control that should be run is for the mRNA pertaining to glycerol-3-phosphate dehydrogenase (G3PDH), the housekeeping enzyme present in all cells. Additional information on these procedures has been previously described (Ullmer *et al.* (1995), Kyveris *et al.* (2002), Sharif *et al.*, (2002), Chidlow *et al.* (2004) and Sharif and Senchyna (2002)).

Donor #	$5HT_{2A}$	$5HT_{2B}$	$5HT_{2C}$	$5HT_3$	$5HT_4$	$5HT_5$	$5HT_6$	$5HT_7$
5HT receptor subtype mRNA signals in human ciliary body								
1	+++	+++	++	+++	+++	+++	–	+++
2	+++	+++	++	++	++	++	–	+++
3	+++	+++	–	–	++	++	–	+++
4	+++	+++	+	+++	++	++	–	+
5	+++	+++	+	+	++	–	–	+++
6	+++	+++	+++	–	+++	++	–	+++
5HT receptor subtype mRNA signals in human ciliary epithelium								
1	+++	–	×	×	×	×	×	×
2	+++	+	+	×	×	×	×	–
3	+++	–	+	×	×	×	×	+
4	+++	+	+	×	×	×	×	+
5HT receptor subtype mRNA signals in human TM cells								
Data from 8 donors	+++	+++	+	–	–	+	–	+
5HT receptor subtype mRNA signals in human optic nerve								
1	–	+	–	–	–	–	–	–
2	+	–	–	×	×	++	+	++
3	–	+++	–	–	+	–	–	–

Fig. (1). Distribution and density of mRNAs for 5-HT receptors and some sub-types of receptors in human ocular tissues determined by RT-PCR. Relative abundance is indicated as follows: - indicates low or absence; + - ++ and +++ indicate increasing abundance. Adapted from Sharif and Senchyna (2006) with permission from the authors.

In situ Hybridization to Localize and Visualize mRNAs for PG Receptors

The *in situ* hybridization (ISH) technique uses a labeled complementary DNA, RNA, or modified nucleic acids strand (*i.e.*, probe) to discretely localize a specific DNA or RNA sequence in a cell or tissue (Ito *et al.*, 1995; Mukhopadhyyay *et al.*, 2001; Schlotzer-Schrehardt *et al.*, 2002) (*e.g.*, Fig. (**2**); top and bottom panels). This process is distinctly different from immunohistochemistry, which localizes proteins in cells or on thin sections of specific tissues. Hence, the specific probes labeled with either radio-isotopes or fluorescent- or antigen-labeled bases (*e.g.*, digoxigenin) can be visualized and quantified in the target cells/tissues using either autoradiography, fluorescence microscopy, or immunohistochemical methods. Two or more transcripts can be visualized simultaneously using radioactive and non-radioactive probes in the same sample of cells/tissue sections.

Tissue Preparation

- Obtain human or animal eyes a few hours post-mortem and keep cool in ice-cold Dexol preservation fluid or ice. Bisect eyeballs equatorially in a laminar flow hood if possible, fix in 4% neutral buffered paraformaldehyde, and then embed in paraffin. If frozen tissue sections are needed, then mount the specimen on microtome chucks using tissue-tec or chilled water.
- Cut 5μm tissue sections from the specimens on a cryostat or a compresstome tissue slicer and collect on slides precoated with 2% APTES (39-aminopropyltriethoxysilane; Sigma, St. Louis, MO). Some of the tissue sections

should be stained with hematoxylin and eosin for future histological examination.

Target	Sequence (5′ to 3′ Direction)	Annealing Temperature (°C)	Expected PCR Product Size (bp)	Accession No.
EP1				
Sense	CGCTATGAGCTGCAGTACCC	55	508	NM_000955
Antisense	CCAGGATCTGGTTCCAGGAG			
EP2				
Sense	CAACCTCATCCGCATGCAC	55	419	NM_000956
Antisense	CTCAAAGGTCAGCCTG			
EP3				
Sense	CGCCTCAACCACTCCTACACA	61	837	NM_000957
Antisense	GCAGACCGACAGCACGCACAT			
EP4				
Sense	TGGTATGTGGGCTGGCTG	55	434	NM_000958
Antisense	GAGGACGGTGGCGAGAAT			
FP				
Sense	CACAAGCTGCCAGACGGAAAAC	55	510	NM_000959
Antisense	TTGTAGAAACACCAGGTCCTCG			
GAPDH				
Sense	ACCACAGTCCATGCCATCAC	58	490	M33197
Antisense	TCCACCACCCTGTTGCTGTA			

	Cornea			Conjunctiva			Sclera		Trabecular Meshwork			
	Epithelium	Keratocytes	Endothelium	Epithelium	Stromal Cells	Vessels	Stromal Cells	Vessels†	Trabecular Cells	Schlemm Canal Cells	Collector Channels	Lens Epithelium
EP1	++	±	±	++	±	+	±‡	+	++	++	++	++
EP2	++	±	±	+*	±*	+*	±	+	+	±	±	+
EP3	±	++	++	±	++*	+	±	+	++	+	+	+
EP4	±	++	++	±	++*	+	±‡	+	++	+	+	+
FP	++	±	±	+*	±*	+*	±	+	+	+	+	+

	Iris				Ciliary Body					Choroid			Retina								
	Epithelium	Muscles	Stromal Cells	Vessels	Epithelium	Muscle	Stromal Cells	Vessels§	Capillaries‖	Stromal Cells	Vessels	Capillaries	RPE	PR#	ONL	INL	PL	GC	NFL	MC	Vessels
EP1	+	+	+	++	++	+	+	+	+	±	+	+	−	++	+	++	±	++	+	−	+
EP2	+	+	±	+	+	±	±	+	+	±	+	++	−	±	±	±	±	+	+	−	+
EP3	−	+	++	±	++	+	+	+	±	+	+	−	−	−	−	−	−	−	−	++	±
EP4	−	+	++	+	++	+	+	+	−	+	+	−	−	±	±	±	+	±	++	−	−
FP	±	++	+	+	++	++¶	+	+	−	+	+	−	−	+	+	+	±	+	+	−	±

Fig. (2). Primers for various PG receptors (mainly EP1-4 and FP) (top panel) and relative distribution and abundance of mRNAs of various PG receptors in human ocular tissues determined by *in situ* immunohistochemistry (lower panel) are shown. The relative abundance of the receptor mRNAs shown in the lower panel is depicted as: - indicates low or absence; + - ++ and +++ indicate increasing abundance. Adapted from Schlötzer-Schrehardt *et al.* (2022) with permission from the authors.

Probe Preparation

- For various prostaglandin receptor mRNA localization studies, appropriate riboprobes should be synthesized from pcDNA I (Invitrogen, San Diego, CA) plasmid vectors containing SP6 and T7 promoters and the full-length human EP1 or FP receptor cDNA. A similar approach should be adopted for the other PG receptors and their subtypes.

- Now, follow the manufacturer's directions to perform the transcription reaction with SP6 (antisense) or T7 (sense) polymerases. Mix the following ingredients: 1 mg linearized plasmid DNA, 2 ml DIG RNA labeling mix, and 2 ml 103-transcription buffer to a final volume of 18 ml. At this point, add RNA polymerase (2 ml; SP6 or T7) to the reaction mixture and incubate for 2 hours at 37°C. Then, use DNAase I (2 ml) to remove the template DNA.
- Now, precipitate the labeled probes and purify from DNA and any unincorporated DIG-UTP. Determination of the labeling efficiency is accomplished semi-quantitatively utilizing a standard DIG-labeled control RNA of known concentration. Based on experience, about 90% of DIG-UTP can be expected to be incorporated into the probe of interest. Using the same procedures as above, sense and antisense FP-receptor probes should be prepared from a plasmid pertaining to the full-length cDNA of the human FP receptor and linearized with NcoI as above.

In situ Hybridization Procedure

- For the ISH, rehydrate the tissue sections, permeabilize in 0.2% Triton X-100, wash in PBS, and then digest with 1 mg/ml proteinase K for 30 minutes at 37°C. Postfix the sections in 4% paraformaldehyde for 10 minutes and wash in PBS and then in 2x SSC (0.3 M NaCl, 30 mM sodium citrate, pH 7.4).
- Hybridize in 50% formamide, 10% dextran sulfate, 53 Denhardt's solution, 100 mg/ml denatured salmon sperm DNA, 0.1% SDS, and 3 ml DIG-labeled antisense or sense probes. Now apply 25 ul of the hybridization solution on to each tissue section. Perform the prehybridization and hybridization procedures at 42°C for 1 hour and overnight, respectively.
- After this, gently wash the slides (5 medium changes) in 23 SSC with 0.1% SDS medium at 48°C and then gently and briefly rinse in PBS buffer. Now, the blocking reagent should be added to tissue sections, incubated for 2 hours at room temperature, and then washed with PBS buffer. The sections should be incubated with antiDIG–AP (alkaline phosphatase) conjugate for 30 minutes, covered with a coverslip, incubated for another 60 minutes, and finally rinsed in PBS buffer.
- Incubate the tissue sections with the AP substrate nitro-blue tetrazolium/5-bromo-4-chloro-3-indolyl-phosphate (NBT/BCIP) for 2 hours (in the dark) to develop the color. Now examine the tissues with a light microscope and take photomicrographs on Ektar, 200 ASA photographic film (Eastman Kodak, Rochester, NY).
- As mentioned above, ISH can also be performed using either a ^{32}P-labeled EP1receptor or ^{32}P-labeled FP receptor probe in the High-Efficiency Hybridization Buffer (Molecular Research, Cincinnati, OH) containing 1% SDS and 0.1 M NaCl overnight at 60°C. The sections should then be rinsed 3 times in

13 SSC/0.1% SDS for 7 minutes at 55°C. Autoradiographic images should then be captured on hyperfilm, ultrafilm, or BioMax MR film (Kodak, Rochester, NY) in X-ray cassettes by apposing the radio-isotope-sensitive films under dim red-light conditions over 1-12 hrs depending on the desired darkness of the images. This is usually ascertained by trial and error to achieve the best results. The films, after the appropriate exposure time, should be developed under red-light conditions according to the manufacturer's instructions to preserve the images on the film. The resultant autoradiograms can then be visualized and annotated with a permanent marker as desired. Later, the same images can be quantified *via* appropriate image analysis machines and software. Note: Too long an exposure of the film to the radiolabeled sections can saturate the film and make the images unusable.

In Vitro Autoradiography to Visualize and Quantify Receptor/Enzyme Proteins

The autoradiographic technique has been utilized for many decades to localize, visualize, and quantify receptor/enzyme/ion-channel/transporter proteins in cells and tissues using radiolabeled transmitter molecules or cognate drugs with high affinity for these proteins. Abundant literature is available describing the use of autoradiography to localize and quantify receptors involved in lowering and controlling intraocular pressure in human and animal ocular tissues (*e.g.*, Tobin *et al.*, 1989; Sharif *et al.*, 1999, 2006a,b). The procedures described below were adapted from the latter sources to illustrate the principle of radioligand-based autoradiography, and other drug receptors have been mapped using the same technology (Sharif, 1989; Sharif and Eglen, 1993; Sharif and Hughes, 1989).

Tissue Preparation

- Whole donor human eyeballs should be acquired within a few hours of death, stored at 4°C in a moist chamber or in ice prior to donor serology testing, and transported from various eye banks. Laboratory animal eyeballs can be enucleated after sacrifice according to the institutional rules and requirements.
- Using Tissue-Tek® OCT embedding medium (SakuraFintek U.S.A., Inc., Torrance, CA), embed the eyeballs on the microtome with the corneal surface facing outwards. If only the front of the eye tissues are the focus of the study, then the globes can be equatorially cut and mounted on the chuck. Likewise, if the retina and optic nerve are the focus of the study, the cut semi-eyeball can be appropriately positioned on the chuck. The embedded eyeballs (full or halves) on the chucks are then frozen at -40°C prior to long-term storage at -80°C as needed. If the sectioning must be performed on the following day, the loaded chucks can be left within the cryostat overnight (-17°C) to equilibrate and allow the eyeball to fully adhere to the chucks.

- Eyeball sectioning should then be performed on a cryostat microtome (*e.g.*, Bright Instrument Co., Ltd., Huntington, England) using a profile-C knife. Duplicate sagittal sections (20 µm) should be collected on 75 x 38 mm glass microscope slides previously coated with 1% gelatin and annotated/labeled with a permanent marker (*e.g.*, #1, #2, *etc.* or Total, NSB, *etc.*). The consecutive adjacent sections should then be collected on the slides at the appropriate position, and the completed slides should be placed sequentially in slide holders. These should be kept frozen in the cryostat and later transferred to a -80°C freezer until needed for experiments. Prior to the experiment, appropriate volumes of solutions of the radioligand to be used should be prepared in separate 10-25 ml plastic tubes using the applicable buffer and other constituents. If total and non-specific binding of the radioligand to the target protein needs to be determined, then one of the tubes with the radioligand must contain an excess (at least 100 to a 1000-fold higher concentration; 1-10 µM final) of the unlabeled ligand (this will define non-specific binding).
- For the autoradiography experiments, the slide holders should be taken out from the freezer and the tissue sections should be allowed to thaw and semi-dry at room temperature. This will ensure tight adherence of the sections to the gelatin coating. The slide holder(s) should then be placed in deep staining dishes containing 50-100 ml of ice-cold 50 mM Tris-HCl buffer (pH 7.4; containing 3 mM calcium chloride, 100 mM sodium chloride, and 5% bovine serum albumen) and placed on a gently rolling table-top platform (shaker) for 1 hr at 23°C in order to remove endogenous PGs and other potential interfering substances from the tissue sections. The slide holder should then be removed, the buffer should be allowed to drain for 5 minutes onto a water-absorbent mat, and the base of the holder should be blotted with tissue paper to remove excess liquid and then left on damp tissue paper at room temperature for 3-5 minutes.
- Individual slides should then be removed, their lower edges should be gently blotted to remove any excess buffer, and then the slides must be placed sequentially and horizontally on metal rods in a plexiglass incubation box. For FP-receptors, for instance, each tissue section should then be carefully covered with 0.5 ml per section of 5 nM [^{3}H]-AL-5848 solution or 10 nM [^{3}H]PGF$_{2\alpha}$ solution in the same buffer containing only 1% BSA (binding buffer) to radiolabel FP-prostaglandin receptors. Incubation should be performed without other additions (for total binding) or with the radioligands plus 0.1 -1µM unlabeled fluprostenol (to determine nonspecific binding on adjacent sections). For the generation of binding inhibition curves, 10 nM - 10 µM of unlabeled cloprostenol, fluprostenol, PHXA85, or latanoprost-free acid should be added to the [^{3}H]-AL-5848-containing or [^{3}H]PGF$_{2\alpha}$-containing solution (Sharif *et al.*, 1999; Davis and Sharif, 1999).

- At the conclusion of the incubation for 2 hrs at 23°C, the receptor binding solutions need to be decanted from the slides into a radioactive waste container, and the bottom edges of the slides must be gently blotted to remove excess liquid. The slides can then be loaded into slide holders and rinsed (2 times) with fresh ice-cold receptor binding buffer (50-100 ml in staining dishes) for 20 min at 23°C on a table-top horizontal rocker/moving platform. The slide holders should then be removed, and the excess liquid should be allowed to drain under gravity onto blotting paper. After gentle shaking of the slide holders to further remove any remaining liquid, place them in front of a cool air stream to dry at room temperature. After vacuum desiccation overnight at 23°C, load slides into X-ray film cassettes along with [^{3}H]-polymer autoradiographic Microscale® radiation standards (Amersham Pharmacia Biotech Inc., Arlington Heights, IL, #RPA510) in a dark room with dim red light (Sharif *et al.*, 1999; Davis and Sharif, 1999).
- Expose the radiolabeled sections on the slides to the tritium-sensitive Hyperfilm® for 3-6 months to generate autoradiographic images once the film is developed in the darkroom under safe light conditions. The developed film(s) can be hung to dry at room temperature in the darkroom. If needed, following the latter procedure, the same radiolabeled sections can be exposed to tritium-sensitive storage phosphor screens (Packard Instrument Company, Inc., Meridan, CT) for 20-30 days at 23°C in the dark in a lead-shielded container. These screens can then be processed to quantify the receptor binding by image analysis (Davis and Sharif, 1999).
- The black/white autoradiographic images depicting the receptor localization in the various ocular tissues on the Hyperfilm should then be annotated according to the slides that were used to generate the images. Using a computerized image analysis system, generate a standard curve relating image darkness (intensity) to the relative "receptor density" using the [^{3}H]-microscale images on the film (Sharif *et al.*, 1999; Davis and Sharif, 1999). Using image procedures, digitally subtract the non-specific binding images from the total binding images to obtain digital images of specific binding to the FP-receptors. Now, select specific tissues of interest from the specific binding images to ascertain the relative receptor densities using the stored standard curve. Examples of images and data that can be obtained from such autoradiographic studies are shown below (Figs. **2** - **5**).
- Similar image analysis procedures can be utilized to construct radioligand concentration-specific binding curves (*e.g.*, receptor saturation analysis) and likewise receptor binding inhibition curves when radioligand displacement experiments using various unlabeled drugs are performed (Figs. **6A** and **6B**).

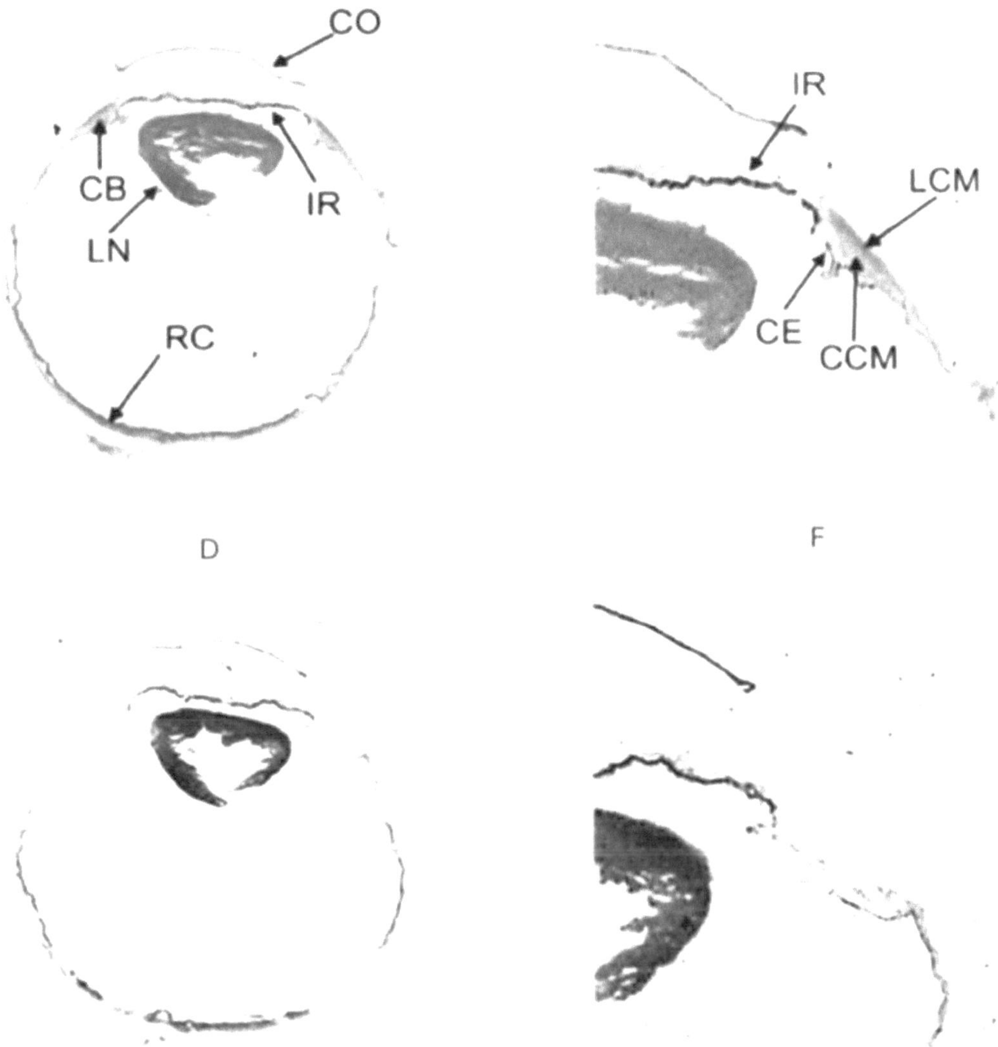

Fig. (3). Autoradiographic localization of FP receptors in human eye sections. Autoradiograms of total and non-specific binding of [^{3}H]-travoprost acid to FP-receptors are shown in thin sections of human eyes. This is a typical collection of images that appear on the Ultrafilm or Hyperfilm after exposure of labeled sections over a 6-month period. These black and white images can then be color-coded using a computerized image analysis machine, and the specific receptor binding is determined by subtracting the non-specific binding images from the total binding. Collective data obtained from multiple donor eyes using such quantitative subtraction image analyses are shown in Figure 4. Adapted from Sharif *et al.* (1999) with permission from the authors.

Tissue region	Specific [^{3}H]AL-5848 binding (digital light units mm^{-2})
Eye from man	
Iris sphincter muscle	14 367 ± 1325
Iris (minus sphincter)	13 261 ± 1187
Retina	3611 ± 1182
Ciliary epithelium/process	3593 ± 673
Lens	2628 ± 698
Longitudinal ciliary muscle	2517 ± 236
Circular ciliary muscle	1861 ± 352
Cornea	966 ± 371
Bovine corpus luteum	
Granulosa cells	115 212 ± 5154
Connective tissue and blood vessels	3268 ± 534

Fig. (4). Quantitative autoradiographic localization and the relative FP-prostaglandin receptor density in tissue sections of post-mortem human donor eyes ascertained using [^{3}H]-Travoprost acid (40 nM [^{3}H]-A--5848) as the radioligand. Example images used to derive these kinds of data are shown in Fig. (**3**. Adapted from Sharif *et al.* (1999) with permission from the authors.

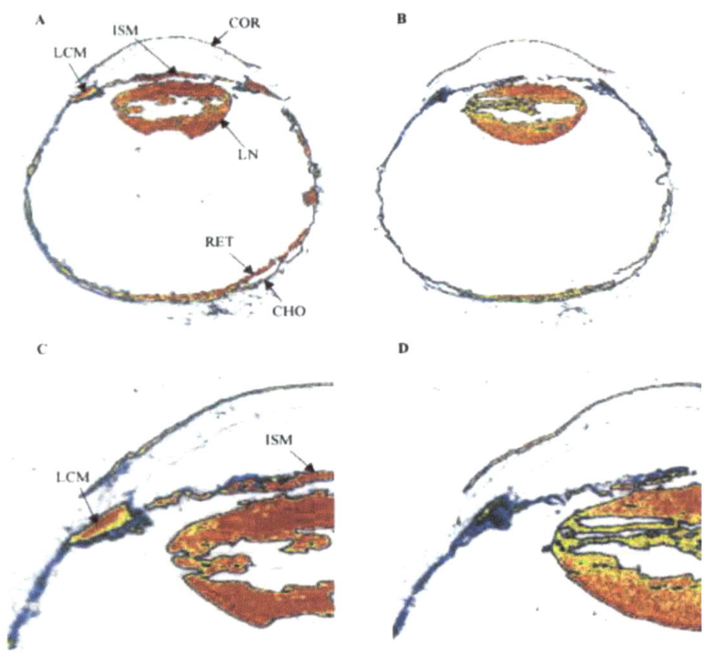

Fig. (5). Pseudo-color coded autoradiographic visualization of FP-receptors in post-mortem human eye tissue sections using 10 nM [^{3}H]PGF$_{2\alpha}$ as the radioligand. (Fig. **5A**) depicts total binding, while (Fig. **5B**) shows nonspecific binding. Enlarged views C (total binding) and D (nonspecific) illustrate low specific binding to the ciliary epithelium and ciliary processes but high binding to the ciliary muscle, for instance. The original black/white autoradiographic images on the Hyperfilm®, after a 6-month exposure to the radiolabeled tissue sections, were captured by the image analysis system (Optiquant®, Agfa Arcus® scanner) and color-coded, per visual spectrum [red being high and blue as low receptor binding /density], for visualization and quantification purposes. COR, cornea; ISM, iris smooth muscle; LCM, longitudinal ciliary muscle; LN, lens; RET, retina; CHO, choroid. Adapted from Davis and Sharif (1999) with permission from the authors.

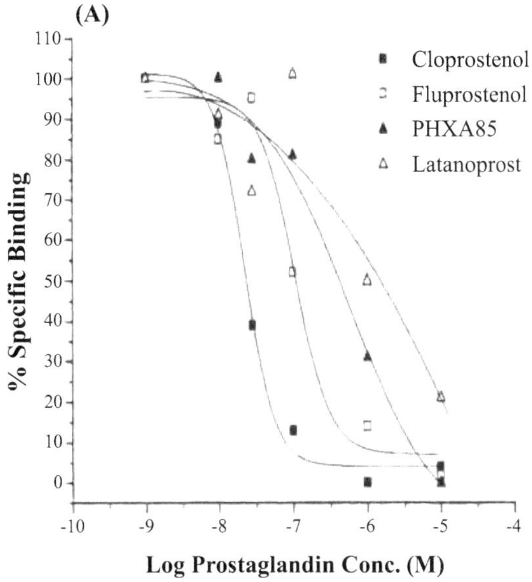

Fig. (6A). Drug concentration-inhibition curves for various ligands displacing 10 nM [^{3}H]PGF$_{2\alpha}$ from FP-receptors on the post-mortem human longitudinal ciliary muscle. Cloprostenol and fluprostenol are potent and high-affinity FP-receptor agonists and are free acid forms of the compounds. PHXA85 is the free acid of the latanoprost, which is the isopropyl ester form. Adapted from Davis and Sharif (1999) with permission from the authors.

Prostaglandin	FP Prostaglandin Affinity (K_i, nM) in Different Human Ocular Tissues and BCLM			
	Longitudinal ciliary Muscle	**Iris sphincter Muscle**	**Neural retina**	**BCLM**
Cloprostenol	13 ± 4 nM (n = 4 donors)	37 ± 18 nM (n = 4 donors)	23 ± 8 nM (n = 4 donors)	32 ± 2 nM
Fluprostenol	98 ± 18 nM (n = 4 donors)	64 nM; 29 nM (n = 2 donors)	56 ± 21 nM (n = 4 donors)	98 ± 9 nM
PHXA85	181 ± 74 nM (n = 4 donors)	203 ± 114 nM (n = 4 donors)	206 ± 55 nM (n = 4 donors)	98 ± 11 nM
Latanoprost	4,500 ± 2,780 nM (n = 4 donors)	431 ± 261 nM (n = 3 donors)	> 450 nM (n = 3 donors)	4,200 ± 790 nM

Fig. (6B). Equilibrium inhibition constants derived from displacing [^{3}H]PGF$_{2\alpha}$ from FP-receptors from eye sections of post-mortem human eyes in Fig. (**6A**) are shown below. Note that the Ki values are inversely related to the affinity of the competing drug for the FP-receptor. BCLM represents the tissue section of bovine corpus luteum, which contains a high density of FP-receptors, and which was used as a positive control tissue and for comparison purposes. Adapted from Davis and Sharif (1999) with permission from the authors.

CONCLUSION

The techniques described in this chapter provide means to determine the localization, distribution, and relative abundance of mRNAs and proteins for receptors/ enzymes/ion channels/transporter proteins of interest in human or animal ocular tissues. As a general guide, the radioligands to be used for such studies should exhibit a relatively high affinity (ideally, the dissociation constant [K_d or IC_{50} or K_i values] to be in the pM to 300 nM range) to obtain good results. For the proteins mentioned above, the ligand can be radio-labeled using ^{3}H, ^{35}S, or ^{32}P, and the specific activity of the final radioligand will dictate the ultimate exposure time of the radiolabeled tissue sections to the radio-isotope-sensitive film or phosphor-screen. However, in the current chapter, the focus was directed to receptors for prostaglandins (Figs. **2-6**) and serotonin (Fig. **1**) since agonist drugs for these have been shown to lower and control IOP in ocular hypertensive monkey and human eyes (Sharif *et al*., 2006b); localization and quantification of other cellular receptors/enzyme/ion-channels/transporters can be similarly ascertained (Sharif, 1989; Sharif and Hughes, 1989; Sharif and Eglen, 1993). Specific conditions to radiolabel such proteins have been described in many literature reports cited below.

REFERENCES

Chidlow, G, Hiscott, PS & Osborne, NN (2004) Expression of serotonin receptor mRNAs in human ciliary body: a polymerase chain reaction study. *Graefes Arch Clin Exp Ophthalmol,* 242, 259-64.
[http://dx.doi.org/10.1007/s00417-003-0785-7] [PMID: 14770316]

Davis, TL & Sharif, NA (1999) Quantitative autoradiographic visualization and pharmacology of FP-prostaglandin receptors in human eyes using the novel phosphor-imaging technology. *J Ocul Pharmacol Ther,* 15, 323-36.
[http://dx.doi.org/10.1089/jop.1999.15.323] [PMID: 10463871]

Ito, T, Suzuki, T, Lim, DK, Wellman, SE & Ho, IK (1995) A novel quantitative receptor autoradiography and *in situ* hybridization histochemistry technique using storage phosphor screen imaging. *J Neurosci Methods,* 59, 265-71.
[http://dx.doi.org/10.1016/0165-0270(94)00212-Y] [PMID: 8531495]

Kyveris, A, Maruscak, E & Senchyna, M (2002) Optimization of RNA isolation from human ocular tissues and analysis of prostanoid receptor mRNA expression using RT-PCR. *Mol Vis,* 8, 51-8.
[PMID: 11951086]

Mukhopadhyay, P, Bian, L, Yin, H, Bhattacherjee, P & Paterson, C (2001) Localization of EP(1) and FP receptors in human ocular tissues by *in situ* hybridization. *Invest Ophthalmol Vis Sci,* 42, 424-8.
[PMID: 11157877]

Schlötzer-Schrehardt, U, Zenkel, M & Nüsing, RM (2002) Expression and localization of FP and EP prostanoid receptor subtypes in human ocular tissues. *Invest Ophthalmol Vis Sci,* 43, 1475-87.
[PMID: 11980863]

Senchyna, M, Kyveris, A, May, C & Sharif, NA (2000) RT-PCR analysis of prostanoid FP receptor mRNA in human pigmented ocular tissues: methodological considerations and results. *Invest Ophthalmol Vis Sci,* 41, S511.

Sharif, NA (1989) Quantitative autoradiography of TRH receptors in discrete brain regions of different mammalian species. *Annals New York Academy of Sciences,* 553, 147-75.
[http://dx.doi.org/10.1111/j.1749-6632.1989.tb46638.x]

Sharif NA, Hughes J. (1989). Neuroanatomical mapping and quantification of peptide and drug receptors by quantitative digital subtraction autoradiography. Brain Imaging: Techniques and Applications. (Sharif NA, Lewis ME; Eds). Ellis Horwood Ltd, Chichester, pp. 36-76
[http://dx.doi.org/10.1016/0196-9781(89)90135-6]

Sharif NA, Eglen RM. (1993). Quantitative Autoradiography: A Tool to Visualize and Quantify receptors, Enzymes, Channels and Second Messenger Systems. In: Molecular Imaging in Neuroscience: A Practical Approach, (Sharif NA, Ed.), pp. 71 138, Oxford University Press

Sharif NA, Senchyna M, Xu SX. (2002). Pharmacological and molecular biological (RT-PCR) characterization of functional TP prostanoid receptors in immortalized human non-pigmented ciliary epithelial cells. *J Ocul Pharmacol Ther, 18*: pp. 141-162

Sharif, NA, Senchyna, M & Xu, SX (2002) Pharmacological and molecular biological (RT-PCR) characterization of functional TP prostanoid receptors in immortalized human non-pigmented ciliary epithelial cells. *J Ocul Pharmacol Ther,* 18, 141-62.
[http://dx.doi.org/10.1089/108076802317373905] [PMID: 12002668]

Sharif, NA & Senchyna, M (2006) Serotonin receptor subtype mRNA expression in human ocular tissues, determined by RT-PCR. *Mol Vis,* 12, 1040-7.
[PMID: 16971896]

Sharif, NA, Davis, TL & Williams, GW (1999) [^{3}H]AL-5848 ([^{3}H]9β-(+)-Fluprostenol). Carboxylic acid of travoprost (AL-6221), a novel FP prostaglandin to study the pharmacology and autoradiographic localization of the FP receptor. *J Pharm Pharmacol,* 51, 685-94.
[http://dx.doi.org/10.1211/0022357991772989] [PMID: 10454045]

Sharif, NA, Kelly, CR, Crider, JY & Davis, TL (2006) Serotonin-2 (5-HT$_2$) receptor-mediated signal transduction in human ciliary muscle cells: role in ocular hypotension. *J Ocul Pharmacol Ther,* 22, 389-401. a
[http://dx.doi.org/10.1089/jop.2006.22.389] [PMID: 17238805]

Sharif, NA, Kelly, CR & McLaughlin, M (2006) Human trabecular meshwork cells express functional serotonin-2A (5HT2A) receptors: role in IOP reduction. *Invest Ophthalmol Vis Sci,* 47, 4001-10. b
[http://dx.doi.org/10.1167/iovs.06-0062] [PMID: 16936116]

Sharif, NA (2018) iDrugs and iDevices discovery and development- preclinical assays, techniques and animal model studies for ocular hypotensives and neuroprotectants. *J Ocul Pharmacol Ther,* 34, 7-39.
[http://dx.doi.org/10.1089/jop.2017.0125] [PMID: 29323613]

Sharif, NA (2021) Therapeutic drugs and devices for tackling ocular hypertension and glaucoma, and need for neuroprotection and cytoprotective therapies. *Front Pharmacol,* 12, 729249.
[http://dx.doi.org/10.3389/fphar.2021.729249] [PMID: 34603044]

Sharif, NA, Odani-Kawabata, N, Lu, F & Pinchuk, L (2023) FP and EP2 prostanoid receptor agonist drugs and aqueous humor outflow devices for treating ocular hypertension and glaucoma. *Exp Eye Res,* 229, 109415.
[http://dx.doi.org/10.1016/j.exer.2023.109415] [PMID: 36803996]

Tobin, AB & Osborne, NN (1989) Evidence for the presence of serotonin receptors negatively coupled to adenylate cyclase in the rabbit iris-ciliary body. *J Neurochem,* 53, 686-91.
[http://dx.doi.org/10.1111/j.1471-4159.1989.tb11758.x] [PMID: 2547897]

Ullmer, C, Schmuck, K, Kalkman, HO & Lübbert, H (1995) Expression of serotonin receptor mRNAs in blood vessels. *FEBS Lett,* 370, 215-21.
[http://dx.doi.org/10.1016/0014-5793(95)00828-W] [PMID: 7656980]

Weinreb, RN, Aung, T & Medeiros, FA (2014) The pathophysiology and treatment of glaucoma: a review. *JAMA,* 311, 1901-11.
[http://dx.doi.org/10.1001/jama.2014.3192] [PMID: 24825645]

CHAPTER 5

Protocol for Generating and Utilizing Ocular Tissue Homogenates for Receptor Binding Studies

Nozhat Choudry[1,*]

[1] *Santen Inc., 6401 Hollis Street, Suite 125, Emeryville, CA-94608, USA*

Abstract: Ocular tissues play a vital role in various physiological processes for visual processing and are critical for understanding ocular diseases and drug development. By homogenizing ocular tissues, researchers can obtain a representative sample of ocular components, allowing for the investigation of receptor binding characteristics. This method provides valuable insights into the molecular interactions between ligands and ocular receptors, aiding in the development of novel therapeutic interventions. The utilization of ocular tissue homogenates offers a practical approach to studying ocular receptor binding and holds significant potential for advancing our understanding of ocular pharmacology and the development of targeted ocular therapies. The role of prostaglandins (PGs) in regulating IOP was studied several years prior to identifying prostaglandin receptors in the eye. Quantitative autoradiography, *in situ* hybridization, immunohistochemistry, and RT-PCR confirmed EP and FP receptors presence in the ciliary epithelium, cornea, conjunctiva, iris sphincter muscle, longitudinal ciliary muscle, retinal ganglion cells, trabecular meshwork, sclera, Muller cells, and optic nerves. For illustrative purposes, the aim of this chapter is to describe the key elements of experimental protocols used to study the pharmacological characteristics and regional distribution of prostaglandin E2 (PGE2) and prostaglandin F2α (PGF2α) receptor binding sites in membranes isolated from bovine iris ciliary body.

Keywords: Bovine, Iris ciliary body, Ocular receptor binding sites, Prostaglandins, Sphincter.

INTRODUCTION

As our population ages, the incidence of devastating eye diseases increases. It has been estimated that more than 65 million people suffer from glaucoma worldwide (Quigley and Broman. Br J Ophthalmol 90:262–267, 2006). In addition, developing treatment programs for these various diseases that could affect our eyesight is also critical. One of the most effective treatments we have is in the development of specific drugs that can be used to target various components of

* **Corresponding author Nozhat Choudry:** Santen Inc., 6401 Hollis Street, Suite 125, Emeryville, CA-94608, USA; Tel: 1 647 272 0887; E-mail: nozhatchoudry@hotmail.com

Najam A. Sharif and Sunny E. Ohia (Eds.)

the mechanisms that lead to ocular disease. Understanding basic principles of the pharmacology of the eye is important if one seeks to develop effective drug treatments. The eye is a complex sense organ that is composed of many unique types of tissues involved in light sensing and the visual transduction cascade. Within these tissues are cells that contain various classes of proteins that can act as receptors for pharmacological drugs to interact with and produce a measurable cellular/signaling response that leads to the final biological response (*e.g.*, tissue contraction/relaxation, transmitter release, and intraocular pressure reduction [IOP]).

The role of prostaglandins (PGs) in regulating IOP was studied several years prior to identifying prostaglandin receptors in the eye. Early studies revealed that topical ocular dosing of many different classes of prostaglandins produces a diverse set of responses, including a biphasic response in terms of IOP: an initial short-term increase in IOP followed by a sustained decrease in IOP (Camras *et al.* 1977; Starr 1971). These were dose-, time- and species-dependent. Prostaglandins are ubiquitous, and the types produced in a given cell are dependent on the expression profile of the prostaglandin synthetic enzymes in that particular cell. Prostaglandins are autocrine or juxtacrine modulators that have diverse pharmacological effects on the central nervous, the cardiovascular, gastrointestinal, and visual systems.

Quantitative autoradiography, *in situ* hybridization, immunohistochemistry, and RT-PCR confirmed EP and FP receptors presence and a differential distribution in the ciliary epithelium, cornea, conjunctiva, iris sphincter muscle, longitudinal ciliary muscle, retinal ganglion cells, trabecular meshwork, sclera, Muller cells, and optic nerves (Anthony *et al.* 2001; Davis and Sharif 1999; Matsuo and Cynader 1992; Ocklind *et al.* 1996; Schlotzer-Schrehardt *et al.* 2002). In the eye, topical ocular prostaglandins (PGs), in particular PGE2 and PGF2 alpha, may induce vasodilation, disruption of the blood-aqueous barrier, and IOP reduction, depending on the species.

The purpose of this chapter is to describe the key elements of experimental protocols to study the characteristics and regional distribution of prostaglandin E_2 (PGE_2) and prostaglandin $F_{2\alpha}$($PGF_{2\alpha}$) in membrane from isolated bovine iris ciliary bodies. Currently, 5 types of prostanoid receptors have been classified based on their affinity for naturally occurring prostanoids (Kennedy I *et al.* 1982; Coleman *et al.* 1984), *i.e.*, PGE_2, $PGF_{2\alpha}$, PGD_2, thromboxane, and prostacyclin. Understanding the specific prostanoid receptor distribution will provide a better understanding of the ocular effects of PGs and their analogs in terms of their on-target and off-target effects. Below are described methods to study the receptor binding characteristics of [^{3}H]-PGE_2 and [^{3}H]-PGF_{2a} to cell membrane homogenates of the bovine iris-ciliary body as originally described by Csukas *et al.* (1993). The same types of procedures can be utilized to dissect human eyeballs and conduct receptor binding experiments to discern the pharmacology of other receptor types in ocular tissues of other species using different radioligands (Chidlow *et al.*, 1995).

Experimental Protocols

Tissue Membrane Preparation

- Obtain freshly isolated bovine eyes transported on ice from the abattoir.
- Dissect the iris ciliary body circumferentially into three parts: sphincter muscle, ciliary body and processes, and the rest of the iris. This is achieved by dissecting out the sphincter and then the ciliary body with attached processes. The rest of the iris will include the blood vessels and the dilator muscle, with some sphincter muscle and ciliary body fragments (Csukas *et al.* 1993).
- Maintain the tissues at 2-4°C and homogenize each tissue separately in 50mM tris buffer at a pH of 7.5, which should contain cyclooxygenase (1μM flurbiprofen), protease (0.43mM PMSF), and 0.01% soybean trypsin inhibitors to remove endogenous PGs. Add 1mM EGTA to the homogenization buffer (Csukas *et al.* 1993).
- Obtain tissue membranes after three-stage high-speed centrifugation (Bhattacherjee *et al.* 1990). Centrifuge the tubes in an ultracentrifuge for 60 min at 120,000 g, discard the supernatant (Chidlow *et al.*,1995), then centrifuge the homogenate at 300g for 10 minutes at 4°C, and aspirate away the supernatant.
- Coarsely mince the pellets and place them in a glass scintillation vial containing 2M sucrose and glass beads and disperse the pellet further to homogeneity as much as possible. This procedure is gentler than using an electrical homogenizer.
- Now add this suspension to fresh ultracentrifuge tubes and gently overlay with fresh buffer solution.
- Centrifuge tubes for 90 min at 120,000 g and isolate the turbid layer formed at the sucrose-buffer interface, which contains the cell membranes, using a Pasteur pipette.
- Transfer the isolated fraction into fresh ultracentrifuge tubes and centrifuge for 1hr at 120,000 g to compact the membranes.
- Now, resuspend the resulting pellet in fresh receptor binding buffer to the appropriate protein concentration or membrane concentration (*e.g.*, 150-400 Mm/ml).

Radioligand Binding Assay

Perform all radioligand binding assays in the binding buffer at 37°C in a shaking water bath (120 strokes/min).

- At this point, supplement the binding buffer with 2.5mM manganese (Mn^{++}) and bovine serum albumin for radioligand-receptor saturation and drug competition studies.
- Now reconstitute membranes in the binding buffer and incubate the aliquoted portions containing 50-300μg of membrane protein with 1- 8 nM [^{3}H]-PGE_2 (200 Ci/mmol) or [^{3}H]-PGF_{2a} (209 Ci/mmol) in a final volume of 500μl in the presence or absence of various concentrations of unlabeled PGE_2 or PGF_{2a} at 37°C for 30 min in a shaking water bath.
- At the end of the incubation period, separate the free radioligand from the bound radioligand using rapid filtration under vacuum through filters (0.45 um, type HA; Millipore) on a filtration manifold.
- To determine the nonspecific radioligand binding to the filters, use blanks that contain 1-8 nM [^{3}H]-PGE_2 or [^{3}H]-PGF_{2a} in 500 ul buffer and no tissue membranes and filter as in step 4. The radioactivity that is retained on the filters in the absence of membranes is subtracted from all other values to account for nonspecific filter binding.
- Now rapidly wash the membrane-radioligand complex that is left in the filters twice with 2 ml ice-cold buffer *via* the filtration process to further remove unbound radioligand. This process of washing/filtration and washing should be completed within 10 sec to prevent radioligand dissociating from the membranes.
- The vacuum filtration should render the filters relatively dry, and now the filter-bound radioactivity can be determined using a liquid scintillation counter (*e.g.*, Model LS-3801 Beckham).
- In order to calculate the specific binding, subtract the nonspecific binding values from the total binding.
- In order to perform radioligand-receptor binding time-course studies, incubate the washed and dispersed tissue membranes with the radioligand of choice (+/- the unlabeled ligand) and then terminate the incubation assay at selected times up to 60-90 min by rapid vacuum filtration as described above.
- For any radioligand dissociation studies, incubate all tube contents for a 30-min period with 1 nM [^{3}H]-PGE_2 in the presence or absence of 1 nM unlabeled PGE_2. At this point, add 1 uM unlabeled PGE_2 to tubes that have tissue membranes and 1 nM [^{3}H]-PGE_2 alone in order to allow the unlabeled compound to displace the radioligand from the EP-receptors.

- The dissociation time period varies between 2-60 min; the assay is terminated by vacuum filtration and the remaining receptor-bound radioligand is determined as described above.
- Any desired radioligand competition assays using a range of unlabeled test compounds at various concentrations (*e.g.*, 1nM-10 uM final) can be performed at 30 min using the previously isolated bovine ICB tissue membranes and a low radioligand concentration (*e.g.*, 1-8 nM final) in the final volume of 500 ul. An example of a typical competition curve derived from such studies is shown in Fig. (**1**). The inhibition constant (*e.g.*, the concentration needed to displace 50% of the radioactivity from the receptors; IC_{50} or K_i) for each unlabeled drug can be determined from the concentration-inhibition curves.
- To perform receptor saturation experiments using Scatchard analysis, the concentration of $[^3H]$-PGE_2 radioligand is varied from 1nM to 50-100 nM final concentration.

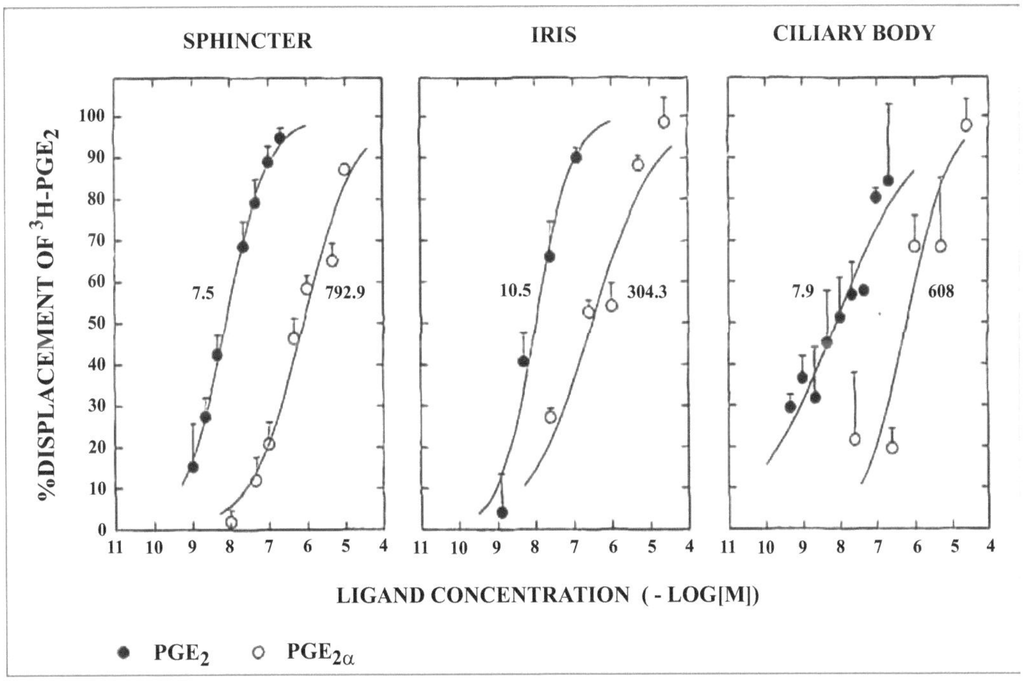

Fig. (1). Competition for $[^3H]$-PGE_2 binding to EP receptors in washed bovine iris, ciliary body, and iris sphincter muscle homogenates by unlabeled PGE_2 and $PGF_{2\alpha}$. Csukas *et al.* (1993).

However, when $[^3H]$-serotonin (5-hydroxytryptamine; 5HT; $[^3H]$-5HT) binding to 5HT1A receptors in rabbit ICB membranes was conducted (Chidlow *et al.*, 1995), typical saturation and competition data (as shown in Figs. **2A** and **2B**) were obtained.

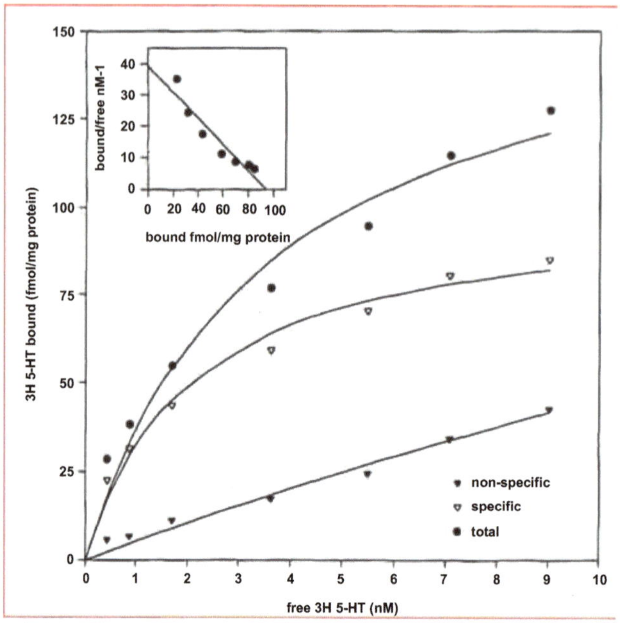

Fig. (2A). Saturation analysis of [^{3}H]-5HT binding to rabbit iris-ciliary body homogenates and Scatchard analysis (inset) to define the dissociation constant and the maximal receptor density present in the tissue under study. Chidlow *et al.* (1995).

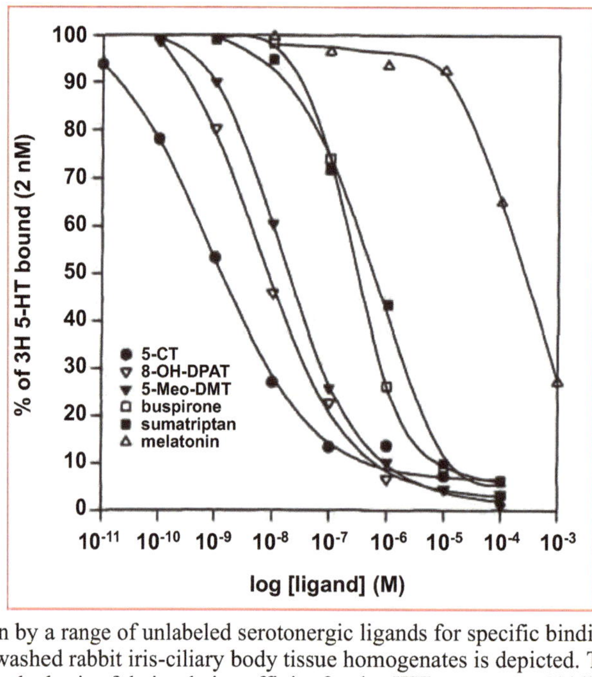

Fig. (2B). Competition by a range of unlabeled serotonergic ligands for specific binding of [^{3}H]-5HT binding to $5HT_{1A}$ receptors in washed rabbit iris-ciliary body tissue homogenates is depicted. These types of data help rank the compounds on the basis of their relative affinity for the $5HT_{1A}$ receptor. Chidlow *et al.* (1995).

Radioligands such as [^{3}H]-PGE$_2$ can be purchased from Amersham Corporation (Arlington Heights, IL), and various unlabeled PGE2, PGF2a and other prostaglandins can be obtained from Cayman Chemicals (Ann Arbor, MI). Other compounds mentioned above can be purchased from Sigma (St. Louis, MO).

There are many other examples of receptor binding studies performed on rabbit and human retinas (Sharif and Xu, 1999a,b) and various other cells and tissues (Sharif *et al.*, 1991, 1994) using the basic techniques and technologies described above. These are also good sources of how to conduct radioligand receptor binding studies on animal and human ocular tissues.

CONCLUSION

In conclusion, the protocols described above are based on original publications cited within this chapter. The protocols described above have endeavored to provide sufficient experimental details. Original publications should be checked, and further literature searches may be of use to find any modifications (*e.g.*, different animal tissues or cultured cells) or refinements to the procedures described herein. The protocols described in this chapter should help provide information on how to generate and utilize ocular tissue homogenates for receptor binding studies.

REFERENCES

Anthony, TL, Lindsey, JD, Aihara, M & Weinreb, RN (2001) Detection of prostaglandin EP(1), EP(2), and FP receptor subtypes in human sclera. *Invest Ophthalmol Vis Sci,* 42, 3182-6.
[PMID: 11726620]

Bhattacherjee, P, Csukas, S & Paterson, CA (1990) Prostaglandin E2 binding sites in bovine iris-ciliary body. *Invest Ophthalmol Vis Sci,* 31, 1109-13.
[PMID: 2162336]

Camras, CB, Bito, LZ & Eakins, KE (1977) Reduction of intraocular pressure by prostaglandins applied topically to the eyes of conscious rabbits. *Invest Ophthalmol Vis Sci,* 16, 1125-34.
[PMID: 924742]

Chidlow, G, De Santis, LM, Sharif, NA & Osborne, NN (1995) Characteristics of [^{3}H]5-hydroxytryptamine binding to iris-ciliary body tissue of the rabbit. *Invest Ophthalmol Vis Sci,* 36, 2238-45.
[PMID: 7558717]

Csukas, S, Bhattacherjee, P, Rhodes, L & Paterson, CA (1993) Prostaglandin E2 and F2 alpha binding sites in the bovine iris ciliary body. *Invest Ophthalmol Vis Sci,* 34, 2237-45.
[PMID: 8389343]

Coleman, RA, Humphrey, PPA, Kennedy, I & Lumley, P (1984) Prostanoid receptors — the development of a working classification. *Trends Pharmacol Sci,* 5, 303-6.
[http://dx.doi.org/10.1016/0165-6147(84)90452-8]

Davis, TL & Sharif, NA (1999) Quantitative autoradiographic visualization and pharmacology of FP-prostaglandin receptors in human eyes using the novel phosphor-imaging technology. *J Ocul Pharmacol Ther,* 15, 323-36.
[http://dx.doi.org/10.1089/jop.1999.15.323] [PMID: 10463871]

Kennedy, I, Coleman, RA, Humphrey, PPA, Levy, GP & Lumley, P (1982) Studies of the characterisation of prostanoid receptors: A proposed classification. *Prostaglandins,* 24, 667-89.
[http://dx.doi.org/10.1016/0090-6980(82)90036-3] [PMID: 6131499]

Matsuo, T & Cynader, MS (1992) Localisation of prostaglandin F2 alpha and E2 binding sites in the human eye. *Br J Ophthalmol,* 76, 210-3.
[http://dx.doi.org/10.1136/bjo.76.4.210] [PMID: 1327095]

Ocklind, A, Lake, S, Wentzel, P, Nistér, M & Stjernschantz, J (1996) Localization of the prostaglandin F2 alpha receptor messenger RNA and protein in the cynomolgus monkey eye. *Invest Ophthalmol Vis Sci,* 37, 716-26.
[PMID: 8603857]

Quigley, HA & Broman, AT (2006) The number of people with glaucoma worldwide in 2010 and 2020. *Br J Ophthalmol,* 90, 262-7.
[http://dx.doi.org/10.1136/bjo.2005.081224] [PMID: 16488940]

Schlötzer-Schrehardt, U, Zenkel, M & Nüsing, RM (2002) Expression and localization of FP and EP prostanoid receptor subtypes in human ocular tissues. *Invest Ophthalmol Vis Sci,* 43, 1475-87.
[PMID: 11980863]

Sharif, NA, Wong, EH, Loury, D, Stefanich, E, Eglen, RM, Michel, A & Whiting, RL (1991) Characteristics of 5HT3 binding sites in rat cerebral cortex, NG108 15 and NCB 20 neuroblastoma cells using [3H]-quipazine and [3H]-GR65630 binding. *British J Pharmacology,* 102, 919-25.

Sharif, NA, Xu, S & Yanni, JM (1994) Histamine receptor subtype affinities, selectivities and potencies of emedastine (Emedine®), a novel H1 selective antagonist, and other ocularly employed antihistamines. *Drug Development Research,* 33, 448-53.

Sharif, NA & Xu, SX (1999) Pharmacological characterization of [^{3}H]-Ifenprodil binding to polyamine binding sites on rabbit and rat retinal homogenates: role in neuroprotection? *J Ocul Pharmacol Ther,* 15, 271-81. a
[http://dx.doi.org/10.1089/jop.1999.15.271] [PMID: 10385136]

Sharif, NA & Xu, SX (1999) Human retina contains polyamine sensitive [^{3}H]-ifenprodil binding sites: implications for neuroprotection? *Br J Ophthalmol,* 83, 236-40. b
[http://dx.doi.org/10.1136/bjo.83.2.236] [PMID: 10396205]

Starr, MS (1971) Further studies on the effect of prostaglandin on intraocular pressure in the rabbit. *Exp Eye Res,* 11, 170-7.
[http://dx.doi.org/10.1016/S0014-4835(71)80020-9] [PMID: 5001095]

CHAPTER 6

Protocols for Visualizing and Quantifying Receptors in Ocular Tissues Involved in Aqueous Humor Inflow and Outflow

Najam A. Sharif[1,*] and **Saima Chaudhry**[2]

[1] *Vice President and Head of Research & Development Nanoscope Therapeutics Inc., 2777 N. Stemmons Fwy, Suite 1102, Dallas, TX-75207, USA*

[2] *Univ N. Texas at Arlington, 701 S Nedderman Dr, Arlington, TX-76019, USA*

Abstract: Glaucomatous optic neuropathy (GON) globally afflicts millions of patients and gradually but progressively robs them of their eyesight over decades of undetected and undiagnosed disease progression. Chronically raised intraocular pressure (IOP), also known as ocular hypertension (OHT), is most significantly associated with the development of GON and is the only modifiable and treatable biomarker for the most prevalent form of glaucoma, open-angle glaucoma (OAG). There continues to be a need to discover and introduce new drugs with good therapeutic indices in the clinical management of OAG. Potential targets are being discovered from genetic studies, but their localization and verification in the target tissues and cells in the anterior chamber (ANC) of the eye need to be determined before embarking on initiating drug discovery campaigns. Several techniques have been developed for target verification. This chapter deals with quantitative autoradiographic procedures to visualize receptor targets for drug candidates and existing marketed medicines treating OHT and OAG.

Keywords: Autoradiography, Drug targets, Enzymes, Immunohistochemistry, Receptors.

INTRODUCTION

Several million people worldwide suffer from neurodegenerative ocular diseases grouped together as glaucoma. The most prevalent form is open-angle glaucoma (OAG), in which ocular hypertension (OHT) caused by excess accumulation of aqueous humor (AQH) in the anterior chamber (ANC) of the eye is the major culprit and risk factor (Weinreb *et al.*, 2014; Sharif, 2021-2023). The elevated intraocular pressure (IOP) damages the delicate retinal structures and the optic

* **Corresponding author Najam A. Sharif:** Vice President and Head of Research & Development Nanoscope Therapeutics Inc., 2777 N. Stemmons Fwy, Suite 1102, Dallas, TX-75207, USA; Tel: +1(817)-565-7686; E-mail: nsharif@nanostherapeutics.com

Najam A. Sharif and Sunny E. Ohia (Eds.)

nerve at the rear of the globe and kills the highly sensitive and critically important retinal ganglion cells (RGCs). These damaging events occur over decades, but once half of the original RGCs have been lost, the connections between the retina and the brain structures involved in visual perception and eyesight are also halved, and the patient starts to notice significant visual impairment (Sharif, 2021-2023). In order to stave off further damage, the elevated IOP has to be reduced using pharmaceuticals, drainage-device implants, or via surgery. The most cost-effective means is topical ocular administration of IOP-lowering medications (Bucolo *et al.*, 2018; Sharif, 2021-2023).

Whilst a number of drugs are available for lowering and controlling IOP (Bucolo *et al.*, 2018; Sharif, 2021; Sharif *et al.*, 2023), they impart significant side effects and their pharmacological and pharmacokinetic properties are somewhat undesirable and should be improved. New drug discovery is an active and important discipline in this endeavor. However, whilst new therapeutic targets are being discovered via genome-wide associated studies, the localization and verification of potential receptors, enzymes, ion channels, and transporters in the ANC of the eye, which may mediate beneficial effects through such proteins, are often lacking. Even though immunohistochemistry (Sharif *et al.*, 2014) is a useful technique to define the distribution of receptors, autoradiography is perhaps easier to perform and is quantitative when coupled with computerized image analysis (Sharif and Hughes, 1989; Sharif and Eglen, 1993; Davis and Sharif, 1999; Sharif *et al.*, 1995, 1988, 1999, 2000, 2001, 2004, 2014; Sharif and Lewis, 1989; Sharif, 1986, 1989, 1996).

Protocols for Performing Prostaglandin Receptor Autoradiography *In Vitro*

Many neurotransmitter and drug receptors have been visualized on thin sections of animal and human postmortem eyes over the years from a basic research perspective. Most studies have simply reported the presence or absence of these target receptor or enzyme proteins (Pilotte *et al.*, 1984). Over the intervening years, the use of powerful image analysis technologies and techniques has successfully permitted quantitative digital subtraction of autoradiographic images to provide high specific receptor binding profiles of radiolabeled molecules in ocular tissues and tissues from other body organs. Additional progress has been made in performing kinetic and drug-concentration-based titration to help determine receptor binding affinities in tissues that are too small to isolate for traditional receptor binding techniques described elsewhere in this book and in many publications (Sharif and Hughes, 1989; Davis and Sharif, 1999; Sharif *et al.*, 2000; Green and Sambrook, 2020; Hansen *et al.*, 2022; Kecheliev *et al.*, 2022; Mikkelsen *et al.*, 2022; Mitsukawa *et al.*, 2022; Murgas *et al.*, 2022; Neuman *et al.*, 2022; Voss *et al.*, 2022; Waldman *et al.*, 2022; Ganaglio *et al.*, 2023;

Krogsback *et al.*, 2023). An example of localizing and quantitative autoradiography is presented below with emphasis on FP-and DP-prostaglandin receptors in human eye sections *in vitro* (Fig. **1**).

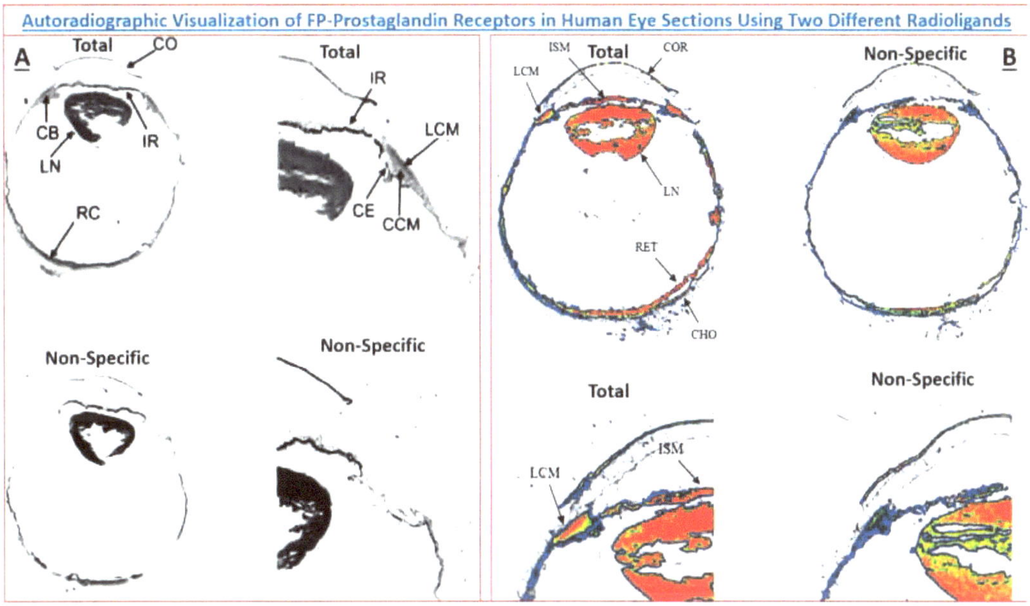

Fig. (1). Visualization of FP-prostaglandin receptors in postmortem human eye sections by autoradiographic means using [^{3}H]-travoprost acid as the radioligand, shown in black and white as images appeared on the tritium-sensitive Hyperfilm (A). In the next panel (B) is the [^{3}H]PGF$_{2\alpha}$ binding to human postmortem eye tissues, where the autoradiographic images have been pseudo-color coded by the Optiquant® software on an Agfa Arcus® scanner image analysis system to show the relative density of the receptors present using the visual spectrum of colors (blue to red: with increasing density). Note the high density of specific binding to the longitudinal ciliary muscle (LCM), iris sphincter muscle (ISM), and retina (RET). The retina is distinguished from the choroid (CHO) in this section as it is pulled away from the choroid during sectioning. Also, note low levels of specific binding to lens (LN). Enlarged views in C (total binding) and D (nonspecific) show weak specific binding to the ciliary epithelium and ciliary process (CP). The cornea (COR) is barely visible in C. Magnifications pertaining to panels A and B, which were 3.5x, while panels C and D were 9.1x of the original images.

- Obtain enucleated postmortem human eye globes within 4-12 hours post-death from local eye banks and keep them on ice.
- Embed a globe in Tissue-Tek O.C.T embedding material and leave it in the cryostat for a few hours to fully freeze.
- Cut tissue sections (20 um) at 17C on a freezing microtome and collect them on gelatinized glass microscope slides. Store slides in a desiccator at -20°C for up to 1 week or when needed for experiments. It is recommended that these sections be used within 1-2 months after cutting.
- For the receptor binding experiments, thaw the slides/sections at room temp (22°C) and then preincubate them by dipping whole racks of slides in sufficient

volume of 50 mM Tris-HCl buffer (pH 7.4) containing 3 mM calcium chloride, 100 mM sodium chloride, and 5% BSA in order to remove endogenous PGs and other potential interfering substances. After 45 min, remove the slide racks and leave them on blotting paper for up to 30 mins in order to ensure that all of the buffer solution has been drained away from the tissue sections. A gentle stream of cool air can help partially dry out the sections.

- While the slides are drying out, prepare two separate vials of the aforementioned buffer containing 10 nM [^{3}H]-PGF2α. Ensure there is a sufficient solution to cover each of the tissue sections that will receive 0.5ml of the radioligand-containing buffer. The vial with the radioligand, which will be used for the "non-specific binding" part of the experiment, should contain 10 μM of unlabeled PGF2α to saturate all the FP-receptors and other no-specific proteins and tissue sections. The vial that will be used to define the "total binding" only has the buffer and no unlabeled PG. For generation of binding inhibition curves, 10 nM – 10 μM of cloprostenol, fluprostenol, PHXA85, or Latanoprost are added to additional vials containing the radioligand. Obviously, for these experiments, many more slides will be required and need to be appropriately prepared.
- For the simpler receptor binding experiments, an appropriate number of slides containing adjacent sections are labeled "Total" or "Non-Specific" with a permanent ink marker and laid out flat on metal rods in a damp plexiglass container at room temperature.
- Now carefully cover each tissue section with 0.5ml of the buffer from the appropriate vial. After a 2-hr incubation at room temperature, pour off the solutions from each slide into containers equipped to receive radioactive solutions. After lightly blotting the edges of the slides, place them in the appropriately labeled slide racks and dip them into dishes containing excess fresh, ice-cold buffer for 10 min, and repeat the process one more time for 10 min with a gentle shaking of the dishes to move the buffer around and remove any excess radioactive material from the slides.
- Decant the radioactive buffer from the dishes, gently blot the slide-racks on a thick mat of paper towels, and then place the slides in front of a fan that gently but quickly dries the sections. Now place the racks of slides into vacuum desiccators and allow the slides and the radiolabeled tissue sections to completely dry overnight.
- The next day, visually check that the tissue sections and slides are completely free of any moisture. Allow slides to dry further as needed.
- Now place the slides horizontally in a specific order that matches the "total binding" and "non-specific binding" labels on the slides and tape them down firmly on the edges to the inside of X-ray cassettes. Also, place [^{3}H]-polymer autoradiographic microscale standards (Amersham Pharmacia Biotech Inc.,

Arlington Heights, IL, #RPA510) alongside one of the slides.

- In dim red light in a darkroom, place a tritium-sensitive Hyperfilm-^{3}H® (Amersham Pharmacia Biotech) on top of the slides, ensuring good contact, and close the X-ray cassette. Place a label on the front of each cassette describing the contents, the date of the experiment, *etc.*, and then store the cassettes in a freezer or in a cool, dry, and dark place at room temperature for 6 months.

In the case of the use of phosphor-imaging technology to capture the autoradiographic images, the slides containing the radiolabeled tissue sections are opposed to storage phosphor screens (Packard Instrument Company, Inc., Meridan, CT) for up to 30 days at room temperature as per the manufacturer's directions.

- After the 6-month exposure of the film to the radiolabeled sections, the cassettes are opened in a dark room (red light), and the Hyperfilm is developed with Kodak D10® developer as directed by the manufacturer. After the final rinse, hang the films to drip dry in the darkroom for several hours.

In the case of the phosphor-imaging, the imaging screens are loaded into the machine, and the images are converted to 8-bit greyscale image files using an Arcus II® digital scanner (AGFA Geafert AG).

- The autoradiographic images (black and white) can be printed on photographic paper as needed. An example is shown in Fig. (**1A**). Pseudo-color-coded images of the autoradiographs can be determined using image analysis systems and can be presented as shown in Fig. (**1B**) and Fig. (**2**).

Data Acquisition and Analysis

- After drying and annotating the Hyperfilms, the autoradiographic images can be scanned via the Agfa scanner into the Optiquant® software package of the Cyclone® phosphor imager (Packard Instrument Company, Inc., Meridan, CT), and some images can be pseudo color-coded. For the image analysis of the phosphor screens, the X-ray film cassettes are opened under subdued incandescent light, and each screen is scanned at 600 dpi using a Cyclone® phosphor imager.
- The resulting grayscale image files are analyzed using the associated Optiquant® software package (Packard Instrument Company, Inc., Meridan, CT) after delineating the autoradiographic standards and specific regions of interest on the eye sections. Table **1** shows an example of the distribution of FP-prostaglandin receptors in various tissues of postmortem human eyes.
- Data output in digital light units (DLU/mm^2) can be imported into Microsoft Excel® for calculation of means and standard errors after outlier analysis by

Dixon's test. The competition curves are then plotted using the Origin® computer program (Microcal, Northampton, MA). Other software packages can also be used for such analyses and graphic representation.

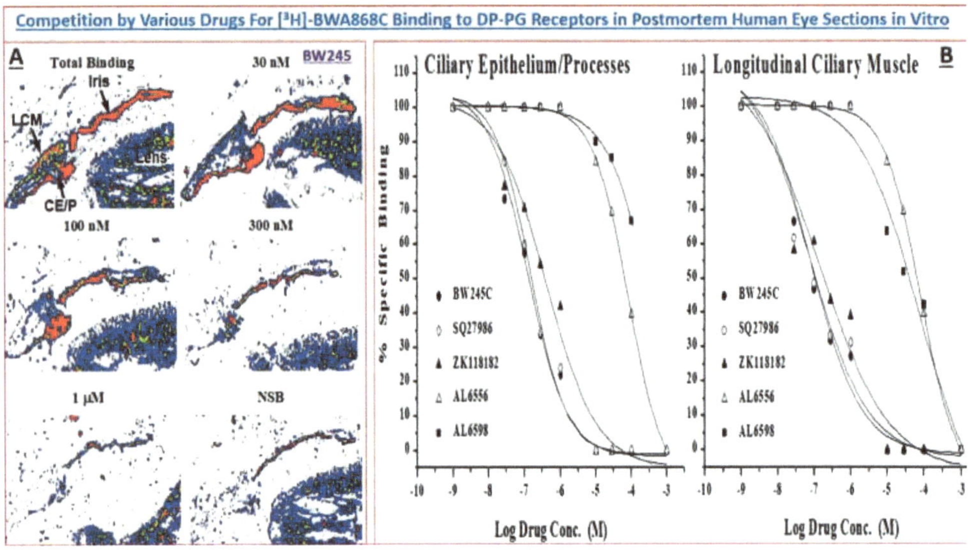

Fig. (2). Competition by numerous DP-receptor agonist drugs for binding to various human postmortem eye tissues using the highly DP-receptor-selective radioligand, [^{3}H]-BWA868A, and quantitative receptor autoradiography methods. Panel A shows the visual and image-analysis determined competition by the potent DP-receptor-selective agonist BW245 in a color-coded format. Panel B depicts the competition curves for a number of drugs in the ciliary epithelium and longitudinal ciliary muscle within the human eye, determined as described in panel A.

Table 1. Quantitative autoradiographic distribution of FP-prostaglandin receptors in human eye sections *in vitro* using [^{3}H]-PGF2α as the radioligand and using phosphor imaging technology. Specific binding (Total minus nonspecific binding) to various tissues was determined using quantitative digital subtraction autoradiography. The units for the relative receptor densities (concentration) are Digital Light Units/mm^2. The % specific binding as a percentage of total binding to FP-receptors was also calculated. SEM, standard error of the mean.

Tissue	n	Total*		Nonspecific		Specific	% Specific
		Mean	SEM	Mean	SEM		
Iris Sphincter Muscle	4	26317	8262	7056	1401	19261	73.2
Longitudinal Ciliary	4	18767	3607	6026	1846	12741	67.9
Retina	4	17966	3718	8422	2030	9544	53.1
Iris (Sphincter Omitted)	4	9436	1065	5660	1184	3776	40.0
Circular Ciliary/Epithelium	4	7337	1250	4782	1218	2554	34.8
Choroid	3	5992	2046	4322	1431	1671	27.9
Cornea	3	6693	1388	5135	989	1558	23.3
Lens	4	15211	3477	13325	3150	1886	12.4

D. Such quantitative autoradiographic imaging techniques have progressed to a level where drug testing and profiling for receptor or enzyme affinities for numerous unlabeled drugs can be performed on the thin tissue sections derived from various organs (Table **2**). Such data can help rank order compounds for progression to animal-based studies of lead compounds.

Table 2. Quantitative autoradiographic determination of the pharmacological properties of the FP-prostaglandin receptor in various tissues of the postmortem human eye using [^{3}H]-PGF2α and various unlabeled compounds competing with its binding to the FP-receptor. LCM, longitudinal ciliary muscle; ISM, iris sphincter muscle; RET, retina; BCLM, bovine corpus luteum (positive control tissue); SEM, standard error of the mean value. The IC_{50}/K_i values are in molar terms. These values are inversely related to receptor affinity parameters. Cloprostenol, fluprostenol, and PHXA85 are the free acid-active forms of the drugs. Latanoprost is the isopropyl ester of PHXA85. These data were obtained from concentration-binding graphs derived from competition experiments (Davis and Sharif, 1999).

Compound	**LCM**		-	**ISM**		-	**RET**		-	**BCLM**	
-	Mean	SEM	-	Mean	SEM	-	Mean	SEM	-	Mean	SEM
Cloprostenol	4.97E-09	1.95E-09	-	1.58E-08	9.17E-09	-	8.68E-09	3.67E-09	-	3.20E-08	1.80E-09
Fluprostenol	5.17E-08	7.64E-09	-	9.26E-08	5.23E-08	-	2.63E-08	1.15E-08	-	9.80E-08	9.20E-09
PHXA85	4.20E-08	4.79E-09	-	1.49E-07	6.44E-08	-	1.04E-07	3.27E-08	-	9.80E-08	1.10E-08
Latanoprost	3.05E-06	1.81E-06	-	2.33E-06	1.61E-06	-	3.43E-08	7.18E-09	-	4.20E-06	7.90E-07

CONCLUSION

The technique of receptor/enzyme autoradiography is now quite mature and has been successfully utilized to image and quantify the regional distribution of such proteins in many organs of the body, including the eye. For radioligand-based imaging, the transmitter or drug molecules for which the target localization is needed must be radioactively labeled without changing their binding and pharmacological properties. Isotopes that have been used include tritium (^{3}H), radioactive iodine (^{125}I), and sulfur (^{35}S). Whilst ^{14}C is also used, the signal from this low-activity isotope requires a much longer time for film or phosphoscreen exposure than the latter. Radioligands using ^{125}I require the shortest film exposure times, sometimes just a few minutes to a few hours, depending on the concentration of the radioligand used. Many methods for specific radioligands are available in the literature and researchers are encouraged to consult those sources as listed in the bibliography.

REFERENCES

Bucolo, C, Platania, CBM, Drago, F, Bonfiglio, V, Reibaldi, M, Avitabile, T & Uva, M (2018) Novel therapeutics in glaucoma management. *Curr Neuropharmacol,* 16, 978-92. [http://dx.doi.org/10.2174/1570159X15666170915142727] [PMID: 28925883]

Davis, TL & Sharif, NA (1999) Quantitative autoradiographic visualization and pharmacology of FP-

prostaglandin receptors in human eyes using the novel phosphor-imaging technology. *J Ocul Pharmacol Ther,* 15, 323-36.
[http://dx.doi.org/10.1089/jop.1999.15.323] [PMID: 10463871]

Gabaglio, M, Prini, P, Zamberletti, E, Rubino, T & Parolaro, D (2023) Assay of GTPγS binding in autoradiography. *Methods Mol Biol,* 2576, 181-8.
[http://dx.doi.org/10.1007/978-1-0716-2728-0_14] [PMID: 36152186]

Green, MR & Sambrook, J (2020) Autoradiography and Phosphorimaging. *Cold Spring Harb Protoc,* 2020, pdb.top100446.
[http://dx.doi.org/10.1101/pdb.top100446] [PMID: 33262238]

Hansen, JY, Shafiei, G, Markello, RD, Smart, K, Cox, SML, Nørgaard, M, Beliveau, V, Wu, Y, Gallezot, JD, Aumont, É, Servaes, S, Scala, SG, DuBois, JM, Wainstein, G, Bezgin, G, Funck, T, Schmitz, TW, Spreng, RN, Galovic, M, Koepp, MJ, Duncan, JS, Coles, JP, Fryer, TD, Aigbirhio, FI, McGinnity, CJ, Hammers, A, Soucy, JP, Baillet, S, Guimond, S, Hietala, J, Bedard, MA, Leyton, M, Kobayashi, E, Rosa-Neto, P, Ganz, M, Knudsen, GM, Palomero-Gallagher, N, Shine, JM, Carson, RE, Tuominen, L, Dagher, A & Misic, B (2022) Mapping neurotransmitter systems to the structural and functional organization of the human neocortex. *Nat Neurosci,* 25, 1569-81.
[http://dx.doi.org/10.1038/s41593-022-01186-3] [PMID: 36303070]

Kecheliev, V, Spinelli, F, Herde, A, Haider, A, Mu, L, Klohs, J, Ametamey, SM & Ni, R (2022) Evaluation of cannabinoid type 2 receptor expression and pyridine-based radiotracers in brains from a mouse model of Alzheimer's disease. *Front Aging Neurosci,* 14, 1018610.
[http://dx.doi.org/10.3389/fnagi.2022.1018610] [PMID: 36248003]

Krogsbaek, M, Larsen, NY, Landau, AM, Sanchez, C & Nyengaard, JR (2023) Changes in hypothalamic mu-opioid receptor expression following acute olanzapine treatment in female rats: Implications for feeding behavior. *J Chem Neuroanat,* 132, 102324.
[http://dx.doi.org/10.1016/j.jchemneu.2023.102324] [PMID: 37557929]

Mikkelsen, JD, Aripaka, SS, Kaad, S, Pazarlar, BA, Pinborg, L, Finsen, B, Varrone, A, Bang-Andersen, B & Bastlund, JF (2023) Characterization of the novel P2X7 eceptor radioligand [^{3}H]JNJ-64413739 in human brain tissue. *ACS Chem Neurosci,* 14, 111-8.
[http://dx.doi.org/10.1021/acschemneuro.2c00561] [PMID: 36535632]

Mitsukawa, K & Kimura, H (2022) Orexin 2 receptor (OX2R) protein distribution measured by autoradiography using radiolabeled OX2R-selective antagonist EMPA in rodent brain and peripheral tissues. *Sci Rep,* 12, 8473.
[http://dx.doi.org/10.1038/s41598-022-12601-x] [PMID: 35589803]

Murgaš, M, Michenthaler, P, Reed, MB, Gryglewski, G & Lanzenberger, R (2022) Correlation of receptor density and mRNA expression patterns in the human cerebral cortex. *Neuroimage,* 256, 119214.
[http://dx.doi.org/10.1016/j.neuroimage.2022.119214] [PMID: 35452805]

Neuman, J, Roeder, N, Richardson, B, Quattrin, T, Hamilton, J & Thanos, PK (2022) High fat diet increases [^{3}H]Flunitrazepam binding in the mouse brain that is dependent on the expression of the dopamine D2 gene. *Neurochem Res,* 47, 3003-11.
[http://dx.doi.org/10.1007/s11064-022-03644-7] [PMID: 35708880]

Pilotte, N, Sharif, NA & Burt, DR (1984) Characterization and autoradiographic localization of TRH receptors in sections of rat brain. *Brain Research,* 293, 372-6.
[http://dx.doi.org/10.1016/0006-8993(84)91246-0]

Sharif, NA, Davis, TL & Williams, GW (1999) [3H]AL-5848 ([3H]9β-(+)-Fluprostenol). Carboxylic acid of travoprost (AL-6221), a novel FP prostaglandin to study the pharmacology and autoradiographic localization of the FP receptor. *J Pharm Pharmacol,* 51, 685-94.
[http://dx.doi.org/10.1211/0022357991772989] [PMID: 10454045]

Sharif, NA & Hughes, J (1989) Discrete mapping of brain mu and delta opioid receptors using selective peptides: quantitative autoradiography, species differences and comparison with kappa receptors. *Peptides,*

10, 499-522.
[http://dx.doi.org/10.1016/0196-9781(89)90135-6]

Sharif, NA, Williams, GW & Davis, TL (2000) Pharmacology and autoradiography of human DP prostanoid receptors using [^{3} H]-BWA868C, a DP receptor-selective antagonist radioligand. *Br J Pharmacol,* 131, 1025-38.
[http://dx.doi.org/10.1038/sj.bjp.0703686] [PMID: 11082108]

Sharif, NA, Kelly, CR, Crider, JY & Davis, TL (2006) Serotonin-2 (5-HT2) receptor-mediated signal transduction in human ciliary muscle cells: role in ocular hypotension. *J Ocul Pharmacol Ther,* 22, 389-401.
[http://dx.doi.org/10.1089/jop.2006.22.389] [PMID: 17238805]

Sharif NA, Eglen RM. (1993). Quantitative Autoradiography: a tool to visualize and quantify receptors, enzymes, channels and second messenger systems. *Molecular Imaging in Neuroscience: A Practical Approach*, (Sharif NA, Ed.), Oxford University Press, pp. 71 138

Sharif, NA, Hunter, JC, Hill, RG & Hughes, J (1988) [125I]-dynorphin (1 8) produces a similar pattern of kappa opioid receptor labelling to [3H]-dynorphin (1—8) and [3H]-etorphine in guinea pig brain: a quantitative autoradiographic study. *Neuroscience Letters,* 86, 272-8.

Sharif, NA, Katoli, P, Scott, D, Li, L, Kelly, C, Xu, S, Husain, S, Toris, C & Crosson, C (2014) FR-190997, a nonpeptide bradykinin B2-receptor partial agonist, is a potent and efficacious intraocular pressure lowering agent in ocular hypertensive cynomolgus monkeys. *Drug Dev Res,* 75, 211-23.
[http://dx.doi.org/10.1002/ddr.21174] [PMID: 24796320]

Sharif, NA, Nunes, JL, Rosenkranz, RP, Eglen, RM & Whiting, RL (1995) Quantitative autoradiography demonstrates selective modulation of brain regional dopamine (D1 & D2) receptor subtypes after chronic manipulation of dietary salt. *Neurochemical Research,* 20, 121-8.

Sharif, NA, Williams, GW, Crider, JY, Xu, SX & Davis, TL (2004) Molecular pharmacology of the ocular hypotensive DP/EP2 class prostaglandin AL-6598 and localization of DP and EP2 receptor sites in human eyes. *J Ocul Pharmacol Ther,* 20, 489-508.
[http://dx.doi.org/10.1089/jop.2004.20.489] [PMID: 15684809]

Sharif NA. (1996). Quantitative Autoradiographic Methods. In: Brain Mapping: The Methods. (A. Toga & J. Mazziotta, Eds.), Chapter 5, Academic Press, New York, pp. 115 144

Sharif, NA (1986) Brain imaging: new approaches to neuronal communication. *Trends Pharmacol Sci,* 7, 46-7. [TIPS].
[http://dx.doi.org/10.1016/0165-6147(86)90246-4]

Sharif, NA & Lewis, ME Brain Imaging: techniques and applications. (1989) Ellis Horwood Ltd. pp 293.

Sharif, NA, Xu, SX, Crider, JY, McLaughlin, M & Davis, TL (2001) Levobetaxolol (Betaxon) and other β-adrenergic antagonists: preclinical pharmacology, IOP-lowering activity and sites of action in human eyes. *J Ocul Pharmacol Ther,* 17, 305-17.
[http://dx.doi.org/10.1089/108076801753162726] [PMID: 11572462]

Sharif, NA (1989) Quantitative autoradiography of TRH receptors in discrete brain regions of different mammalian species. *Annals New York Academy of Sciences,* 553, 147-75.
[http://dx.doi.org/10.1111/j.1749-6632.1989.tb46638.x]

Sharif, NA (2022) Targeting of signal transduction pathway components to mitigate selected ocular disorders. *Acta Scientific Ophthalmology,* 5, 3-17.

Sharif, NA (2021) Therapeutic drugs and devices for tackling ocular hypertension and glaucoma, and need for neuroprotection and cytoprotective therapies. *Front Pharmacol,* 12, 729249.
[http://dx.doi.org/10.3389/fphar.2021.729249] [PMID: 34603044]

Sharif, NA (2023) Identifying new drugs and targets to treat rapidly elevated intraocular pressure for angle closure and secondary glaucomas to curb visual impairment and prevent blindness. *Exp Eye Res,* 232, 109444.

[http://dx.doi.org/10.1016/j.exer.2023.109444] [PMID: 36958427]

Voss, JH, Al-Hroub, H, Gedschold, R, Dietrich, JM, Gaffal, E, Toma, M, Kehraus, S, König, GM, Brust, P, Fleischmann, BK, Wenzel, D, Deuther-Conrad, W & Müller, CE (2022) Imaging of $G\alpha_q$ proteins in mouse and human organs and tissues. *Pharmaceutics,* 15, 57.
[http://dx.doi.org/10.3390/pharmaceutics15010057] [PMID: 36678686]

Waldman, L, Richardson, B, Hamilton, J & Thanos, P (2022) Chronic oral olanzapine treatment but not haloperidol decreases [^{3}H] MK-801 binding in the rat brain Independent of dietary conditions. *Neurosci Lett,* 781, 136657.
[http://dx.doi.org/10.1016/j.neulet.2022.136657] [PMID: 35483503]

Weinreb, RN, Aung, T & Medeiros, FA (2014) The pathophysiology and treatment of glaucoma: a review. *JAMA,* 311, 1901-11.
[http://dx.doi.org/10.1001/jama.2014.3192] [PMID: 24825645]

CHAPTER 7

Protocols for Prostaglandin Receptor Localization in Eye Tissues Using Immunohistochemistry

Ursula Schlötzer-Schrehardt[1,*]

[1] *Department of Ophthalmology, Friedrich-Alexander University Erlangen-Nürnberg, Schwabachanlage 6, 91054 Erlangen, Germany*

Abstract: This chapter describes the detailed protocols for light and electron microscopic immunolocalization of prostaglandin (PG) receptors in ocular cells and tissues using immunofluorescence labeling of frozen sections, immunoperoxidase labeling of paraffin sections, and immunogold labeling of ultrathin sections. Unlike Western blotting analysis, immunohistochemistry allows for fine mapping of protein localization in intact tissues and cells, including assessment of relative abundance using image analysis software programs. Precise receptor subtype distribution is important for understanding mechanisms of action of therapeutic PG analogs, for identifying targets for novel treatments using subtype-specific high-affinity receptor agonists, and for improving safety profiles and minimizing potential side effects of anti-glaucoma pharmacotherapies.

Keywords: Trabecular meshwork, Anterior segment, EP receptor, FP receptor, Glaucoma, Human eye, Immunohistochemistry, Prostaglandin receptors.

INTRODUCTION

Prostaglandins (PGs) are arachidonic acid-derived lipid mediators that regulate a great variety of cellular functions by acting on specific G-protein-linked cell surface receptors expressed in the majority of mammalian cells. The prostanoid receptor subfamily comprises nine known members, including DP1-2 (PGD_2 receptors), EP1–4 (PGE_2 receptors), FP ($PGF_{2\alpha}$ receptor), IP (prostacyclin I2 receptor), and TP (thromboxane A_2 receptor), which are classified according to the prostanoid ligand that binds with greatest affinity (Coleman *et al.* 1994). Activation of these receptors by their respective ligands results in an elevation (DP-, EP2-, EP4-, and IP-receptors) or reduction (EP3-receptors) of cAMP or in the production of intracellular inositol phosphates that, in turn, raise intracellular

* **Corresponding author Ursula Schlötzer-Schrehardt:** Department of Ophthalmology, Friedrich-Alexander University Erlangen-Nürnberg, Schwabachanlage 6, 91054 Erlangen, Germany; Tel: +49-0131-8534433; E-mail: ursula.schloetzer-schrehardt@uk-erlangen.de

Najam A. Sharif and Sunny E. Ohia (Eds.)

Ca^{2+} concentrations (EP1, FP- and TP-receptors) (Sharif *et al.* 2023). These changes in cAMP and Ca^{2+} trigger downstream signal transduction pathways, such as phosphorylation and activation of various kinases, transducing prostanoid receptor activation into biological effects. The precise roles of prostanoid receptors in physiologic and pathologic conditions depend on multiple factors, including cellular context, receptor expression profile, ligand affinity, and coupling to various signal transduction pathways. This complexity is highlighted by the diverse and often opposing effects of PGs, which, for example, commonly act as pro-inflammatory mediators but can also have anti-inflammatory properties in certain settings (Hata and Breyer 2004).

In the eye, PG receptors have been implicated in the regulation of inflammatory processes, immune responses, blood flow, and intraocular pressure (IOP) (Doucette and Walter 2017). FP, DP, and EP receptor subtypes have been identified in virtually all human ocular tissues, including cornea, sclera, conjunctiva, trabecular meshwork, Schlemm's canal, ciliary body and ciliary muscle, iris, lens, choroid and retina (Woodward *et al.* 1997; Mukhopadhyay *et al.* 1997, 2001; Kamphuis *et al.* 2004; Schlötzer-Schrehardt *et al.* 2002; Biswas *et al.* 2004; Doucette and Walter 2017) using molecular biologic and immunohistochemical methods (Fig. **1**). FP receptors were found abundantly in the ciliary muscle, particularly the circular portion, and ciliary epithelium, as well as in dilator and sphincter muscles of the iris. EP1-4 receptor transcripts and proteins were found to be widely expressed in many ocular cell types, predominantly corneal epithelium, endothelium and keratocytes, trabecular endothelium, iris epithelium, vascular endothelium and stromal cells, and ciliary epithelium. DP receptors were also localized at high concentrations to the epithelium of the ciliary processes, ciliary muscle, iris tissue, choroid, and retina using quantitative autoradiography (Sharif *et al.* 2005). The TP receptor was also found to be expressed in the trabecular meshwork (Kamphuis *et al.* 2001). Prostaglandin receptor expression in ocular tissues may be altered by certain stimuli, including elevated IOP (Schneemann *et al.* 2002) and in certain pathological conditions (Singh *et al.* 2023; Ueta *et al.* 2011).

Topically administered PGs and their analogs have been shown to significantly lower IOP and have thus evolved as first-line drugs in glaucoma therapy. Classical PG analogs like latanoprost lower IOP *via* the FP receptor, principally by increasing aqueous outflow facility through the uveoscleral pathway by the activation of matrix metalloproteinases and extracellular matrix turnover in the ciliary muscle and sclera (Sharif *et al.* 2023). However, FP receptor agonists may also cause ocular side effects, such as conjunctival hyperemia as well as iris and periorbital skin darkening. Moreover, the effect of FP receptor agonists on the conventional outflow pathway and on trabecular endothelial cells has been less clear. In fact, FP and EP2 receptor agonists have been shown to exert opposing effects on trabecular cell contraction, myofibroblast transformation, and collagen deposition (Kalouche *et al.* 2016). More recently, a novel dual FP/EP3 receptor agonist, sepetaprost (ONO-9054 or DE-126), and a selective non-PG prostanoid EP2 receptor agonist, omidenepag isopropyl (OMDI), have also demonstrated robust IOP-reducing activities by enhancing both the uveoscleral and the conventional trabecular outflow pathways (Yamagishi-Kimura *et al.* 2022; Sharif *et al.* 2023).

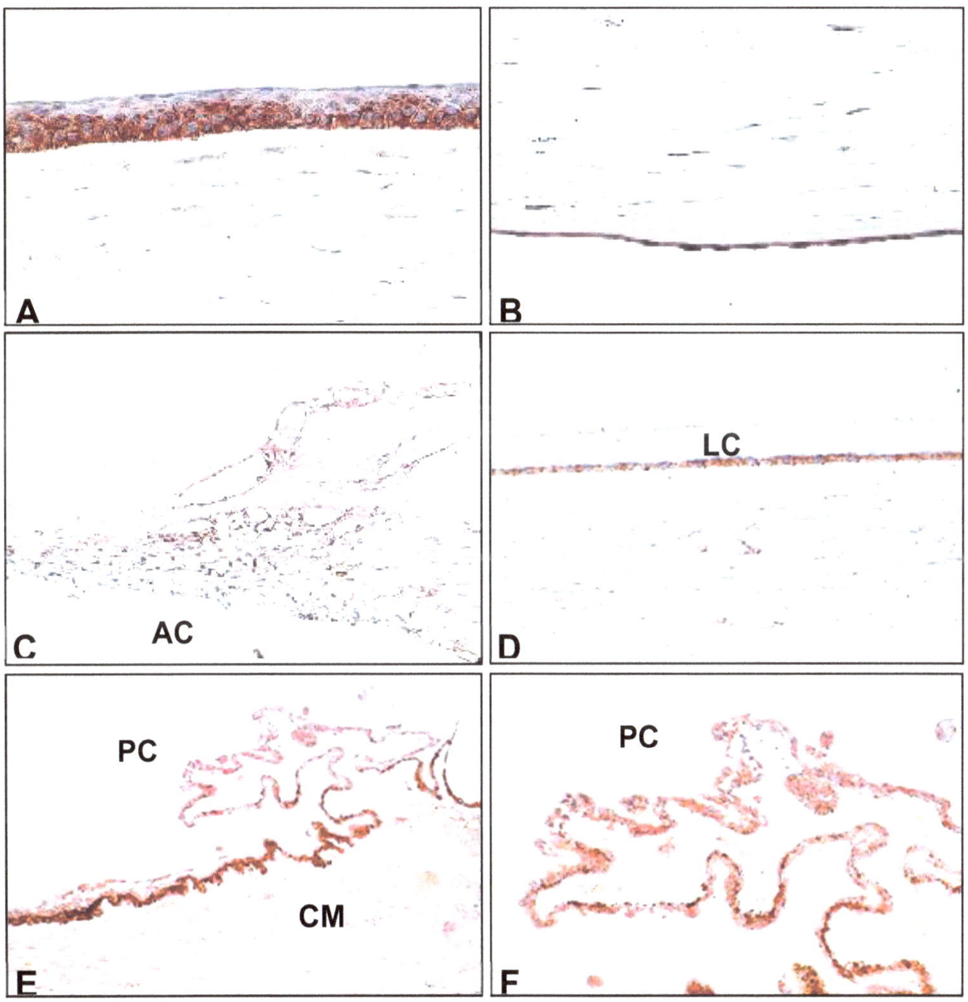

Fig. (1). Immunolocalization of the EP1 receptor in paraffin-embedded sections of human anterior segment tissues. Positive immunoreactions can be seen in the corneal epithelium (**A**), the corneal endothelium (**B**), the trabecular meshwork, Schlemm's canal, collector channels and intrascleral aqueous veins (**C**), the lens epithelium (**D**), the ciliary muscle and the ciliary epithelium (**E,F**); (AC, anterior chamber; CM, ciliary muscle; LC, lens capsule; PC, posterior chamber).

Since PG receptor agonists may exert differential effects on ocular cells (Wang *et al.* 2013), the expression and localization of PG receptor subtypes in the eye have been of great clinical and scientific interest. Precise receptor subtype distribution is important for understanding mechanisms of action of therapeutic PG analogs, for identifying targets for novel treatments using subtype-specific high-affinity receptor agonists, and for improving safety profiles and minimizing potential side effects (Matsou and Anastasopoulos 2018; Angeli & Supuran 2019). Therefore, the purpose of this chapter is to describe the detailed protocols for light and electron microscopic immunolocalization of PG receptors in ocular cells and tissues using immunofluorescence labeling of frozen sections, immunoperoxidase labeling of paraffin sections, and immunogold labeling of ultrathin sections as previously performed (Schlötzer-Schrehardt *et al.* 2002). The preparation of ocular tissues for (immuno)histologic examination requires special handling (Torczynski 1981). Unlike Western blotting analysis, immunohistochemistry allows for fine mapping of protein localization in intact tissues and cells, including assessment of relative abundance using image analysis software programs.

EXPERIMENTAL PROTOCOLS

The following procedures were performed in compliance with the principles of the Declaration of Helsinki for experiments involving human tissues and samples and were approved by the institutional ethics committee of the Friedrich-Alexander University Erlangen-Nürnberg.

Tissue Collection and Preparation

Note: Whole human donor eyes not suitable for corneal transplantation were obtained from the Erlangen Cornea Bank within 24 hours postmortem after receiving informed written consent from the relatives of the donor.

- Keep globes in a refrigerator until preparation. When handling human donor eyes, always wear gloves. Autoclave the dissection tools beforehand.
- Clean the outer surface of eyeballs from extraocular connective, muscle, and adipose tissue using forceps, scissors, and sterile scalpels on a sterile OP-towel.

Note: Tissue marking dyes can be used to mark the eyes for orientation purposes (Fig. **2**).

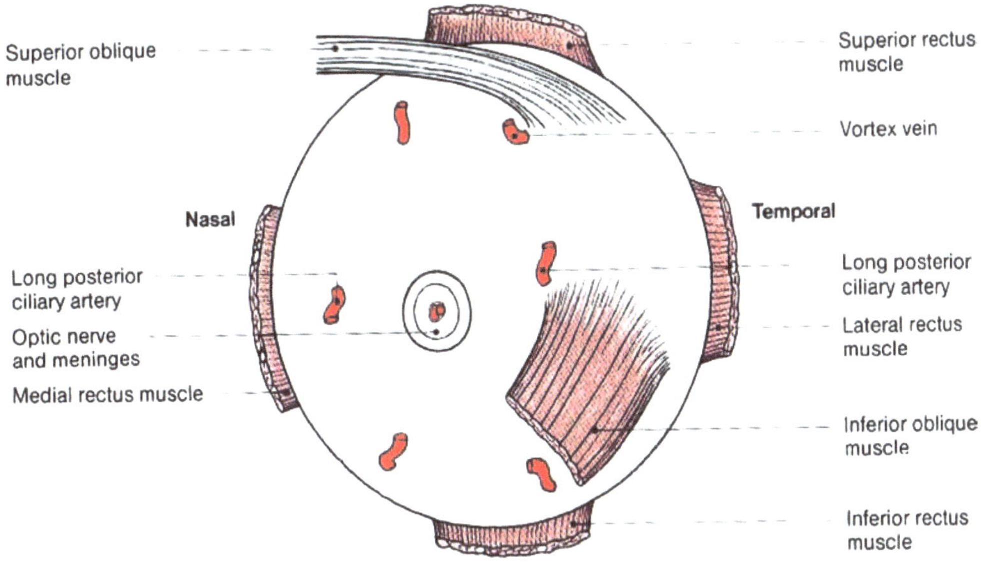

Fig. (2). Orientation of the right globe from behind (from G.O.H. Naumann, D.J. Apple: Pathology of the Eye, 1986).

Immunofluorescence Labeling of Frozen Sections

Preparation of Cryosections

- Bisect the native donor eyes along the equatorial plane behind the ora serrata with a PTFE-coated, single-edge steel razor blade (Ted Pella, Inc).
- Immerse the anterior and posterior halves in 90 mm Petri dishes containing 10 ml cold sterile Dulbecco's Balanced Salt Solution (DPBS) each.
- Fill both semi-cups with ~2ml sterile DPBS containing protease inhibitor cocktail 100x (Sigma-Aldrich).
- Dissect the zonules with Vannas scissors and remove the lens from the anterior segment under a dissecting microscope (Fig. **3**).
- Remove any vitreous from the eyecup using micro-scissors and cotton-swabs.
- Cut the anterior segment into four quadrants with a razor blade and straighten the edges (Fig. **3**).
- Immerse the pieces of anterior segment tissues into cryomolds (Tissue-Tek®) filled with optimal cutting temperature medium (O.C.T. compound, Tissue-Tek®), arrange the orientation of the tissue, and mark the future plane of sectioning on the mold. Make sure the tissue piece is fully embedded in the medium.
- Use long forceps to immerse the molds in isopentane precooled in liquid nitrogen for a few seconds until the embedding medium turns white.

- Store the frozen specimens tightly wrapped in aluminum foil and plastic bags at -80°C.
- Prepare tissue specimens of the posterior eyecup accordingly.
- Place a sample block on the stage of a cryostat in an orientation that enables sectioning along the sagittal anteroposterior axis of the eye, *i.e.* from the cornea to the retina.
- Section sample blocks in 30μm thickness steps until reaching a complete tissue level.
- Switch to desired section thickness ranging from 6 to 10 μm.
- Collect tissue sections by attaching them to glass slides coated with gelatine or poly-L-lysine.
- Air dry the frozen sections for 15 min.
- Store cryosections on glass slides at 4°C for same-day processing or at -20 or -80°C for future processing.

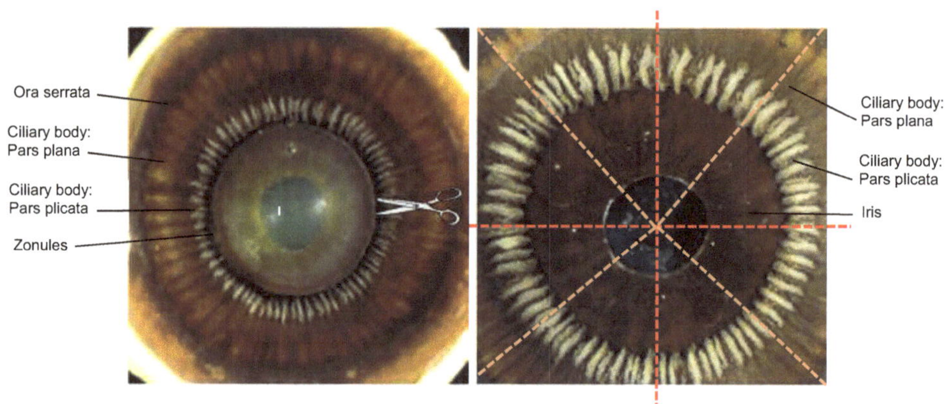

Fig. (3). Macroscopic image of the anterior eyecup as viewed from behind before and after dissection of the lens. The dashed lines indicate planes of sectioning.

Immunofluorescence Labeling and Imaging

- Fix sections with cold acetone for 10 min at 4°C.
- Air dry sections and draw an aqueous barrier circle around tissue sections using a PAP pen (Dako).
- Incubate tissue sections in phosphate-buffered saline (PBS, with Ca^{2+} and Mg^{2+}) at room temperature for 5 min.
- Block unspecific binding sites with a blocking solution consisting of 10% (v/v) normal serum in PBS for 30 min at room temperature.
- Incubate sections in primary antibodies diluted in PBS 1:200 – 1:500 overnight at 4°C in a dark and humid chamber.

Note: Affinity-purified rabbit polyclonal antibodies raised against synthetic peptides specific for FP and EP receptor subtypes were provided by Rolf M. Nüsing, Institute of Clinical Pharmacology, Pharmazentrum Frankfurt, University Hospital Frankfurt, Germany. The antibodies were tested using Western blot analysis to determine their specificity and cross-reactivity (Morath R *et al.* 1999). Alternatively, polyclonal rabbit antibodies against PG receptor subtypes can be obtained from commercial sources.

- Rinse tissue sections three times with PBS.
- Incubate sections with Alexa 488- or Alexa 555-conjugated secondary antibodies (Molecular Probes) diluted in PBS 1:300 for 30 min at room temperature.
- Rinse tissue sections three times with PBS.
- Perform nuclear counterstaining with propidium iodide (0.5 μg/ml), DAPI (1 μg/ml) or Hoechst 33342 (0.2 μg/ml) (Sigma-Aldrich) for 10 min at room temperature.
- Rinse tissue sections three times with PBS.
- Pipette one drop of mounting medium (Vectashield) over tissue sections and cover with a glass coverslip.

Note: Slides are now ready for imaging or can be stored at 4°C for up to 1 month. It is recommended to take images within 24 hours after mounting because tissue sections retain their fluorescent properties for a limited period only. Many ocular tissues exhibit autofluorescence, which should be verified on a control slide without fluorescent stain.

- Acquire images using a standard fluorescence microscope or a confocal microscope.
- Fluorescence intensity values of staining reactions can be quantitatively analyzed on at least three images/specimens after correcting for negative control background using ImageJ or comparable software programs.
- Include appropriate negative control experiments, *i.e.* replace the primary antibody with PBS, equimolar concentrations of an isotype-specific control antibody, or primary antibody preadsorbed with synthetic peptides.
- Include appropriate positive controls, *e.g.* brain or kidney sections expressing all EP receptors (Morath R *et al.* 1999).

Immunohistochemistry of Paraffin-Embedded Sections

Preparation of Paraffin Sections

- Immerse the globes in 150-200 ml 4% paraformaldehyde in PBS at 4°C overnight.

Note: Globes should not be opened before fixation, nor should fixative be injected into the ocular cavity.

- Rinse tissues three times with PBS.
- Bisect the donor eyes along the sagittal (anteroposterior) axis using a razor blade.
- Dehydrate the eyecups by passing them through a series of increasing ethanol concentrations at room temperature: 30%, 50%, 70%, 90%, and 100% ethanol for 60 min each.
- Clear tissues with xylene for 4 hours at room temperature.

Note: All steps must be performed in the fume cupboard.

- Infiltrate the tissues in three changes of melted paraffin at 56°C for 2.5 hours each.
- Use forceps to transfer the tissues to the well of a metallic embedding mold by placing the section plane on the bottom.
- Fill the mold with melted paraffin and solidify the paraffin blocks with the help of an embedding machine.
- Mount the paraffin block on the microtome.
- Cut paraffin sections at 4-5 µm thickness.
- Pick up the sections using small brushes and transfer them into the histology bath containing deionized water at 56°C to allow sections to stretch.
- Dip a glass slide (Superfrost Plus, Thermo Scientific) into the histology bath, allowing the tissue section to adhere to its surface.
- Dry the slides in an oven at 56°C for 1 hour up to overnight.

Immunoenzyme Labeling and Imaging

- Place glass slides in glass staining racks.
- Deparaffinize the sections by two successive xylene baths, 5 min each.
- Rehydrate the sections by passing through decreasing concentrations of ethanol: 2 changes of 100% ethanol, 5 min each, 2 changes of 96% ethanol, 5 min each, followed by 80%, 70%, and 50% ethanol for 5 min each, and deionized water for 5 min.
- For antigen retrieval, transfer the slides into PMP staining jars with a lid filled with 10 mM sodium citrate buffer (pH 6.0).
- Heat slides in the microwave partially covered with a lid for ~1 min until boiling is initiated and sub-boil for 10 min.
- Cool slides on bench top for 20 min.
- Wash the slides in deionized water for 5 min two times.
- Immerse slides in PBS-T (0.1% Tween 20 in PBS) for 5 min.
- Draw a circle around each section using a PAP pen.

Note: From this point forward, transfer the slides into a humidity chamber. Wash the slides in the glass staining dish.

- Block endogenous peroxidase and alkaline phosphatase with 100-200 µl BLOXALL® (Vector Laboratories) for 10 min.
- Wash the slides in PBS-T for 5 min.
- Incubate sections with blocking buffer (10% normal serum in PBS-T) for 30 min at room temperature.
- Block sections with a drop of avidin for 15 min, rinse briefly in PBS-T, and block sections with a drop of biotin for 15 min at room temperature (Avidin/Biotin blocking kit; Vector Laboratories).
- Wash the slides in PBS-T for 5 min.
- Incubate sections in primary antibodies diluted in PBS-T 1:200 – 1:500 overnight at 4°C.
- Wash the slides in PBS-T for 5 min.
- Incubate sections with biotinylated secondary antibodies (VECTASTAIN® Elite ABC Kit) for 60 min at room temperature.
- Wash slides in PBS-T for 5 min.
- Incubate for 60 min with prepared VECTASTAIN Elite ABC reagent.
- Wash slides in PBS-T for 5 min.
- Incubate in a peroxidase substrate solution (AEC peroxidase substrate; Vector Laboratories) for ~10-30 min until desired staining intensity develops.
- Briefly rinse in deionized water.
- Counterstain in Meyer's hemalum (Sigma-Aldrich) for 10 min.
- Rinse in tap water for 5 min.
- Mount sections in aqueous mounting media (Aquatex®, Sigma-Aldrich) by avoiding trapping air bubbles.
- Store slides in a cardboard folder and acquire images using a standard light microscope.

Immunogold Labeling of Resin-Embedded Sections

Preparation of Ultrathin Resin Sections

- Immerse small blocks of tissue (~5x5 mm) in 4% paraformaldehyde and 0.1% glutaraldehyde in 0.1M cacodylate buffer (pH 7.4) for 2-5 hours at 4°C (for preparation, see 2.1.6)
- Rinse in three changes of 0.1M cacodylate buffer containing 3.7% sucrose at 4°C for 20 min each.
- Dehydrate specimens in 30% ethanol at 4°C for 30 min, in 50% ethanol at 0°C (on ice) for 1 hour, and in two changes of 70% ethanol at -20°C for 1 hour and overnight.

- Immerse specimens in a 1:1 mixture of 70% ethanol and LR White resin (medium grade, Science Services) for 1 hour at 4°C.
- Immerse specimens in 3 changes of pure LR White for 1 hour at 4°C, then for 1 hour at room temperature, and finally on a rotator overnight.
- Transfer specimens in gelatin capsules (Science Services) completely filled with fresh LR White, close the cap tightly to avoid large air bubbles at the top, and polymerize the resin at 45-50°C for 24 hours.
- Prepare ultrathin sections (60-80 nm thickness) from the resin blocks using an ultramicrotome, transfer sections onto nickel grids (hexagonal 200 mesh grids; Science Services), and air dry in a grid storage box.

Immunogold Labeling and Imaging

- Incubate sections on grids successively on drops (10 µl) of Tris-buffered saline (TBS) for 5 min, 0.05 M glycine in TBS for 30 min, two changes of TBS for 2 min each, and a mixture of 0.5% ovalbumin and 0.5% fish gelatin (Sigma-Aldrich) in TBS for 30 min at room temperature.
- Incubate sections in primary antibodies diluted 1:200 – 1:500 in TBS-ovalbumin overnight at 4°C in a humid chamber.
- Rinse sections 5 times in TBS-ovalbumin-gelatin for 5 min each.
- Incubate sections in 10 nm gold-conjugated secondary antibody (Abcam) diluted 1:30 in TBS-ovalbumin for 1 hour at room temperature.
- Rinse sections 5 times in TBS-ovalbumin for 2 min each.
- Rinse sections 5 times in TBS for 2 min each.
- Air dry grids and stain with 4% aqueous uranyl acetate for 3 min.
- Examine sections with a transmission electron microscope.

CONCLUSION

The protocols described above endeavor to provide sufficient details for reliable light and electron microscopic immunostaining of PG receptors (or any other antigens of interest). This will help scientists save time, effort, and antibody costs during the application of these techniques. Since there is a need for the development of novel anti-glaucoma or anti-inflammatory pharmacotherapies with enhanced efficacy, sustained effects, and improved safety profile, a better understanding of PG receptor distribution in ocular tissues may contribute to designing more specific PG receptor agonists to modulate aqueous outflow and IOP as well as inflammatory responses.

REFERENCES

Angeli, A & Supuran, CT (2019) Prostaglandin receptor agonists as antiglaucoma agents (a patent review 2013 – 2018). *Expert Opin Ther Pat,* 29, 793-803. [http://dx.doi.org/10.1080/13543776.2019.1661992] [PMID: 31462124]

Biswas, S, Bhattacherjee, P & Paterson, CA (2004) Prostaglandin E2 receptor subtypes, EP1, EP2, EP3 and EP4 in human and mouse ocular tissues—a comparative immunohistochemical study. *Prostaglandins Leukot Essent Fatty Acids,* 71, 277-88.
[http://dx.doi.org/10.1016/j.plefa.2004.03.021] [PMID: 15380814]

Coleman, RA, Smith, WL & Narumiya, S (1994) International Union of Pharmacology classification of prostanoid receptors: properties, distribution, and structure of the receptors and their subtypes. *Pharmacol Rev,* 46, 205-29.
[PMID: 7938166]

Doucette, LP & Walter, MA (2017) Prostaglandins in the eye: Function, expression, and roles in glaucoma. *Ophthalmic Genet,* 38, 108-16.
[http://dx.doi.org/10.3109/13816810.2016.1164193] [PMID: 27070211]

Hata, AN & Breyer, RM (2004) Pharmacology and signaling of prostaglandin receptors: Multiple roles in inflammation and immune modulation. *Pharmacol Ther,* 103, 147-66.
[http://dx.doi.org/10.1016/j.pharmthera.2004.06.003] [PMID: 15369681]

Kalouche, G, Beguier, F, Bakria, M, Melik-Parsadaniantz, S, Leriche, C, Debeir, T, Rostène, W, Baudouin, C & Vigé, X (2016) Activation of Prostaglandin FP and EP2 Receptors Differently Modulates Myofibroblast Transition in a Model of Adult Primary Human Trabecular Meshwork Cells. *Invest Ophthalmol Vis Sci,* 57, 1816-25.
[http://dx.doi.org/10.1167/iovs.15-17693] [PMID: 27082296]

Kamphuis, W, Schneemann, A, van Beek, LM, Smit, AB, Hoyng, PF & Koya, E (2001) Prostanoid receptor gene expression profile in human trabecular meshwork: a quantitative real-time PCR approach. *Invest Ophthalmol Vis Sci,* 42, 3209-15.
[PMID: 11726624]

Kamphuis, W, Schneemann, A, Shichi, H, Broersma, L & Hoyng, P (2004) Immunolocalization of prostanoid EP receptor isotypes in human trabecular meshwork. *Curr Eye Res,* 29, 17-26.
[http://dx.doi.org/10.1080/02713680490513155] [PMID: 15370363]

Matsou, A & Anastasopoulos, E (2018) Investigational drugs targeting prostaglandin receptors for the treatment of glaucoma. *Expert Opin Investig Drugs,* 27, 777-85.
[http://dx.doi.org/10.1080/13543784.2018.1526279] [PMID: 30227753]

Morath, R, Klein, T, Seyberth, HW & Nüsing, RM (1999) Immunolocalization of the four prostaglandin E2 receptor proteins EP1, EP2, EP3, and EP4 in human kidney. *J Am Soc Nephrol,* 10, 1851-60.
[http://dx.doi.org/10.1681/ASN.V1091851] [PMID: 10477136]

Mukhopadhyay, P, Geoghegan, TE, Patil, RV, Bhattacherjee, P & Paterson, CA (1997) Detection of EP2, EP4, and FP receptors in human ciliary epithelial and ciliary muscle cells. *Biochem Pharmacol,* 53, 1249-55.
[http://dx.doi.org/10.1016/S0006-2952(97)00011-7] [PMID: 9214685]

Mukhopadhyay, P, Bian, L, Yin, H, Bhattacherjee, P & Paterson, C (2001) Localization of EP(1) and FP receptors in human ocular tissues by *in situ* hybridization. *Invest Ophthalmol Vis Sci,* 42, 424-8.
[PMID: 11157877]

Schlötzer-Schrehardt, U, Zenkel, M & Nüsing, RM (2002) Expression and localization of FP and EP prostanoid receptor subtypes in human ocular tissues. *Invest Ophthalmol Vis Sci,* 43, 1475-87.
[PMID: 11980863]

Schneemann, A, Hoyng, PFJ & Kamphuis, W (2002) Effects of elevated pressure on prostanoid receptor gene expression levels in human trabecular meshwork. *Ophthalmic Res,* 34, 314-8.
[http://dx.doi.org/10.1159/000065606] [PMID: 12381894]

Sharif, NA, Davis, TL & Williams, GW (2005) Ocular hypotensive DP-class prostaglandin receptor affinities determined by quantitative autoradiography on human eye sections. *J Ocul Pharmacol Ther,* 21, 121-32.
[http://dx.doi.org/10.1089/jop.2005.21.121] [PMID: 15857278]

Sharif, NA, Odani-Kawabata, N, Lu, F & Pinchuk, L (2023) FP and EP2 prostanoid receptor agonist drugs

and aqueous humor outflow devices for treating ocular hypertension and glaucoma. *Exp Eye Res,* 229, 109415.
[http://dx.doi.org/10.1016/j.exer.2023.109415] [PMID: 36803996]

Singh, S, Rao, BS & Basu, S (2023) Altered Prostaglandin E Receptor Subtype 3 Expression in Lacrimal Glands of Patients with Chronic Stevens-Johnson Syndrome. *Ocul Immunol Inflamm,* 31, 343-7.
[http://dx.doi.org/10.1080/09273948.2022.2028286] [PMID: 35113749]

Torczynski, E (1981) Preparation of ocular specimens for histopathologic examination. *Ophthalmology,* 88, 1367-71.
[http://dx.doi.org/10.1016/S0161-6420(81)34877-5] [PMID: 7033857]

Ueta, M, Sotozono, C, Yokoi, N, Inatomi, T & Kinoshita, S (2011) Prostaglandin E receptor subtype EP3 expression in human conjunctival epithelium and its changes in various ocular surface disorders. *PLoS One,* 6, e25209.
[http://dx.doi.org/10.1371/journal.pone.0025209] [PMID: 21966456]

Yamagishi-Kimura, R, Honjo, M & Aihara, M (2022) The Roles Played by FP/EP3 Receptors During Pressure-lowering in Mouse Eyes Mediated by a Dual FP/EP3 Receptor Agonist. *Invest Ophthalmol Vis Sci,* 63, 24.
[http://dx.doi.org/10.1167/iovs.63.2.24] [PMID: 35147658]

Wang, JW, Woodward, DF & Stamer, WD (2013) Differential effects of prostaglandin E2-sensitive receptors on contractility of human ocular cells that regulate conventional outflow. *Invest Ophthalmol Vis Sci,* 54, 4782-90.
[http://dx.doi.org/10.1167/iovs.13-12363] [PMID: 23766471]

Woodward, DE, Regan, JW, Lake, S & Ocklind, A (1997) The molecular biology and ocular distribution of prostanoid receptors. *Surv Ophthalmol,* 41 (Suppl. 2), S15-21.
[http://dx.doi.org/10.1016/S0039-6257(97)80003-3] [PMID: 9154272]

OCULAR CELL TYPES AND SOURCES FOR ISOLATION AND CHARACTERIZATION

CHAPTER 8

Isolation and Use of Trabecular Meshwork Cells

Najam A. Sharif[1,*] and **Saima Chaudhry**[2]

[1] *Vice President and Head of Research & Development Nanoscope Therapeutics Inc., 2777 N. Stemmons Fwy, Suite 1102, Dallas, TX-75207, USA*

[2] *Univ N. Texas at Arlington, 701 S Nedderman Dr. Arlington, TX-76019, USA*

Abstract: As described elsewhere in the book, ocular hypertension (OHT) is a major risk factor for the development and progression of open-angle, closed-angle, and secondary forms of glaucoma. OHT or elevated intraocular pressure (IOP) is caused when the major aqueous humor (AQH)-drainage pathway, the trabecular meshwork (TM), and Schlemm's canal (SC) are slowly occluded by progressive deposition of extracellular matrix in and around the latter structures. In order to study the structure and function of the TM, most researchers isolate this tissue from different species, including from post-mortem human eyes, and either use the whole tissue (*e.g.*, in contraction/relaxation assays) or isolate individual single cells and propagate them under tissue culture conditions. These cells can then be used for studying the morphological, biochemical, and pharmacological changes induced by various insults to simulate OHT/glaucomatous disease states or in response to compounds of interest utilizing various functional readouts.

Keywords: Functional assays, Intrinsic activity, Intraocular pressure, Ocular hypertension, Potency, Prostaglandin, Trabecular meshwork.

INTRODUCTION

Trabecular meshwork (TM), in conjunction with Schlemm's canal (SC), represents the major outflow drainage pathway for aqueous humor (AQH) in the anterior chamber of the eye (ANCe). Under normal circumstances, there is an equal volume of AQH produced by the ciliary body and exiting the ANCe to maintain a steady intraocular pressure (IOP) (Acott *et al.*, 2020). This ensures that the AQH provides the tissue lining the ANCe nourishment, oxygen, and anti-microbial substances to ensure homeostasis and good health of all those tissues and their cells. The constant IOP at normal levels (14-21 mmHg) also ensures a steady shape of the eyeball. However, in advancing age and under pathological

* **Corresponding author Najam A. Sharif:** Vice President and Head of Research & Development Nanoscope Therapeutics Inc., 2777 N. Stemmons Fwy, Suite 1102, Dallas, TX-75207, USA; Tel: +1(817)-565-7686; E-mail: nsharif@nanostherapeutics.com

conditions, as in different forms of glaucoma, the TM and the juxtacanalicular area experience an abnormal deposition of the extracellular matrix, which clogs these tissues and slow down the AQH egress from the ANCe (Rhee *et al.*, 2003; Weinreb *et al.*, 2014). As the AQH production continues, accumulating AQH fluid in the ANCe raises the IOP. Whilst this happens slowly and can take decades to manifest, even small increases in IOP can begin to damage the retinal ganglion cells and their axons (which form the optic nerve), leading to vision loss. There is a direct correlation between elevation of IOP and RGC loss and visual impairment (Heill *et al.*, 2002; Kass *et al.*, 2002). Therefore, it is important to diagnose and treat the OHT with pharmaceutical, device, or surgical interventions (Weinreb *et al.*, 2014; Sharif, 2018, 2021) to lower and control the IOP.

Since the TM is the key tissue providing resistance to AQH drainage (Acott *et al.*, 2020), it has been and continues to be the major tissue of interest linking OHT/glaucoma to visual impairment and for studying effects of glaucomatous insults on the cell morphology, biochemistry, and pharmacology. These cells have also been successfully used to profile compounds of interest that may possess IOP-lowering activities (Sharif *et al.*, 2018, 2021). Primary TM cells have been isolated from the eyes of many mammalian species, cultured, and propagated over at least a few passages for the latter purposes (Keller *et al.*, 2013, 2018). In some cases, the cells have been immortalized, and these have proven useful for receptor characterization in a functional assay system (Pang *et al.*, 1994). This chapter aims to provide guidance on the isolation and culturing of primary TM cells, as recently detailed in a consensus publication (Keller *et al.*, 2018). Readers are highly encouraged to consult the latter paper and the bibliography therein for an excellent background and other important aspects of the current topic.

Procedures for TM Isolation

Most researchers isolate TM cells from whole globes or anterior segments of the eye of a variety of animals and post-mortem human subjects. Corneal transplant corneal rim discards can also be utilized. Storage of tissues is preferably performed on ice in a humidified container with phosphate-buffered saline (PBS) or in Optisol, a specialized fluid that maintains corneal health. Post-mortem human eyeballs can be obtained from local eye banks under strict quality and safety conditions and should be carefully handled and placed in ice or brought to the lab in corneal transplant-solution. They must be serologically tested and worked on in a biological safety laminar flow hood. Isolated eyeballs of large animals such as cattle and pigs can be obtained fresh from local abattoirs and brought back to the lab in/on ice. Non-human primate tissue is often only obtained from the institutional animal husbandry department (vivarium) under strict IUCUC regulations. All eyeballs and tissues derived from the latter species should be handled carefully and under stringent safety procedures as they may contain a variety of infectious viruses, bacteria, and perhaps even fungi. As such, researchers are encouraged to sterilize the eyeballs using ethanol (at least 70%) and/or an iodine-based antiseptic fluid to get rid of any infective agents. However, before dissection begins, ensure that the sterilizing fluids are removed by a series of rinses with sterile PBS. Since newly isolated cell viability and yield are time-dependent, the time elapsed from eyeball harvesting to tissue and cell isolation should be minimized as much as possible.

- Equatorially bisect the whole eyeballs using fresh, clean, and sharp scissors, a scalpel, or a single-edged razor blade.
- Under a well-illuminated binocular dissecting microscope, carefully dissect away ciliary processes, iris, and lens. In this case, cutting the anterior segment into many radial wedges in order to observe a flatter tissue surface and see the positioning of the TM/SC is deemed useful.
- Under the dissecting microscope, tip upwards the cut surface to see the SC and the TM. Now, isolate the TM from the tissue wedges using the techniques described in detail by Keller *et al.* (2018). The pooled TM tissue from several donor eyes can then be used to isolate the TM cells for culturing purposes.

TM Cell Isolation Procedures

- Place the dissected TM tissue strips (*e.g.*, each 2–5 mm in length, cumulatively about 25–35 mm as per the circumference of the human TM) into one well of a six-well culture plate and then carefully add the culture medium. Smaller 16 mm well plates can be used if necessary, but in this case, only 4–6 TM strips are placed in each well.
- Maintain the TM cultures undisturbed at 37°C in the humidified and 5% CO_2-controlled incubator for 1–2 weeks so that TM cells can migrate out of the TM explants and attach to the bottom of the well.
- As the TM cells migrate out, the TM strips should be moved into new plates to harvest more TM cells. The culture medium should be carefully changed every 3–5 days without disturbing the tissue strips. The TM cells obtained from a single individual (animal or human donor eye) should be described as cell strains.
- Unfortunately, a common issue encountered during the harvest of TM cells from the incubated TM explants is that the latter float up from the bottom of the plate well, especially when the culture medium is changed, and the cells can die. A remedy utilized to obviate this problem is to coat the culture plates with collagen or gelatin such that the cells and tissue strips can attach to the well-bottom surface and remain attached. Another solution for this problem is to place a sterile coverslip on top of the TM implant such that the tissue remains in contact

with the bottom of the well. TM cells may migrate and attach to the coverslip, in which case remove the coverslip and place it in a separate culture-plate well with the culture medium to encourage these cells to proliferate. Yet another approach is to put the TM strip(s) onto the bottom of a dry well of a 6-well plate for a few minutes (15 min) to permit them to adhere to the plastic surface and then carefully add a small amount of the culture medium (~1 ml) to submerge the TM strips. Carefully add more medium after the tissue attachment has occurred so that the tissues are not disturbed. Of course, the key is to not let the tissue strips dry out during these early stages, so a balance needs to be struck between tissue attachment and medium addition.

- Addition of high-quality bacterial collagenase (10 mg/ml) and/or dispase (10 mg/ml) (*e.g.* Fisher, Cat. #17-104-019 or Worthington Cat. #4188), with lowest possible amount of low tryptic and caseinase activity, for up to 30 min (37 °C with rotation) to the culture medium prior to placement of the TM explants in culture, may be used to encourage TM cells to migrate out from the tissue more easily. After this process, the TM cells attached to the plate surface can be propagated to increase the overall yield.
- Following the tissue digestion procedure, the TM tissue strips should be pelleted by centrifugation at low speed (*e.g.*, 1500g) and then carefully resuspended into fresh culture medium and placed into a single well of a 6-well culture dish as described above.
- As a standardized procedure, TM cells obtained from animal tissues are isolated and cultured as described for human TM above. For example, porcine TM cells isolated from 10-20 eyes are pooled and propagated to reduce data variability when used in experiments. However, as with human TM cell isolation, pig TM cells can also be isolated and cultured from individual animals if gender and genetic variations need to be accounted for and to increase the overall n-values of samples of animal tissue employed in specific experimental paradigms (Rhee *et al.*, 2003; Keller and Acott, 2013).
- When culturing the TM cells, use a standardized culture medium. For example, a medium composed of a mixture of Dulbecco's Modified Eagle's Medium (DMEM) contains low glucose (*e.g.*, 1 mg/L), antibiotics [0.5% gentamicin or penicillin (100 units/ml), streptomycin (100 µg/ml)], 2 mM L-glutamine, and 10% fetal bovine serum (FBS). To ensure optimal growth and propagation of TM cells, different FBS lots should be evaluated. The one that yields the best results should then be utilized in future TM isolation and cell culture endeavors.
- Use 20% FBS supplementation to culture medium when the isolated TM cells are isolated from the eyeballs of older (> 60 years old) human donors. Also, fibroblast growth factors (bFGF/FGF-2, 250 ng/ml) added to the culture medium can enhance cell propagation/growth (Polansky *et al.*, 1979, 1984). To reduce fungal contamination, use 1% amphotericin B in the culture medium, especially

when TM cells are obtained from animal eyes. With experience, some researchers use DMEM containing a 1:1 mix of low glucose and high glucose.

- When TM cell cultures attain confluence, the FGF can be removed, and the serum concentration can be decreased down to as low as 1% final. Whilst a medium containing FBS helps expand TM cells, these cells can be maintained in a medium with low or no serum for up to I month, although this is not encouraged. However, the removal of FBS and the inherent growth factors obviously occurs for a brief period when the culture medium is removed and replaced with a warm incubation buffer in order to conduct experiments on the TM cells.
- When TM cells reach 70-90% confluency, they can be removed by the traditional trypsinization procedure using 0.05% trypsin/0.5 mM EDTA made in buffer or in fresh medium lacking FBS and other additives. Fibroblasts detach from the culture plates or flasks faster than TM cells after light trypsinization within 30s–1 min of adding the 0.05% trypsin/0.5 mM EDTA solution. In this manner, cultures of TM cells can be enriched by removing the fibroblasts before the TM cells begin detaching.

The procedure to passage TM cells uses a traditional method of trypsinization (*e.g.*) to reduce cell-matrix and cell-cell adhesions and to aid cell detachment from the plates, ready for centrifuging. When passaging the cell cultures, fibroblasts detach quite fast, but TM cells need a longer incubation (3–5 min) with the trypsin. Hence, by varying the time of exposure of cell cultures to the trypsin, enrichment of TM cells from contaminating fibroblasts can be achieved since the fibroblasts can be simply washed away following light trypsinization. Once trypsinized, TM cells at 70–90% confluence are generally split 1:3 to maintain appropriate cell densities. TM cells appear to require paracrine factors from surrounding cells for growth, so splitting cells at lower cell densities may result in slow or no growth. Once initial isolates are trypsinized (passage 1), cells are considered "secondary" cultures and should be referred to as "normal" TM cells, not "primary" TM cells. TM cells have a finite number of doublings and begin to change in appearance after 6–8 passages. By passage 9 or 10, they can no longer be described as TM cells since they start to develop senescence features such as vacuoles, increased size, and reduced doubling time. Major changes in gene expression patterns are also observed (Hernandez *et al.*, 1987). For this reason, it is generally not recommended to use TM cells from human eyes at greater than 7 passages. For TM cells derived from animal sources, the recommended passage number is often decreased. For instance, porcine TM cells are typically used within 5 passages. Since the duration of passaging of individual cell strains depends upon the initial number of cell isolates, it is critical to visually monitor all cultures for senescence features no matter the passage number.

CONCLUSION

The importance of the TM in mediating AQH efflux from the anterior chamber of the eye to regulate IOP is well established. Due to the heterogeneity of the cells in the TM, it is important to understand and define the properties (morphological as well as functional) of the isolated TM cells. It appears that the smooth muscle-like cells within the TM outnumber the endothelial-like cells, and thus, collections of cells isolated and passaged most likely will be the former types. Understanding the biochemical and pharmacological properties of the TM cells can aid in characterizing IOP-lowering agents and defining their potential mechanism(s) of action (Sharif *et al.*, 2003; 2006).

REFERENCES

Acott, TS, Vranka, JA, Keller, KE, Raghunathan, V & Kelley, MJ (2021) Normal and glaucomatous outflow regulation. *Prog Retin Eye Res,* 82, 100897.
[http://dx.doi.org/10.1016/j.preteyeres.2020.100897] [PMID: 32795516]

Heijl, A, Leske, MC, Bengtsson, B, Hyman, L, Bengtsson, B & Hussein, M (2002) Reduction of intraocular pressure and glaucoma progression: results from the Early Manifest Glaucoma Trial. *Arch Ophthalmol,* 120, 1268-79.
[http://dx.doi.org/10.1001/archopht.120.10.1268] [PMID: 12365904]

Hernandez, MR, Weinstein, BI, Schwartz, J, Ritch, R, Gordon, GG & Southren, AL (1987) Human trabecular meshwork cells in culture: morphology and extracellular matrix components. *Invest Ophthalmol Vis Sci,* 28, 1655-60.
[PMID: 3654139]

Kass, MA, Heuer, DK, Higginbotham, EJ, Johnson, CA, Keltner, JL, Miller, JP, Parrish, RK, II, Wilson, MR & Gordon, MO (2002) The Ocular Hypertension Treatment Study: a randomized trial determines that topical ocular hypotensive medication delays or prevents the onset of primary open-angle glaucoma. *Arch Ophthalmol,* 120, 701-13.
[http://dx.doi.org/10.1001/archopht.120.6.701] [PMID: 12049574]

Keller, KE & Acott, TS (2013) The juxtacanalicular region of ocular trabecular meshwork: a tissue with a unique extracellular matrix and specialized function. *J Ocul Biol,* 1, 3.
[PMID: 24364042]

Keller, KE, Bhattacharya, SK, Borrás, T, Brunner, TM, Chansangpetch, S, Clark, AF, Dismuke, WM, Du, Y, Elliott, MH, Ethier, CR, Faralli, JA, Freddo, TF, Fuchshofer, R, Giovingo, M, Gong, H, Gonzalez, P, Huang, A, Johnstone, MA, Kaufman, PL, Kelley, MJ, Knepper, PA, Kopczynski, CC, Kuchtey, JG, Kuchtey, RW, Kuehn, MH, Lieberman, RL, Lin, SC, Liton, P, Liu, Y, Lütjen-Drecoll, E, Mao, W, Masis-Solano, M, McDonnell, F, McDowell, CM, Overby, DR, Pattabiraman, PP, Raghunathan, VK, Rao, PV, Rhee, DJ, Chowdhury, UR, Russell, P, Samples, JR, Schwartz, D, Stubbs, EB, Tamm, ER, Tan, JC, Toris, CB, Torrejon, KY, Vranka, JA, Wirtz, MK, Yorio, T, Zhang, J, Zode, GS, Fautsch, MP, Peters, DM, Acott, TS & Stamer, WD (2018) Consensus recommendations for trabecular meshwork cell isolation, characterization and culture. *Exp Eye Res,* 171, 164-73.
[http://dx.doi.org/10.1016/j.exer.2018.03.001] [PMID: 29526795]

Pang, IH, Shade, DL, Clark, AF, Steely, HT & DeSantis, L (1994) Preliminary characterization of a transformed cell strain derived from human trabecular meshwork. *Curr Eye Res,* 13, 51-63.
[http://dx.doi.org/10.3109/02713689409042398] [PMID: 8156826]

Polansky, JR, Weinreb, RN, Baxter, JD & Alvarado, J (1979) Human trabecular cells. I. Establishment in tissue culture and growth characteristics. *Invest Ophthalmol Vis Sci,* 18, 1043-9.

[PMID: 383640]

Polansky, JR, Wood, IS, Maglio, MT & Alvarado, JA (1984) Trabecular meshwork cell culture in glaucoma research: evaluation of biological activity and structural properties of human trabecular cells *in vitro*. *Ophthalmology,* 91, 580-95.
[http://dx.doi.org/10.1016/S0161-6420(84)34241-5] [PMID: 6540429]

Rhee, DJ, Tamm, ER & Russell, P (2003) Donor corneoscleral buttons: a new source of trabecular meshwork for research. *Exp Eye Res,* 77, 749-56.
[http://dx.doi.org/10.1016/j.exer.2003.07.008] [PMID: 14609563]

Sharif, NA (2018) iDrugs and iDevices discovery and development- preclinical assays, techniques and animal model studies for ocular hypotensives and neuroprotectants. *J Ocul Pharmacol Ther,* 34, 7-39.
[http://dx.doi.org/10.1089/jop.2017.0125] [PMID: 29323613]

Sharif, NA (2021) Therapeutic drugs and devices for tackling ocular hypertension and glaucoma, and need for neuroprotection and cytoprotective therapies. *Front Pharmacol,* 12, 729249.
[http://dx.doi.org/10.3389/fphar.2021.729249] [PMID: 34603044]

Sharif, NA, Kelly, CR & Crider, JY (2003) Human trabecular meshwork cell responses induced by bimatoprost, travoprost, unoprostone, and other FP prostaglandin receptor agonist analogues. *Invest Ophthalmol Vis Sci,* 44, 715-21.
[http://dx.doi.org/10.1167/iovs.02-0323] [PMID: 12556403]

Sharif, NA, Kelly, CR & McLaughlin, M (2006) Human trabecular meshwork cells express functional serotonin-2A (5HT2A) receptors: role in IOP reduction. *Invest Ophthalmol Vis Sci,* 47, 4001-10.
[http://dx.doi.org/10.1167/iovs.06-0062] [PMID: 16936116]

Stamer, WD, Seftor, REB, Williams, SK, Samaha, HAM & Snyder, RW (1995) Isolation and culture of human trabecular meshwork cells by extracellular matrix digestion. *Curr Eye Res,* 14, 611-7.
[http://dx.doi.org/10.3109/02713689508998409] [PMID: 7587308]

Tamm, ER (2009) The trabecular meshwork outflow pathways: Structural and functional aspects. *Exp Eye Res,* 88, 648-55.
[http://dx.doi.org/10.1016/j.exer.2009.02.007] [PMID: 19239914]

Tripathi, RC & Tripathi, BJ (1982) Human trabecular endothelium, corneal endothelium, keratocytes, and scleral fibroblasts in primary cell culture. A comparative study of growth characteristics, morphology, and phagocytic activity by light and scanning electron microscopy. *Exp Eye Res,* 35, 611-24.
[http://dx.doi.org/10.1016/S0014-4835(82)80074-2] [PMID: 6185354]

Weinreb, RN, Aung, T & Medeiros, FA (2014) The pathophysiology and treatment of glaucoma: a review. *JAMA,* 311, 1901-11.
[http://dx.doi.org/10.1001/jama.2014.3192] [PMID: 24825645]

CHAPTER 9

Protocols for TM Cell Replacement Using Differentiated TM-Like Induced Pluripotent Stem Cells (iPSC)

Mary J. Kelley[1,*] and **Ted S. Acott**[1]

[1] *Department of Ophthalmology, Casey Eye Institute Oregon Health & Science University Portland, Oregon, USA*

Abstract: Induced pluripotent stem cells are differentiated into TM-like iPSCs and transplanted into a cell depletion glaucomatous cell loss model. This restores the capability of this cell loss-perfused human anterior segment model to respond to a 2X pressure challenge with a normal IOP homeostatic response. Glaucomatous anterior segments cannot adequately respond to a 2x pressure challenge. Herein, we present protocols for working with human iPSCs, differentiating iPSCs into TM-like iPSCs, establishing the saponin TM cell depletion perfusion model for cell loss in the anterior segment, testing IOP homeostatic response, transplanting TM-like iPSCs into perfused human anterior segments, and evaluating transplanted cell integration. These protocols should facilitate similar studies on glaucomatous anterior segments and translation of these approaches to treat glaucomatous TM cell loss and their compromised IOP homeostatic response.

Keywords: Glaucoma cell loss, Intraocular pressure homeostasis, Induced pluripotent stem cells (iPSCs), Stem cell differentiation, TM cell replacement.

INTRODUCTION

Some years ago, a putative trabecular meshwork (TM) stem cell population was identified anterior to the filtering TM beneath Schwalbe's line inserted into the peripheral cornea, a region called the "TM insert". (Acott, *et al.*, 1989) Resting human anterior segments exhibited low levels of cell division in this insert region, and treatment with laser trabeculoplasty approximately doubled this division rate within the first 24 hours. Pulse-chase studies showed that approximately 50% of the freshly divided cells then migrated out and repopulated the laser burn sites (Acott *et al.*, 1989).

* **Corresponding author Mary J. Kelley:** Department of Ophthalmology, Casey Eye Institute Oregon Health & Science University Portland, Oregon, USA; E-mail: kelleyma@ohsu.edu

Najam A. Sharif and Sunny E. Ohia (Eds.)

Alvarado *et al.* (1981, 1984) and Grierson and Howe (1987) assessed TM cell density in electron micrographs and found a significant loss of cellularity with age and a much more pronounced TM cell loss in age-matched glaucomatous TMs. Abu-Hassan *et al.* (2015) developed a saponin detergent-based TM cell depletion model for glaucomatous loss in the anterior segment and found that a 30% TM cell depletion knocked out the intraocular pressure (IOP) homeostatic response to a 2x pressure challenge (Acott *et al.*, 2014, 2016, 2021). Raghunathan *et al.* (2018) showed that glaucomatous anterior segments are also unable to mount an IOP homeostatic response to a 2x pressure challenge. When Abu-Hassan *et al.* (2015) added TM cells back to the saponin cell depletion model, the IOP homeostatic response was restored.

Based on the putative insert stem cell population and the glaucomatous cell loss with associated loss of IOP homeostatic responsiveness, Kelley *et al.* (2009) proposed that stem cells could be added to glaucomatous eyes and might restore IOP homeostatic capability. Following up on this hypothesis, a method for differentiating human iPSCs from TM-like iPSCs and then transplanting them into the saponin TM cell depletion human anterior segment model was established (Abu-Hassan, 2015). After transplantation and attachment of these TM-like iPSCs into the saponin TM cell depletion model, the IOP homeostatic response to a 2x pressure challenge was restored (Abu-Hassan, 2015). Variations of these studies by others have been conducted by using different models and efficacy assessments (Du *et al.*, 2012, 2013; Zhu *et al.*, 2016, 2017).

Experimental Protocols

Preparation of iPSC Embryoid Bodies (EBs)

a. Human iPS cells may be obtained from WiCell Laboratories or from other sources online. Previously, we obtained fibroblasts derived from dermal foreskin (catalog designation: *DF6-9-9T.B,* WiCell Laboratories).
b. The human iPS cells were grown and maintained as per the company's instructions.
c. For control cells, normal adult human dermal fibroblasts were procured from the American Type Culture Collection (ATCC) and cultured according to the supplier's instructions. We also isolated and grew standard TM cultures and used donated HUVEC cells (a gift from Dr. Nabil Alkayed, Oregon Health & Science University, Portland, Oregon) and embryoid bodies (EBs) we generated from iPSCs. Other control cell cultured lines may be necessary for the investigator's experiments.

Generation of Embryoid Bodies:

a) *First, prepare extracellular matrix (ECM) derived from TM cultures*:

1. Grow human TM primary cultures in 6-well plates for 7 days using a standard TM growth medium to produce an extensive ECM.
2. Remove the TM cells by treating the cultures with 0.1% saponin for 1 hour, followed by washing extensively with PBS.
3. The ECM is then incubated for several days in PBS prior to use. No cells should be visible after this time, but it is best to check the surface under a microscope to make sure all the TM cells have been removed.
4. The ECM plates may be wrapped tightly with parafilm and stored for several months frozen at -20 degrees C.

b) *Second, prepare the conditioned medium (CM):*

1. Prepare TM cell cultures in T-75 flasks using serum-free TM medium (DMEM high/low glucose medium-1:1, 1% antibiotic/anti-mycotic).
2. When the incubated TM cell cultures (37 degrees C and 5% CO_2) are confluent or nearly so, collect the conditioned medium (CM) after 48 hours. Centrifuge the CM at 15,000 xg for 15 minutes.
3. Use the TM cell-conditioned medium as a part of DiffMedium in the differentiation of the EBs below.
4. The CM may be stored in sterile tubes at -20 degrees C for several months until ready for use.

c) *To generate the embryoid bodies (EBs)* to be differentiated to TM-like iPSCs on a large scale, detach medium-sized undifferentiated iPS cell colonies from 6-well plates by treating them with Accutase (Innovative Cell Technologies) as suggested by the manufacturer.

1. This procedure will generate uniform small-size EBs.
2. Transfer the detached cells to AggreWell plates (Stem Cell Technologies) and add AggreWell medium (Stem Cell Technologies) for 24 hours.
3. Transfer the EBs from the AggreWell plates to 6-well plates and initiate differentiation (Fig. **1**).

Differentiation of EBs

a) Differentiation is initiated by culturing the EBs on TM-cell derived ECM in DiffMedium, concocted by a mixture of:

1. standard TM cell growth medium (25%):

a.) medium-glucose Dulbecco's Modified Essential Medium-[DMEM; Gibco], a 1:1 mix of high and low glucose media.

b.) 10% Fetal Bovine Serum [Hyclone/Thermo Scientific]

c.) 1% Antibiotic/Anti-mycotic [100X; Life Technologies]

1. AggreWell medium (50%) [Stem Cell Technologies]

3) TM cell conditioned medium (CM) (25%)
   a. The EBs are grown on the TM cell-derived ECM with the DiffMedium. The DiffMedium should be changed every other day, and the EBs should be maintained in culture for 30 days.
   b. After 30 days, the differentiated cells are cultured in 100% TM cell growth medium and passaged 1:3 with trypsin, as performed with TM cells for up to 7 passages.

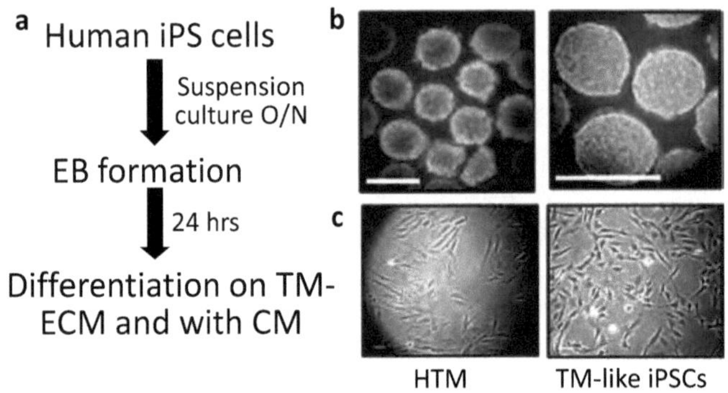

Fig. (1). Growth of EBs to differentiated TM-like iPSCs, comparison with the beginning culture of HTM in lower panels.

Validation of Differentiation:

a. To validate the differentiation of EBs into TM-like iPSCs, use Western blotting, immunohistochemistry, and quantitative RT-PCR. An example is shown below in Fig. (**2**). We compared mature normal human TM cells, HTM-like iPSCs, and iPSCs using 4 stem cell markers (Nanog, OCT ¾, SOX2, and KLF4) with these 3 cell types to distinguish stem characteristics. Other stem cell markers may be possible to use. We also used mature HTM cell markers CH3L1, α-3 integrin, Wnt1, and AQP1 to distinguish mature TM cell characteristics.
b. Use DAPI, a blue nuclear stain, to make sure that the cells are actually present. Note that the iPSCs are normally very small in comparison to the HTM cells.
c. Loading controls:
   1. α-tubulin works well for Western immunoblots.
   2. 18S ribosomal subunit works well for mRNA gels.
      d) *Western immunoblotting*:
         1. Grow human TM cells, iPSCs, and TM-like iPSCs on 6-well plates until confluent.
         2. Collect cell lysates using a RIPA buffer mixed with a protease inhibitor cocktail (Sigma-Aldrich).
         3. Measure protein concentration using a BCA kit from Pierce Biotechnology (Thermo Scientific) or other protein assay.

4. Add 0.1 M dithiothreitol to the lysates and boil the samples for 15 minutes.
5. Add equal amounts of protein (20 μg) per lane in SDS-PAGE gels.
6. Run gels at 120 volts for 90 minutes.
7. Wet transfer gels at 4 degrees C to polyvinylidene fluoride (PVDF) membranes.
8. Use 5% non-fat dry milk as a blocking buffer.
9. Primary antibodies at 1:1000 dilution in PBS with 0.05% Tween generally work well for the antibodies we used.
10. Secondary antibodies of rabbit and mouse work well with the biomarkers we used. (Rockland Immunochemicals)
11. Dilute the secondary antibodies in PBS and incubate for 1 hr at room temperature.

e) *Immunohistochemistry:*

1. Human TM, iPSCs, and TM-like cells may be grown on Lab-Tec II CC2-coated glass chamber slides (Nagle Nunc, Inc.) until 60-80% confluent.
2. The cells may then be fixed with 4% paraformaldehyde and permeabilized with 0.3% Triton X100 in PBS.
3. Slides may be blocked in 5% normal goat serum in PBS.
4. Primary antibodies for the cell markers can be added at a 1:200 dilution.
5. Alexa Fluor 488-and 595-conjugated secondary antibodies work well at a 1:500 dilution.
    a. *Quantitative RT-PCR:*
        1. Human TM, iPSCs, and TM-like iPSCs may be grown on 6-well plates until confluent.

2) The cells are then harvested, and total RNA is extracted with Trizol (Life Technologies) using the manufacturer's suggestions.

3) Reverse transcription is then performed using SuperScript III First-Strand Synthesis System (Invitrogen) according to the manufacturer's instructions.

4) Primers for Wnt1, CHI3L1, α3-integrin, AQP1, KLF4, NANOG, SOX2, and OCT 3/4 can be designed for use with the Integrated DNA Technologies website (www.idtdna.com).

5) Primer sequences are available there.

6) Ribosomal RNA (18S) may be used as a housekeeping gene.

7) The DNA Engine quantitative RT-PCR machine (Bio-Rad) or other qRT-PCR machine and RT^2 SYBR Green qPCR master mixes (Qiagen) may be used for real-time PCR by following the manufacturer's instructions.

8) To quantify the relative mRNA levels standardized to the measured iPS cell counts, the threshold cycle (C_t) can be determined for each sample and used for this purpose.

9) To verify size, the samples may then be run on agarose gels.

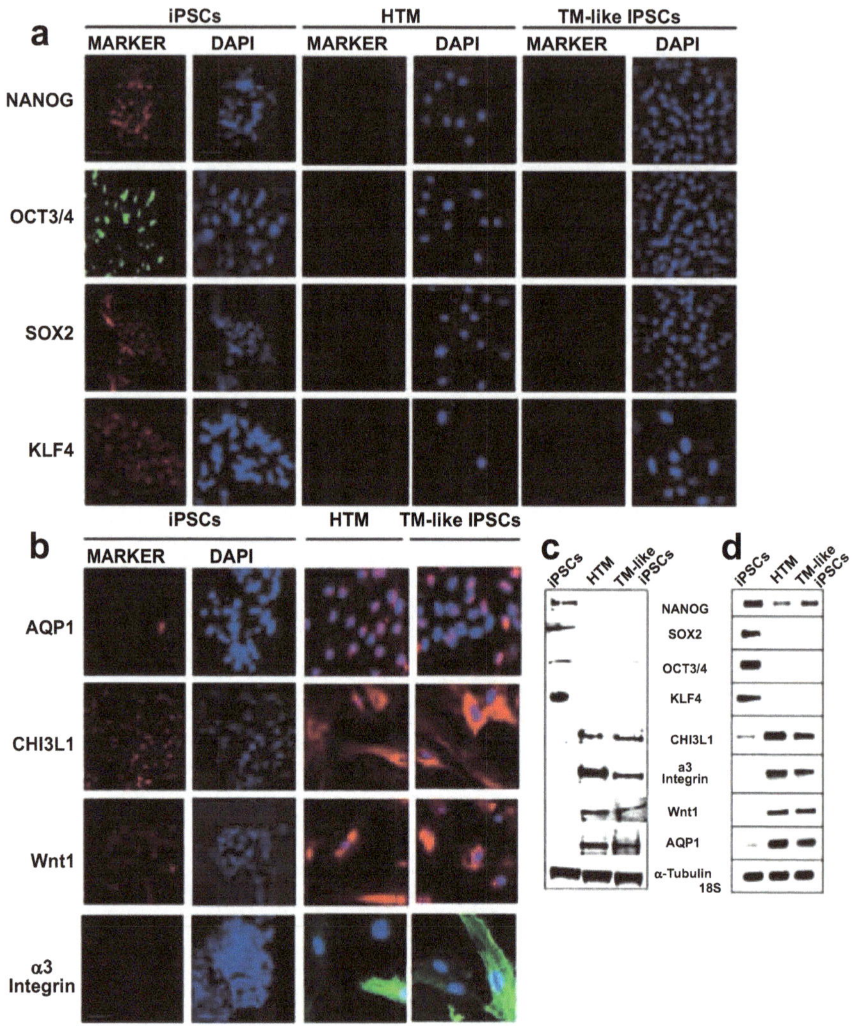

Fig. (2). Biomarker expression comparison between iPSCs, mature human TM cells (HTM), and differentiated TM-like iPSCs. A) *Immunohistochemical comparison* of levels of four stem cell markers, NANOG, OCT ¾, SOX2, and KLF4, by these three cell types. Cell nuclei are stained with DAPI (blue). All panels are exactly the same size with a scale bar=100 μm. B) TM cell markers as expressed by iPSCs, HTM, and TM-like iPSCs. DAPI nuclear stain is blue; all panels are the exact same size, and scales are identical with the white scale bars=100 μm. C) *Western immunoblot* showing levels of these two groups of proteins, and D) gels from *quantitative RT-PCR analysis* showing levels of mRNA expression for these genes. Loading controls are α-tubulin for the Western immunoblots and the 18S ribosomal subunit for mRNA gels.

Preparation for the Development of the Saponin Glaucomatous Cell Loss Anterior Segment Perfusion Model:

a) Prepare human anterior segments by bisecting whole globes with a single-edge razor blade or a sharp scalpel under sterile conditions.
b) Discard the posterior segment and all of the structures within the anterior segment except for the TM, Schlemm's Canal, cornea, and a thin rim of sclera.
c) The scleral rim will be used to clamp the anterior segment into place in the flow cell; do not cut too closely so that it cannot clamp the anterior segment. This will be determined by the dimensions of the engineered flow cell and the anterior segment and refined by experience.
d) The anterior segment should then be placed in a 6-well plate with serum-free standard TM medium for 5-7 days to recover from post-mortem effects prior to using it for transplantation.
e) In the anterior segment perfusion system described herein, constant pressure is used. After the recovery from post-mortem effects, human anterior segments are perfused at 1x pressure (8.8 mm Hg) for 48 hours. This is to stabilize a baseline flow with gravimetric flow analysis (i.e., weigh the reservoir bottle at several intervals per day to measure the fluid loss). The 1x flow for baseline should be approximately 2.5-3 μl/min.
f) Prepare the saponin detergent solution of 0.01% saponin in a serum-free TM growth medium (medium-glucose DMEM with 1% Antibiotic/Anti-mycotic) (Fig. **3**).

Preparation for Transplantation of Differentiated TM-Like iPSC into Saponin Model and Labeling of Cells:

a. Transplantation of all cell types, experimental and controls, is conducted in the same fashion.
b. Harvest the cells to be transplanted with trypsin and rinse thoroughly with PBS.
c. Label the cells to be transplanted with 3 μl of Q-Dot nanoparticles (Qtracker 655 Cell Labeling Kit; Life Technologies) so that they can be distinguished from the endogenous cells.
d. Label controls as well, as the transplantation studies may be conducted separately for each cell type.
e. For the labeling procedure, incubate the nanoparticles with the cells to be transplanted for 1 hr at 37 degrees C.
f. Wash the cells thoroughly with PBS to eliminate excess nanoparticles not taken up by the cells.
g. Verify nanoparticle uptake and count cell numbers by fluorescence microscopy.

a. The flow chamber in use should be in an incubator at 37 degrees C and 5% CO_2 and kept under sterile conditions.
b. Replace the perfusion medium by flowing in the saponin 0.01% solution for 7 minutes for human anterior segments. This will remove approximately 30% of the TM cells.
c. Rinse out the saponin solution and replace it with the serum-free TM growth medium again. Restart the flow at 1x pressure (8.8 mg Hg) and re-establish the baseline for 24 hours.

Testing for Loss of IOP Homeostatic Response to 2x Sustained Pressure Challenge

a. Increase perfusion pressure to 2x (17.6 mm Hg) for both saponin-treated and control anterior segments for 48 hours.
b. After this time, stop the flow and invert the flow chamber so that the cornea is no longer facing up.
c. Inject 300,000 labeled cells into the flow line whether you are using TM-iPSCs or control cells in this perfusion (such as fibroblasts, HUVEC cells, EBs, no cells, or others) and perfuse them in at 0.5 mm Hg for 2 hours.
d. After 2 hours, stop the flow and allow the cells to attach overnight. Leave the flow chamber inverted during this time.
e. Subsequent to the overnight attachment of the transplanted cells, turn the flow chamber right-side up and resume the flow at 1x pressure for 24 hours.
f. Now that the labeled cells are attached to the TM, test for recovery of the IOP homeostatic response by increasing the pressure to 2x.
g. Assess the IOP homeostatic capability by continuing the 2x perfusion pressure over several days prior to terminating the experiment.
h. Make a graph of normalized flow vs. time. If the normalized flow does not increase significantly over time, but appears more flattened, the anterior segment did not have a restored IOP homeostatic response. (**Saponin treatment**)This eye mimics a glaucomatous eye, which cannot restore IOP homeostasis (Fig. **4**).
i. If the normalized flow continues an upward trend over time, the anterior segment has restored the IOP homeostatic response. (**Normal**) This anterior segment is functioning as a normal anterior segment with a positive IOP homeostatic response (Fig. **4**).
j. Restoration of the IOP homeostatic response is the only known way to properly assess the functioning of an anterior segment.
k. Transplantation of TM-like iPSCs in the TM cell depletion model for cell loss in an anterior segment restores the IOP homeostatic response to a 2x pressure challenge after saponin treatment (Fig. **5**).

1. Statistical significance may be assessed by One-Way ANOVA with Dunnett's Multiple Testing Correction, unpaired t-tests, or other means to determine the statistical significance of the experiment.

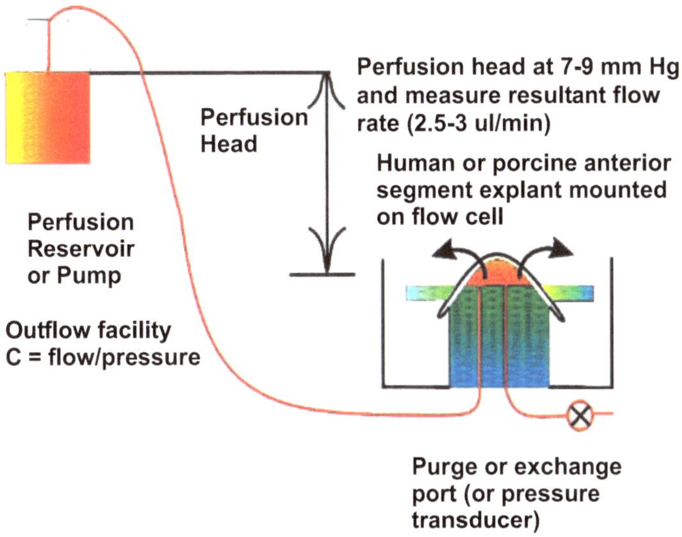

Fig. (3). Anterior segment perfusion system. A perfusion reservoir with serum-free growth medium with a perfusion head at approximately 8.8 mm Hg is placed in an incubator above the engineered plastic flow cell. The reservoir and the flow cell are connected by tubing such that media can flow through the flow cell to the TM and exit *via* Schlemm's Canal. The simplified outflow facility is C=flow/pressure (µl/min/mmHg). The anterior segment is mounted cornea side up on the top of the flow cell and clamped in place by a clamping ring on the rim of the sclera. For the saponin TM-depleted model for cell loss, saponin solution temporarily replaces the media, thereby killing TM cells and resulting in the lack of a proper IOP homeostatic response to a 2x pressure challenge. The IOP homeostatic response may be restored by attachment and integration of either TM cells or TM-like iPSCs.

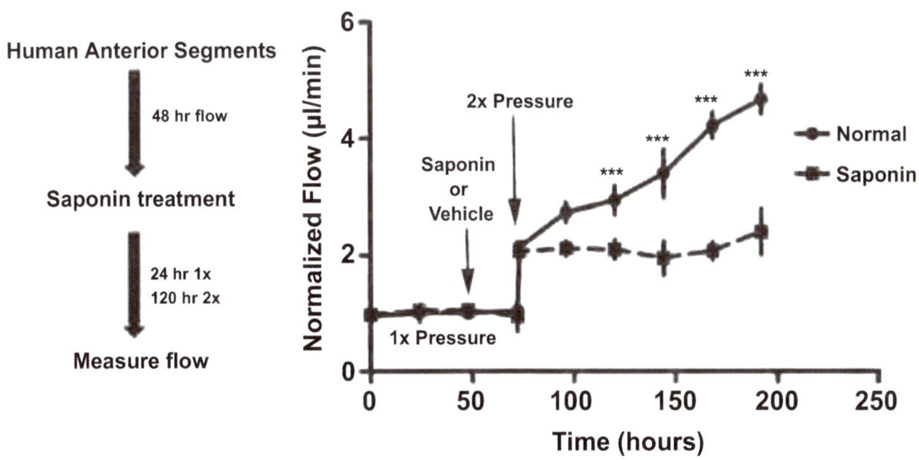

Fig. (4). Saponin impairs the normal IOP homeostatic response to a 2x pressure challenge.

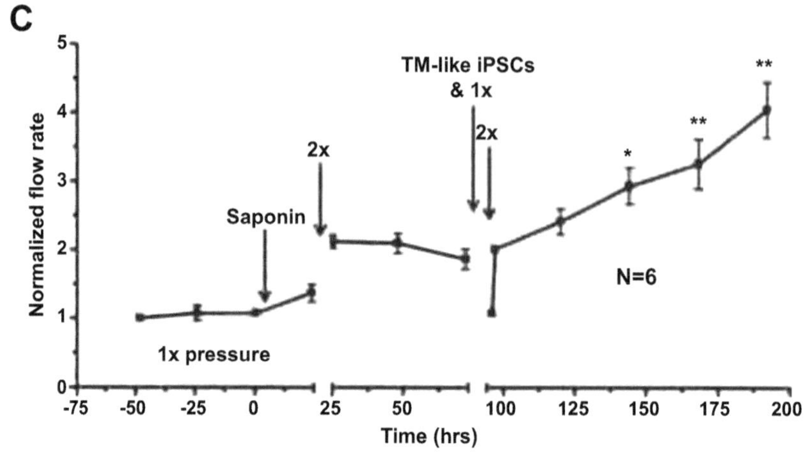

Fig. (5). Transplantation of TM-like iPSCs in the TM depletion model for cell loss restores the IOP homeostatic response previously lost by saponin treatment, killing TM cells.

Note the flow rate continues to rise over time as the resistance to flow decreases in response to a 2x pressure challenge.

Assessing the Integration of Transplanted TM-Like iPSCs

a. The 300,000 QDot-labeled differentiated TM-like iPSCs should now be attached and integrated into the TM. Frontal sections of the TM will now show that the transplanted TM-like iPSCs are found even at the deepest level of TM, the juxtacanalicular (JCT) layer. The QDots are fluorescent and come in various colors, so these should be visible with a fluorescent microscope.
b. CD44 labels the cell membranes of the cell surfaces, and QDot-containing transplanted cells may be carefully scanned through z-stacks on confocal microscopy to define the CD44-QDot labeled cell surfaces. Lines may be drawn around them to identify the transplanted cells.

CONCLUSION

Generation of differentiated TM-like iPSCs from iPSCs may be achieved using TM-derived ECM and conditioned medium, along with specialized medium. The TM cell depletion anterior segment perfusion model for TM cell loss and measuring for a positive IOP homeostatic response is the most definitive method to determine TM functionality. The IOP homeostatic response to the 2x pressure challenge is lost after saponin treatment, as approximately 30% of the TM cells are killed. However, it is regained after successful transplantation and integration into the TM with the addition of either TM cells or TM-like iPSCs.

ACKNOWLEDGEMENTS

NEI grants EY031071 (MJK), EY021800 (MJK), EY008274 (TSA), EY003279 (TSA), EY025721 (TSA), EY030238 (TSA), EY010572 (TSA); Lewis Rudin Glaucoma Prize (MJK), Glaucoma Research Foundation Shaffer Award (MJK), and an unrestricted grant from Research to Prevent Blindness Foundation to the Casey Eye Institute, Oregon Health & Science University.

REFERENCES

Abu-Hassan, DW, Li, X, Ryan, EI, Acott, TS & Kelley, MJ (2015) Induced pluripotent stem cells restore function in a human cell loss model of open-angle glaucoma. *Stem Cells,* 33, 751-61.
[http://dx.doi.org/10.1002/stem.1885] [PMID: 25377070]

Samples, JR, Bradley, JMB, Bacon, DR, Bylsma, SS, Van Buskirk, EM & Acott, TS (1989) Trabecular repopulation by anterior trabecular meshwork cells after laser trabeculoplasty. *Am J Ophthalmol,* 107, 1-6.
[http://dx.doi.org/10.1016/0002-9394(89)90805-2] [PMID: 2912110]

Acott, TS, Kelley, MJ, Keller, KE, Vranka, JA, Abu-Hassan, DW, Li, X, Aga, M & Bradley, JM (2014) Intraocular pressure homeostasis: maintaining balance in a high-pressure environment. *J Ocul Pharmacol Ther,* 30, 94-101.
[http://dx.doi.org/10.1089/jop.2013.0185] [PMID: 24401029]

Acott, TS, Kelley, MJ & Keller, KE (2016) IOP Homeostasis - Why most people do not ever develop glaucoma. In: Knepper, P.A., Samples, J.R., (Eds.), *Glaucoma Research and Clinical Advances 2016-2018* Kugler Publications, Amsterdam, The Netherlands 87-98.

Acott, TS, Vranka, JA, Keller, KE, Raghunathan, V & Kelley, MJ (2021) Normal and glaucomatous outflow regulation. *Prog Retin Eye Res,* 82, 100897.
[http://dx.doi.org/10.1016/j.preteyeres.2020.100897] [PMID: 32795516]

Alvarado, J, Murphy, C, Polansky, J & Juster, R (1981) Age-related changes in trabecular meshwork cellularity. *Invest Ophthalmol Vis Sci,* 21, 714-27.
[PMID: 7298275]

Alvarado, J, Murphy, C & Juster, R (1984) Trabecular meshwork cellularity in primary open-angle glaucoma and nonglaucomatous normals. *Ophthalmology,* 91, 564-79.
[http://dx.doi.org/10.1016/S0161-6420(84)34248-8] [PMID: 6462622]

Du, Y, Roh, DS, Mann, MM, Funderburgh, ML, Funderburgh, JL & Schuman, JS (2012) Multipotent stem cells from trabecular meshwork become phagocytic TM cells. *Invest Ophthalmol Vis Sci,* 53, 1566-75.
[http://dx.doi.org/10.1167/iovs.11-9134] [PMID: 22297497]

Du, Y, Yun, H, Yang, E & Schuman, JS (2013) Stem cells from trabecular meshwork home to TM tissue *in vivo. Invest Ophthalmol Vis Sci,* 54, 1450-9.
[http://dx.doi.org/10.1167/iovs.12-11056] [PMID: 23341019]

Grierson, I & Howes, RC (1987) Age-related depletion of the cell population in the human trabecular meshwork. *Eye (Lond),* 1, 204-10.
[http://dx.doi.org/10.1038/eye.1987.38] [PMID: 3653434]

Kelley, MJ, Rose, AY, Keller, KE, Hessle, H, Samples, JR & Acott, TS (2009) Stem cells in the trabecular meshwork: Present and future promises. *Exp Eye Res,* 88, 747-51.
[http://dx.doi.org/10.1016/j.exer.2008.10.024] [PMID: 19061887]

Raghunathan, VK, Benoit, J, Kasetti, R, Zode, G, Salemi, M, Phinney, BS, Keller, KE, Staverosky, JA, Murphy, CJ, Acott, T & Vranka, J (2018) Glaucomatous cell derived matrices differentially modulate non-glaucomatous trabecular meshwork cellular behavior. *Acta Biomater,* 71, 444-59.
[http://dx.doi.org/10.1016/j.actbio.2018.02.037] [PMID: 29524673]

Zhu, W, Gramlich, OW, Laboissonniere, L, Jain, A, Sheffield, VC, Trimarchi, JM, Tucker, BA & Kuehn, MH (2016) Transplantation of iPSC-derived TM cells rescues glaucoma phenotypes *in vivo*. *Proc Natl Acad Sci USA,* 113, E3492-500.
[http://dx.doi.org/10.1073/pnas.1604153113] [PMID: 27274060]

Zhu, W, Jain, A, Gramlich, OW, Tucker, BA, Sheffield, VC & Kuehn, MH (2017) Restoration of Aqueous Humor Outflow Following Transplantation of iPSC-Derived Trabecular Meshwork Cells in a Transgenic Mouse Model of Glaucoma. *Invest Ophthalmol Vis Sci,* 58, 2054-62.
[http://dx.doi.org/10.1167/iovs.16-20672] [PMID: 28384726]

CHAPTER 10

Protocols to Isolate and Characterize Ciliary Muscle Cells and Schlemm's Canal Cells and Detect Matrix Metalloproteases

Shahid Husain[1,*]

[1] *Department of Ophthalmology, Storm Eye Institute, Medical University of South Carolina, 167 Ashley Ave, Charleston, SC-29425, USA*

Abstract: Ocular hypertension and the ensuing glaucomatous optic neuropathy occur when the aqueous humor drainage system within the anterior chamber of the eye, trabecular meshwork (TM), and its associated Schlemm's canal (SC) system become clogged due to the abnormally deposited excess extracellular matrix components. A similar series of events plague the ciliary muscle (CM) bundles in the uveoscleral pathway for AQH drainage. In order to study pathological events and endogenous chemicals associated with the latter tissues, isolated cells of TM, SC, and CM have proven useful. This chapter provides a brief and simple description of protocols to 1) isolate and characterize ciliary smooth muscle cells, 2) isolate and characterize Schlemm's canal cells, and 3) measure enzyme activities and expression pattern of matrix metalloproteases (MMPs) secreted from the isolated ocular cells using zymography and Western blotting. These studies are important for the characterization of the biochemical pharmacology of the drugs that activate specific receptors and enzymes that mediate the aqueous humor outflow from the anterior chamber of the eye to lower the IOP.

Keywords: Ciliary muscle cells, Glaucoma, Intraocular pressure, MMPs, Zymography.

INTRODUCTION

Ocular hypertension (OHT) is a major risk factor associated with open-angle and closed-angle glaucoma. OHT or elevated intraocular pressure (IOP) develops when excess aqueous humor (AQH) accumulates in the anterior chamber of the eye due to the partial occlusion of the trabecular meshwork (TM) and the associated Schlemm's canal (SC) and the AQH drainage pathway between ciliary muscle (CM) bundles. In order to better understand the pathological factors and

* **Corresponding author Shahid Husain:** Department of Ophthalmology, Storm Eye Institute, Medical University of South Carolina, 167 Ashley Ave, Charleston, SC-29425, USA; Tel: +843-792-2792; Fax: +843-792-1155; E-mail: husain@musc.edu

Najam A. Sharif and Sunny E. Ohia (Eds.)

events involved in the aforementioned occlusive processes, studies conducted on isolated TM, SC, and CM cells are necessary. Furthermore, the potential mechanisms of action of potential IOP-lowering agents can be determined using such cell isolates. TM cell isolation is described in Chapter 8 of this book; therefore, the current chapter will focus on the other cell types.

Isolation and Characterization of Ciliary Smooth Muscle Cells

Ciliary smooth muscle cell cultures were established from post-mortem human eyes (donors age range, 45–89 years), and human tissue in this study conformed to the tenets of the Declaration of Helsinki. The human eyeballs should be obtained within 24-72 hours after death and kept moist in ice. The following procedures are recommended for the isolation of human (or animal) ciliary smooth muscle (SM) cells.

- Upon arrival of human eyes in the laboratory, ciliary muscles should be immediately dissected with the aid of a dissecting microscope under sterile conditions. Briefly, the eyes must be equatorially bisected and the posterior half should be removed. The anterior half of the eye can then be placed in a sterile Petri dish. The zonules can be cut and the lens removed.
- To remove the ciliary muscle, carefully insert one branch of fine forceps in the supraciliary or suprachoroidal space of the specimen and gently pull the ciliary muscle tissue away from the underlying sclera. This also allows detachment from the scleral spur. The ciliary muscle can be recognized as a broad, pale, and circular band, which should then be cleaned and cut into small pieces (1 to 2 mm) with a fine pair of scissors under the dissecting microscope.
- In order to isolate the ciliary SM cells, place the cut ciliary muscle pieces in DMEM-199 culture medium containing 2 mg/mL collagenase type IA, 10% FBS, and 50 μg/mL gentamicin in a sterile 25-50 ml plastic tube and incubate for 1 to 2 hours at 37°C with occasional gentle mixing/shaking. The major parts of the explants should be dispersible into single cells or groups of cells after this time.
- Centrifuge the contents of the tube at 200*g* for 10 minutes and discard the supernatant. Next, resuspend the pelleted cells in fresh DMEM-199 medium supplemented with 10% FBS, 100 U/mL penicillin, 100 μg/mL streptomycin, and 0.25 μg/mL amphotericin B to help cells stabilize and the future cell cultures to be free of any potential contamination.
- A suspension of the cells from above should be incubated in 100 mm tissue culture Petri dishes for 1 hour at 37°C in a 5% CO_2 humidified incubator to allow the contaminating fibroblasts to attach to the bottom of the dish.
- After this time, the floating non-adherent cells (ciliary SM cells) can now be transferred to another Petri dish and incubated at 37°C in a 5% CO_2 humidified

incubator to allow them to attach and proliferate. As mentioned above, the DMEM-199 medium should contain 1% FBS, 100 U/mL penicillin, 100 µg/mL streptomycin, and 0.25 µg/mL amphotericin B.

- Replace the culture medium after 3 days and check the morphology of the cells under the phase contrast microscope to ensure cells look healthy and uniform as much as possible (see Husain *et al.*, 2002; Fig. **1**).
- When the ciliary SM cells are 80-90% confluent (within 3-5 days), these cells should then be passaged using 0.05% trypsin and 0.02% EDTA to detach the cells; the medium should be diluted with fresh medium to stop trypsin activity and centrifuged in appropriate tubes. The supernatant is aspirated, the cells are washed and spun down, the pellet is resuspended in a fresh growth medium, and the cells are replated using a split ratio of 1:4 (Husain *et al.*, 2002).

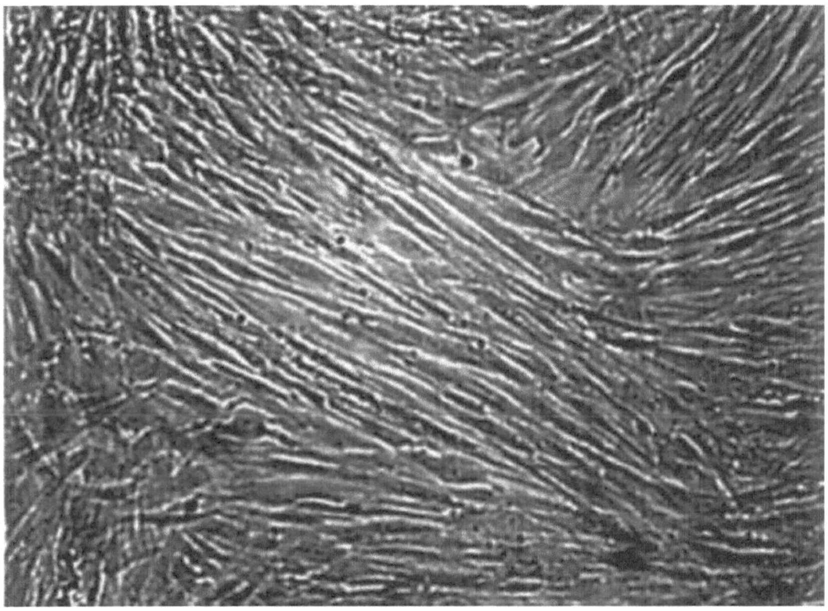

Fig. (1). Phase contrast image of normal human ciliary muscle (HCM) cells. HCM cells have typical hill-and-valley arrangement of growth as described and shown earlier. (Husain, Kaddour-Djebbar *et al.* 2002).

Characterization of Ciliary Smooth Muscle Cells by Immunocytochemistry

- In order to confirm that the isolated and cultured human ciliary SM cells are not contaminated with fibroblasts, characterize the cells using specific antibodies as described by Husain *et al.*, (2002).
- Briefly, culture the cells to 70-80% confluency on sterile glass microscope slides with individual chambers and carefully fix them with ice-cold methanol for 15 minutes. After this time, carefully and gently rinse with phosphate-buffered saline (PBS) buffer 3 times with a 5-minute interval between each wash.

- Now, incubate them with primary anti-α-actin (at a dilution of 1:50), anti-SM myosin (at a dilution of 1:50), or anti-desmin (at a dilution of 1:20) antibodies. Primary antibodies are to be diluted in PBS with 1% goat serum. The cells should be incubated with primary antibodies for 2 hours at 24°C or overnight at 4°C.
- After the above incubation step, carefully and gently wash the cells 3 times with PBS with a 5-minute interval between each wash step.
- Now, incubate the cells with fluorescein-conjugated secondary antibodies (at a dilution of 1:100) for 60 minutes at 24°C, after which they should be gently rinsed with PBS 3-5 times with an interval of 5 minutes between each wash.
- Now, carefully remove the chambers from the slides without touching or disturbing the cells.
- Using slide coverslip mounting material, carefully mount the cells for microscopic examination using a fluorescence microscope (*e.g.*, Axiophot; Carl Zeiss, Oberkochen, Germany). Run negative controls in parallel using goat serum instead of the primary antibodies.

The specific antibody staining should yield positive staining with anti-α-actin antibodies, showing typical straight, uninterrupted, cable-like fibers that align with the length of each cell, as shown in Fig. (**2**) (Husain *et al.*, 20002). Additional identification of ciliary SM cells can be determined with positive staining for the intermediate filament protein desmin and SM-myosin (heavy chain). Overall, this protocol provides a simple and reproducible procedure by which pure ciliary smooth muscle cells can be isolated at a large scale in a short period of time. The following Table **1** describes the use of ciliary muscle cells for biological assays in ocular research.

Table 1. Use of human ciliary smooth muscle cells for biological assays in ocular research.

Cells	Biological Assays
Human Ciliary Smooth Muscle Cells	Enzyme expression and activities of matrix metalloproteinases
Human Ciliary Smooth Muscle Cells	Enzyme activities of histone acetylases and deacetylases
Human Ciliary Smooth Muscle Cells	Measuring secretion of cytokines (e,g. interleukins, tumor necrosis factor-α, interferon-γ, and others)
Human Ciliary Smooth Muscle Cells	Measuring signaling pathways mediators such as second messenger cAMP, inositol phosphates, cGMP, intracellular Ca^{2+}, natriuretic peptides, and transcriptional factors.

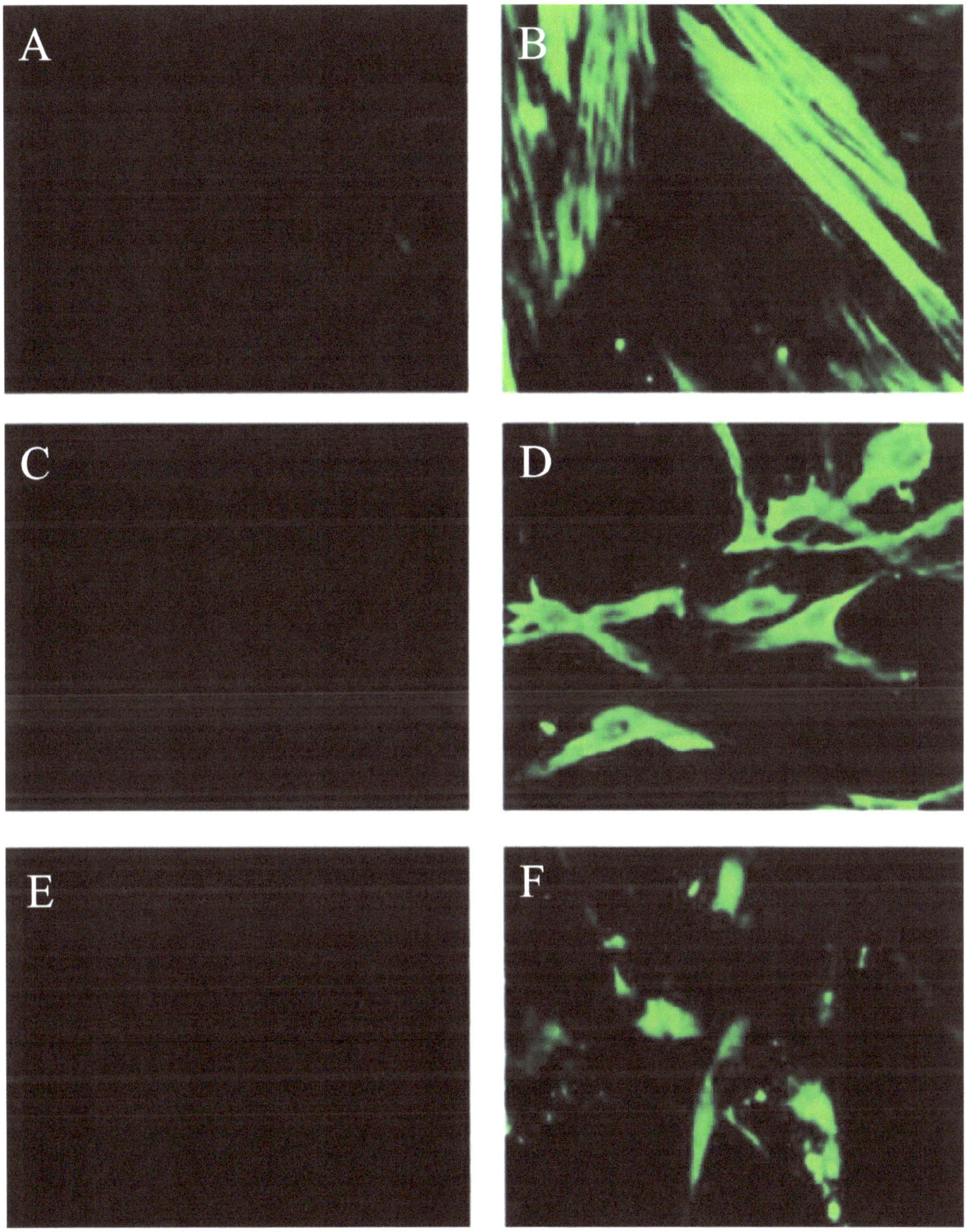

Fig. (2). Immunostaining of α-smooth muscle actin (**A**), Smooth muscle (**SM**)-myosin (**B**), and Desmin (**C**) using selective antibodies for each marker. The negative control (**A, C, E**) showed no positive immunostaining. Phase contrast image of normal human ciliary muscle (HCM) cells as shown earlier. (Husain, Kaddour-Djebbar *et al.* 2002).

Isolation and Characterization of Schlemm's Canal Cells

Isolation, establishment, and characterization of human Schlemm's canal (SC) cells can be accomplished using post-mortem normal human eyes (without any ocular history; donors age range, 45–89 years) obtained from regional eye banks, preferably within 24 hrs of death. Below are some methods and conditions to permit this task using procedures described by Stamer *et al.* (1998). Perform as many of the procedures described below in a sterile environment to reduce the risk of infection of the tissue cultures.

- Coat several pieces of sterile nylon monofilament suture of 1-2 cm in length with sterile 2% gelatin and dry in a vented laminar flow hood (sterile environment) if possible.
- Obtain the eyeballs from the eye bank and keep them in ice until ready to perform the dissection. In a laminar flow hood, scrape the conjunctival tissues from the limbus using a sharp scalpel blade and place the eyeball for 5-15 minutes in 2.0% povidone-iodine (Betadine) (Escalon Ophthalmic, Skillman, NJ) prepared using phosphate-buffered saline (PBS).
- After this time, rinse the eyeballs with sterile (if possible) ice-cold PBS at least 3 times to remove betadine. Then, remove the cornea and about 4mm of the scleral rim from the eyeball and excise the tissue into small radial symmetrical wedge-shaped pieces.
- Under a dissecting microscope, insert a piece of the gelatin-coated suture into the lumen of SC through the visible opening on the cut edge of the tissue and advance it into the canal as shown in the publication by Stamer *et al.* (1998).
- In a laminar flow hood, place the cannulated tissue wedges in cell culture medium (Dulbecco's modified Eagle's medium [DMEM] containing 10% fetal bovine serum, 100 units/ml penicillin G sodium, and 100 µg/ml streptomycin sulfate) in sterile 6-12-well culture plates and maintain at 37°C in an incubator with humidified air containing 5% CO_2 for 3 weeks.
- In a laminar flow hood, view the cannulated tissue wedges under a dissecting microscope and cut small pieces using a sterile scalpel blade. Make a curvilinear incision using a 1.5-mm 15-degree beaver blade 1 mm posterior and parallel to Schwalbe's line, which projects towards the posterior side of the suture material within the SC. Such a cut typically produces a flap of TM that can be gently retracted with a pair of fine-toothed forceps in order to expose the suture. At this point, the suture thread should be carefully removed with a second pair of sterile fine-toothed forceps.
- One by one, carefully and slowly remove the suture threads from each of the tissue wedges, gently rinse in sterile PBS, and place one or two suture threads covered in SC cells in one gelatin-coated 6-well plate or into a 60 mm Petri dish containing the cell culture medium.

- Alternatively, remove SC cells from the suture threads by exposing them to a 0.2-0.25% % trypsin-EDTA solution in a Petri dish for over 5 minutes. After this digestion procedure, a complete culture medium should be added to quench trypsin and stop its actions, and the incubation should be continued at 37°C in an incubator containing humidified air containing 5% CO_2.
- Monitor these cultures over time for cell morphology and potential contamination. Allow cultures to attain 80-90% confluency before trypsinization and passaging at a 1:4 ratio.

Characterization of Schlemm's Canal Cells by Immunocytochemistry

Use immunohistochemical methods to confirm the identity of SC cells that have endothelial cell-like features and bear biomarkers such as von Willebrand factor-receptor complex (vWF), CD44, CD55, and vascular endothelial cadherin.

- Grow cells on chamber slides with up to 80% confluency. Rinse them with PBS and fix them with 4% paraformaldehyde over 15 minutes at room temperature.
- Gently rinse the cell chambers/cells 3 times with PBS, followed by treatment with 0.2% Triton X-100 detergent for 3 minutes to permeabilize them, and then rinse 3 times with PBS at 5-minute intervals.
- Block the cells with 5% BSA for 1 hour at 24°C, and then wash them with PBS 3 times with 5-minute intervals.
- Incubate cells with primary antibodies to vWF complex, anti-CD44, anti-CD55, or anti-vascular endothelial cadherin at a 1:100 dilution in 0.2% BSA for 3 hours at 24°C or overnight at 4°C and then wash with PBS 3 times with 5-minute intervals. Incubate additional cells with 0.2% BSA instead of the primary antibody to serve as negative controls.
- Incubate cells with appropriate AlexaFlour 488 conjugated secondary antibody at a 1:400 dilution at 24°C for 1 hour. The chambers are removed from the glass chamber slides carefully without touching the cells.
- Finally, mount the cells using a gel mounting medium and with coverslips. View the immunostaining using a fluorescence microscope (*e.g.*, Axiophot; Carl Zeiss, Oberkochen, Germany).

Matrix Metalloproteinases in Ocular Cells/ Tissues

Tissues represent dynamic environments in which resident cells interact reciprocally with each other and the adjoining matrix. Coordinated enzymatic activity of matrix metalloproteinases (MMPs) controls the tissue architecture in all organs. At present, >28 MMPs have been found in vertebrates, of which 24 genes have been identified in human subjects (Murphy and Nagase 2008; Bassiouni *et al.*, 2021). MMPs include gelatinases, collagenases, stromelysins, membrane-bound forms (MT-MMP), and various others (Brew, Dinakarpandian, *et al.* 2000; Sternlicht and Werb 2001). Some MMPs (*e.g.*, MMP-2) are constantly expressed, while most others are induced and are tissue-specific. Soluble MMPs are secreted as pro-enzymes (latent forms), which need to be activated before their enzymic activity is realized. Plasmin (which activates proMMP-1, -3, -7, -9, -10, and -13), urokinase-type plasminogen activator (uPA), and tissue-type plasminogen activator (tPA) activate the latent MMPs (Mignatti and Rifkin 1993), which occurs extracellularly and is mediated by various already-activated MMPs. For example, MMP-2 activates proMMP-1, -9, and -13, while MMP-3 activates proMMP-1, -7, -8, -9, and -13,. Tissue inhibitors of MMPs (TIMPs) modulate extracellular matrix degradation (Brew *et al.*, 2000; Cayetano-Salazar *et al.*, 2022).

MMPs have many physiological and pathological functions, including angiogenesis, inflammation, wound healing, embryogenesis, tumor metastasis, arthritis, and cardiovascular disease (Werb 1997; Nagase and Woessner 1999; Brew *et al.* 2000, Sternlicht and Werb 2001; Moracho *et al.*, 2022). From the ocular perspective, MMPs are involved in the breakdown of the blood-retinal barrier, age-related macular degeneration, corneal wound healing, uveitis, ocular angiogenesis, and corneal epithelial barriers, retinal ganglion cell degeneration, and aqueous humor dynamics (Gabelt and Kaufman 1989; Bradley *et al.* 1998; Sternlicht and Werb 2001; Zhang *et al.* 2004; Husain *et al.* 2005; Zaidi *et al.*, 2020).

Matrix Metalloproteinases (MMPs) and Aqueous Humor Dynamics in Glaucoma

Much published literature points to an involvement of MMPs in the regulation of intraocular pressure (IOP) in glaucoma patients and in animal models of such ocular hypertension by promoting aqueous humor outflow at the trabecular meshwork and ciliary muscle levels (Weinreb *et al.*, 1997; Husain *et al.* 2005; Husain and Crosson 2008).

IOP represents a balance between aqueous humor (AQH) generation by the ciliary processes and AQH drainage through the trabecular (conventional outflow) and ciliary muscle (uveoscleral outflow) routes. The increased IOP in open-angle glaucoma patients is due to an increased AQH outflow resistance caused by abnormally enhanced deposition of extracellular matrix (ECM) in the AQH outflow routes, primarily the uveoscleral pathway (Tamm, 2013). Several investigations have shown that MMPs play a critical role in regulating AQH outflow and IOP under physiological and pathophysiological conditions (Samples *et al.*, 1993; Parshley *et al.*, 1996; Bradley *et al.*, 1998; Ocklind, 1998; Husain *et al.*, 2005; Husain and Crosson, 2008).

MMP Activity Measurement by Zymography

In order to measure the enzymic activity of MMPs in ocular cells *in vitro*, they have to be cultured in serum-free medium for 16 hours, followed by the addition of test drugs for various times ranging from 4-72 hours as previously described (Husain *et al.*, 2005; Zaidi *et al.*, 2020). After this time, the media and/or cell lysates should be harvested, labeled, and stored (preferably at -80°C) until analyzed for MMPs.

- For measuring MMPs' activity in the medium, it should be concentrated at least 10-fold using an ultrafiltration centrifugal concentrator (10-30 kDa cutoff; Centricon; Amicon Beverly, MA), and then all samples must be adjusted in concentration by a 10:1 factor (Husain *et al.*, 2005).
- Rinse the cells with ice-cold PBS and lyse them using a lysis buffer solution of the following composition: 50 mM Tris-HCl buffer [pH 8.0] containing 100 mM NaCl, 1% Nonidet P-40, 0.1% SDS, 1 mM EDTA, 50 mM NaF, 0.5% deoxycholate, 50 µg/mL aprotinin, 5 mM PMSF, and 10 µg/mL leupeptin for 30 minutes on ice.
- Now, mix the samples of cell lysates or media samples with zymogram PAGE sample buffer in a 1:1 ratio, keeping them on ice until being heated (60-90ºC for 3-10 mins) prior to loading onto zymogram gels.
- Load equal volume (*i.e.*, 30-40 µL) of the medium or equal amount of protein (*i.e.*, 5-15 µg) from cell lysates on 10% SDS-PAGE gels that contain 1 mg/mL gelatin or casein under non-reducing conditions for 40-60 minutes at a low voltage (*e.g.*, 100 Volts) at a low temperature (*e.g.*, 4ºC).
- Following the electrophoresis process, wash the gels twice in 50 mM Tris-HCl buffer (pH 7.5) that contains 2.5% Triton X-100 with slow shaking for 30 minutes.
- After this step, transfer the gels to a Petri dish containing the activation buffer (50 mM Tris-HCl [pH 7.5], 150 mM NaCl, and 10 mM $CaCl_2$) and maintain for 18 hours at 37°C in order to allow enzyme-based degradation of the substrate.
- Now, stain the gels with Coomassie blue R-250 dye for 4-6 hours at 24°C (room temperature).
- After this time, subject the gels to a destaining solution (*i.e.*, 10% Acetic Acid and 25% Ethanol) over 24-72 hours.
- Gelatin or casein digestion at the position of the active enzyme can be observed as a clear area with a uniformly dark-staining gel (Husain *et al.*, 2005).
- The relative density of the digested substrate areas can now be measured by computerized densitometry and normalized against the total cellular protein.

Measurement of Matrix Metalloproteinases (MMPs) Expression by Western Blotting

The following procedure can be used to measure the changes in the expression pattern of MMPs. Purified MMP (each isoform) should be run in parallel with the below procedures as a positive control to identify each isoform of MMP.

- Culture the cells in serum-free medium for 16 hours, followed by the addition of test compound various times, and then collect the medium and/or cell lysates and store at -80°C before the sample analysis.
- Concentrate the medium at least 10-fold using an ultrafiltration centrifugal concentrator (10-30 kDa cutoff; Centricon; Amicon Beverly, MA) and dilute all samples to a final concentration ratio of 10:1.
- Both cell lysates and media samples should be mixed with SDS-PAGE sample buffer in a 1:1 ratio or at a higher ratio, depending upon the experimental conditions. All samples should now be heated as per the manufacturer's recommendation (*i.e.*, 60-90ºC for 3-10 mins).
- Samples are now loaded and separated on 10% SDS-PAGE for the separation of proteins. Equivalent volumes (*i.e.*, 40 μL) of the medium or equal amount of protein from cell lysates (*i.e.*, 5-15 μg) are loaded onto 10% SDS-polyacrylamide gels (PAGE), and the proteins are separated at 125-150 volts for 45-60 minutes at 24ºC/room temperature.
- Carefully remove the gels from the electrophoresis unit and keep them in Petri dishes containing transfer buffer for 15 minutes with slow shaking to remove SDS from the gels.
- Now, set the gels in the protein transfer assembly along with nitrocellulose membranes, blotting paper, and blotting pads for 2-3 hours at 24ºC or overnight at 4ºC.
- Nitrocellulose membranes can be removed and blocked with 5% Non-Fat milk or using 3% BSA in TBS for 1 hour at 24ºC.
- Following the blocking process, probe the membranes with anti-MMP antibodies (1:1000 or as per the recommendation of the antibody supplier) in 0.1% BSA or 0.1% milk overnight at 4°C.
- After the above step, wash the membranes with 0.5% TBST buffer 3 times with an interval of 5 minutes with gentle shaking.
- After the washing process, probe the membranes with the appropriate secondary antibodies (*e.g.*, horse radish peroxide-conjugated antibodies) at a 1:3000 ratio in 0.1% BSA or 0.1% milk for 1 hour at 24ºC. Then, wash the membranes 5 times with 5 minutes intervals to decrease non-specific binding, followed by further washing for 5 minutes with TBS buffer.
- At this point, the protein bands can be visualized using the ECL reagents using Bio-Rad Versadoc.

- The band intensities should be quantitated by computerized densitometry and normalized with respect to total cellular protein. This normalization process is necessary to correct for differences in the number of cells used in each assay.

CONCLUSION

Ciliary muscle and Schlemm's canal cells are important players in the process of AQH outflow from the anterior chamber of the eye to regulate and control IOP. Screening of potential IOP-reducing compounds can be performed on such cells to gain a better understanding of the biochemical pharmacology of the associated receptors and enzymes within these cells (Sharif *et al.*, 2003, 2006, 2016; Ellis *et al.*, 2010). It is hoped that the cell isolation procedures and uses described in this chapter meet the researcher's and readers' needs.

ACKNOWLEDGEMENTS

This study was supported by NIH/NEI grant EY-034514.

REFERENCES

Abdul, Y, Akhter, N & Husain, S (2013) Delta-opioid agonist SNC-121 protects retinal ganglion cell function in a chronic ocular hypertensive rat model. *Invest Ophthalmol Vis Sci,* 54, 1816-28.
[http://dx.doi.org/10.1167/iovs.12-10741] [PMID: 23404122]

Bassiouni, W, Ali, MAM & Schulz, R (2021) Multifunctional intracellular matrix metalloproteinases: implications in disease. *FEBS J,* 288, 7162-82.
[http://dx.doi.org/10.1111/febs.15701] [PMID: 33405316]

Bradley, JM, Vranka, J, Colvis, CM, Conger, DM, Alexander, JP, Fisk, AS, Samples, JR & Acott, TS (1998) Effect of matrix metalloproteinases activity on outflow in perfused human organ culture. *Invest Ophthalmol Vis Sci,* 39, 2649-58.
[PMID: 9856774]

Brew, K, Dinakarpandian, D & Nagase, H (2000) Tissue inhibitors of metalloproteinases: evolution, structure and function. *Biochim Biophys Acta Protein Struct Mol Enzymol,* 1477, 267-83.
[http://dx.doi.org/10.1016/S0167-4838(99)00279-4] [PMID: 10708863]

Cayetano-Salazar, L, Nava-Tapia, DA, Astudillo-Justo, KD, Arizmendi-Izazaga, A, Sotelo-Leyva, C, Herrera-Martinez, M, Villegas-Comonfort, S & Navarro-Tito, N (2022) Flavonoids as regulators of TIMPs expression in cancer: Consequences, opportunities, and challenges. *Life Sci,* 308, 120932.
[http://dx.doi.org/10.1016/j.lfs.2022.120932] [PMID: 36067841]

Ellis, DZ, Sharif, NA & Dismuke, WM (2010) Endogenous regulation of human Schlemm's canal cell volume by nitric oxide signaling. *Invest Ophthalmol Vis Sci,* 51, 5817-24.
[http://dx.doi.org/10.1167/iovs.09-5072] [PMID: 20484594]

Gabelt, BAT & Kaufman, PL (1989) Prostaglandin F2α increases uveoscleral outflow in the cynomolgus monkey. *Exp Eye Res,* 49, 389-402.
[http://dx.doi.org/10.1016/0014-4835(89)90049-3] [PMID: 2792235]

Husain, S, Abdul, Y & Crosson, CE (2012) Preservation of retina ganglion cell function by morphine in a chronic ocular-hypertensive rat model. *Invest Ophthalmol Vis Sci,* 53, 4289-98.
[http://dx.doi.org/10.1167/iovs.12-9467] [PMID: 22661469]

Husain, S & Crosson, CE (2008) Role of PKCepsilon in PGF2alpha-stimulated MMP-2 secretion from

human ciliary muscle cells. *J Ocul Pharmacol Ther,* 24, 268-77.
[http://dx.doi.org/10.1089/jop.2008.0014] [PMID: 18462068]

Husain, S, Jafri, F & Crosson, CE (2005) Acute effects of PGF2alpha on MMP-2 secretion from human ciliary muscle cells: a PKC- and ERK-dependent process. *Invest Ophthalmol Vis Sci,* 46, 1706-13.
[http://dx.doi.org/10.1167/iovs.04-0993] [PMID: 15851572]

Husain, S, Kaddour-Djebbar, I & Abdel-Latif, AA (2002) Alterations in arachidonic acid release and phospholipase C-beta(1) expression in glaucomatous human ciliary muscle cells. *Invest Ophthalmol Vis Sci,* 43, 1127-34.
[PMID: 11923256]

Husain, S, Zaidi, SAH, Singh, S, Guzman, W & Mehrotra, S (2021) Reduction of Neuroinflammation by δ-Opioids *Via* STAT3-Dependent Pathway in Chronic Glaucoma Model. *Front Pharmacol,* 12, 601404.
[http://dx.doi.org/10.3389/fphar.2021.601404] [PMID: 33628191]

Mignatti, P & Rifkin, DB (1993) Biology and biochemistry of proteinases in tumor invasion. *Physiol Rev,* 73, 161-95.
[http://dx.doi.org/10.1152/physrev.1993.73.1.161] [PMID: 8419965]

Moracho, N, Learte, AIR, Muñoz-Sáez, E, Marchena, MA, Cid, MA, Arroyo, AG & Sánchez-Camacho, C (2022) Emerging roles of MT-MMPS in embryonic development. *Dev Dyn,* 251, 240-75.
[http://dx.doi.org/10.1002/dvdy.398] [PMID: 34241926]

Murphy, G & Nagase, H (2008) Progress in matrix metalloproteinase research. *Mol Aspects Med,* 29, 290-308.
[http://dx.doi.org/10.1016/j.mam.2008.05.002] [PMID: 18619669]

Nagase, H & Woessner, JF, Jr (1999) Matrix Metalloproteinases. *J Biol Chem,* 274, 21491-4.
[http://dx.doi.org/10.1074/jbc.274.31.21491] [PMID: 10419448]

Ocklind, A (1998) Effect of latanoprost on the extracellular matrix of the ciliary muscle. A study on cultured cells and tissue sections. *Exp Eye Res,* 67, 179-91.
[http://dx.doi.org/10.1006/exer.1998.0508] [PMID: 9733584]

Parshley, DE, Bradley, JM, Fisk, A, Hadaegh, A, Samples, JR, Van Buskirk, EM & Acott, TS (1996) Laser trabeculoplasty induces stromelysin expression by trabecular juxtacanalicular cells. *Invest Ophthalmol Vis Sci,* 37, 795-804.
[PMID: 8603864]

Samples, JR, Alexander, JP & Acott, TS (1993) Regulation of the levels of human trabecular matrix metalloproteinases and inhibitor by interleukin-1 and dexamethasone. *Invest Ophthalmol Vis Sci,* 34, 3386-95.
[PMID: 8225873]

Sharif NA, Crider JY, Husain S, Kaddour-Djebbar I, Ansari HR, Abdel-Latif AA. Human ciliary muscle responses to FP-class prostaglandin analogs: phosphoinositide hydrolysis, intracellular Ca2+ mobilization and MAP kinase activation. J. Ocular Pharmacology & Therapeutics 19: 437-455 (2003).

Sharif NA, Crider JY, Kelly CR, Davis TL. (2006). Serotonin-2 (5HT2) receptor-mediated signal transduction in human ciliary muscle cells: role in ocular hypotension. J. Ocular Pharmacology & Therapeutics 22: 389-401.

Sharif NA, Patil R, Li L, Husain S. (2016). Human ciliary muscle cell responses to kinins: activation of ERK1/2 and pro-matrix metalloproteinases secretion. World J. Ophthalmology 6: 20-27.

Stamer, WD, Roberts, BC, Howell, DN & Epstein, DL (1998) Isolation, culture, and characterization of endothelial cells from Schlemm's canal. *Invest Ophthalmol Vis Sci,* 39, 1804-12.
[PMID: 9727403]

Sternlicht, MD & Werb, Z (2001) How matrix metalloproteinases regulate cell behavior. *Annu Rev Cell Dev Biol,* 17, 463-516.

[http://dx.doi.org/10.1146/annurev.cellbio.17.1.463] [PMID: 11687497]

Tamm, ER (2013) Functional morphology of the outflow pathways of aqueous humor and their changes in open angle glaucoma. *Ophthalmologe,* 110, 1026-35.
[http://dx.doi.org/10.1007/s00347-012-2670-4] [PMID: 24231909]

Weinreb, RN, Kashiwagi, K, Kashiwagi, F, Tsukahara, S & Lindsey, JD (1997) Prostaglandins increase matrix metalloproteinase release from human ciliary smooth muscle cells. *Invest Ophthalmol Vis Sci,* 38, 2772-80.
[PMID: 9418730]

Werb, Z (1997) ECM and cell surface proteolysis: regulating cellular ecology. *Cell,* 91, 439-42.
[http://dx.doi.org/10.1016/S0092-8674(00)80429-8] [PMID: 9390552]

Zaidi, SAH, Guzman, W, Singh, S, Mehrotra, S & Husain, S (2020) Changes in Class I and IIb HDACs by δ-Opioid in Chronic Rat Glaucoma Model. *Invest Ophthalmol Vis Sci,* 61, 4.
[http://dx.doi.org/10.1167/iovs.61.14.4] [PMID: 33263714]

Zaidi, SAH, Thakore, N, Singh, S, Guzman, W, Mehrotra, S, Gangaraju, V & Husain, S (2020) Histone Deacetylases Regulation by δ-Opioids in Human Optic Nerve Head Astrocytes. *Invest Ophthalmol Vis Sci,* 61, 17.
[PMID: 32915982]

Zhang, X, Cheng, M & Chintala, SK (2004) Kainic acid-mediated upregulation of matrix metalloproteinase-9 promotes retinal degeneration. *Invest Ophthalmol Vis Sci,* 45, 2374-83.
[http://dx.doi.org/10.1167/iovs.03-1239] [PMID: 15223820]

CHAPTER 11

A Protocol for Primary Culture of Non-Pigmented Ciliary Epithelium Cells

Mohammad Shahidullah[1,*] and **Nicholas Delamere**[1]

[1] *Department of Physiology and Department of Ophthalmology & Vision Science, College of Medicine, University of Arizona, 1501 N Campbell Avenue, Tucson, AZ 85724, USA*

Abstract: Here, we provide a methodology for routine primary culture of porcine non-pigmented ciliary epithelium (NPE), a cell type that plays a critical role in AH formation. Using fresh eyes from adult pigs, the dissection protocol allows us to obtain the entire ring of NPE as a ruffled sheet of cells attached to the vitreous. Dispersal of the cells for initial culture is made possible by treatment with collagenase and hyaluronidase. We describe the seeding density, time to confluence, and trypsinization protocol for NPE cells established in primary culture. Comparison of the freshly isolated and cultured NPE cells includes analysis of several proteins known to be characteristic of the NPE. This includes measuring the expression of xenobiotic transporters (PgP, BCRP, MRP4, MRP 2, MRP1), connexins (Cx-43 and Cx-50), sodium-hydrogen exchangers, and carbonic anhydrases. The diffusion barrier property of cultured NPE monolayers is also examined. Prior to the development of this technique in 2007, experts in the field did not believe it was feasible to culture and propagate NPE. Our success hinged on being able to seed freshly isolated NPE cells at a sufficiently high density. This, in turn, hinged upon being able to isolate a relatively large quantity of NPE cells, first by isolating the entire ciliary ring from each eye, then by dispersion of cells by enzyme treatment of the cell-to-vitreous body attachment.

Keywords: Ciliary body, Non-pigmented ciliary epithelium, Pigmented ciliary epithelium, Porcine eye, Primary culture.

INTRODUCTION

Glaucoma is a neurodegenerative eye disease in which the hallmark pathological lesion is the deterioration and death of ganglion cells, the neurons that transmit visual information from the retina to the brain. The underlying causes of glaucoma appear to be multifactorial and are poorly understood. However, the most common form of the disorder, primary open-angle glaucoma, is associated

* **Corresponding author Mohammad Shahidullah:** Department of Physiology and Department of Ophthalmology & Vision Science, College of Medicine, University of Arizona, 1501 N Campbell Avenue, Tucson, AZ 85724, USA; E-mail: shahidua@arizona.edu

Najam A. Sharif and Sunny E. Ohia (Eds.)

with abnormally high fluid pressure within the eye (ocular hypertension). Because lowering intraocular pressure (IOP) is the most effective way to reduce the rate of glaucomatous vision loss (Kass, Heuer *et al.* 2002), there is considerable interest in the dynamics of aqueous humor (AH) flow through the eye. Normal IOP reflects a perfect balance between aqueous humor formation and drainage, and high IOP commonly results from inadequate aqueous humor exit (Acott, Vranka *et al.* 2021). IOP-lowering medications either slow AH formation or improve drainage. The continuous flow of AH through the anterior chamber of the eye is critically important. It supplies nutrition to the avascular tissues of the eye, removes metabolic wastes, and establishes the IOP required for the structural rigidity and optical alignment of the eye.

Here, we describe a technique for the primary culture of non-pigmented ciliary epithelium (NPE), a cell type that plays a critical role in AH formation. The site of AH production is the ciliary body (CB), a ring-like structure situated between the retina and the iris root. The base of the CB contains the ciliary muscles, forms the ciliary ring, and connects to the choroid. Closest to the retina is a flattened zone of the CB, the *pars plana*, which is the anchor point for the Zonules of Zinn that hold the lens in place and keep it under some degree of tension (Bassnett 2021). However, most of the CB, the *pars plicata*, is an elaborate arrangement of highly vascularized radial projections called the ciliary processes (CP). The stroma and leaky capillary network inside each CP are covered by the double layer of ciliary epithelial cells, the NPE, and the pigmented epithelium (PE), which are connected by gap junctions at their apical surfaces (Shahidullah and Delamere 2014, Li, Shan *et al.* 2018). The NPE faces the aqueous humor, and the PE layer faces the stroma. AH secretion is a metabolically active process whereby fluid from the stroma passes across the PE-NPE bilayer into the posterior chamber of the eye (Edelman, Sachs *et al.* 1994, Civan and Macknight 2004).

NPE cells are specialized. They have the physiological characteristics and morphology of a fluid-transporting epithelium, including extensive invaginations in the basolateral membranes facing the AH, tight junctions between the apical membranes, abundant mitochondria, and well-developed rough endoplasmic reticulum (Tormey 1966, Schlötzer-Schrehardt, Müller *et al.* 1990, Wolosin, Chen *et al.* 1993). The PE and NPE coordinate as a functional unit to secrete AH (McLaughlin, Zellhuber-McMillan *et al.* 2004), and the NPE plays a particularly important role because it is the source of almost all the Na, K-ATPase activity that provides the driving force (Shahidullah, Wilson *et al.* 2003). Na, K-ATPase is highly enriched in NPE cells. The cells express multiple Na, K-ATPase isoforms at the basolateral surface, which faces the AH (Martin-Vasallo, Ghosh *et al.* 1989, Ghosh, Hernando *et al.* 1991, Coca-Prados, Fernández-Cabezudo *et al.* 1995, Shahidullah, Tamiya *et al.* 2007). In order to develop remedies to slow AH secretion and lower intraocular pressure for the treatment of glaucoma, it would obviously be useful to understand the individual contribution of NPE and PE to AH formation. While there have been several studies in this area (Tormey 1966, Shi, Zamudio *et al.* 1996, Patil, Han *et al.* 2001, Do and Civan 2009), questions remain. Thus, establishing protocols for the primary culture of PE and NPE would be useful. It turns out that PE cells, which are thought to be developmentally related to retinal pigment epithelium (Coca-Prados, Fernández-Cabezudo *et al.* 1995), are comparatively easy to grow in primary culture (Helbig, Korbmacher *et al.* 1988, Helbig, Korbmacher *et al.* 1989, Coca-Prados, Ghosh *et al.* 1992, Bode, Hamel *et al.* 1993, Shahidullah and Wilson 1999, Fleisher, McGahan *et al.* 2000, Hochgesand, Dunn *et al.* 2001). In contrast, NPE cells are developmentally related to the neural retina (Coca-Prados, Fernández-Cabezudo *et al.* 1995), and obtaining primary cultures of NPE monolayers has proved to be difficult. For many years, it was believed that NPE cells could not be grown *in vitro*. However, after more than 10 years of trial and error, we were able to isolate NPE cells from the porcine eye and establish the cells in primary culture (Shahidullah and Delamere 2006), forming monolayers that retain many of the *in vivo* NPE characteristics (Shahidullah, Tamiya *et al.* 2007). In this chapter, we describe in detail the protocol for porcine eye dissection, isolation of NPE in bulk, and culturing the cells in monolayers.

EXPERIMENTAL PROTOCOLS

The use of animals in the following procedure was approved by the Institutional Animal Care and Use Committee (IACUC) of the University of Arizona and complied with the Association for Research in Vision and Ophthalmology guidelines on the use of animals in research.

Preparation of the Porcine Eye for Dissection

Fresh eyes from young adult pigs (6-10 months; usual slaughter weight of 280 lbs. or more) were collected from a local abattoir and transported to the lab on ice. The eyes were enucleated from the carcasses along with reasonable remnants of extraocular muscles, avoiding undue pressure that might negatively affect internal structures. In the lab, the remnants of extraocular muscles and fat were trimmed away using a pair of surgical scissors and a pair of rat tooth forceps. The eyes were washed with Dulbecco's phosphate-buffered saline containing calcium and magnesium (Gibco™ 14040133) that also contained a high concentration of Gentamicin (400 µg/ml) (Sigma, Cat # G1397) and then placed in serum-free DMEM (Gibco, Cat # 12430-062) containing 200 µg/ml Gentamicin in a biological safety cabinet for subsequent dissection. The washing and storing of eyes in an antibiotic-containing medium minimizes the chances of bacterial contamination.

Dissection of the Eye

Trimmed, cleaned, and antibiotic-soaked eyes were placed cornea side down in the concave depression of a plasticine cup molded to the approximate curvature of the eye. This holds the eye in place while it is dissected open from the posterior pole. Using a sharp scalpel, two incisions were made at right angles to one another through the middle of the optic nerve, extending on both sides to 3- 4 mm away from the corneoscleral junction. The incisions should be deep enough to span just the thickness of the sclera, choroid, and retina with minimum penetration into the underlying vitreous. These incisions created 4 flaps that were folded backward to expose the intact vitreous body (Fig. **1A**). This was followed by everting the cornea by pulling the cut scleral flaps backward while at the same time gently pushing the cornea inward with the index finger (Fig. **1B**), causing the intact vitreous body to protrude with its base still attached to the pars plana of the ciliary body. The dissection procedure has been described in our earlier publications (Shahidullah and Delamere, 2006; Shahidullah, Tamiya *et al*., 2007).

Isolation of the NPE

The NPE sheet was isolated as a ring of cells attached to the vitreous body. One of the scleral flaps of the dissected eye (above) was firmly held with a pair of rat tooth forceps in the left hand, and the protruding vitreous was gently pushed sideways from the pars plana using the back of a pair of curved forceps held in the right hand. This caused the vitreous to become separated from the eye (Fig. **1C**). Because the entire ring of NPE remains attached to the vitreous, it too is separated from the eye (Fig. **1D**), while the PE cell layer remains attached to the ciliary body. The NPE is obtained as a ring formed by the ruffled sheet of cells that previously covered the peaks and valleys of the ciliary processes. With practice and using fresh eyes, the NPE obtained in this manner shows little evidence of contamination with pigment. Electron microscopic examination of the NPE ring revealed no detectable contamination with PE (Shahidullah and Delamere 2006).

Dispersion and Initial Culture of the NPE

Most of the vitreous was trimmed away from the NPE ring using fine scissors although some vitreous remained attached to the cells. The ring was cut into 1-2 mm pieces and transferred to an ice-cold centrifuge tube containing serum-free High Glucose DMEM (Gibco, Cat # 12430-062) and 100 μg/ml Gentamicin. By trial and error, we determined that pooling tissue pieces from 5-7 fresh eyes was sufficient to establish the NPE cells in culture. If the eyes are not fresh enough, it is difficult to obtain the entire NPE ring free of pigment or PE contamination, as shown in Fig. (**1D**). In these instances, we needed more than 7 eyes since only the pigment-free pieces of the rings were collected instead of the whole ring from each eye. To disperse the cells, the pieces of the NPE ring were transferred to a 100 mm petri dish containing 15 ml of 0.15 to 0.25% collagenase A (Sigma, Cat # C2674-500MG) and 300-500 U/ml of hyaluronidase (Sigma, Cat # H3884-500MG) in a buffer comprising (mM) NaCl 66.7, KCl 6.7. HEPES 10, and $CaCl_2$ 4.8 with the pH adjusted to 7.4. Since the collagenase and hyaluronidase are non-sterile products, these constituents were dissolved in the buffer solution and sterilized by passing through a 2.0 μm syringe filter before use. The Petri dish containing the pieces of NPE ring immersed in the enzyme-containing medium was then placed on a rotary shaker for 5-7 min in a CO_2 incubator at 37°C. The Petri dish was then removed from the shaker, and the collagenase and hyaluronidase were neutralized with an excess amount (5-7 ml) of a mixture of newborn calf serum (NCS) (Sigma, Cat # N4637-500ML) and fetal bovine serum (FBS) (Gibco, Cat # 10082-147) (1:1). The purpose of the collagenase treatment was to digest the collagen of the NPE basement membrane, while the hyaluronidase treatment was carried out to aid dispersion of the NPE cells from the vitreous. Using a sterile smooth, rounded tip, Pasteur pipette fitted with a dropper bulb, the enzyme-treated fragments of the tissue were picked up and transferred to 2 sterile centrifuge tubes (15 ml size), each containing 10 ml of High Glucose DMEM (GIBCO cat # 12430-062) containing 20% of a mixture of NCS and fetal bovine serum (FBS) (1:1) and 100 U/ml Gentamicin. The fragments were gently triturated using the Pasteur pipette, avoiding bubble formation. The suspension of cells dispersed in this manner was centrifuged for 10 min at 670 × g at 4°C. Then, the supernatant was discarded, and the cell pellet was redispersed in 2 ml of complete culture medium (DMEM + 10% FBS + 100 IU Gentamicin/ml). The cells prepared in this way were then incubated at 37°C in a scant amount of the complete medium (3.5-4 ml) in a 25 cm^2 tissue culture-treated flask, which was placed in a humidified (90-95%) incubator supplied with 5% CO_2 for 3-4 days without changing the medium. After this, the medium was changed every alternate day. In 8 to 9 days, there were many isolated colonies of confluent cells. At this stage, the cells were trypsinized and propagated. The entire lot of cells after trypsinization was again seeded in a 25 cm^2 flask and this lot of cells was designated as the first passage. The medium was changed the next day and then every alternate day.

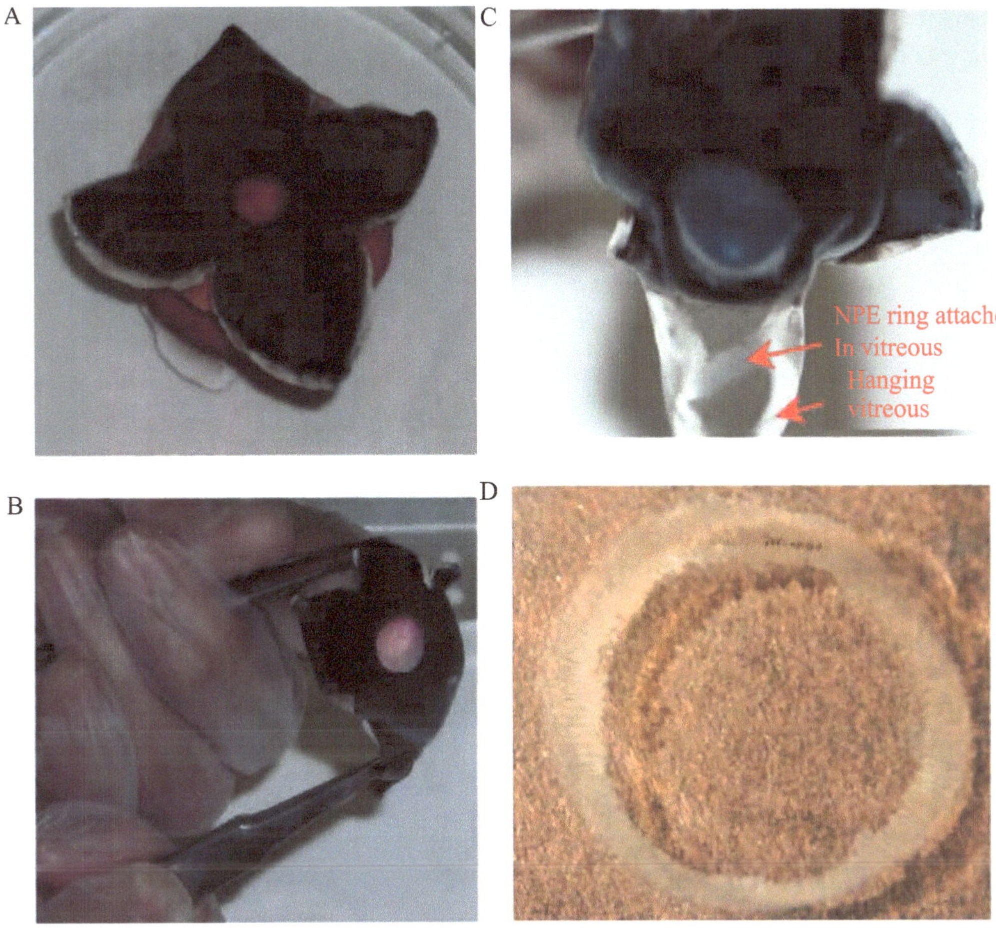

Fig. (1). Dissection of the porcine eye to isolate the intact NPE layer. (**A**) Crosswise cuts through the posterior of the globe allow the eye to be opened by folding the resultant four flaps of the sclera. (**B**) Everting the cornea was accomplished by pulling the scleral flaps backward and, at the same time, pushing the cornea inward with the index finger. (**C**) The ring of NPE remained attached to the vitreous when the vitreous was gently pushed sideways and separated from the pars plana. (**D**) The isolated intact ring of the NPE layer. Note that the NPE ring isolated from the porcine eye showed no detectable contamination by PE cells or pigment granules. Adapted from Shahidullah *et al.*; Current Eye Research 32:511-522, 2007, with permission from Taylor and Francis.

Trypsinization and Propagation of the Cultured NPE

Trypsinization was done when the cells reached a confluent stage (95% confluence or above). The cells were washed 2-3 times, each with 10 ml of a sterile calcium-free and magnesium-free Dulbecco's Phosphate Buffered Saline (Sigma, Cat # D8537), and then incubated for 3-4 min with 5 ml of Gibco™ Trypsin-EDT solution (0.25%, 1×) (Gibco, Cat #25200056) at 37°C. The cells were easily detached by gently shaking the flask 3-4 times, then the trypsin was neutralized by adding 5 ml of a mixture of NCS and FBS (1:1). The cells suspension was centrifuged, the supernatant was discarded, and the pellet was resuspended in 2-5 ml of the complete medium and seeded in culture flasks at high density (5×10^4 cells/cm^2). The medium was changed the next day and then every alternate day. At this seeding density, confluent monolayers were usually obtained in 5 days. We propagated the NPE cells up to the 10th passage without any obvious signs of changing cell morphology as observed by light microscopy or alteration in growth characteristics (time to reach confluence). Images of confluent monolayers of 1st and 7th passage NPE cells are shown in Fig. (**2**). The initial cell isolation and culture methods were published earlier (Shahidullah and Delamere 2006, Shahidullah, Tamiya *et al.* 2007). In this article, we describe a slightly modified and mature protocol that we developed over time.

A

B

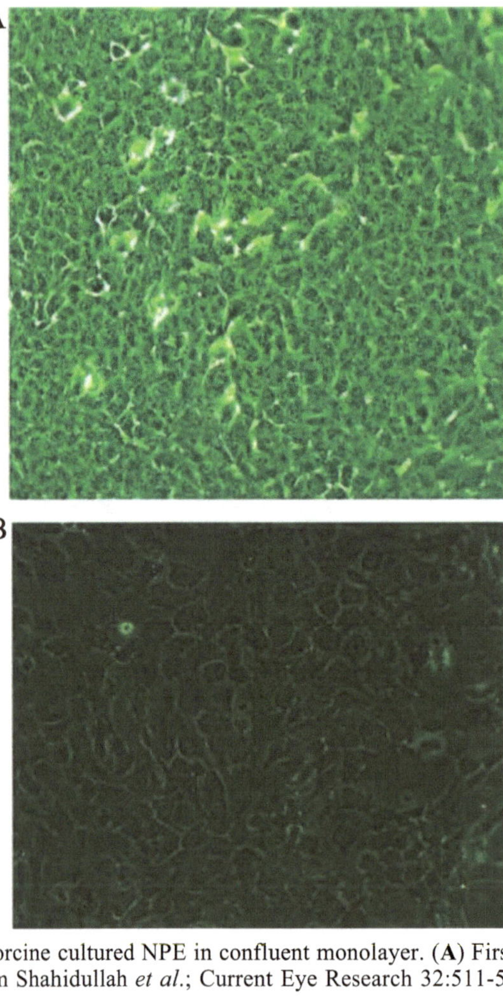

Fig. (2). Photographs of porcine cultured NPE in confluent monolayer. (**A**) First passage and (**B**) Seventh passage cells. Adapted from Shahidullah *et al.*; Current Eye Research 32:511-522, 2007, with permission from Taylor and Francis.

CHARACTERIZATION OF THE CULTURED NPE CELLS

In keeping with its role in aqueous humor secretion, the NPE is highly enriched in Na, K-ATPase and expresses three different isoforms (α1, α2, and α3) at the basolateral surface (Ghosh, Hernando *et al.* 1991, Shahidullah, Tamiya *et al.* 2007). The NPE is also the principal component of the blood-aqueous barrier (BAB). More specifically, the NPE layer is an active biological barrier that expresses membrane proteins that protect the eye by actively transporting toxins and xenobiotics out of the aqueous humor and into the ciliary process stroma, where they are removed by the blood. The physical blood-aqueous barrier is formed by tight junctions between the lateral sides of the NPE (Raviola and Raviola 1978, Cunha-Vaz 1979, Freddo 2001). By restricting diffusion, the BAB enables aqueous humor to have a composition quite unlike the blood serum from which it is formed (Shahidullah, Al-Malki *et al.*, 2011; Ermolaev, Novikov *et al.*, 2016). For example, the concentration of protein in aqueous humor is very low. The active chemical barrier is formed by the expression of multi-substrate organic molecule transporters at the NPE basolateral and apical surfaces. For example, organic anion transporters OAT1 and OAT3 are localized on the NPE basolateral surface (Gao, Huber *et al.* 2005), while the multidrug transporter MRP2 is situated on the NPE apical surface. Working in coordination, these and other transport mechanisms shift organic molecules across the NPE, clearing potentially harmful molecules from the aqueous humor (Pelis, Shahidullah *et al.* 2009; Lee, Shahidullah *et al.* 2015). This is extremely important for the protection of the very long-lived cells in the avascular tissues of the eye - the lens, trabecular meshwork, and corneal endothelium. For the purpose of AH formation, the NPE and PE function as a syncytium with solute passing between the cells *via* gap junctions (Civan and Macknight 2004). For xenobiotic transport, however, the NPE is equipped to function alone, with uptake transporters on the basolateral side and efflux transporters positioned on the apical surface so at to shift cargo toward the blood (Pelis, Shahidullah *et al.*, 2009; Lee, Shahidullah *et al.*, 2015).

We characterized the primary cultured porcine NPE in terms of the expression of important functional proteins expressed by the native tissue. In the original reports on the isolation and culture methodology, we confirmed robust expression of α1, α2, and α3 Na, K-ATPase isoforms, the tight junction protein ZO1 important for the formation of BAB, and all 3 isoforms of nitric oxide (NO) synthase (nNOS, eNOS, iNOS) (Shahidullah, Tamiya *et al.* 2007). NO signaling leads to the inhibition of Na, K-ATPase activity in porcine NPE (Shahidullah and Delamere 2006) and is known to regulate AH secretion (Kiel, Reitsamer *et al.* 2001, Shahidullah, Yap *et al.* 2005). Subsequently (as described below), we have shown that the cultured NPE displays other important characteristics consistent with its *in vivo* function.

Cultured NPE Cells Grown on Permeable Support form a Diffusion Barrier

Transepithelial movement of fluorescein-labeled dextran was measured across cultured NPE passage 4 cells grown to confluence on Transwell® permeable supports (Costar, 3450). Fluorescein dextran (4000 kDa) (Fl-dextran) was added to the bathing solution on either side of the monolayer (apical or basal), and its appearance in the bathing medium on the opposite side was determined using a fluorimeter. As shown in Fig. (**3**), the cultured porcine NPE forms a monolayer that restricts paracellular diffusion.

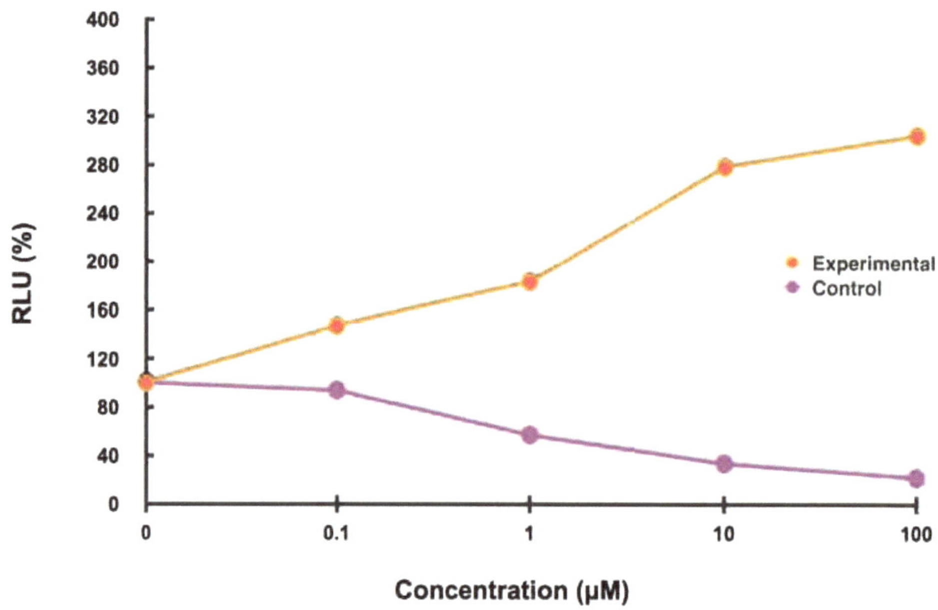

Fig. (3). Fl-dextran does not leak across the NPE monolayer (passage 4 cells) cultured on a permeable support. (Unpublished data).

Cultured Porcine NPE Cells Express Xenobiotic Transporters

We used RT-PCR to examine the expression of major xenobiotic transporters by cultured porcine NPE and also compared the expression of these transporters in human CB tissue. As shown in Fig. (**4**), both human CB and cultured porcine NPE express P-glycoprotein (Pgp), breast cancer resistance protein (BCRP), and multidrug resistance proteins MRP1, MRP2, and MRP4.

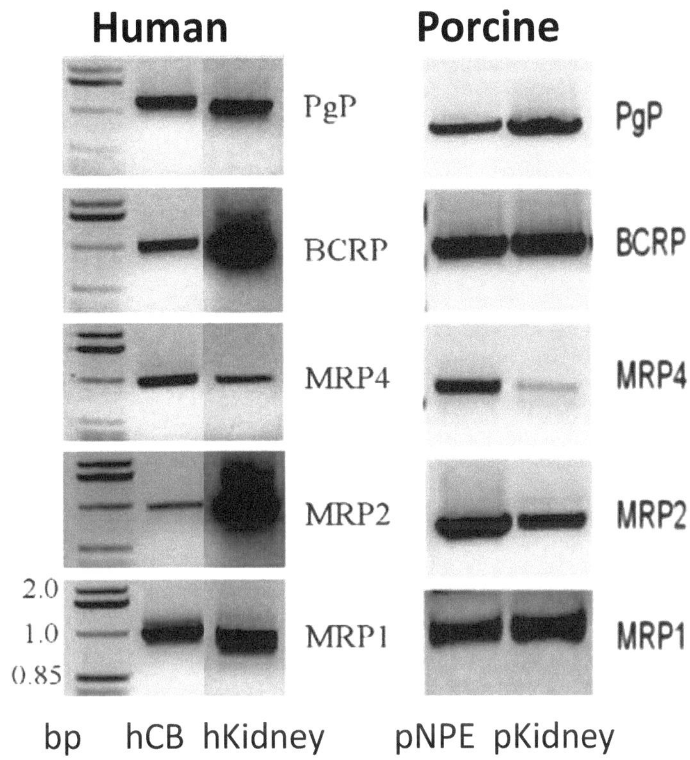

Fig. (4). mRNA (RT-PCR) expression of ABC transporters, MRP1, MRP2, MRP4, BCRP and P-gp in the human ciliary body (hCB)(left panel) and in the cultured porcine NPE (pNPE, right panel). Human or porcine kidney cortex was used as positive control. Unpublished data.

Cultured Porcine NPE Expresses Connexin 43 and Connexin 50

The NPE and PE cell layers are able to work in a coordinated manner to form aqueous humor because connexin proteins form gap junctions between the two cell layers (Wang, Do *et al.* 2010, Li, Shan *et al.* 2018). Gap junctions also connect adjacent cells (McLaughlin, Zellhuber-McMillan *et al.* 2004). The NPE *in vivo* expresses two different connexin, connexin 43 and connexin 50. Gap junctions appear critical to the mechanism of fluid formation. In an Ussing chamber study, it was shown that a gap junction blocker, heptanol (3.5 mM), significantly reduced fluid flow across the porcine iris-ciliary body (Law, Candia *et al.* 2009). Here, we used Western blot analysis to confirm similar expression of connexin 43 (Fig. **5A**) and connexin 50 (Fig. **5B**) in cultured and native porcine NPE.

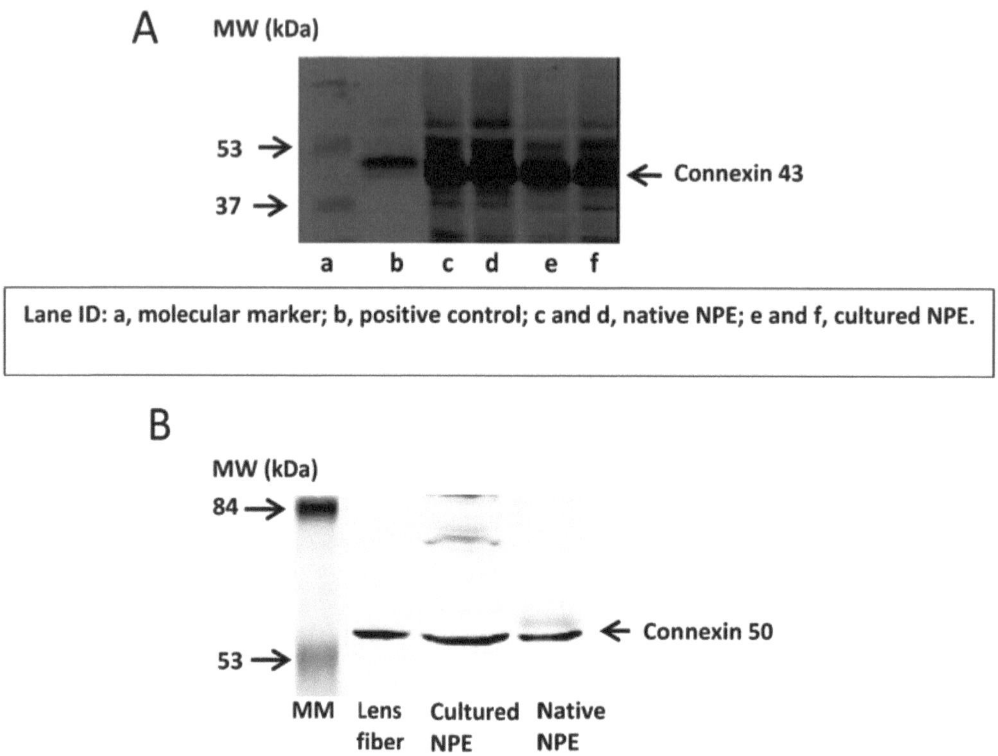

Fig. (5). Western blot detection of connexin 43 (Panel A) and connexin 50 (Panel B) in freshly isolated porcine NPE and in cultured porcine NPE (4th passage). Glutathione-S-transferase fusion protein containing the cytoplasmic carboxy-terminal tail of Connexin 43 (GST-Cx43) and porcine lens fibers were used as positive controls for connexin 43 and connexin 50, respectively. 60 mg of protein was loaded into each lane. Adapted from Shahidullah and Delamere; Exp Eye Res. 2014; 118: 20–29 with permission from Elsevier.

Cultured Porcine NPE Expresses NHE1, NHE4, AE2, and Carbonic Anhydrases II and IV

Sodium hydrogen exchangers (NHE), carbonic anhydrases, and chloride-bicarbonate exchangers are known to be critical to the mechanism of aqueous humor secretion (McLaughlin, Peart *et al.* 1998, Avila, Seidler *et al.* 2002, Civan and Macknight 2004, Shahidullah, To *et al.* 2009). Importantly, immunolocalization studies indicate robust expression of NHE1 and NHE4 in the NPE layer of the intact porcine eye and also in cultured porcine NPE (Shahidullah, Mandal *et al.* 2009). Similarly, immunolocalization and RT-PCR studies confirmed the expression of carbonic anhydrase II, carbonic anhydrase IV, and the chloride bicarbonate exchanger AE2 in the NPE layer of the intact eye as well as cultured porcine NPE (Shahidullah, To *et al.* 2009).

DISCUSSION AND CONCLUSION

Here, we provide a methodology for routine primary culture of porcine NPE. Prior to the development of this technique in 2007 (Shahidullah and Delamere 2006, Shahidullah, Tamiya *et al.* 2007), experts in the field did not believe it was feasible to propagate NPE. Our success hinged on being able to seed freshly isolated NPE cells at a sufficiently high density. This, in turn, hinged upon being able to isolate a relatively large quantity of NPE cells, first by isolating the entire ciliary ring from each eye, then by dispersion of cells by enzyme treatment of the cell-to-vitreous body attachment. For reference purposes, readers are informed of the existence of an immortalized cell-line of NPE cells that faithfully represents the primary cell culture of NPE (Coca-Prados and Wax, 1986). This cell-line has been utilized for studies on signal transduction, receptor pharmacology and screening of compounds for functional activity measuring cAMP generation (Crider *et al.*, 1998).

ACKNOWLEDGEMENTS

The authors would like to thank the Swift Company, Louisville, Kentucky, and the University of Arizona Meat Laboratory for supplying fresh pig eyes. The authors are thankful to Dr. Ryan Pelis for RT-PCR studies to detect the efflux transporters in the human ciliary body and porcine NPE. This work was supported by NIH grant R01EY029171.

REFERENCES

Acott, TS, Vranka, JA, Keller, KE, Raghunathan, V & Kelley, MJ (2021) Normal and glaucomatous outflow regulation. *Prog Retin Eye Res,* 82, 100897.
[http://dx.doi.org/10.1016/j.preteyeres.2020.100897] [PMID: 32795516]

Avila, MY, Seidler, RW, Stone, RA & Civan, MM (2002) Inhibitors of NHE-1 Na+/H+ exchange reduce mouse intraocular pressure. *Invest Ophthalmol Vis Sci,* 43, 1897-902.
[PMID: 12036996]

Bassnett, S (2021) Zinn's zonule. *Prog Retin Eye Res,* 82, 100902.
[http://dx.doi.org/10.1016/j.preteyeres.2020.100902] [PMID: 32980533]

Bode, DC, Hamel, LT & Wax, MB (1993) Distinct profiles of phosphodiesterase isozymes in cultured cells derived from nonpigmented and pigmented ocular ciliary epithelium. *J Pharmacol Exp Ther,* 267, 1286-91.
[PMID: 8263791]

Civan, MM & Macknight, ADC (2004) The ins and outs of aqueous humour secretion. *Exp Eye Res,* 78, 625-31.
[http://dx.doi.org/10.1016/j.exer.2003.09.021] [PMID: 15106942]

Coca-Prados M, Wax MB. (1986). Transformation of human ciliary epithelial cells by simian virus 40: induction of cell proliferation and retention of beta 2-adrenergic receptors. Proc Natl Acad Sci (USA). 83(22):8754-8758.

Coca-Prados, M, Fernández-Cabezudo, MJ, Sánchez-Torres, J, Crabb, JW & Ghosh, S (1995) Cell-specific expression of the human Na+,K(+)-ATPase beta 2 subunit isoform in the nonpigmented ciliary epithelium. *Invest Ophthalmol Vis Sci,* 36, 2717-28.

[PMID: 7499094]

Coca-Prados, M, Ghosh, S, Gilula, NB & Kumar, NM (1992) Expression and cellular distribution of the al gap junction gene product in the ocular pigmented ciliary epithelium. *Curr Eye Res,* 11, 113-22. [http://dx.doi.org/10.3109/02713689209000061] [PMID: 1374005]

Crider JY, Griffin BW, Sharif NA. (1998). Prostaglandin-stimulated adenylyl cyclase activity via a pharmacologically defined EP2 receptor in human nonpigmented ciliary epithelial cells. J Ocul Pharmacol Ther. 14(4):293-304.

Cunha-Vaz, J (1979) The blood-ocular barriers. *Surv Ophthalmol,* 23, 279-96. [http://dx.doi.org/10.1016/0039-6257(79)90158-9] [PMID: 380030]

Do, CW & Civan, MM (2009) Species variation in biology and physiology of the ciliary epithelium: Similarities and differences. *Exp Eye Res,* 88, 631-40. [http://dx.doi.org/10.1016/j.exer.2008.11.005] [PMID: 19056380]

Edelman, JL, Sachs, G & Adorante, JS (1994) Ion transport asymmetry and functional coupling in bovine pigmented and nonpigmented ciliary epithelial cells. *Am J Physiol Cell Physiol,* 266, C1210-21. [http://dx.doi.org/10.1152/ajpcell.1994.266.5.C1210] [PMID: 8203485]

Ermolaev, AP, Novikov, IA, Mel'nikova, LI, Griboedova, IG & Avetisov, KS (2016) Elemental composition of aqueous humour and blood serum at various levels of intraocular pressure. *Vestn Oftalmol,* 132, 43-8. [http://dx.doi.org/10.17116/oftalma2016132643-48] [PMID: 28121298]

Fleisher, LN, McGAHAN, MC & Ferrell, JB (2000) Rabbit pigmented ciliary epithelium produces interleukin-6 in response to inflammatory cytokines. *Exp Eye Res,* 70, 271-9. [http://dx.doi.org/10.1006/exer.1999.0787] [PMID: 10712813]

Freddo, TF (2001) Shifting the paradigm of the blood-aqueous barrier. *Exp Eye Res,* 73, 581-92. [http://dx.doi.org/10.1006/exer.2001.1056] [PMID: 11747359]

Gao, B, Huber, RD, Wenzel, A, Vavricka, SR, Ismair, MG, Remé, C & Meier, PJ (2005) Localization of organic anion transporting polypeptides in the rat and human ciliary body epithelium. *Exp Eye Res,* 80, 61-72. [http://dx.doi.org/10.1016/j.exer.2004.08.013] [PMID: 15652527]

Ghosh, S, Hernando, N, Martín-Alonso, JM, Martin-Vasallo, P & Coca-Prados, M (1991) Expression of multiple Na^+, K^+-ATPase genes reveals a gradient of isoforms along the nonpigmented ciliary epithelium: Functional implications in aqueous humor secretion. *J Cell Physiol,* 149, 184-94. [http://dx.doi.org/10.1002/jcp.1041490203] [PMID: 1660898]

Helbig, H, Korbmacher, C, Kühner, D, Berweck, S & Wiederholt, M (1988) Characterization of exchange in cultured bovine pigmented ciliary epithelium. *Exp Eye Res,* 47, 515-23. [http://dx.doi.org/10.1016/0014-4835(88)90091-7] [PMID: 3181332]

Helbig, H, Korbmacher, C, Wohlfarth, J, Coca-Prados, M & Wiederholt, M (1989) Electrical membrane properties of a cell clone derived from human nonpigmented ciliary epithelium. *Invest Ophthalmol Vis Sci,* 30, 882-9.
[PMID: 2470692]

Hochgesand, DH, Dunn, JJ & Crook, RB (2001) Catecholaminergic regulation of Na-K-Cl cotransport in pigmented ciliary epithelium: differences between PE and NPE. *Exp Eye Res,* 72, 1-12. [http://dx.doi.org/10.1006/exer.2000.0927] [PMID: 11133177]

Kass, MA, Heuer, DK, Higginbotham, EJ, Johnson, CA, Keltner, JL, Miller, JP, Parrish, RK, II, Wilson, MR & Gordon, MO (2002) The Ocular Hypertension Treatment Study: a randomized trial determines that topical ocular hypotensive medication delays or prevents the onset of primary open-angle glaucoma. *Arch Ophthalmol,* 120, 701-13. [http://dx.doi.org/10.1001/archopht.120.6.701] [PMID: 12049574]

Kiel, JW, Reitsamer, HA, Walker, JS & Kiel, FW (2001) Effects of nitric oxide synthase inhibition on ciliary blood flow, aqueous production and intraocular pressure. *Exp Eye Res,* 73, 355-64.

[http://dx.doi.org/10.1006/exer.2001.1050] [PMID: 11520110]

Law, CS, Candia, OA & To, CH (2009) Inhibitions of chloride transport and gap junction reduce fluid flow across the whole porcine ciliary epithelium. *Invest Ophthalmol Vis Sci,* 50, 1299-306.
[http://dx.doi.org/10.1167/iovs.08-1888] [PMID: 18824735]

Lee, J, Shahidullah, M, Hotchkiss, A, Coca-Prados, M, Delamere, NA & Pelis, RM (2015) A renal-like organic anion transport system in the ciliary epithelium of the bovine and human eye. *Mol Pharmacol,* 87, 697-705.
[http://dx.doi.org/10.1124/mol.114.096578] [PMID: 25661037]

Li, SKL, Shan, SW, Li, HL, Cheng, AKW, Pan, F, Yip, SP, Civan, MM, To, CH & Do, CW (2018) Characterization and Regulation of Gap Junctions in Porcine Ciliary Epithelium. *Invest Ophthalmol Vis Sci,* 59, 3461-8.
[http://dx.doi.org/10.1167/iovs.18-24682] [PMID: 30025101]

Martin-Vasallo, P, Ghosh, S & Coca-Prados, M (1989) Expression of Na,K-ATPase alpha subunit isoforms in the human ciliary body and cultured ciliary epithelial cells. *J Cell Physiol,* 141, 243-52.
[http://dx.doi.org/10.1002/jcp.1041410203] [PMID: 2553750]

McLaughlin, CW, Peart, D, Purves, RD, Carré, DA, Macknight, AD & Civan, MM (1998) Effects of HCO3- on cell composition of rabbit ciliary epithelium: a new model for aqueous humor secretion. *Invest Ophthalmol Vis Sci,* 39, 1631-41.
[PMID: 9699552]

McLaughlin, CW, Zellhuber-McMillan, S, Macknight, ADC & Civan, MM (2004) Electron microprobe analysis of ouabain-exposed ciliary epithelium: PE-NPE cell couplets form the functional units. *Am J Physiol Cell Physiol,* 286, C1376-89.
[http://dx.doi.org/10.1152/ajpcell.00248.2003] [PMID: 14761890]

Patil, RV, Han, Z, Yiming, M, Yang, J, Iserovich, P, Wax, MB & Fischbarg, J (2001) Fluid transport by human nonpigmented ciliary epithelial layers in culture: a homeostatic role for aquaporin-1. *Am J Physiol Cell Physiol,* 281, C1139-45.
[http://dx.doi.org/10.1152/ajpcell.2001.281.4.C1139] [PMID: 11546649]

Pelis, RM, Shahidullah, M, Ghosh, S, Coca-Prados, M, Wright, SH & Delamere, NA (2009) Localization of multidrug resistance-associated protein 2 in the nonpigmented ciliary epithelium of the eye. *J Pharmacol Exp Ther,* 329, 479-85.
[http://dx.doi.org/10.1124/jpet.108.149625] [PMID: 19201990]

Raviola, G & Raviola, E (1978) Intercellular junctions in the ciliary epithelium. *Invest Ophthalmol Vis Sci,* 17, 958-81.
[PMID: 100466]

Schlötzer-Schrehardt, U, Müller, HG, Wirtz, PM & Naumann, GO (1990) Desmosomal-mitochondrial complexes in human nonpigmented ciliary and retinal pigment epithelia. *Invest Ophthalmol Vis Sci,* 31, 664-9.
[PMID: 2335434]

Shahidullah, M., W. H. Al-Malki and N. A. Delamere (2011). Mechanism of Aqueous Humor Secretion, Its Regulation and Relevance to Glaucoma, Glaucoma - Basic and Clinical Concepts. S. Rumelt, InTech; Available from: http://www.intechopen.com/articles/show/title/mechanism-of-aqueous-humor-secretion-its-regulation-and-relevance-to-glaucoma

Shahidullah, M & Delamere, NA (2006) NO donors inhibit Na,K-ATPase activity by a protein kinase G-dependent mechanism in the nonpigmented ciliary epithelium of the porcine eye. *Br J Pharmacol,* 148, 871-80.
[http://dx.doi.org/10.1038/sj.bjp.0706795] [PMID: 16770322]

Shahidullah, M & Delamere, NA (2014) Connexins form functional hemichannels in porcine ciliary epithelium. *Exp Eye Res,* 118, 20-9.

[http://dx.doi.org/10.1016/j.exer.2013.11.004] [PMID: 24262135]

Shahidullah, M, Mandal, A & Delamere, NA (2009) Responses of sodium-hydrogen exchange to nitric oxide in porcine cultured nonpigmented ciliary epithelium. *Invest Ophthalmol Vis Sci,* 50, 5851-8. [http://dx.doi.org/10.1167/iovs.09-3453] [PMID: 19608532]

Shahidullah, M, Tamiya, S & Delamere, NA (2007) Primary culture of porcine nonpigmented ciliary epithelium. *Curr Eye Res,* 32, 511-22. [http://dx.doi.org/10.1080/02713680701434899] [PMID: 17612967]

Shahidullah, M, To, CH, Pelis, RM & Delamere, NA (2009) Studies on bicarbonate transporters and carbonic anhydrase in porcine nonpigmented ciliary epithelium. *Invest Ophthalmol Vis Sci,* 50, 1791-800. [http://dx.doi.org/10.1167/iovs.08-2487] [PMID: 19011010]

Shahidullah, M & Wilson, WS (1999) Atriopeptin, sodium azide and cyclic GMP reduce secretion of aqueous humour and inhibit intracellular calcium release in bovine cultured ciliary epithelium. *Br J Pharmacol,* 127, 1438-46. [http://dx.doi.org/10.1038/sj.bjp.0702681] [PMID: 10455294]

Shahidullah, M, Wilson, WS, Yap, M & To, C (2003) Effects of ion transport and channel-blocking drugs on aqueous humor formation in isolated bovine eye. *Invest Ophthalmol Vis Sci,* 44, 1185-91. [http://dx.doi.org/10.1167/iovs.02-0397] [PMID: 12601048]

Shahidullah, M, Yap, M & To, C (2005) Cyclic GMP, sodium nitroprusside and sodium azide reduce aqueous humour formation in the isolated arterially perfused pig eye. *Br J Pharmacol,* 145, 84-92. [http://dx.doi.org/10.1038/sj.bjp.0706156] [PMID: 15711584]

Shi, XP, Zamudio, AC, Candia, OA & Wolosin, JM (1996) Adreno-cholinergic modulation of junctional communications between the pigmented and nonpigmented layers of the ciliary body epithelium. *Invest Ophthalmol Vis Sci,* 37, 1037-46. [PMID: 8631619]

Tormey, JM (1966) The ciliary epithelium: an attempt to correlate structure and function. *Trans Am Acad Ophthalmol Otolaryngol,* 70, 755-66. [PMID: 5970712]

Wang, Z, Do, CW, Valiunas, V, Leung, CT, Cheng, AKW, Clark, AF, Wax, MB, Chatterton, JE & Civan, MM (2010) Regulation of gap junction coupling in bovine ciliary epithelium. *Am J Physiol Cell Physiol,* 298, C798-806. [http://dx.doi.org/10.1152/ajpcell.00406.2009] [PMID: 20089928]

Wolosin, JM, Chen, M, Gordon, RE, Stegman, Z & Butler, GAD (1993) Separation of the rabbit ciliary body epithelial layers in viable form: identification of differences in bicarbonate transport. *Exp Eye Res,* 56, 411-27. [http://dx.doi.org/10.1006/exer.1993.1054] [PMID: 8500555]

CHAPTER 12

Anterior Segment Scleral Fibroblasts and Protocols for Ocular Cell Isolation and Characterization for Glaucoma Studies

Veluchamy A. Barathi[1,*]

[1] *Translational Pre-Clinical Model Platform, Singapore Eye Research Institute, ACP in Ophthalmology & Visual Sciences, DUKE-NUS Graduate Medical School, Department of Ophthalmology, Yong Loo Lin School of Medicine, National University of Singapore, Singapore 119077, Singapore*

Abstract: Scleral fibroblasts (SF) are crucial in maintaining and remodeling the extracellular matrix of the sclera, which is vital for preserving the structural integrity and biomechanical properties of the eye. Investigating the behavior and characteristics of SF is essential for understanding the development of various ocular conditions. This chapter provides an overview of the protocols for isolating and characterizing SF, with a specific focus on their relevance to glaucoma research on the anterior segment.

The initial step in studying SF involves isolating them from either animal models or post-mortem human eyes. Sterile conditions are maintained during the dissection and enzymatic digestion of scleral tissue using collagenase or trypsin. The resulting cells are then cultured in an appropriate growth medium supplemented with serum and antibiotics. Immunocytochemistry is employed to characterize the isolated SF, and flow cytometry can be used to analyze cell-surface markers associated with the SF phenotype. Co-culture experiments provide valuable insights into the interactions between SF and other cell types relevant to glaucoma, such as retinal ganglion cells or trabecular meshwork cells. *In vitro* models can be developed to mimic glaucomatous conditions by subjecting SF to mechanical stress or cyclic stretching, enabling the study of their response to elevated intraocular pressure. Secretome analysis techniques, such as ELISA or multiplex immunoassays, can be employed to examine the factors secreted by SF cultures, providing insights into their role in modulating glaucoma-related processes. In conclusion, these protocols serve as a valuable resource for researchers investigating SF in the context of glaucoma research on the anterior segment.

[*] **Corresponding author Veluchamy A. Barathi:** Translational Pre-Clinical Model Platform, Singapore Eye Research Institute, ACP in Ophthalmology & Visual Sciences, DUKE-NUS Graduate Medical School, Department of Ophthalmology, Yong Loo Lin School of Medicine, National University of Singapore, Singapore 119077, Singapore; Tel: +65 65767275; E-mails: ophvab@nus.edu.sg, amutha.b.veluchamy@seri.com.sg

Najam A. Sharif and Sunny E. Ohia (Eds.)

Keywords: Cell culture, Characterization, Cell proliferation, Co-culture, Extracellular matrix, Flow cytometry, Isolation, Immunocytochemistry, Scleral fibroblasts, Viability assays.

INTRODUCTION

Glaucoma is a progressive optic neuropathy characterized by the degeneration of retinal ganglion cells (RGCs) and corresponding visual field loss. It is one of the leading causes of irreversible blindness worldwide, affecting millions of individuals (Mélik PS *et al.*, 2020). Despite extensive research, the underlying mechanisms of glaucoma pathogenesis remain incompletely understood (Razeghinejad R *et al.*, 2020). However, recent studies have suggested the involvement of various ocular cell types, including scleral fibroblasts, in the development and progression of glaucoma (Wong, T. Y. *et al.*, 2014; Downs JC., 2015; Pitha I, *et al.*, 2018; Minnelli C *et al.*, 2023).

The anterior segment of the eye plays a crucial role in maintaining ocular homeostasis and proper visual function. Among the various cell types present in the anterior segment, scleral fibroblasts have gained significant attention in recent years due to their involvement in the pathogenesis of glaucoma, a leading cause of irreversible blindness worldwide. Scleral fibroblasts are responsible for maintaining the structural integrity of the sclera and regulating extracellular matrix (ECM) remodeling, which can directly impact intraocular pressure (IOP) and optic nerve health (Soma, T., *et al.*, 2017). They are responsible for synthesizing and remodeling the ECM, which provides mechanical support to the ocular tissues (Downs JC., 2015; Wang, W., *et al.*, 2017). In glaucoma, alterations in scleral fibroblast behavior and ECM remodeling have been observed, leading to changes in scleral biomechanics and potentially contributing to the development of elevated IOP and retinal ganglion cells (RGC) degeneration (Agarwal R *et al.*, 2019; Iomdina EN *et al.*, 2020; Boote C. *et al.*, 2020). An area of key importance is the ability of FP-receptor-class prostaglandins to release matrix metalloproteinases from SF to help digest ECM in the uveoscleral outflow pathway to lower IOP in the treatment of glaucoma (Weinreb et al., 2004; Sharif *et al.*, 2023).

To better understand the molecular mechanisms underlying glaucoma and the involvement of scleral fibroblasts, it is essential to isolate and characterize these cells effectively. Several protocols have been developed to isolate ocular cells from the anterior segment, including the sclera. These protocols involve the enzymatic digestion of ocular tissues, followed by cell isolation and culture techniques tailored to the specific cell type of interest.

In this chapter, we will discuss the various protocols available for the isolation and characterization of scleral fibroblasts, focusing on the anterior segment of the eye. We will explore the different enzymatic digestion methods, the selection of appropriate culture media and conditions, and the characterization techniques commonly used to assess fibroblast phenotype, viability, proliferation, and ECM production. Additionally, we will highlight the importance of quality control measures to ensure the reliability and reproducibility of the isolated cells.

Understanding the molecular and cellular changes in scleral fibroblasts associated with glaucoma can provide valuable insights into the pathogenesis of the disease. This knowledge may lead to the identification of novel therapeutic targets for the prevention or treatment of glaucoma, as well as the development of tissue engineering strategies aimed at restoring scleral homeostasis and preserving visual function.

EXPERIMENTAL PROTOCOLS

The following procedures were performed in compliance with the guidelines of the Canadian Council on Animal Care for the Use of Experimental Animals and the Statement for the Use of Animals in Ophthalmic and Visual Research from the Association for Research in Vision and Ophthalmology (ARVO).

ISOLATION OF SCLERAL FIBROBLASTS

Materials

Enucleated eyes from human or animal donors

Dulbecco's modified Eagle's medium (DMEM)

Fetal bovine serum (FBS)

Penicillin-streptomycin solution

Trypsin-EDTA solution

Phosphate-buffered saline (PBS)

Sterile surgical instruments (scalpel, forceps, scissors)

70% ethanol

Tissue culture plates or dishes

Cell culture incubator (37°C, 5% CO_2)

Cell Culture Vessels

Use tissue culture-treated plastic dishes or flasks for seeding the isolated cells. These vessels are designed to support cell attachment and growth.

Culture Medium

Prepare a suitable culture medium to support the growth and maintenance of scleral fibroblasts. The specific composition of the medium may vary depending on the desired experimental conditions or protocols. A commonly used medium for fibroblast culture is Dulbecco's Modified Eagle Medium (DMEM) or a similar basal medium. The medium should be supplemented with fetal bovine serum (FBS) and antibiotics.

Fetal Bovine Serum (FBS)

Add FBS to the culture medium as a source of essential nutrients, growth factors, and hormones necessary for cell proliferation and survival. The recommended concentration of FBS can vary, but it is typically around 10-20% (vol/vol) for fibroblast culture.

Antibiotics

Include antibiotics in the culture medium to prevent bacterial or fungal contamination. Commonly used antibiotics are penicillin and streptomycin, which provide broad-spectrum coverage. The concentrations of antibiotics can vary, but a typical concentration is 100 units/mL of penicillin and 100 µg/mL of streptomycin.

Incubation Conditions

Maintain the cultured cells in a controlled environment with specific temperature and atmospheric conditions. The standard conditions for scleral fibroblast culture include:

Temperature

Set the incubator to a defined temperature, usually 37°C (98.6°F). This temperature closely mimics the physiological conditions of the human body.

Humidity

Ensure a humidified atmosphere within the incubator. The humidity level should be kept high to prevent excessive evaporation and desiccation of the cells.

Carbon Dioxide (CO_2) Concentration

Maintain a carbon dioxide level of 5% in the incubator. This concentration helps to maintain pH balance in the culture medium, as well as provides an optimal environment for cell growth.

Overall, these culture conditions provide a suitable environment for scleral fibroblasts to adhere, proliferate, and maintain their characteristic properties. Regular monitoring, feeding, and passage of the cells are required to ensure their healthy growth and viability.

Preparation

Sterilize surgical instruments and work area with 70% ethanol.

Prepare DMEM supplemented with 10% FBS and 1% penicillin-streptomycin solution and pre-warm it in the cell culture incubator.

Eye Dissection

Place the enucleated eye in a sterile dish.

Rinse the eye with PBS to remove any external contaminants.

Use a scalpel and scissors to carefully remove the cornea and iris, exposing the sclera.

Cut the sclera into small pieces (1-2 mm) using scissors and forceps.

Tissue Digestion

Transfer the scleral tissue pieces to a sterile tissue culture plate.

Add a sufficient amount of trypsin-EDTA solution to cover the tissue pieces and incubate at 37°C for 30-60 minutes to allow digestion.

Gently agitate the plate every 10-15 minutes to enhance tissue dissociation.

Cell Isolation

After the incubation period, gently pipette the digested tissue suspension to break up the tissue clumps.

Transfer the suspension to a new sterile tube and centrifuge at low speed (*e.g.*, 200-300 × g) for 5 minutes to pellet the cells.

Discard the supernatant and resuspend the cell pellet in DMEM supplemented with 10% FBS.

CELL CULTURE

Plate the cells in tissue culture plates or dishes at a density of approximately 5,000-10,000 cells/cm^2.

Incubate the plates in a cell culture incubator at 37°C with 5% CO_2.

Maintain the cells in DMEM supplemented with 10% FBS and 1% penicillin-streptomycin solution, and change the medium every 2-3 days.

Allow the cells to reach confluency before passaging or using them for further experiments.

Characterization of Scleral Fibroblasts

Once the scleral fibroblasts have been isolated, they can be characterized using various techniques. Here are a few common methods:

Morphological Analysis

Observe the cells under an inverted phase-contrast microscope to assess their morphology, including spindle-shaped fibroblast-like appearance (Fig. **1**).

Cell Proliferation Assay

Assess the proliferative capacity of the scleral fibroblasts using assays such as the MTT (3-(4,5-dimethylthiazol-2-yl)-2,5-diphenyltetrazolium bromide) assay or BrdU (bromodeoxyuridine) incorporation assay (Fig. **2**).

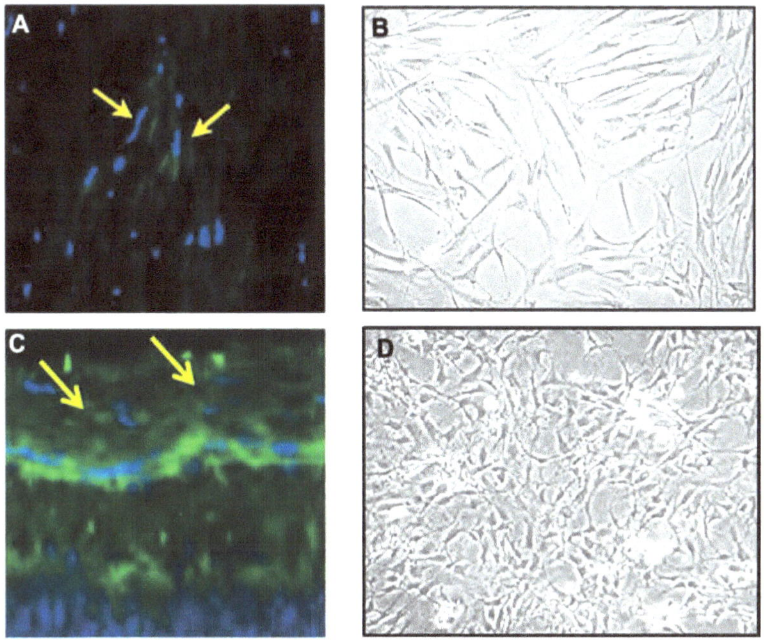

Fig. (1). Morphology of scleral fibroblasts in tissue and culture conditions.
1A: Human scleral tissue (magnification 200X). Arrow indicates scleral fibroblasts.
1B: Human scleral fibroblasts in culture condition.
1C: Mouse scleral tissue (magnification 200X). Arrow indicates scleral fibroblasts.
1D: Mouse Scleral fibroblasts in culture condition

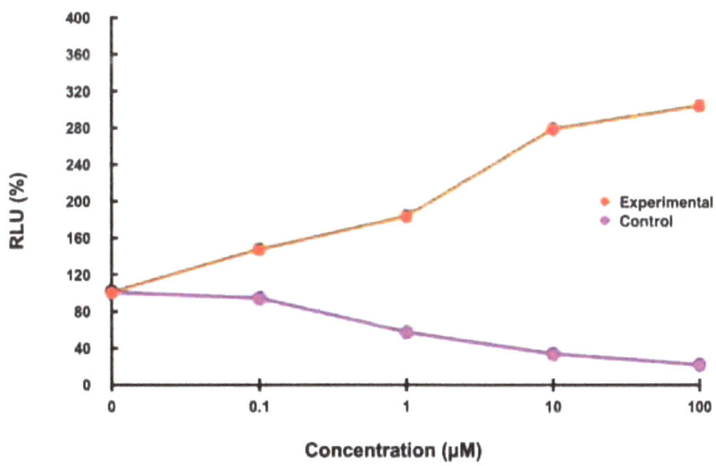

Fig. (2). Scleral fibroblast cell proliferation.
BrdU (Bromodeoxyuridine / 5-bromo-2'-deoxyuridine) is an analog of the nucleoside thymidine used in the BrdU assay to identify proliferating cells. BrdU labeling was performed from primary SF cell cultures to identify cell proliferation in experimental and control cells. BrdU incorporation is a measure of DNA synthesis rate reflecting the rate of cell proliferation.

Follow the manufacturer's instructions to perform the chosen assay.

MTT Assay

Prepare a stock solution of MTT (3-(4,5-dimethylthiazol-2-yl--2,5-diphenyltetrazolium bromide) in phosphate-buffered saline (PBS) at a concentration of 5 mg/mL.

Plate the scleral fibroblasts in a 96-well plate at the desired density (*e.g.*, 5,000 cells per well) and incubate them under suitable conditions (*e.g.*, 37°C, 5% CO_2) for attachment.

Treat the cells with different experimental conditions or treatments as required.

After the desired treatment period, add MTT solution to each well at a final concentration of 0.5 mg/mL.

Incubate the plate for 2-4 hours at the appropriate temperature (*e.g.*, 37°C) to allow the conversion of MTT to formazan crystals by metabolically active cells.

Carefully remove the culture medium from the wells without disturbing the formed formazan crystals.

Add a suitable solvent (*e.g.*, dimethyl sulfoxide or DMSO) to each well to dissolve the formazan crystals.

Gently shake the plate or pipette up and down to ensure complete dissolution of the formazan crystals.

Measure the absorbance of the resulting solution at a wavelength around 570 nm using a microplate reader.

The absorbance is directly proportional to the number of metabolically active cells, and the values can be used to assess the proliferative capacity of the scleral fibroblasts.

BrdU Incorporation Assay

Plate the scleral fibroblasts in a suitable culture vessel (*e.g.*, 24-well plate or chamber slides) at the desired density and incubate them under appropriate conditions for attachment.

Treat the cells with different experimental conditions or treatments as required.

Add BrdU (bromodeoxyuridine) to the culture medium at a suitable concentration (*e.g.*, 10 μM) and incubate the cells for a specific period of time (*e.g.*, 1-4 hours).

After the incubation period, carefully remove the culture medium from the wells.

Fix the cells with a suitable fixative (*e.g.*, 4% paraformaldehyde) for 15-20 minutes at room temperature.

Wash the cells with PBS to remove any residual fixative.

Permeabilize the cells by incubating them with a permeabilization buffer (*e.g.*, 0.1% Triton X-100 in PBS) for 10-15 minutes at room temperature.

Block non-specific binding sites by incubating the cells with a blocking solution (*e.g.*, 1% bovine serum albumin in PBS) for 1 hour at room temperature.

Incubate the cells with an anti-BrdU antibody diluted in a blocking solution for the recommended time and temperature according to the manufacturer's instructions.

Wash the cells with PBS to remove unbound primary antibodies.

Incubate the cells with a suitable secondary antibody conjugated to a fluorescent dye (*e.g.*, Alexa Fluor) diluted in the blocking solution for the recommended time and temperature.

Wash the cells with PBS to remove unbound secondary antibodies.

Mount the cells with a mounting medium containing a nuclear counterstain (*e.g.*, DAPI).

Visualize the cells using a fluorescence microscope.

Immunocytochemistry

Materials

Scleral fibroblasts

Cell culture medium

Phosphate-buffered saline (PBS)

Fixative (*e.g.*, 4% paraformaldehyde)

Permeabilization buffer (*e.g.*, 0.1% Triton X-100 in PBS)

Blocking solution (*e.g.*, 1% bovine serum albumin in PBS)

Primary antibodies against fibroblast markers (*e.g.*, vimentin, fibronectin)

Secondary antibody conjugated to a fluorophore (*e.g.*, Alexa Fluor)

Mounting medium containing a nuclear counterstain (*e.g.*, DAPI)

Microscope slides

Coverslips

Pipettes and pipette tips

Incubator

Humidified chamber or slide rack

Fluorescence microscope

Protocol

Plate the scleral fibroblasts in a suitable culture vessel (*e.g.*, 24-well plate or chamber slides) at the desired density and incubate them under appropriate conditions for attachment and growth.

When the cells have reached the desired confluency or experimental time point, carefully aspirate the culture medium from the wells.

Rinse the cells with PBS to remove any residual medium or debris.

Fix the cells by adding an appropriate volume of fixative (*e.g.*, 4% paraformaldehyde) directly to the wells or culture vessel. Incubate for 15-20 minutes at room temperature.

Carefully remove the fixative and wash the cells with PBS to remove any residual fixative.

Permeabilize the cells by adding permeabilization buffer (*e.g.*, 0.1% Triton X-100 in PBS) to each well or culture vessel. Incubate for 10-15 minutes at room temperature.

Remove the permeabilization buffer and wash the cells with PBS.

Block non-specific binding sites by adding blocking solution (*e.g.*, 1% bovine serum albumin in PBS) to each well or culture vessel. Incubate for 1 hour at room temperature or according to the recommended time by the manufacturer.

Dilute the primary antibody against the target protein in the blocking solution. Add the diluted primary antibody to each well or culture vessel. Incubate for the recommended time and temperature as specified by the manufacturer.

After the incubation, carefully remove the primary antibody solution and wash the cells with PBS to remove the unbound antibody.

Dilute the secondary antibody conjugated to a fluorophore (*e.g.*, Alexa Fluor) in a blocking solution. Add the diluted secondary antibody to each well or culture vessel. Incubate for the recommended time and temperature specified by the manufacturer.

Remove the secondary antibody solution and wash the cells with PBS to remove the unbound antibody.

If desired, counterstain the nuclei by adding a mounting medium containing a nuclear counterstain (*e.g.*, DAPI) to each well or culture vessel.

Carefully place a coverslip over the cells, taking care to avoid trapping air bubbles.

Allow the mounting medium to dry, and seal the edges of the coverslip with nail polish or an appropriate sealant.

Place the slides in a slide rack or a humidified chamber to prevent drying.

Visualize the immunostained cells using a fluorescence microscope. Adjust the microscope settings (*e.g.*, excitation and emission wavelengths) according to the fluorophores used (Fig. **3**).

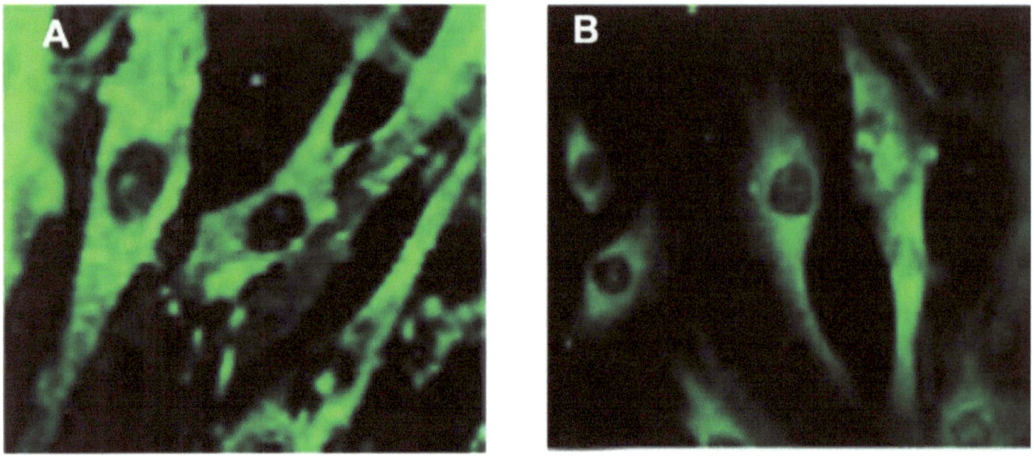

Fig. (3). Immunocytochemistry images of scleral fibroblasts in culture.
3A: Immunocytochemistry of human scleral fibroblasts, which are stained by fibroblast marker (in Green).
3B: Immunocytochemistry of mouse scleral fibroblasts, which are stained by fibroblast marker (in Green).

Note: The specific concentrations and incubation times may vary depending on the antibodies and protocols recommended by the manufacturers. It is always important to refer to the antibody datasheet and manufacturer's instructions for optimal conditions.

Protocols for Scleral Fibroblasts and Extracellular Matrix (ECM) Production

This may vary depending on the specific experimental design and desired outcomes. However, here we provided a general outline of the protocols involved in isolating scleral fibroblasts and promoting ECM production.

Isolation and Culture of Scleral Fibroblasts

Tissue Collection

Obtain fresh scleral tissue from a suitable animal model (*e.g.*, rabbits, mice, or pigs) or human donors. Follow ethical guidelines and obtain necessary approvals.

Work in a sterile environment using a laminar flow hood.

Tissue Processing

Rinse the scleral tissue with a sterile phosphate-buffered saline (PBS) solution to remove any blood or debris.

tructions for the transfer apparatu

Trim the tissue into small pieces (approximately 1-2 mm in size) using sterile scissors or a scalpel.

Enzymatic Digestion

Prepare a collagenase solution by dissolving collagenase type II or IV in Dulbecco's Modified Eagle's Medium (DMEM) supplemented with antibiotics (*e.g.*, penicillin/streptomycin).

Transfer the scleral tissue pieces into a sterile container and add enough collagenase solution to cover the tissue.

Incubate the tissue-collagenase mixture at 37°C for 2-4 hours with gentle agitation (*e.g.*, on a shaker) to allow enzymatic digestion.

Cell Isolation

After the incubation period, transfer the tissue-collagenase mixture into a sterile centrifuge tube and add an equal volume of DMEM to stop the enzymatic digestion.

Centrifuge the tube at a low speed (*e.g.*, 200-300 × g) for 5 minutes to pellet the cells.

Discard the supernatant and resuspend the cell pellet in DMEM supplemented with fetal bovine serum (FBS) and antibiotics.

Count the cells using a hemocytometer or an automated cell counter, and adjust the cell suspension concentration as required.

Cell Culture

Plate the isolated scleral fibroblasts in tissue culture dishes or flasks pre-coated with extracellular matrix proteins (*e.g.*, collagen or fibronectin) or use tissue culture-treated plates without coating.

Maintain the cells in a suitable culture medium, such as DMEM supplemented with FBS (10% v/v) and antibiotics.

Culture the cells at 37°C in a humidified incubator with 5% CO_2.

Replace the medium every 2-3 days and subculture the cells upon reaching confluence using standard trypsinization techniques.

Promoting ECM Production

Substrate Selection

Depending on your experimental needs, choose a suitable substrate for promoting ECM production. This can include tissue culture plastic, specialized culture inserts, or three-dimensional scaffolds.

ECM Stimulation

Treat the scleral fibroblasts with specific growth factors or cytokines known to promote ECM synthesis and deposition. Commonly used factors include transforming growth factor-beta (TGF-β), fibroblast growth factor (FGF), or platelet-derived growth factor (PDGF).

Determine the optimal concentration and duration of stimulation for your experimental setup through pilot experiments or previous literature.

ECM Analysis

Assess ECM production using various techniques such as immunofluorescence staining, Western blotting, or quantitative polymerase chain reaction (qPCR).

Immunostain the cultured cells using specific antibodies against ECM proteins (*e.g.*, collagen I, collagen III, or fibronectin) to visualize their expression and distribution.

Analyze the protein expression levels by Western blotting or enzyme-linked immunosorbent assay (ELISA).

Measure mRNA levels using qPCR to evaluate the transcriptional changes in ECM-related genes.

To Detect Scleral Fibroblasts Using Western Blotting

To detect scleral fibroblasts using Western blotting, you will need to follow a series of protocols. Here is a step-by-step guide

Sample Collection and Protein Extraction

Obtain scleral tissue samples from the desired experimental subjects or patients.

Cut the scleral tissue into small pieces and homogenize it in a suitable lysis buffer. The lysis buffer should contain protease and phosphatase inhibitors to prevent protein degradation.

Incubate the homogenized samples on ice for 30 minutes to allow complete cell lysis and protein extraction.

Centrifuge the lysates at high speed (*e.g.*, 12,000 x g) for 15 minutes at 4°C to pellet cell debris. Collect the supernatant containing the protein lysate.

Protein Quantification

Determine the protein concentration in the lysates using a suitable protein quantification method, such as the Bradford assay or BCA assay. This step ensures that you load equal amounts of protein in each lane of the gel.

SDS-PAGE Gel Electrophoresis

Prepare a denaturing polyacrylamide gel for SDS-PAGE according to the desired protein size range. Generally, 8-12% acrylamide gels are suitable for most proteins.

Mix the protein lysates with an appropriate volume of loading buffer containing a reducing agent (*e.g.*, β-mercaptoethanol or DTT) and denature the samples by heating them at 95°C for 5 minutes.

Load equal amounts of denatured protein (based on the protein quantification) into each well of the gel.

Run the gel at a constant voltage until the protein bands have sufficiently separated. The duration and voltage depend on the gel percentage and apparatus being used.

Protein Transfer

After electrophoresis, carefully transfer the separated proteins from the gel to a nitrocellulose or PVDF membrane using a semi-dry or wet transfer apparatus. Ensure the transfer is performed in a cold room or at 4°C to maintain protein integrity.

Use an appropriate transfer buffer (*e.g.*, Towbin's buffer, Tris-glycine buffer) and follow the manufacturer's instructions for the transfer apparatus.

Membrane Blocking

Block the transferred membrane by incubating it in a blocking solution (*e.g.*, 5% non-fat dry milk or BSA) for 1-2 hours at room temperature or overnight at 4°C. This step prevents the non-specific binding of antibodies to the membrane.

Primary Antibody Incubation

Dilute the primary antibody against the scleral fibroblast-specific marker according to the manufacturer's instructions. Common markers for fibroblasts include vimentin or fibronectin.

Incubate the membrane with the primary antibody solution overnight at 4°C or for 2-3 hours at room temperature with gentle shaking.

Washing

Wash the membrane several times (3-5 times) with a suitable washing buffer (*e.g.*, PBS-T or TBST) to remove unbound primary antibodies. Each wash step should be for 5-10 minutes with gentle agitation.

Secondary Antibody Incubation

Prepare a secondary antibody solution conjugated to an enzyme, such as horseradish peroxidase (HRP), according to the manufacturer's instructions.

Incubate the membrane with the secondary antibody solution for 1-2 hours at room temperature with gentle shaking.

Washing

Wash the membrane again with the washing buffer, as described in step 7.

Visualization and Detection

Use an appropriate detection method, such as chemiluminescence or fluorescence, based on the secondary antibody used.

Apply the detection reagents (*e.g.*, ECL substrate) to the membrane according to the manufacturer's instructions.

Capture the chemiluminescent or fluorescent signal using an imaging system or X-ray film.

Data Analysis

Analyze the Western blot image to quantify the protein bands of interest using suitable software or densitometry techniques.

Compare the protein expression levels between samples, including scleral fibroblasts, and analyze the data statistically if applicable.

Detecting Scleral Fibroblasts using an Enzyme-Linked Immunosorbent Assay (ELISA)

Detecting scleral fibroblasts using an enzyme-linked immunosorbent assay (ELISA) involves a series of steps that include sample preparation, coating the ELISA plate, incubation with primary and secondary antibodies, and detection of the signal. Here is a detailed protocol for detecting scleral fibroblasts *via* ELISA.

Sample Preparation

- Obtain the scleral fibroblast samples. These can be cell lysates or tissue homogenates.
- Ensure that the samples are properly stored and handled to maintain protein integrity.
- Centrifuge the samples at a suitable speed and duration to remove any debris or insoluble components. Collect the supernatant containing the protein of interest.

Coating the ELISA Plate

- Prepare a suitable coating buffer (*e.g.*, phosphate-buffered saline, PBS) at the desired pH (typically pH 7.2-7.4).
- Dilute the protein samples in the coating buffer to an appropriate concentration (typically 1-10 μg/mL) depending on the expected concentration of the target antigen.
- Add the diluted samples to the wells of a microplate (ELISA plate) and incubate overnight at 4°C or for a few hours at room temperature to allow the protein to adhere to the plate surface.
- After the incubation, aspirate the protein solution from the wells and wash the plate multiple times with a suitable wash buffer (*e.g.*, PBS with 0.05% Tween-20) to remove any unbound proteins.

Blocking

- Prepare a blocking buffer (*e.g.*, PBS containing 1% bovine serum albumin, BSA) to prevent non-specific binding of antibodies.
- Add the blocking buffer to each well and incubate for 1-2 hours at room

temperature or overnight at 4°C.

- After incubation, aspirate the blocking buffer and wash the plate as described in step 2d.

Primary Antibody Incubation

- Dilute the primary antibody specific for scleral fibroblasts in a suitable antibody diluent (*e.g.*, PBS with 1% BSA).
- Add the diluted primary antibody to the wells and incubate for 1-2 hours at room temperature or overnight at 4°C to allow binding of the primary antibody to the target antigen.
- Aspirate the primary antibody solution and wash the plate as described in step 2d.

Secondary Antibody Incubation

- Prepare a secondary antibody solution conjugated to an enzyme such as horseradish peroxidase (HRP) or alkaline phosphatase (AP).
- Dilute the secondary antibody in the antibody diluent.
- Add the diluted secondary antibody to the wells and incubate for 1-2 hours at room temperature.
- Aspirate the secondary antibody solution and wash the plate as described in step 2d.

Detection

- Prepare a suitable substrate solution for the enzyme conjugated to the secondary antibody. The choice of substrate depends on the enzyme used (*e.g.*, HRP substrate like TMB or AP substrate like p-nitrophenyl phosphate, PNPP).
- Add the substrate solution to each well and incubate for the appropriate time period, usually 10-30 minutes, at room temperature in the dark.
- Stop the enzymatic reaction by adding a stop solution appropriate for the substrate used (*e.g.*, sulfuric acid for TMB or sodium hydroxide for PNPP).
- Measure the absorbance or color development using a microplate reader at the appropriate wavelength for the substrate used.

Data Analysis

- Determine the absorbance or color intensity of each well using the microplate reader.
- Compare the absorbance or color intensity of the wells containing the samples with the standards or controls to quantify the presence of scleral fibroblasts.
- Perform appropriate statistical analysis to interpret the results.

Note: It is important to optimize the concentrations of the primary antibody, secondary antibody, and substrate solution, as well as the incubation times and temperatures, for the specific assay conditions and reagents used. The protocol provided serves as a general guideline and may require adjustments based on the specific requirements of the antibodies and reagents used in your experiment.

Assessing Extracellular Matrix (ECM) Production Using Quantitative Polymerase Chain Reaction (qPCR)

Assessing extracellular matrix (ECM) production using quantitative polymerase chain reaction (qPCR) involves measuring the expression levels of ECM-related genes. Here is a detailed protocol for performing qPCR to assess ECM production

RNA Extraction

- Collect the cells or tissue samples of interest and homogenize them in a suitable RNA extraction reagent, such as TRIzol or a commercial RNA extraction kit, following the manufacturer's instructions.
- Centrifuge the homogenate to separate the aqueous phase containing RNA from the organic phase.
- Transfer the aqueous phase to a fresh tube and add an equal volume of isopropanol to precipitate the RNA.
- Mix gently and incubate the sample at room temperature for 10 minutes.
- Centrifuge the sample at high speed to pellet the RNA.
- Discard the supernatant and wash the RNA pellet with 75% ethanol.
- Air-dry the RNA pellet and dissolve it in nuclease-free water.
- Measure the RNA concentration and assess its quality using a spectrophotometer or a dedicated RNA analyzer.

cDNA Synthesis

- Use a reverse transcription kit to synthesize complementary DNA (cDNA) from the RNA template. Follow the manufacturer's instructions for the specific kit used.
- Prepare a reaction mixture containing RNA, reverse transcriptase enzyme, oligo(dT) primers or random primers, dNTPs, and reaction buffer.
- Incubate the reaction mixture at an appropriate temperature and duration for reverse transcription (usually 42-55°C for 30-60 minutes).
- Inactivate the reverse transcriptase enzyme by heating the reaction mixture at a higher temperature (*e.g.*, 70-85°C for 5 minutes).

Primer Design

- Design specific primers for the target ECM-related genes of interest. Primers should be specific to the gene of interest and avoid regions of potential genomic DNA contamination.
- Ensure that the primers have similar melting temperatures (Tm) and minimal secondary structures or primer-dimer formation.
- Verify the primer specificity by performing a BLAST search against the target sequence.

qPCR Setup

- Prepare a master mix containing the qPCR reagents, including DNA polymerase, dNTPs, buffer, and fluorescent dyes (*e.g.*, SYBR Green or TaqMan probes), following the manufacturer's instructions.

- Add the cDNA template, specific primers, and the master mix to individual wells of a qPCR plate or PCR tubes. Include negative controls (no-template control and no-reverse transcriptase control) for each primer pair.
- Seal the plate or tubes and centrifuge briefly to ensure proper mixing.

qPCR Amplification

- Place the qPCR plate or tubes in a real-time PCR instrument.
- Perform qPCR amplification with the appropriate cycling conditions, including denaturation, annealing, and extension steps. The cycling parameters and conditions depend on the specific instrument and the primers used.
- Collect fluorescence data during each amplification cycle to monitor the accumulation of PCR products.

Data Analysis

- Analyze the qPCR data using the software provided by the PCR instrument or dedicated analysis software.
- Determine the cycle threshold (Ct) values, which represent the cycle number at which the fluorescence signal exceeds a predefined threshold.
- Calculate the relative gene expression levels using the $2^{-\Delta\Delta Ct}$ method or other appropriate methods, normalizing to reference genes or internal controls.
- Perform statistical analysis to assess the significance of the differences in gene expression levels between samples.

Note: Ensure proper experimental controls, such as negative controls and reference genes, and replicate samples to ensure reliable and accurate qPCR results. It is essential to optimize the primer concentrations, annealing temperatures, and other experimental conditions for each specific gene and experimental setup.

Co-culture Experiments

Co-culture experiments involving the interaction between scleral fibroblasts (SF) and other cell types relevant to glaucoma, such as retinal ganglion cells (RGCs) or trabecular meshwork cells (TMCs), can provide valuable insights into the cellular crosstalk and molecular mechanisms underlying glaucoma pathology. Here is a detailed protocol for performing co-culture experiments:

Cell Culture

- Culture SF, RGCs, and TMCs separately in appropriate culture media supplemented with necessary growth factors, cytokines, and supplements following standard cell culture protocols.
- Maintain the cells at suitable conditions, including temperature, humidity, and CO_2 levels, as recommended for each cell type.
- Passage the cells when they reach confluence or as per their growth characteristics.

Co-culture Setup

- Determine the appropriate cell ratio for co-culturing SF with RGCs or TMCs based on the specific research objectives and previous studies.
- Prepare culture vessels (plates, inserts, or chambers) suitable for co-culture experiments, ensuring compatibility with the cell types and assay requirements.
- Seed SF and the respective target cells (RGCs or TMCs) separately in their respective culture vessels according to the desired cell ratio.
- Allow the cells to adhere and stabilize for a specified duration (*e.g.*, 24-48 hours) before initiating co-culture.

Direct Co-culture

- Combine SF and the respective target cells by physically mixing them together in the same culture vessel.
- Maintain the cells in co-culture media formulated to support the growth requirements of both cell types. Optimize the composition and formulation of the co-culture media based on the specific experimental goals.
- Incubate the co-culture at appropriate conditions as recommended for the respective cell types.

Indirect Co-culture (Transwell or Inserts)

- Seed SF and the respective target cells in separate culture vessels (*e.g.*, plates or flasks).
- Place inserts or transwell membranes with appropriate pore sizes in the wells of a culture plate.
- Seed SF in the upper compartment of the insert and the target cells in the lower compartment.
- Add co-culture media to both compartments, allowing for the exchange of soluble factors without direct cell-to-cell contact.
- Incubate the co-culture at suitable conditions, ensuring proper gas exchange and maintaining sterility.

Monitoring Co-culture

- Regularly monitor the co-culture system under a microscope to observe cell morphology, proliferation, and interaction between SF and target cells.

- Perform periodic medium changes as required to maintain cell viability and optimize experimental conditions.
- Consider time points appropriate for the specific research objectives to collect samples or perform assays.

Sample Collection and Analysis

- At the desired time points, carefully collect co-culture samples for analysis, which can include cell harvesting, RNA/protein extraction, or specific functional assays.
- Perform downstream assays such as qPCR, Western blotting, immunofluorescence staining, enzyme-linked immunosorbent assay (ELISA), or functional assays relevant to glaucoma pathology.
- Analyze and interpret the results, comparing co-culture samples with monocultures of SF, RGCs, or TMCs as controls.

Controls and Experimental Considerations

- Include appropriate controls, such as monocultures of SF, RGCs, or TMCs, to assess cell-specific effects and account for potential artifacts.
- Consider technical replicates and biological replicates to ensure the reproducibility and reliability of the co-culture experiments.
- Optimize the cell seeding densities, co-culture duration, and culture conditions to achieve the desired outcomes and minimize potential confounding factors.
- Adhere to ethical guidelines and regulations for working with human or animal-derived cells, if applicable.

Note: It is important to adapt and modify the protocol based on the specific cell types, research objectives, and available resources. The co-culture conditions, medium composition, and duration may require optimization to achieve the desired cellular interactions and obtain meaningful results.

In vitro models to mimic glaucomatous conditions

Developing *in vitro* models to mimic glaucomatous conditions by subjecting scleral fibroblasts (SF) to mechanical stress or cyclic stretching can provide insights into the cellular and molecular responses of SF to elevated intraocular pressure. Here is a detailed protocol for developing such an *in vitro* model:

Cell Culture

- Culture SF in appropriate culture media supplemented with necessary growth factors, cytokines, and supplements following standard cell culture protocols.

- Maintain SF at suitable conditions, including temperature, humidity, and CO_2 levels, as recommended for the cell type.
- Passage the cells when they reach confluence or as per their growth characteristics.

Mechanical Stress/Stretching Setup

- Select an appropriate system for applying mechanical stress or cyclic stretching to the SF culture. This can include specialized stretching devices, custom-built systems, or commercially available systems.
- Follow the manufacturer's instructions or design a suitable setup that allows controlled application of mechanical stress or cyclic stretching to the SF culture.
- Consider the desired parameters, such as magnitude, frequency, and duration of the mechanical stress or stretching, based on previous studies and the specific objectives of your research.

Mechanical Stress/Stretching Protocol

- Seed SF in appropriate culture vessels (*e.g.*, plates, culture inserts) at desired densities to ensure optimal cell confluence.
- Place the SF culture vessels within the mechanical stress or stretching setup.
- Apply the desired mechanical stress or cyclic stretching according to the established parameters. This can involve applying compressive or tensile forces or cyclic stretching using mechanical actuators or computer-controlled systems.
- Ensure proper alignment and attachment of the SF culture vessels to the mechanical stress or stretching setup to enable uniform and controlled stress application.

- Initiate the mechanical stress or stretching protocol for the specified duration, which can range from minutes to hours or even days, depending on the experimental requirements.

Control Group

- Include a control group of SF that is cultured under normal static conditions without any mechanical stress or stretching.
- Maintain the control group under the same culture conditions (*e.g.*, temperature, humidity, CO_2 levels) as the mechanically stressed or stretched SF.

Monitoring and Sampling

- Monitor the SF culture during the mechanical stress or stretching period using appropriate microscopy techniques to assess cell morphology, alignment, and response to the applied mechanical stimuli.

- Consider sampling SF at various time points during and after the mechanical stress or stretching period to study immediate and prolonged cellular responses.
- Collect samples for downstream analysis, which may include RNA/protein extraction, immunofluorescence staining, biochemical assays, or functional assays relevant to glaucoma pathology.

Analysis

- Perform appropriate assays to analyze the cellular and molecular responses of SF to mechanical stress or stretching. This can include gene expression analysis, protein expression analysis, immunostaining, cytokine profiling, or functional assays such as cell contractility or ECM remodeling assays.
- Compare the results of mechanically stressed or stretched SF with the control group to identify specific responses associated with elevated intraocular pressure mimicked by mechanical stress or stretching.

Controls and Experimental Considerations

- Include appropriate controls, such as SF cultured under static conditions, to account for the effects of mechanical stress or stretching on SF responses.
- Consider technical replicates and biological replicates to ensure the reproducibility and reliability of the experiments.
- Optimize the parameters of the mechanical stress or stretching, such as magnitude, frequency, and duration, to achieve relevant glaucomatous conditions and minimize potential confounding factors.
- Adhere to ethical guidelines and regulations for working with human or animal-derived cells, if applicable.

Note: This protocol serves as a general guideline, and it may require adjustments based on the specific equipment, SF culture conditions, and experimental objectives.

CONCLUSION

This chapter has provided detailed protocols for the isolation, culture, and characterization of scleral fibroblasts. These protocols serve as valuable tools for researchers interested in investigating the cellular and molecular mechanisms underlying scleral remodeling. By understanding the behavior and characteristics of scleral fibroblasts, researchers can gain insights into the pathogenesis of ocular disorders and develop novel therapeutic strategies.

These protocols provide a starting point for studying scleral fibroblasts and their involvement in glaucoma research. Depending on the specific research objectives, additional techniques and approaches may be employed to gain further insights into the cellular and molecular mechanisms underlying glaucoma pathogenesis.

ACKNOWLEDGEMENTS

The authors would like to thank Weon Sung Rhan for her technical support.

REFERENCES

Gupta, SK, Agarwal, R, Agarwal, P, Saxena, R, Agrawal, S & Agrawal, P (2009) Current concepts in the pathophysiology of glaucoma. *Indian J Ophthalmol,* 57, 257-66.
[http://dx.doi.org/10.4103/0301-4738.53049] [PMID: 19574692]

Boote, C, Sigal, IA, Grytz, R, Hua, Y, Nguyen, TD & Girard, MJA (2020) Scleral structure and biomechanics. *Prog Retin Eye Res,* 74, 100773.
[http://dx.doi.org/10.1016/j.preteyeres.2019.100773] [PMID: 31412277]

Downs, JC (2015) Optic nerve head biomechanics in aging and disease. *Exp Eye Res,* 133, 19-29.
[http://dx.doi.org/10.1016/j.exer.2015.02.011] [PMID: 25819451]

Iomdina, EN, Tikhomirova, NK, Bessmertny, AM, Serebryakova, MV, Baksheeva, VE, Zalevsky, AO, Kotelin, VI, Kiseleva, OA, Kosakyan, SM, Zamyatnin, AA, Jr, Philippov, PP & Zernii, EY (2020) Alterations in proteome of human sclera associated with primary open-angle glaucoma involve proteins participating in regulation of the extracellular matrix. *Mol Vis,* 26, 623-40.
[PMID: 32913388]

Mélik Parsadaniantz, S, Réaux-le Goazigo, A, Sapienza, A, Habas, C & Baudouin, C (2020) Glaucoma: A Degenerative Optic Neuropathy Related to Neuroinflammation? *Cells 25,* 9, 535.
[http://dx.doi.org/10.3390/cells9030535]

Minnelli, C, Piva, F, Cecati, M, Armeni, T, Mobbili, G, Galeazzi, R, Melecchi, A, Cristaldi, M, Corsaro, R & Rusciano, D (2023) Meldonium Inhibits Cell Motility and Wound-Healing in Trabecular Meshwork Cells and Scleral Fibroblasts: Possible Applications in Glaucoma *Pharmaceuticals (Basel) 15,* 16, 594.
[http://dx.doi.org/10.3390/ph16040594]

Pitha, I, Oglesby, E, Chow, A, Kimball, E, Pease, ME, Schaub, J & Quigley, H (2018) Rho-Kinase Inhibition Reduces Myofibroblast Differentiation and Proliferation of Scleral Fibroblasts Induced by Transforming Growth Factor β and Experimental Glaucoma. *Transl Vis Sci Technol,* 7, 6.

[http://dx.doi.org/10.1167/tvst.7.6.6]

Razeghinejad, R, Lin, MM, Lee, D, Katz, LJ & Myers, JS (2020) Pathophysiology and management of glaucoma and ocular hypertension related to trauma. *Surv Ophthalmol,* 65, 530-47. [http://dx.doi.org/10.1016/j.survophthal.2020.02.003] [PMID: 32057763]

Sharif NA, Odani-Kawabata N, Lu F, Pinchuk L. (2023). FP and EP2 prostanoid receptor agonist drugs and aqueous humor outflow devices for treating ocular hypertension and glaucoma. Exp Eye Res. 229:109415.

Soma, T (2017) Importance of scleral fibroblasts for ocular tissue engineering. *Nippon Ganka Gakkai Zasshi,* 121, 106-17.

Wong, T. Y., et al. (2014). The epidemiology of age-related eye diseases in Asia. *The B J of Ophth, 98*(6), 674-679

Wang, W (2017) Changes of collagen types and metalloproteinase expression in the sclera of the experimental myopia guinea pig. *J Glaucoma,* 26, 689-97.

Weinreb RN, Lindsey JD, Marchenko G, Marchenko N, Angert M, Strongin A. (2004). Prostaglandin FP agonists alter metalloproteinase gene expression in sclera. Invest Ophthalmol Vis Sci. 45(12): 4368-4377.

CHAPTER 13

Protocols for Isolation and Characterization of Human Corneal Epithelial and Conjunctival Epithelial Cells

Hanna Rao[1,*] and **Najam A. Sharif**[2]

[1] *Department of Arts and Science, McMaster University, Hamilton, Ontario, Canada*

[2] *Vice President and Head of Research & Development, Nanoscope Therapeutics Inc. 2777 N. Stemmons Fwy, Suite 1102, Dallas, TX-75207, USA*

Abstract: The eye is a specialized organ composed of many types of tissues and cells. Since the ocular surface is the first point of contact with light entering the eye, environmental airborne materials, and topically applied medications, it is important to understand the features of these cells and their physiopathology. Furthermore, such characteristics and receptor/enzyme/transporter profiles of the cells can serve as targets for drug discovery and development to treat such eye disorders and/or to show the potential risks of ocular irritation and inflammation associated with certain medications. This is particularly important with respect to corneal and conjunctival epithelial cells and mast cells, which are involved in the disease mechanisms associated with dry eye syndrome, ocular allergies, and ocular surface pain. The isolated cells can also be used to study the mechanisms of actions of certain drugs such as anti-histamines, mast cell stabilizers, and steroids. This chapter aims to provide protocols to isolate, propagate, and study cells obtained from human cadaveric donor tissues. Potential ways to immortalize human corneal epithelial cells will also be described.

Keywords: Conjunctival cells, Corneal epithelial cells, Human corneal cells, Mast cells, Protocols.

INTRODUCTION

The corneal epithelium is composed of multiple layers of cells that cooperatively work together to help maintain the transparency and overall integrity of the cornea. These cells protect the eye from airborne dust, pollen, fungal spores, bacteria, viruses, and radiation. These cells can actively participate in mediating allergic and inflammatory responses and the actions of the adjoining conjunctiva. Conjunctival mast cells are a type of immune cell found in the conjunctiva, which

* **Corresponding author Hanna Rao:** Department of Arts & Science, McMaster University, 16 Dromore Crescent, Hamilton, Ontario, Canada; Tel: (905) 462 6618; E-mail: hxnnnarao@gmail.com

Najam A. Sharif and Sunny E. Ohia (Eds.)

is the clear tissue that covers the white part of the eye and lines the inner surface of the eyelids. Mast cells are a crucial part of the immune system and play a role in various ocular surface disorders (Abelson and Schaefer, 1993; Cook *et al.*, 1998). Histamine and other mediators released by mast cells trigger allergic responses such as itching, redness, and swelling of the conjunctiva, leading to a condition known as allergic conjunctivitis. Recent findings on the role of cytokines released by mast cells have heightened interest in the role of mast cells in allergic conditions (Abelson and Schaefer, 1993; Kahn *et al.*, 1993; Bradding, 1996; Sharif *et al.*, 1996; Cook *et al.*, 1998; Sharif, 2020).

Described below are procedures to isolate, characterize, and immortalize cells derived from human ocular surface tissues, including human corneal epithelial cells, human conjunctival mast cells, and epithelial cells (Cook *et al.*, 1998). The primary cells and immortalized cell line(s) can be used in mechanistic studies on ocular toxicity, irritation, and inflammation, and the latter provides a model to examine mechanistically the effect of mast cell-derived mediators on ocular surface epithelial cells and fibroblasts (Wiernas *et al.*, 1998; Sharif *et al.*, 1998a,b; Offord *et al.*, 1999; Sharif and Wiernas, 2010). Cells isolated from the human ocular surface tissues can be invaluable in exploring mechanisms of action of therapeutic drugs to treat diseases such as dry eye, allergic reactions, and pain associated with the latter or that induced by certain medicines, foreign objects, airborne pollutants, bacteria, and viruses (Abelson and Schafer, 1993; Sharif *et al.*, 1997; Yanni *et al.*, 1999; Sharif, 2020). Such cellular characterization and utility can lead to the discovery of new drugs to treat ocular surface disorders.

EXPERIMENTAL PROTOCOLS

Generally, it is recommended that the described procedures below be performed in a laminar flow-hood under sterile conditions using sterilized reagents and instruments as supplied by the manufacturers. Instructions provided should be followed to ensure the success of the experiments. Researchers are encouraged to consult original cited papers for possible additional guidance and to confirm the conditions and study procedures. Some key publications to consult include the following:

Sharif *et al.*, 1997; Yanni *et al.*, 1999; Offord *et al.*, 1999; Sharif and Wiernas, 2010.

PREPARATION, CHARACTERIZATION, AND IMMORTALIZATION OF PRIMARY CULTURES OF HUMAN CORNEAL EPITHELIAL CELLS

Cell Isolation and Characterization

- Obtain human donor eyes after death (ensure proper consent has been obtained). Dissect the cornea aseptically and rinse in phosphate-buffered saline (PBS).
- Treat with dispase at 10U/ml in 50% Hanks buffered salts and keratinocyte growth medium (KGM) at 4°C for 24-48 hrs (prepare KGM by adding 30μg/ml bovine pituitary extract, 0.5μg/ml hydrocortisone, 5μg/ml insulin, 10μg/ml transferrin, 10ng/ml murine epidermal growth factor, 0.05μg/ml amphotericin B, and 50μg/ml gentamicin to keratinocyte basal medium (KBM) that contains 0.15 mM calcium chloride. KBM, growth factors additives, and antibiotics can be purchased from Clonetics, San Deigo, CA, or Biofluids, Rockville, MD)
- Remove epithelium after incubation by gently sweeping across the tissue with a sharp scalpel blade (if possible sterile).
- To generate individual cells, triturate the tissue and then wash in Dulbecco's modified Eagles medium that contains 10% fetal bovine serum by using low-speed centrifugation-resuspension procedure.
- Resuspend the cell pellet in KGM and plate it into T25 flasks that have been previously coated with 0.1% gelatin type A (can be purchased from Sigma; Fluka Chemie AG, Buchs, Switzerland)
- Incubate at 37°C in a humidified atmosphere of 95% O_2 and 5% CO_2 and change the medium after 24hrs and then every 2 days thereafter.

Cell Immortalization

- Grow primary cultures of human corneal epithelial (P-CEPI) cells to subconfluence in KGM.
- Infect the cells 8 days after isolation with a high-titer recombinant retroviral vector pZIPSVU19, which contains the Bgll-Hpal frag-ment of SV40 T antigen and the neomycin selection marker from Moloney virus (details seen in Mace *et al.*, 1996; Pfeifer *et al.*, 1995; Offord *et al.*, 1999). The process is briefly described in the next few steps.
- Generate a high-titer virus through transfection of pZIPSVU19 into ecotropic and amphotropic packaging cell lines Psi2 and PA137, respectively, followed by coculture of the two cell lines to allow "ping-pong " infection to produce a high-titer virus.
- Infect the P-CEPI cells with 105 to 107 CFU recombinant SV40 virus in the presence of 8 /ng/ml polybrene for 2 hours. (Because of a truncated origin of replication, no SV40 can be subsequently produced in the immortalized cell

line).

- After immortalization, the human corneal epithelial (CEPI) cells subculture can produce up to 20 independent CEPI from several donors. Twenty independent CEPI cell lines from several donors can be generated. The CEPI population 17 (CEPI-17) has been shown to grow well and cloned at passage 15 by seeding the cells at very low density (100 cells per 6cm dish).
- Clones should be trypsinized and propagated separately.

Growth Conditions

- Cells should be seeded on 0.1% gelatin-coated flasks (Costar culture dishes, Integra Bioscience AG, Wallisellen, Switzerland; Gelatin type A, Sigma).
- Prepare growth medium, KGM, from KBM alone or KBM containing 0.15 mM calcium chloride with the addition of 30 μg/ml bovine pituitary extract, 0.5 μg/ml hydrocortisone, 5μg/ml insulin, 10 μg/ml transferrin, 10 ng/ml murine epidermal growth factor, 10,000 U/ml penicillin, and 10,000 μ/ml streptomycin.
- Subculture the cells by rinsing them with PBS and then incubate them in dispase (2.4U/ml in 1:1 ratio with KBM) for up to 1 hour until the cells detach by washing in KBM by centrifugation and plating in gelatin-coated flasks at 37°C in 5% CO.

Karotype and Isozyme Analysis

- Karotypes can be examined for Giemsa-banded chromosomes.
- To calculate the phenotype frequency, product enzymes such as the following can be used: lactate dehydrogenase, glucose-6-phosphate dehydrogenase, phosphoglucomutase-1, phosphoglucomutase-3, esterase D, malic enzyme, mitochondrial, adenylate kinase, and glyoxalase-1.

Test the tumorigenicity of the CEPI-17-CL4 cells by subcutaneous injection of at least 2 x 10^6 cells in 100 ml culture medium into the intracapsular region of 10 athymic BALB/C nude mice.

Virus or Mycoplasma Contamination

CEPI-17-CL4 cells can be analyzed for mycoplasma contamination by specific enzyme-linked immunosorbent assay (Boehringer Mannheim, Mannheim, Germany) and for hepatitis C virus RNA, hepatitis B vims, and human immunodeficiency virus-1 DNA by reverse transcription-polymerase chain reaction (RT-PCR; Anawa Biomedical Services & Products, Zurich, Switzerland).

Immunohistochemistry

- Using indirect immunofluorescence staining of cultured cells, the expression of epithelial cell-specific markers, such as cytokeratins, can be investigated.
- Culture CEPI-17-CL4 cells on plastic slides (Nunc, Life Technologies Trading AG, Basel, Switzerland), fix in cold methanol-acetone (1:1), and then wash with TNP buffer (0.05 M Tris [pH 8.6], 1.8%NaCl, 0.2% PEG 2000).
- Block nonspecific binding by incubating the cells with 1% bovine serum albumin (BSA) in TNP buffer for 30 minutes at room temperature.
- Incubate the cells for 1 to 2 hours at room temperature with the first antibody diluted in TNP-BSA. Use a series of nonconjugated antibodies directed against different keratin (K) isoforms, including anti-K3 (AE5), K4, K7, K8, K13, K14, K17, K18, and K19, as well as anti-vimentin, anti-SV40 large T antigen, or mouse serum as the negative control.
- After 3 washings with TNP, incubate the cells for 1 hour at room temperature with a fluorescein isothiocyanate-goat anti-mouse/rabbit IgG conjugate (Biosys, Compiegne, France) diluted 1:250 in TNP-BSA and centrifuged.
- After 3 washes with TNP, fix the slides and analyze them by fluorescence microscopy.

ISOLATION AND PURIFICATION OF CONJUNCTIVAL MAST CELLS

- Obtain human conjunctival tissue from local biobanks with permission from organ and tissue donors. Tissue acquisition, characterization, and storage protocols should be approved by your institution.
- Collect aseptically upper and lower bulbar conjunctivas within 8-12 hours of death and transport in corneal tissue preservation medium (Dexsol; Chiron Ophthalmics, Irvine, CA).
- When you obtain the cadaveric conjunctival tissues, resuspend in mast cell culture medium (RPMI 1640 supplemented with 20% fetal calf serum, 2.5 mM L-glutamine, 400 μg/ml streptomycin, 20 μg/ml gentamicin, and 5 μg/ml amphotericin) for 4 to 5 days and store at 4°C until four to eight sets have been received. This number of tissues is found routinely to yield enough mast cells and epithelial cells to conduct one experiment.
- Transfer to Petri dishes and equilibrate at 37°C overnight. Blot and weigh to determine the amount of enzyme required for digestion. Use hyaluronidase and collagenase to digest the tissue.
- Perform the digestion process (37°C for 30 minutes on a rotating shaker) at a low concentration of enzymes (two digestions at 200 U/g in a 10-ml final volume), followed by digestion at a high concentration of enzymes (three to six digestions at 2000 U/g in a 10-ml final volume). Follow each digestion by washing the tissue in TGCM (Tyrode physiological salt solution {TG} plus

gelatin consisting of 137mM NaCl, 2.6 mM KCl, 0.35 mM NaH_2PO_4, 11.9 mM $NaHCO_3$ 5.5 mM glucose, 1g/l gelatin {adjusted to pH 7.4} add $CaCl_2$ and $MgCl_2$) over a 100µm nylon-mesh filter to collect the freed cells.

- Centrifuge the freed cells and resuspend in TG, then pool and layer over two single-density 10-ml Percoll gradients (density, 1.041g/ml), and centrifuge for 20 minutes at 800g. After centrifugation, harvest the top layers of the gradients (epithelial cells) and wash and resuspend in keratinocyte growth medium (without hydrocortisone; concentration, 1 X 10^6 cells/ml). Then transfer to a collagen-fibronectin coated, 24-well plate (0.5 ml/well) for culturing at 37°C.
- Change the medium every 48 hours until confluence. Determine the purity by cytokeratin staining using FACS analysis.
- Wash the pelleted cells from the gradients (mast cells) and resuspend to a concentration of 1 X 10^6 cells/ml in mast cell culture medium, then transfer to a 24-well plate (0.5 ml/well) and equilibrate at 37°C.
- After the cells have equilibrated, remove them from the plate with gentle flushing and scraping and suspend in TG. Wash the cells and resuspend them in 1 ml TG and layer over a two-step Percoll gradient (densities of 1.08 g/ml on top of 1.123 g/ml). Centrifuge this gradient for 20 minutes at 800g.
- Harvest the mast cells from the interface of the two Percoll densities and wash and resuspend in TGCM for further studies.
- Evaluate the morphology of the purified mast cells by electron microscopy using an Electron Microscopy Unit, and differentiate other cells on cytospins using Wright's stain.

ISOLATION, PURIFICATION, AND CHARACTERIZATION OF HUMAN CONJUNCTIVAL EPITHELIAL CELLS

Isolation of Cells

- Human conjunctival tissues from palpebral, fornix, and bulbar regions should be aseptically dissected from post-mortem donors obtained from various eye banks within 12 hours of death and transported in ice-cold sterile Dexol corneal preservation medium. Dexol is composed of a buffered tissue culture medium containing dextran, chondroitin sulfate, Gentamicin, and phenol red indicator.
- The tissues from different donors are rinsed in phosphate-buffered saline (PBS) before being treated with Dispase (10 units/ml) in 50% Hanks buffered salts and keratinocyte growth medium (KGM) at 4°C for 24-48 hours. KGM is prepared by adding bovine pituitary extract (30 ug/ml), hydrocortisone (0.5 pg/ml), amphotericin B (0.05 ug/ml)/gentamicin (50 ug/ml), insulin (5 pg/ml), transferrin (10 ug/ml), and 0.05 mM $CaCl_2$ added to keratinocyte basal medium.
- After this incubation period, the slightly yellow conjunctival epithelium should be removed with a scalpel from the white connective tissue containing blood

vessels under a dissecting microscope. The epithelium is gently triturated to generate individual cells and washed in Dulbecco's modified Eagle's medium (DMEM) containing 10% fetal bovine serum using a low speed (500 xg for 5 min) centrifugation and re-suspension procedure.

- The cell pellet should be resuspended in low calcium (0.05 mM) KGM, plated into T75 flasks (previously coated with collagen type IV), and incubated at 37°C under a humidified atmosphere of 95% air/5% C02. The medium is changed 24 h later and then every 2 days thereafter. The cells become confluent in approximately 10 days, at which point they should be sub-cultured.
- The cells are rinsed with PBS and incubated with Dispase for about 20 min until the cells detach. The Dispase is removed from the cell suspension by a centrifugation/resuspension procedure as described above, and the cells are plated on 24-well or 48-well culture plates. These plates were previously coated with an FNC matrix, which contained fibronectin, collagen, and bovine serum albumin.
- The number of cells to be utilized for the signal transduction studies is typically as follows: 10,000 ± 2,000 cells/well for the cAMP assays and 20,000 ± 3,600 cells/well for phosphoinositide (PI) turnover assays. Other studies can be run parallel with measurements of the release of pro-inflammatory agents from similarly isolated human conjunctival mast cells for possible correlative purposes.

Immunostaining for Characterization of Conjunctival Epithelial Cells

- Fix cells in 5% formalin-phosphate-buffered saline (PBS) for 25 min and wash in 0.02% saponin in PBS at 23 °C.
- Add centrifuge monoclonal antibodies (20-500 ug/ml stock solutions) at 1/2, 1/10, 1/25, 1/50, and 1/100 dilutions to the cells for lh at 23°C after which time the cells should be washed in saponin-PBS buffer for 45 min.
- Following this treatment, centrifuged goat anti-mouse-FITC antibody at l/50th dilution should be incubated with the cells for 45 min at 23°C, and then washed for 45 min and mounted in 2% N-propyl gállate (an anti-oxidant and anti-photobleaching agent) in 95% glycerol-PBS (pH 8-8.5). The monoclonal antibodies to be used are AE1, AE3, AE5, GFAP, desmin, factor-VIII, 8.13, and neurofilament. An example of such immuno-staining is shown in Fig. (**1**).
- The cells can then be photographed on a Leitz epifluorescence microscope using Kodak Ektachrome PI600 film (800 ASA). Some cells can also be fixed in 10% formalin, washed, and then stained in a 10% Giemsa staining solution. The slides are then dried and mounted in Permount for morphological analyses under light-microscopic conditions. In most cases, two determinations should be made for each antibody dilution, and the experiments should be performed at least

twice with cells from two different donors to confirm the reproducibility of staining.

- The harvested cultured HPCE cells can then be utilized for functional assays in order to determine the presence of active receptors for various mast cell mediator chemicals such as prostaglandins, histamine, bradykinin, and platelet-activating factor (PAF). Examples of concentration-response studies and results obtained from the use of these cells are illustrated in Figs. (**2** and **3**).

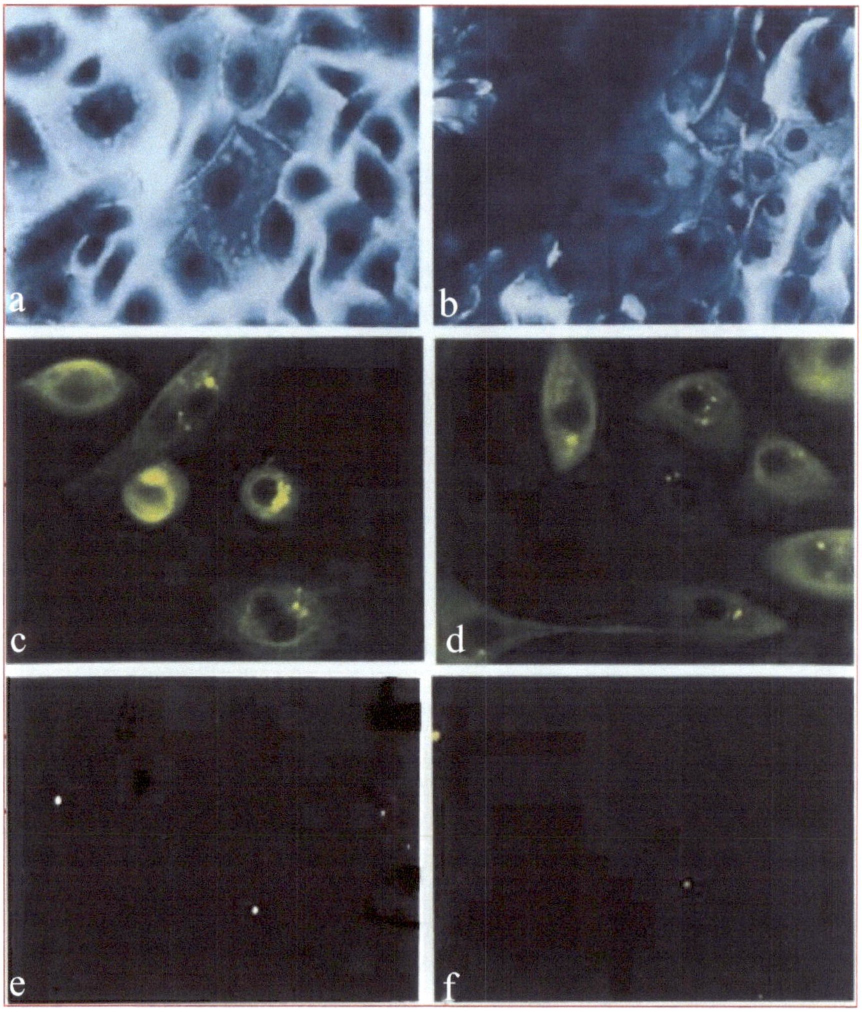

Fig. (1). Immunohistochemistry of isolated human primary conjunctival epithelial cells (HPCE). Giemsa-staining of primary HCE cells showed epithelial cell morphology in undifferentiated (Fig. la) and differentiated (Fig. lb) cultures of cells. The semi-confluent HCE cell cultures were deemed immuno-positive for epithelial cell cytokeratins (AE1, AE3) and AE5 (Figs. **1c** and **1d**). However, there was no binding of monoclonal antibodies to desmin and GFAP (Figs. **le, 1f**) and of factor-VIII and neurofilament to the HPCE cell cultures.

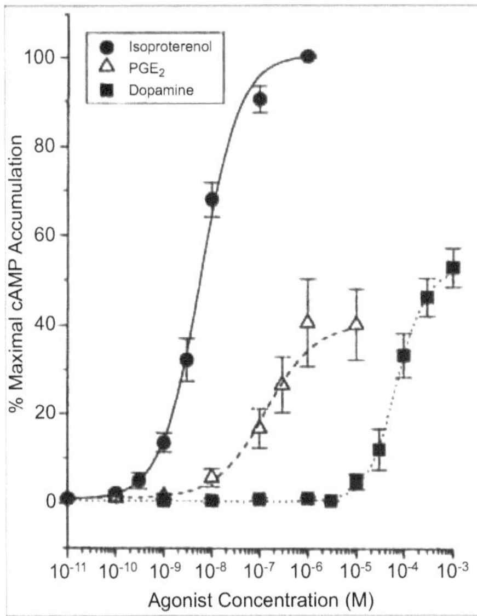

Fig. (2). The stimulation of cAMP production in HPCE cells by various receptor agonists is shown. The concentration-response dependency for each of dopamine, PGE_2, and isoproterenol is displayed. While isoproterenol stimulated beta-adrenergic receptors and maximally increased intracellular cAMP, both dopamine and PGE_2 sub-maximally activated their receptors and behaved as partial agonists in these isolated cells.

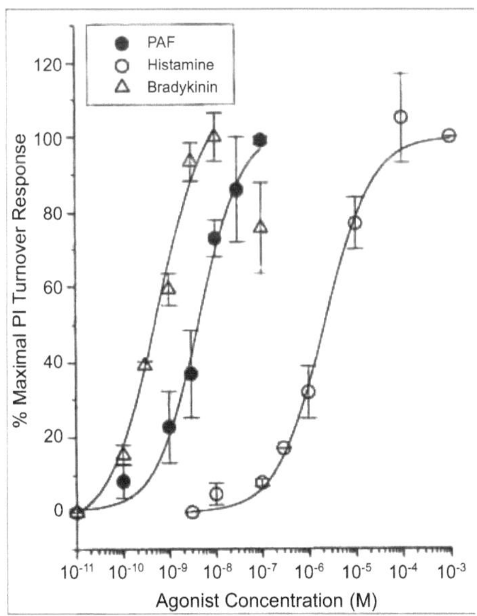

Fig. (3). Inositol phosphate generation through phospholipase C-mediated phosphoinositide turnover by various compounds that stimulate bradykinin, histamine, and platelet-activating factor receptors on HPCE cells is shown. The differential relative potencies (EC50s) of these compounds are readily apparent from the concentration-response curves.

CONCLUSION

Inflammation studies involving primary and immortalized human corneal and conjunctival epithelial cells can help researchers understand the cellular and molecular mechanisms involved in ocular allergies and inflammation. They can be used to investigate the inflammatory response to different stimuli, such as mast cell mediators, cytokines, pathogens, or irritants, and evaluate the efficacy of anti-inflammatory drugs or treatments (Abelson and Schaefer, 1993; Sharif, 2020). By using immortalized human corneal epithelial cells, researchers can perform various experiments to evaluate the potential toxic effects of substances or drugs on the cornea and conjunctiva. These studies are crucial for assessing the safety and potential risks of new ocular medications, cosmetic products, contact lens solutions, or other substances that may come into contact with the eye. The protocols described above are well-established techniques of isolating and culturing cells that have been successfully utilized for the study of the growth of human epithelial cells from multiple origins, such as human mammary epithelial cells and human urothelial cells (Offord *et al.*, 1999). The immortalized CEPI-17 cell line provides several advantages over primary cells, such as a constant and reproducible supply, consistency in behavior, and the ability to propagate and expand for multiple experiments. However, it is important to note that immortalized cell lines may differ from primary cells in certain aspects, and findings should be validated in relevant *in vivo* models or primary cell cultures when possible. Overall, immortalized human corneal epithelial cells offer a valuable *in vitro* model for ocular toxicity and inflammation studies, allowing researchers to gain insights into the effects of various substances or treatments on the cornea and potentially contribute to the development of safer and more effective ocular therapies.

Understanding the role of conjunctival mast cells and human primary conjunctival epithelial (HPCE) cells is important in the diagnosis and treatment of allergic eye conditions. Antihistamine eye drops and other medications that block the action of mast cell mediators are often used to alleviate the symptoms of allergic conjunctivitis (Abelson and Schaefer, 1993; Sharif *et al.*, 1996; Yanni *et al.*, 1999; Sharif, 2020). In the protocols detailed above, the goal was to purify conjunctival mast cells to study whether activation of these cells can provide the necessary cytokine signaling to cause changes in conjunctival epithelium, fibroblast, corneal epithelial cells, and keratocytes. It is important to note that the specific protocols and reagents used for the isolation of conjunctival mast cells and epithelial cells can vary depending on the research goals and available resources. Researchers often optimize these methods based on their specific requirements, and readers are encouraged to perform a PubMed search to obtain the most current publications on the topics covered in this chapter.

REFERENCES

Abelson, MB & Schaefer, K (1993) Conjunctivitis of allergic origin: Immunologic mechanisms and current approaches to therapy. *Surv Ophthalmol,* 38 (Suppl.), 115-32.
[http://dx.doi.org/10.1016/0039-6257(93)90036-7] [PMID: 7901917]

Bradding, P (1996) Human mast cell cytokines. *Clin Exp Allergy,* 26, 13-9.
[http://dx.doi.org/10.1111/j.1365-2222.1996.tb00051.x] [PMID: 8789538]

Cook, EB, Stahl, JL, Miller, ST, Gern, JE, Sukow, KA, Graziano, FM & Barney, NP (1998) Isolation of human conjunctival mast cells and epithelial cells: tumor necrosis factor-α from mast cells affects intercellular adhesion molecule 1 expression on epithelial cells. *Invest Ophthalmol Vis Sci,* 39, 336-43.
[PMID: 9477991]

Kahn, CR, Young, E, Lee, IH & Rhim, JS (1993) Human corneal epithelial primary cultures and cell lines with extended life span: *in vitro* model for ocular studies. *Invest Ophthalmol Vis Sci,* 34, 3429-41.
[PMID: 7693609]

Offord, EA, Sharif, NA, Macé, K, Tromvoukis, Y, Spillare, EA, Avanti, O, Howe, WE & Pfeifer, AM (1999) Immortalized human corneal epithelial cells for ocular toxicity and inflammation studies. *Invest Ophthalmol Vis Sci,* 40, 1091-101.
[PMID: 10235542]

Mace K, Harris CC, Lipsky MM, *et al.* (1996). Human hepatocytes. In: Freshney RI, Freshney MG. eds. *Culture of Immortalized Cells*. London: Wiley-Liss; pp. 161-181.6

Pfeifer, AMA, Mace, K, Tromvoukis, Y & Lipsky, MM (1995) Highly efficient establishment of immortalized cells from adult human liver. *Methods Cell Sci,* 17, 83-9.
[http://dx.doi.org/10.1007/BF00986655]

Sharif, NA, Xu, SX, Miller, ST, Gamache, DA & Yanni, JM (1996) Characterization of the ocular antiallergic and antihistaminic effects of olopatadine (AL-4943A), a novel drug for treating ocular allergic diseases. *J Pharmacol Exp Ther,* 278, 1252-61.
[PMID: 8819509]

Sharif, NA, Crider, JY, Griffin, BW, Davis, TL & Howe, WE (1997) Pharmacological analysis of mast cell mediator and neurotransmitter receptors coupled to adenylate cyclase and phospholipase C on immunocytochemically-defined human conjunctival epithelial cells. *J Ocul Pharmacol Ther,* 13, 321-36.
[http://dx.doi.org/10.1089/jop.1997.13.321] [PMID: 9261768]

Sharif, NA, Wiernas, TK, Griffin, BW & Davis, TL (1998) Pharmacology of [^{3}H]-pyrilamine binding and the histamine-induced phosphoinositide turnover, Ca2+-mobilization and cytokine release from human corneal epithelial cells. *Br J Pharmacol,* 125, 1336-44.
[http://dx.doi.org/10.1038/sj.bjp.0702194] [PMID: 9863665]

Sharif, NA, Wiernas, TK, Howe, WE, Griffin, BW, Offord, EA & Pfeifer, AMA (1998) Human corneal epithelial cell functional responses to inflammatory agents and their antagonists. *Invest Ophthalmol Vis Sci,* 39, 2562-71.
[PMID: 9856766]

Sharif, NA & Wiernas, TK (2010) Platelet-activating factor-induced intracellular signaling and release of cytokines and prostaglandin E2 in immortalized human corneal epithelial cells. *J Ocul Pharmacol Ther,* 26, 21-30.
[http://dx.doi.org/10.1089/jop.2009.0102] [PMID: 20187806]

Sharif, NA (2020) Discovery to launch of anti-allergy (Emadine; Patanol/Pataday/Pazeo) and anti-glaucoma (Travatan; Simbrinza) ocular drugs, and generation of novel pharmacological tools such as AL-8810. *ACS Pharmacol Transl Sci,* 3, 1391-421.
[http://dx.doi.org/10.1021/acsptsci.0c00137] [PMID: 33344909]

Wiernas, TK, Davis, TL, Griffin, BW & Sharif, NA (1998) Effects of bradykinin on signal transduction, cell proliferation, and cytokine, prostaglandin E_2 and collagenase-1 release from human corneal epithelial cells.

Br J Pharmacol, 123, 1127-37.
[http://dx.doi.org/10.1038/sj.bjp.0701700] [PMID: 9559896]

Yanni, JM, Weimer, LK, Sharif, NA, Xu, SX, Gamache, DA & Spellman, JM (1999) Inhibition of histamine-induced human conjunctival epithelial cell responses by ocular allergy drugs. *Arch Ophthalmol,* 117, 643-7.
[http://dx.doi.org/10.1001/archopht.117.5.643] [PMID: 10326962]

OCULAR CELL-BASED *IN VITRO* ASSAYS TO DETERMINE PHARMACOLOGICAL PROPERTIES OF KEY RECEPTORS/ENZYMES/CHANNELS AND FOR SCREENING COMPOUNDS

CHAPTER 14

Overview and Examples of Drug Screening in Cell- and Tissue-Based Assay Systems: Screening Funnels for *In Vitro* and *In Vivo* Studies

Najam A. Sharif[1,*] and **Saima Chaudhry**[2]

[1] *Vice President and Head of Research & Development Nanoscope Therapeutics Inc., 2777 N. Stemmons Fwy, Suite 1102, Dallas, TX-75207, USA*

[2] *Univ N. Texas at Arlington, 701 S Nedderman Dr, Arlington, TX-76019, USA*

Abstract: Chronically elevated intraocular pressure (IOP) is a hallmark of open-angle glaucoma, the most prevalent form of this neurodegenerative eye disease around the world. Although a number of drugs have been approved for lowering and controlling IOP, there continues to be an unmet medical need for superior therapeutics that exhibit better pharmacodynamics and can overcome the significant compliance issues associated with current medicines. As such, it is necessary to continue drug discovery research using both *in vitro* and *in vivo* screening methods. In terms of the former, several cell- and tissue-based assay systems have been developed and implemented in compound screening paradigms that rely on a variety of readouts to assess receptor binding affinity, functional potency, and relative selectivity. In the current chapter, an overview of many functional assay systems using cultured cells or intact tissues derived from ocular tissues involved in ocular hypertension will be presented.

Keywords: CAMP, CGMP, Enzymes, Gaseous transmitters, Inositol phosphates, Receptors.

INTRODUCTION

Glaucoma is an insidious thief of sight, being an asymptomatic neurodegenerative retinal/optic nerve disease that affects millions of people worldwide. One form of glaucoma in which a strong association has been built between the etiology of the disease process and chronically elevated intraocular pressure (IOP) is open-angle glaucoma (OAG) (Weinreb *et al.*, 2014; Sharif, 2018, 2020, 2021; Sharif *et al.*, 2023). Even though many drugs have been introduced into the medical manage-

* **Corresponding author Najam A. Sharif:** Vice President and Head of Research & Development Nanoscope Therapeutics Inc., 2777 N. Stemmons Fwy, Suite 1102, Dallas, TX-75207, USA; Tel: +1(817)-565-7686; E-mail: nsharif@nanostherapeutics.com

Najam A. Sharif and Sunny E. Ohia (Eds.)

ment of OAG and ocular hypertension (OHT) (Bucolo *et al.*, 2018; Sharif, 2021), they have some serious side effects that limit their life-long use to lower and control IOP. These untoward issues have a major effect on the patient's compliance to administer the prescribed eyedrop medications. Thus, there is still an unmet medical need to find and market new drugs that have a better therapeutic index than the existing treatment modalities. In order to screen and characterize new potential drug candidates, a number of *in vitro* assays need to be utilized using isolated cells from the anterior chamber of the eye tissues involved in regulating IOP, such as trabecular meshwork (TM), ciliary muscle (CM), ciliary epithelial cells (CEPI), and perhaps even Schlemm's canal cells, although the latter are more difficult to obtain (Sharif, 2018; Ellis *et al.*, 2010). Data from such cost-effective assay systems allows to profile many compounds and progress them, based on their rank orders of receptor affinities and functional potencies, to *in vivo* studies, which are more expensive and labor-intensive when implemented in screening funnel formats (Sharif, 2018; Figs. **1A** and **1B**).

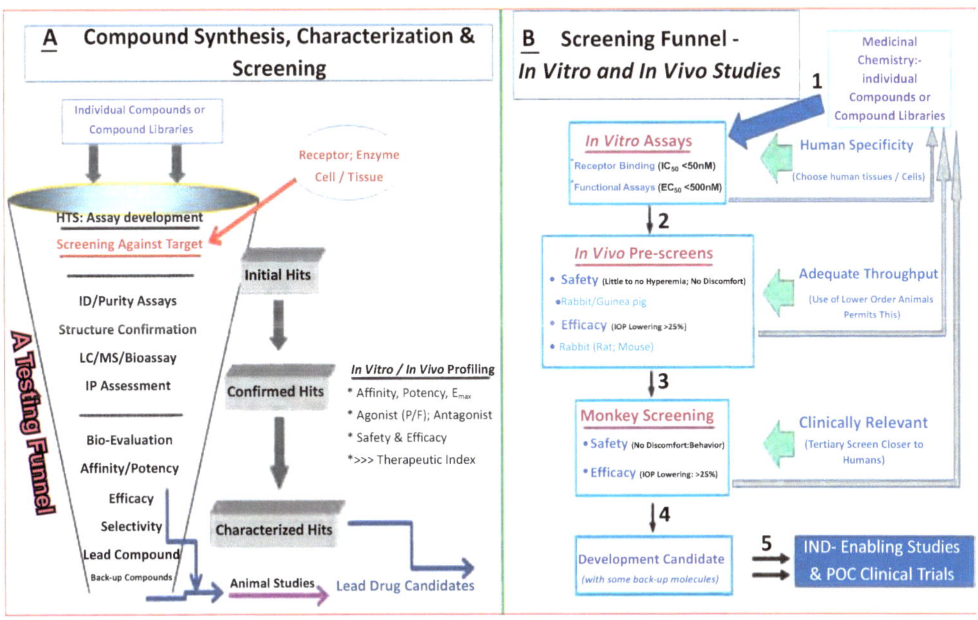

Fig. (1). Screening funnels with stage-gate parameter definition in cellular and *in vivo* studies.

Neurotransmitters, hormones, steroids, and a host of cyto- and chemokines produce their effects via specific receptors, ion channels, and transporters located in cell membranes of tissues and on intracellular organelles. Activation of transmembrane components of these proteins generates intracellular second messengers such as cAMP, cGMP, inositol phosphates, diacylglycerol, Ca^{2+}, and gaseous transmitters such as nitric oxide and hydrogen sulfide that modulate the activity of cytoplasmic proteins, lipids and other cellular components via phosphorylation/dephosphorylation, acetylation, and glycation (see Sharif, 2018; 2021; Fig. **2**). Active modulation of genetic machinery via transcription factors, various chaperones, and secretome/exosome-mediated release of growth factors and microRNAs is also very important in cellular communication, as well as in providing intervention points to mitigate diseases associated with these molecules. The direct transfer of many of the aforementioned chemicals between neighboring cells can also occur via nanotunnels, and this represents a novel mechanism of cellular communication. For now, this chapter outlines methods used to ascertain the functional activity (potency and efficacy [intrinsic activity]) of test compounds in cell- and tissue-based assay systems using second messengers and cell/ tissue contraction/relaxation readouts in a screening funnel arrangement (Sharif, 2018, 2020, 2021, 2023; Figs. **1** & **2**). Those compounds that meet or exceed the *in vitro* criteria and requirements in terms of receptor/enzyme/ion-channel/transporter affinity, functional potency, and intrinsic activity can then be tested in a series of *in vivo* models. The animal-based studies encompass testing for ocular irritation and overall ocular safety by audio and visual observations (*e.g.*, in guinea pigs and rabbits) and for *in vivo* efficacy in terms of IOP lowering in rodents/rabbits/dogs/monkeys using the criteria set to progress from lower phylogenetic animals to the higher ones in order to reduce cost and labor-intensiveness (Fig. **1B**).

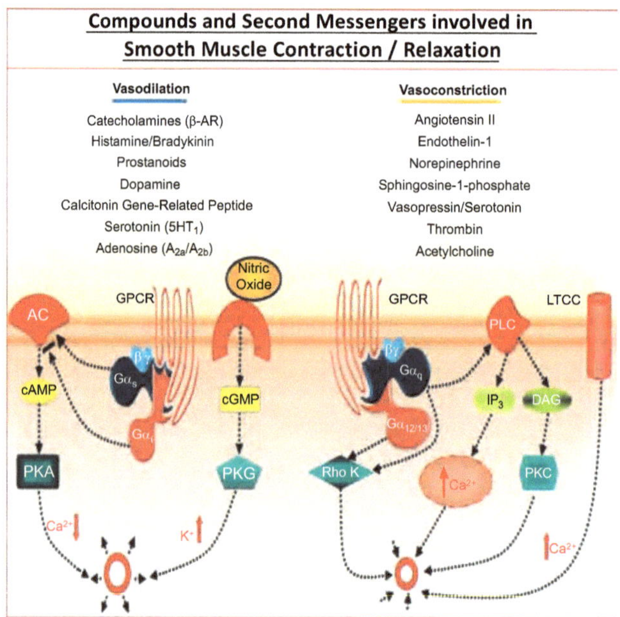

Fig. (2). Examples of neurotransmitters and drugs that can contract or relax the smooth muscle of blood vessels and other tissues.

Protocols for Measuring cAMP and cGMP

It is well-known that cell surface receptors that couple through the Gs or Gi guanine nucleotide couple downstream to the adenylate cyclase or guanylate cyclase to generate or suppress the production of cAMP or cGMP, respectively. Historically, the first step is to raise antibodies against each cAMP and create a procedure from scratch. However, with the advent of enzyme-linked immunosorbent assay (ELISA) kits and other sensitive readouts, generating antibodies in one's laboratory is no longer necessary. Some examples of the use of these assay kit methods are reported in detail (Crider *et al.*, 2001; Katoli *et al.*, 2010; Sharif, 2018), and readers are encouraged to consult these. Examples of data that can be obtained for receptor ligands that activate the production of cAMP in isolated and cultured non-pigmented ciliary epithelial cells in response to DP and EP2 prostaglandin receptor agonists are shown in Fig. (**3**) (Crider *et al.*, 2001; Sharif *et al..*, 2004). In terms of cGMP generation in human TM cells, activators of soluble guanylate cyclase, such as YC-1, are quite effective (Katoli *et al.*, 2010; Sharif *et al.*, 2014; Fig. **4**).

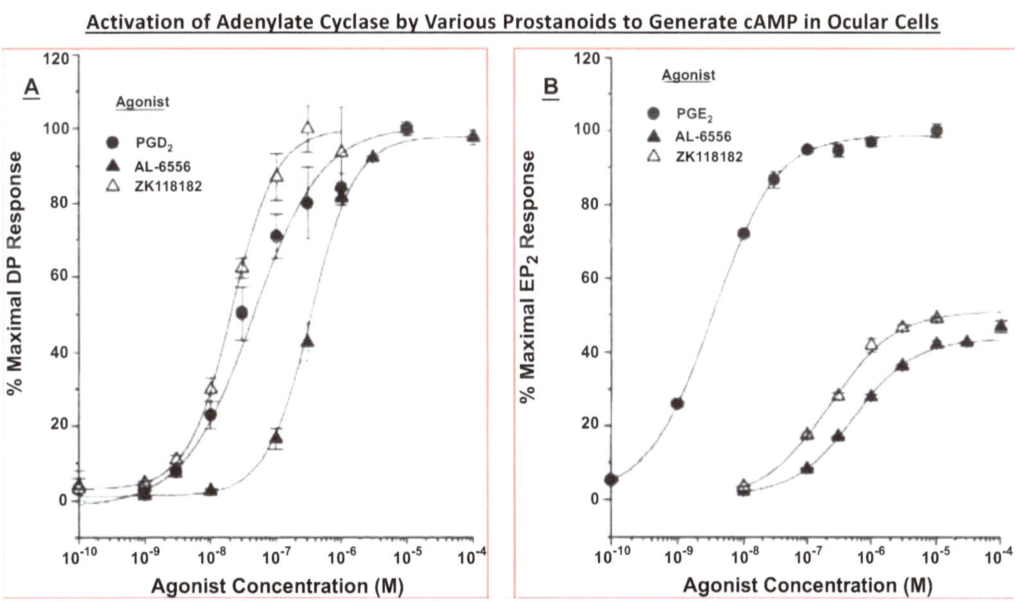

Fig. (3). Examples of data that can be obtained from studying the activation of adenylate cyclase to generate cAMP in human non-pigmented ciliary epithelial cells in culture. Compounds show differences in their potency and intrinsic activity when stimulating cAMP production in NPCE cells via DP- and EP2-prostanoid receptors. The concentration-response curves allow easy discrimination between the activity profiles of compounds allowing rank ordering of the latter agents for *in vivo* studies.

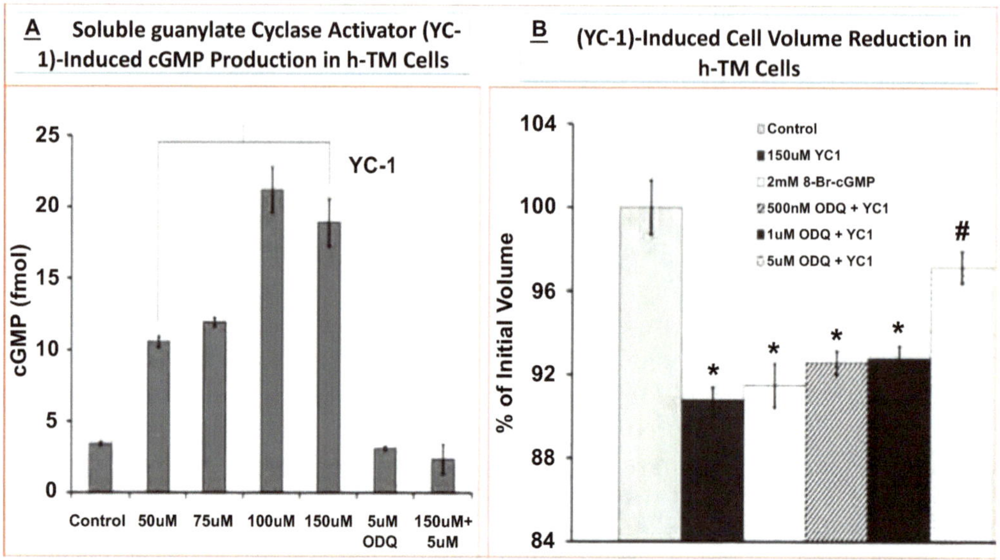

Fig. (4). Drug screening using the generation of cGMP and changes in cell volume using isolated and cultured human TM cells as indices of enzyme activation *in vitro*.

Protocols for Measuring Intracellular Inositol Phosphates and Ca^{2+}-mobilization

As mentioned in the Introduction, many endogenous and exogenously added compounds to cells and tissues interact with specific receptors to activate phospholipase C, which hydrolyses membrane phosphoinositides (PIs) to liberate inositol phosphates (IPs) and diacylglycerol (DAG) into the cytoplasm. Whilst the IPs stimulate the release of intracellular Ca^{2+}, DAG activates various kinases to phosphorylate different kinds of cellular proteins to induce their downstream actions. These can be hormones, prostaglandins or cytokine release, or cell/tissue contraction-relaxation. If [^{3}H]-myo-inositol is allowed to be incorporated into the cell membranes of isolated hCM or hTM cells by an overnight incubation, then the [^{3}H]-IPs generated by activating FP- or bradykinin-receptors can be isolated and measured by ion-exchange chromatography (Sharif and Xu, 1996; Sharif *et al.*, 2003, 2008; Sharif, 2020; Fig. **5A**). The intracellular Ca^{2+}, which is released from the endoplasmic reticulum in seconds by the IPs, can be measured in living cells in real time using a number of different fluorophores as described before (Griffin *et al.*, 1999; Kelly *et al.*, 2003; Sharif *et al.*, 2003, 2009, 2014, Fig. **6A**).

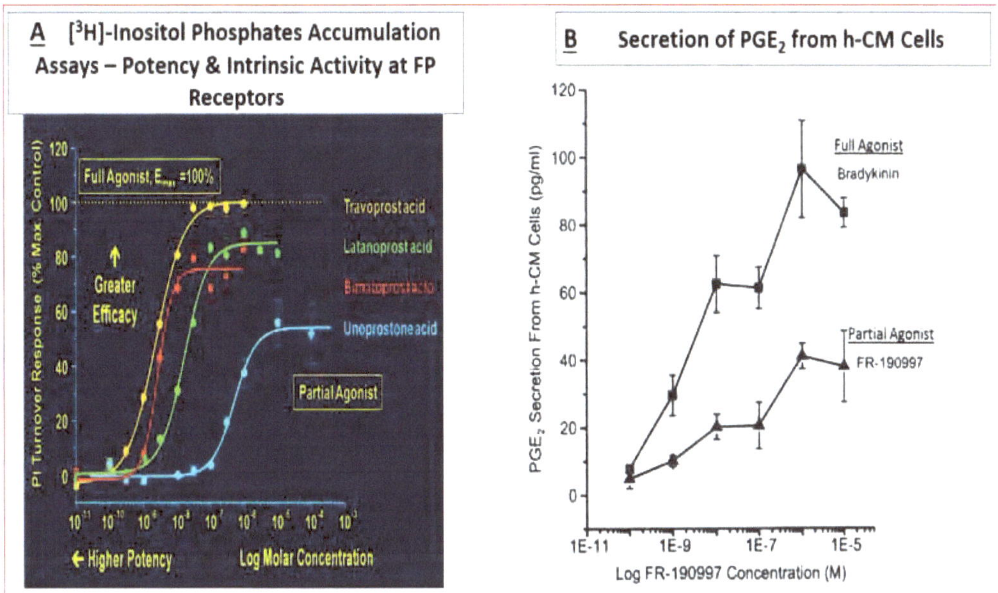

Fig. (5). The accumulation of [^{3}H]-IPs and release of endogenous PGE_2 by FP-receptor agonists and bradykinin receptor agonists is shown. The parameters from such studies can be used for potency and *in vitro* efficacy determinations for the test compounds. Full agonists and partial agonists can be readily differentiated.

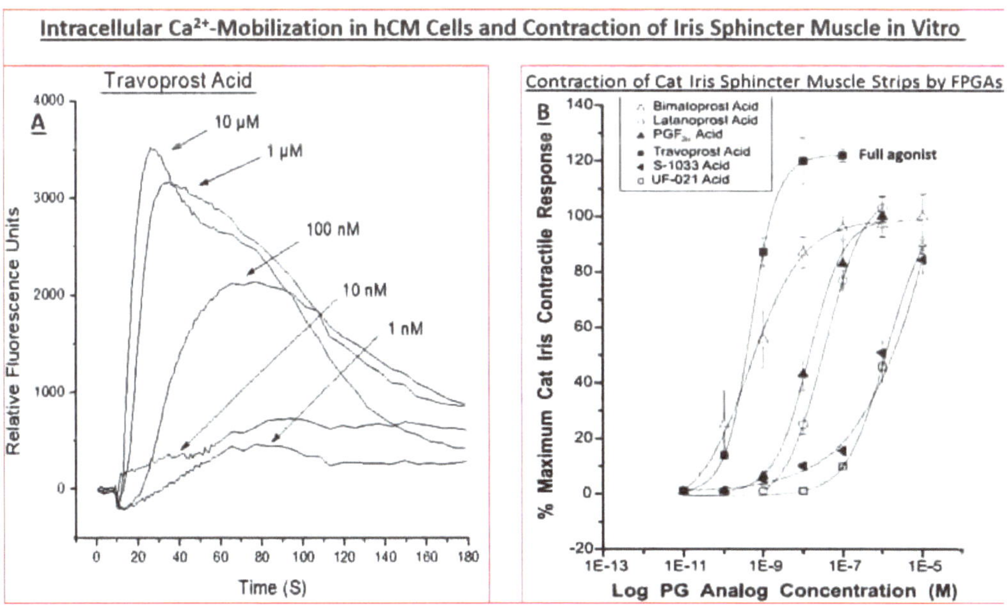

Fig. (6). The FP-receptor agonist (travoprost acid)-induced intracellular Ca2+-mobilization in human CM cells (A) and the ability of many different FP-receptor agonists to cause contraction of cat iris sphincter smooth muscle (B) are depicted. These types of data are helpful in ranking test compounds based on their functional potency and intrinsic activity (Emax).

Protocols for Measuring the Release and Activities of Enzymes in Ocular Cells

As is abundantly clear, external signaling compounds and triggers mediate their actions inside the cells by promoting the production of second messengers that, in turn, are involved in hormone or enzyme release, *etc.* (Figs. **2** - **5**). In terms of IOP-lowering, several classes of compounds such as FP- and EP-2 prostanoid receptor agonists, serotonin-2, and bradykinin-2 receptor agonists increase the production and secretion of matrix metalloproteinases (MMPs) into the extracellular space in and around the TM and SC in the ANC of the eye in order to digest collagens, fibronectin, and other cell debris. This activity results in enhanced drainage of excess AQH, thus lowering IOP. Studies to mechanistically explore the release of MMPs and investigate mitogen-activated kinase (MAP kinase) functionality have been reported, and the full methods are described in detail (Husain *et al.*, 2005; Sharif *et al.*, 2003, 2009, 2014, 2016; (Figs. **7A** and **7B**).

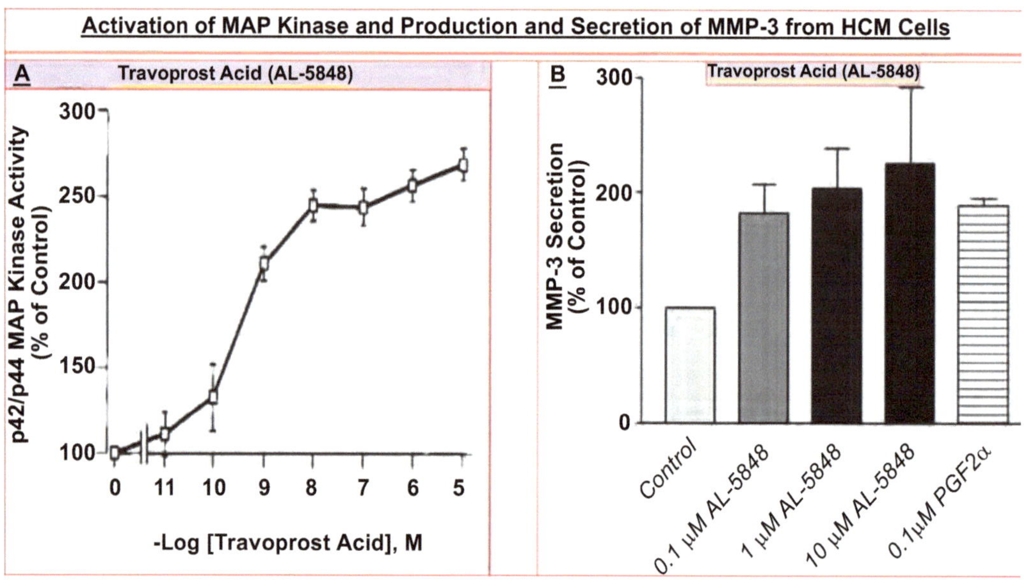

Fig. (7). The ability of compounds to stimulate MAP kinase activity (A) and MMP-3 secretion (B) from human CM cells *in vitro* by the FP-receptor agonist, travoprost-free acid, is displayed. These types of assay systems using cells in culture provide valuable information about the functional activity of test compounds.

Protocols for Measuring the Production of Endogenous Prostaglandins and Stimulating Smooth Muscle Contraction

The downstream actions of receptor activation by neurotransmitters and drugs include stimulated cyclooxygenase-2 activity, which results in the generation and release of endogenous prostaglandins (PGs). FP-receptor agonists such as latanoprost and bradykinin and their non-peptide agonists (*e.g.* FR-190997) promote PGE_2 release from human CM cells (that can be measured by ELISA assays), which further enhances the release of MMPS to increase AQH outflow from the TM and across the CM to lower IOP (Fig. **5B**; Sharif *et al.*, 2014). Likewise, many types of PGs stimulate the contraction of smooth muscles, including the iris sphincter, CM and TM (Fig. **6B**), to release various endogenous molecules, which finally lower IOP. The tissue contraction is quantifiable and can be utilized to rank compounds on the basis of their potency and intrinsic activity (Fig. **1**; Ohia *et al.*, 2018; Sharif *et al.*, 2008).

Protocols for Studying Cell Morphology and Cell Volume Changes

As can be imagined, when the test compounds that lower and control IOP activate their cognate receptors, the cells and tissues respond by inducing signal transduction inside the cells and by changing their shape. Using confocal microscopy, it is possible to label cells in culture with specific dyes and reagents that light up specific cellular proteins and other cytoplasmic components. Using such techniques, it is possible to monitor, record, and calculate intracellular changes in pH, cell volume (Dismuke *et al.*, 2009; Ellis *et al.*, 2010; and cell shapes (Ramachandran *et al.*, 2011; Fig. **8**), and these quantitative parameters can provide insights into the mechanism of action of ocular hypotensive compounds of interest and can be used to rank order test compounds.

Protocols to Assess the Effectiveness of Compounds in Enhancing Outflow Facility

As has been discussed above, several classes of drugs (*e.g.*, FP- and EP2-receptor agonists) lower and control IOP by promoting the drainage of AQH from the ANC of the eye via conventional (TM / SC) and unconventional (uveoscleral) pathways. Other classes of compounds that are efficacious ocular hypotensive agents that work in laser-induced elevated IOP monkey model of OHT are bradykinin-2 receptor agonists (*e.g.*, FR-190997) and serotonin-2A-2C receptor agonists (*e.g.*, cabergoline). A useful *in vitro* model to study and demonstrate the ocular hypotensive activity of drug candidates is the *in vitro* organ culture of ANC segments of the bovine, porcine, and human eyes (Sharif *et al.*, 2009, 2014; Fig. **9**).

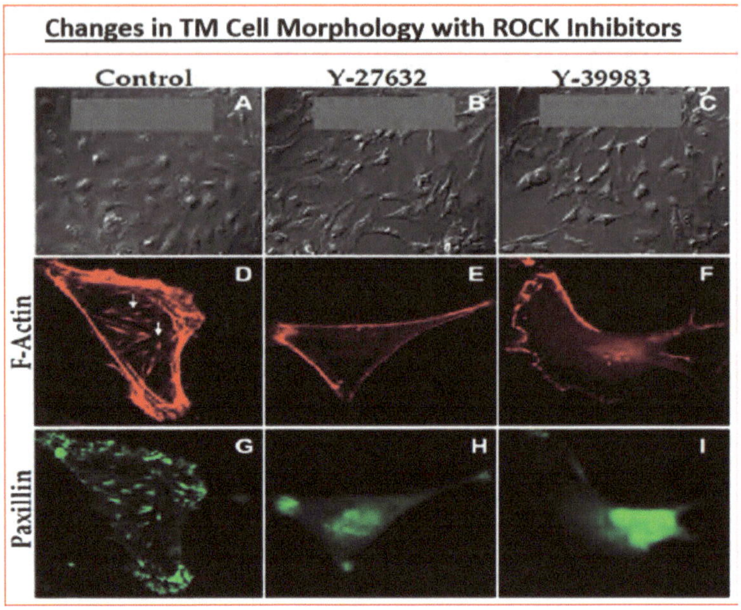

Fig. (8). Morphological and intracellular protein marker changes induced by test compounds can be visualized and quantitated by high-content screening paradigms via confocal microscopy. Shown above are the changes induced by two different rho kinase inhibitors, relative to vehicle controls, in the cell shape and the localization and disposition of F-actin and paxillin in cultured human TM cells.

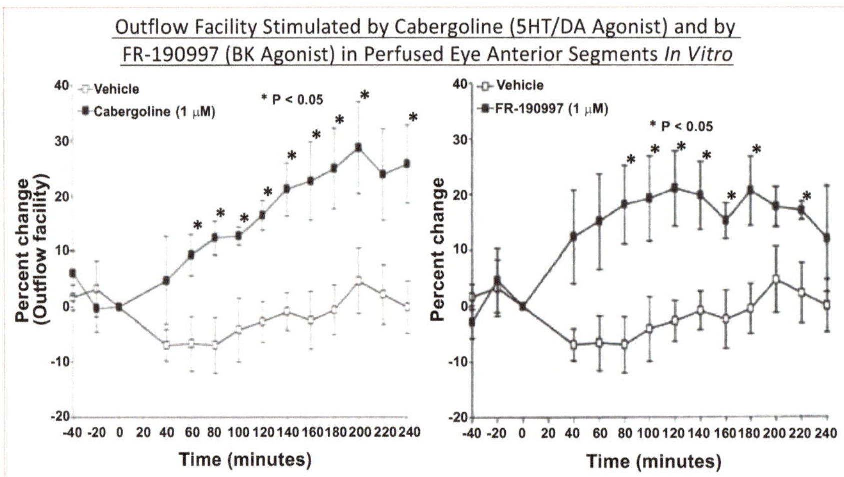

Fig. (9). The mechanism of action of drugs that target OHT and glaucoma can be studied using *in vitro* model systems using ANC segments of the eyes of animals and postmortem humans. If the drugs increase the outflow facility of the perfusate in these systems, then the compounds are deemed to be able to stimulate AQH outflow from the TM/SC drainage system in the intact eye to lower IOP. Above are two different classes of drugs that enhanced the outflow facility in porcine anterior eye segments. Since the effect requires over an hour to significantly increase the outflow of the perfusate suggests that protein synthesis (*e.g.*, production and release of MMPs) may be necessary to mediate this stimulatory action of the compounds.

CONCLUSION

Many different *in vitro* assay and model systems have been developed and deployed for drug screening and progressing them down the screening funnel towards testing in animal models of OHT and glaucoma. The use of second messengers, cell/tissue shape and contraction/relaxation changes, secretion of enzymes, prostaglandins, and hormones as tools for monitoring receptor or enzyme activation by test compounds has been extremely useful in drug discovery and characterization. The incredible complexity associated with intracellular and intercellular communication and the plethora of signaling molecules involved (Figs. **10** and **11**) offers great opportunities to utilize them for screening purposes and also as points of intervention to mitigate OHT and glaucoma at the ANC of the eye level. The astounding fast pace of new genetic association discoveries with disease mechanisms of OHT/OAG will also offer new targets for finding novel therapeutic modalities to treat unfortunate patients afflicted with these eye disorders. Additionally, the advent of new techniques and technologies to help in the drug discovery processes (Fig. **12**) will also be extremely useful in these endeavors.

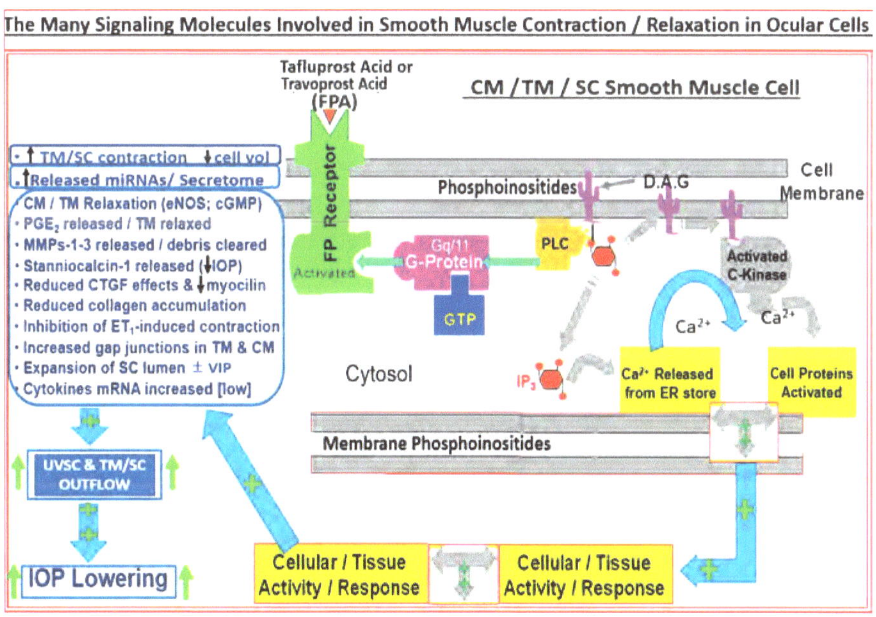

Fig. (10). The complexity of the intracellular and extracellular molecules and activities needed to accomplish IOP lowering by FP-receptor agonist prostaglandins such as travoprost is illustrated. Generation of second messenger molecules (IPs, Ca^{2+}, nitric oxide), MMPs release, hormone (*e.g.* stanniocalcin; vasoactive intestinal peptide (VIP)) and low levels of cytokine release, digestion of extracellular matrix, smooth muscle contraction/relaxation, and down-regulation of collagen/fibronectin (and perhaps myocilin) deposition and endothelin actions all appear to contribute to the final biological response of IOP reduction.

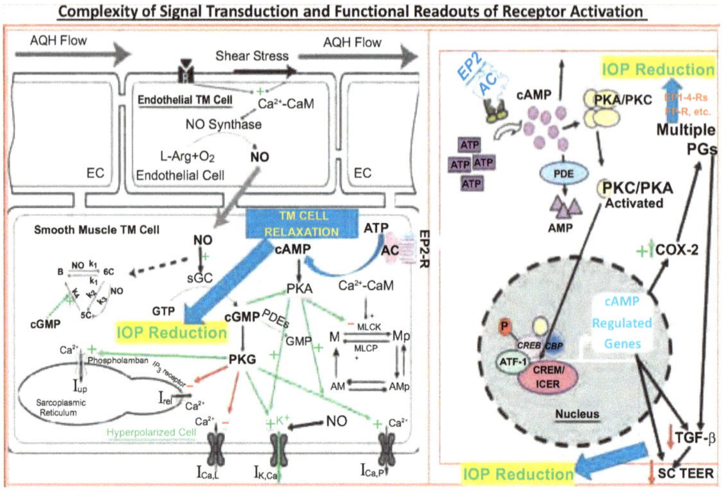

Fig. (11). The remarkable complexity and involvement of multiple signaling molecules and extracellular factors in promoting AQH outflow from the ANC segment of the eye to lower IOP are readily evident from this pictogram. The many possible functional readouts that can used to measure prostanoid receptor activation in human CM/TM cells, especially via the EP2 receptor, are illustrated. As in Fig. 10, the IOP reduction observed due to FP PG receptor activation is an amalgamation and amplification of multiple signaling events at many levels inside the target cells of the key tissues in the ANC segment of the eye.

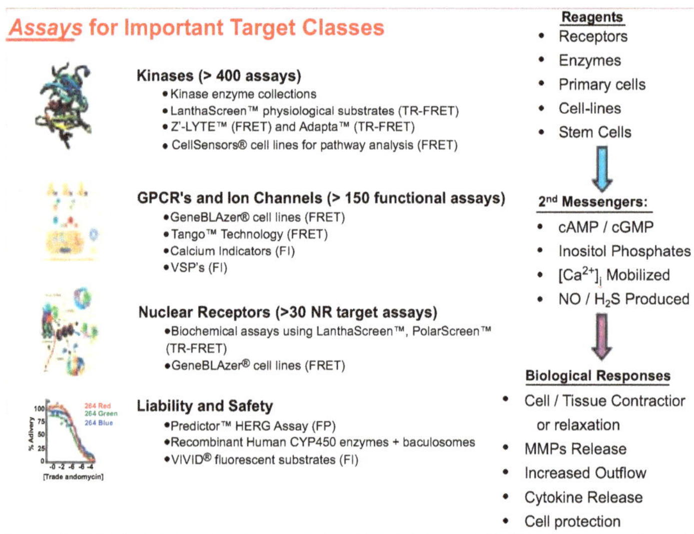

Fig. (12). Along with the complexity and multiplicity of factors and events needed to elicit ocular hypotensive activity of drug candidates shown in Figs. (**9** and **10**) come the many technologies and techniques to measure the functional readouts of receptor activation using *in vitro* assay systems shown here. When implemented into high-throughput screening formats (Fig. **1**), compound screening using the assays and instruments shown above can greatly reduce the time and cost of finding suitable lead compounds to progress toward testing for efficacy in animal models of OHT and glaucoma. Testing for off-target effects of compounds in terms of safety is also possible. It is important to use *in vitro* assays in order to derive a good therapeutic index for the lead and backup compounds of interest.

REFERENCES

Bucolo, C, Platania, CBM, Drago, F, Bonfiglio, V, Reibaldi, M, Avitabile, T & Uva, M (2018) Novel therapeutics in glaucoma management. *Curr Neuropharmacol,* 16, 978-92.
[http://dx.doi.org/10.2174/1570159X15666170915142727] [PMID: 28925883]

Crider, JY & Sharif, NA (2001) Functional pharmacological evidence for EP2 and EP4 prostanoid receptors in immortalized human trabecular meshwork and N-PCE cells. *J Ocul Pharmacol Ther,* 17, 35-46.
[http://dx.doi.org/10.1089/108076801750125658] [PMID: 11322636]

Dismuke, WM, Sharif, NA & Ellis, DZ (2009) Human trabecular meshwork cell volume decrease by NO-independent soluble guanylate cyclase activators YC-1 and BAY-58-2667 involves the BKCa ion channel. *Invest Ophthalmol Vis Sci,* 50, 3353-9.
[http://dx.doi.org/10.1167/iovs.08-3127] [PMID: 19234350]

Ellis, DZ, Sharif, NA & Dismuke, WM (2010) Endogenous regulation of human Schlemm's canal cell volume by nitric oxide signaling. *Invest Ophthalmol Vis Sci,* 51, 5817-24.
[http://dx.doi.org/10.1167/iovs.09-5072] [PMID: 20484594]

Griffin, BW, Williams, GW, Crider, JY & Sharif, NA (1997) FP prostaglandin receptors mediating inositol phosphates generation and calcium mobilization in Swiss 3T3 cells: a pharmacological study. *J Pharmacol Exp Ther,* 281, 845-54.
[http://dx.doi.org/10.1016/S0022-3565(24)36681-9] [PMID: 9152393]

Husain, S, Jafri, F & Crosson, CE (2005) Acute effects of PGF2alpha on MMP-2 secretion from human ciliary muscle cells: a PKC- and ERK-dependent process. *Invest Ophthalmol Vis Sci,* 46, 1706-13.
[http://dx.doi.org/10.1167/iovs.04-0993] [PMID: 15851572]

Katoli, P, Sharif, NA, Sule, A & Dimitrijevich, SD (2010) NPR-B natriuretic peptide receptors in human corneal epithelium: mRNA, immunohistochemistochemical, protein, and biochemical pharmacology studies. *Mol Vis,* 16, 1241-52.
[PMID: 20664698]

Kelly, CR, Williams, GW & Sharif, NA (2003) Real-time intracellular Ca2+ mobilization by travoprost acid, bimatoprost, unoprostone, and other analogs via endogenous mouse, rat, and cloned human FP prostaglandin receptors. *J Pharmacol Exp Ther,* 304, 238-45.
[http://dx.doi.org/10.1124/jpet.102.042556] [PMID: 12490597]

Ohia, SE, Njie-Mbye, YF, Robinson, J, Mitchell, L, Mckoy, M, Opere, CA & Sharif, NA (2018) Serotonin-2B/2C receptors-mediate bovine ciliary muscle contraction: role in IOP regulation. *J Ocul Pharmacol Ther,* 34, 70-5.
[http://dx.doi.org/10.1089/jop.2017.0123] [PMID: 29364761]

Ramachandran, C, Patil, RV, Combrink, K, Sharif, NA & Srinivas, SP (2011) Rho-Rho kinase pathway in the actomyosin contraction and cell-matrix adhesion in immortalized human trabecular meshwork cells. *Mol Vis,* 17, 1877-90.
[PMID: 21850162]

Sharif, NA & Xu, SX (1996) Pharmacological characterization of bradykinin receptors coupled to phosphoinositide turnover in SV40-immortalized human trabecular meshwork cells. *Exp Eye Res,* 63, 631-7.
[http://dx.doi.org/10.1006/exer.1996.0157] [PMID: 9068370]

Sharif, NA, Crider, JY, Husain, S, Kaddour-Djebbar, I, Ansari, HR & Abdel-Latif, AA (2003) Human ciliary muscle cell responses to FP-class prostaglandin analogs: phosphoinositide hydrolysis, intracellular Ca2+ mobilization and MAP kinase activation. *J Ocul Pharmacol Ther,* 19, 437-55.
[http://dx.doi.org/10.1089/108076803322473006] [PMID: 14583136]

Sharif, NA, Kaddour-Djebbar, I & Abdel-Latif, AA (2008) Cat iris sphincter smooth-muscle contraction: comparison of FP-class prostaglandin analog agonist activities. *J Ocul Pharmacol Ther,* 24, 152-63.
[http://dx.doi.org/10.1089/jop.2007.0076] [PMID: 18355130]

Sharif, NA, Katoli, P, Scott, D, Li, L, Kelly, C, Xu, S, Husain, S, Toris, C & Crosson, C (2014) FR-190997, a

nonpeptide bradykinin B2-receptor partial agonist, is a potent and efficacious intraocular pressure lowering agent in ocular hypertensive cynomolgus monkeys. *Drug Dev Res,* 75, 211-23.
[http://dx.doi.org/10.1002/ddr.21174] [PMID: 24796320]

Sharif, NA, McLaughlin, MA, Kelly, CR, Katoli, P, Drace, C, Husain, S, Crosson, C, Toris, C, Zhan, GL & Camras, C (2009) Cabergoline: Pharmacology, ocular hypotensive studies in multiple species, and aqueous humor dynamic modulation in the Cynomolgus monkey eyes. *Exp Eye Res,* 88, 386-97.
[http://dx.doi.org/10.1016/j.exer.2008.10.003] [PMID: 18992242]

Sharif, NA, Odani-Kawabata, N, Lu, F & Pinchuk, L (2023) FP and EP2 prostanoid receptor agonist drugs and aqueous humor outflow devices for treating ocular hypertension and glaucoma. *Exp Eye Res,* 229, 109415.
[http://dx.doi.org/10.1016/j.exer.2023.109415] [PMID: 36803996]

Sharif, NA, Patil, R, Li, L & Husain, S (2016) Human ciliary muscle cell responses to kinins: Activation of ERK1/2 and pro-matrix metalloproteinases secretion. *World J Ophthalmol,* 6, 20-7.
[http://dx.doi.org/10.5318/wjo.v6.i3.20]

Sharif, NA, Williams, GW, Crider, JY, Xu, SX & Davis, TL (2004) Molecular pharmacology of the ocular hypotensive DP/EP2 class prostaglandin AL-6598 and localization of DP and EP2 receptor sites in human eyes. *J Ocul Pharmacol Ther,* 20, 489-508.
[http://dx.doi.org/10.1089/jop.2004.20.489] [PMID: 15684809]

Sharif, NA (2018) iDrugs and iDevices discovery and development- preclinical assays, techniques and animal model studies for ocular hypotensives and neuroprotectants. *J Ocul Pharmacol Ther,* 34, 7-39.
[http://dx.doi.org/10.1089/jop.2017.0125] [PMID: 29323613]

Sharif, NA (2020) Pharmacodynamic Evaluation: Ocular Pharmacology. In: Hock, F.J., Gralinski, M.R., (Eds.), *Drug Discovery and Evaluation: Methods in Clinical Pharmacology.*Springer Publishing Company.
[http://dx.doi.org/10.1007/978-3-319-68864-0_54]

Sharif, NA (2022) Targeting of signal transduction pathway components to mitigate selected ocular disorders. *Acta Scientific Ophthalmology,* 5, 3-17.

Sharif, NA (2021) Therapeutic drugs and devices for tackling ocular hypertension and glaucoma, and need for neuroprotection and cytoprotective therapies. *Front Pharmacol,* 12, 729249.
[http://dx.doi.org/10.3389/fphar.2021.729249] [PMID: 34603044]

Sharif, NA (2023) Identifying new drugs and targets to treat rapidly elevated intraocular pressure for angle closure and secondary glaucomas to curb visual impairment and prevent blindness. *Exp Eye Res,* 232, 109444.
[http://dx.doi.org/10.1016/j.exer.2023.109444] [PMID: 36958427]

Weinreb, RN, Aung, T & Medeiros, FA (2014) The pathophysiology and treatment of glaucoma: a review. *JAMA,* 311, 1901-11.
[http://dx.doi.org/10.1001/jama.2014.3192] [PMID: 24825645]

CHAPTER 15

Protocol for Studying Ocular Cell Relaxation / Contraction by Cell Impedance

Thomas R. Vollmer[1], **Amy Chen**[1], **Ganesh Prasanna**[1] and **Christopher W. Wilson**[1,*]

[1] *Department of Ophthalmology, Novartis Institute of Biomedical Research, 22 Windsor St. Cambridge, MA-02452, USA*

Abstract: Pharmacological control of cellular contractility is a validated mechanism for the modulation of aqueous humor outflow and, thus, modulation of intraocular pressure (IOP). Label-free cellular impedance assays monitor the change in electron flow in response to environmental conditions, allowing the detection of responses to a diverse number of cellular stimuli, including the administration of biological or pharmacological agents that affect the actin cytoskeleton. The impedance assay has several differentiating factors compared to other cell-based assays, including the advantage of time-resolved dynamic measurements from living adherent cells. Numerous reports have described the utility of impedance assays in the characterization of the mechanism of action of individual ligands or small molecules. In addition, these assays are applied in screening campaigns designed to identify new pathways with phenotypes of interest. This chapter describes protocols and considerations for designing, validating, executing, and analyzing cellular impedance assays for the purpose of evaluating effects on cell contractility. The focus here is aimed at cells of the conventional aqueous outflow pathway, but the principles are broadly applicable outside of this field.

Keywords: Cell culture, Contractility, Intraocular pressure, Impedance, Relaxation, Screening.

INTRODUCTION

Cell-based electrical impedance is assessed by plating adherent cells on specialized culture vessels with gold electrodes and applying a continuous current at various frequencies. Cell membranes impede the applied electrical current moving from the electrode into the cell media, and the magnitude of the impedance can be quantified and represented mathematically. This enables indirect measurement of the state of cell morphology, which is a dynamic pheno-

* **Corresponding author Christopher W. Wilson:** Department of Ophthalmology, Novartis Institute of Biomedical Research, 22 Windsor St. Cambridge, MA-02452, USA; Tel: +1-617-871-5316; E-mail: chris.wilson@novartis.com

type of cellular response to the environment. Owing to the non-invasive and real-time nature of the measurements, numerous applications for the technology have been described, including assessment of cytotoxicity (Xing *et al.*, 2005), cell adhesion and migration (Scrace *et al.*, 2013), characterization of GPCR agonists and antagonists (Doijen *et al.*, 2019), assessment of cell-cell junctions and barrier function (Benson *et al.*, 2013), and screening of compound libraries for a variety of readouts (Thieulent *et al.*, 2020, Vollmer *et al.*, 2020). Of note, many of the above phenotypes and readouts are dependent on the state and behavior of the actin cytoskeleton.

A number of approved pharmacological treatments that lower IOP exert their effects through regulation of cell contractility and the actin cytoskeleton, including the Rho kinase inhibitors (Tanna and Johnson, 2018). Taken together, cytoskeletal modulation has been validated as an effective IOP-lowering mechanism. In the pursuit of additional compounds and targets that regulate the cytoskeleton, impedance platforms have been used to evaluate effects of numerous cell contractile and relaxing agents, as well as to understand the effects of Wnt signaling and cadherins (Stamer *et al.*, 2010, Ramachandran *et al.*, 2011a, Ramachandran *et al.*, 2011b, Wang *et al.*, 2013, Cavet *et al.*, 2015, Webber *et al.*, 2018).

The purpose of this chapter is to provide key experimental considerations and a framework for executing and interpreting cellular impedance assays. Two major commercial systems are available: the xCELLigence Real-Time Cell Analysis platform (xCELLigence RTCA, Agilent) and the Electric Cell-substrate Impedance Sensing (ECIS) platform (Applied Biophysics). Although experiments can be performed with manual manipulation, the quality, reproducibility, and scale of data obtained can be improved through the use of automated liquid handling instruments where possible. High-throughput screening is attainable with impedance platforms, as evidenced by our recent report describing a screen of a small library of ~4000 compounds over a few weeks, using a 384-well format and with multiple compound concentrations and replicates (Vollmer *et al.*, 2020). The methods described here were developed using the xCelligence real-time cell analysis (RTCA) high-throughput screening (HTS) platform (Agilent Technologies Inc., California), but conceptually are broadly applicable to other platform types.

CELL SELECTION

For high-throughput compound screening, we recommend selecting immortalized cell lines derived from the tissue of interest (*e.g.*, Normal trabecular meshwork 5 (NTM5), an SV40-immortalized cell line generated at Alcon (Texas, USA) prior to the acquisition of Alcon by Novartis in 2011). The use of primary cells is limiting for high-throughput screens with hundreds or thousands of compounds due to scarcity of material, potential for donor-to-donor variability, cell-type heterogeneity, and passage number limitations. Cell behavior may drift with increased passaging, so we would advise characterizing cells and ensuring maintenance of assay windows with passage number. However, smaller-scale screens and orthogonal confirmation studies can be carried out using primary cells derived from multiple donors. Primary TM cells should be validated for identity by assessing Myocilin protein production *via* a Western blot of whole cell lysates and conditioned media following prolonged (3 – 7 day) steroid treatment, per community recommendations (Keller *et al.*, 2018). Ciliary muscle cells and Schlemm's Canal or surrogate commercially available endothelial cells such as human umbilical vein endothelial cells (HUVEC) may also be used and should be characterized according to current best principles (Tamm *et al.*, 1991; Perkumas and Stamer, 2012).

LIQUID HANDLING AND AUTOMATION

RTCA HTS instruments use 384-well gold-electrode coated microplates; the control unit for this model has 4 ports, which enables connection of up to 4 instruments that can be operated simultaneously and independently. There are many high-throughput liquid handlers that can accommodate 384-well cell dispensing, plate-washing, and compound addition; we recommend that users consider taking advantage of automation where possible to reduce the variability in volumes dispensed or aspirated as well as the potential for human error while enabling swift administration of treatments. Overall, experiment quality will be significantly improved through the use of robotic liquid handling. We understand that not all laboratories will have access to liquid handling instruments, so as an alternative, the use of manual or electronic multi-channel pipettes is possible. While single-channel pipettes may be used, readers are advised that this may contribute to higher assay variability and diminished reproducibility. Impedance instruments with a lower throughput are also available, such as the ECIS platform, and can also be considered.

INSTRUMENT SETTINGS

Impedance instruments may have a variety of frequency settings, which affect the types of measurements that can be inferred, such as cell-cell contacts or cell density (Doijen *et al.*, 2019). While the RTCA platform uses a fixed frequency (10,000 Hz) coupled with disposable plates, ECIS platforms enable the use of multiple frequencies ranging from 100 to 64,000 Hz. Responses to stimuli may vary according to the frequency selected, so method development should be explored to address this variability when using a device with multiple frequency options in order to determine optimal parameters for the measurement of choice.

ADDITIONAL VARIABLES THAT INFLUENCE IMPEDANCE MEASUREMENTS

Depending on the phenotype of interest, several criteria can be used to optimize impedance measurements. In pharmacological screening assays, assay windows and measurement variations can determine the robustness and quality of the assay, which can be measured by the Z factor, also referred to as Z' (Zhang *et al.*, 1999)). It is common to use positive control compounds to evaluate assay parameters. Further, the magnitude of response (V_{max}) and measured compound potency (EC_{50}) can also be affected by assay conditions. These responses may be influenced by other variables such as cell seeding density, serum components, the addition of defined extracellular matrix, cell loss during washing steps, and tolerability to compound solvents such as DMSO. Notably, serum may contain high levels of contractile agents such as sphingosine-1-phosphate (Chrisman *et al.*, 2003), and appropriate consideration of potential assay confounders should be given in the initial stages of assay development. Below, we provide examples of optimization approaches that may be taken prior to running comprehensive experiments. Depending on the desired application, researchers may consider the inclusion of the following steps and assays as appropriate. We advise using at least n = 2 replicate wells for each condition to instill confidence in measurements.

EXPERIMENTAL PROTOCOLS

Assessment of Cell Density Effects

Optimizing Cell Density in Impedance for the Assessment of Vmax, EC50, and Z'

- Set up the RTCA instrument in a cell culture incubator (typically 37 °C + 5% CO_2, adjust as needed for hypoxic conditions) and confirm functionality using the test plate provided by the manufacturer.
- Warm media to 37 degrees C; ensure media used throughout is prewarmed prior to addition to minimize temperature fluctuations.
- Dispense 20 μL of appropriate cell culture medium (in our application, low glucose Dulbecco's Modified Eagle Medium (DMEM) supplemented with 10% fetal bovine serum (FBS) and 1% penicillin-streptomycin (PS); if using a different cell type, use the appropriate media that supports cell viability and growth) to each well of a 384-well xCelligence E-plate either using a multichannel pipettor or a suitable automated liquid handling system (as an

example, the Multidrop Combi Reagent Dispenser (ThermoFisher Scientific, Massachusetts, USA)).

- Briefly centrifuge plates at low speed (<1000 x g, 5 minutes) to remove bubbles at the bottom of wells using a plate attachment in a swinging bucket rotor (*e.g.*, Eppendorf, Germany). Place plates onto RTCA instrument electrodes to record pre-cell impedance measurement, which will be subtracted from subsequent measurements; if bubbles are not removed, this can influence baseline impedance readings. In the RTCA software, check the 'Messages' tab to see if any wells have been flagged for having measurements out of range. If needed, clean RTCA instrument electrodes until messages clear. In some cases, E-plate wells can contribute to aberrant measurements, and this cannot be overcome with electrode cleaning; these data points should be flagged or removed from downstream analysis.
- Dissociate cells to be used from culture flasks, using an agent such as Trypsin/EDTA or other detachment media appropriate for the cell type of interest.
- Count cells, ideally using an automated counter (*e.g.*, ViCell, Beckman Coulter, California, USA). Calculate the volume of cells needed to seed different cell densities per well. An example would be covering a range of densities from 500 – 8,000 cells per well (Fig. **3**).
- Remove the E-plate from the RTCA instrument and dispense cells in 30 µL of appropriate culture medium using a multichannel pipettor or an automated liquid dispenser (if using automation to dispense cells, select a low-speed setting to prevent cell shearing).
- Allow cells to settle for 10 to 15 minutes at room temperature before returning to the incubator to prevent uneven plating caused by convection at 37 °C.
- Plate E-plate(s) back onto the RTCA electrode and set the program to record impedance measurements every 15 minutes as cells adhere overnight. Raw impedance measurements should increase over time as cells adhere, but maximal measurements will differ according to cell seeding density, as indicated in Fig. (**1**).
- After an overnight incubation (approximately 16 hours), manually inspect the Cell Index curves to ensure cells have attached.
- Prepare compound treatments at X-fold greater concentrations such that the final delivered concentration would be 1X. For example, if the starting media volume is 50 µL, the compound can be delivered with 10 µL of 6X the desired final concentration (60 uM to deliver a final concentration of 10 uM). When preparing treatments, ensure 10 – 25% more volume than needed to account for pipetting dead-volume. Compounds should be dissolved in recommended solvents. When performing concentration-response experiments, prepare dilution series in a master plate and dilute compounds in solvent/vehicle prior to

adding to cell media, so all compounds have an equivalent vehicle concentration.

- Add diluted compounds to E-plates using a suitable liquid handler (*e.g.*, Biomek FX, Beckman Coulter, USA). An advantage of using high-throughput liquid handling is rapid addition (> 1 minute), and plates can be returned to the RTCA instrument within 2 to 3 minutes to avoid asynchronous responses. We would advise the use of an electronic multichannel pipettor if liquid handlers are unavailable.
- In the impedance software, set impedance measurements to record at 1-minute intervals for 4 hours, after which measurements can be recorded every 15 minutes for the subsequent 16 – 18 hours.
- Within the RTCA software, impedance measurements are normalized by dividing the measurement at the post-treatment timepoint of interest by an untreated baseline time-point measurement (for example, 30 minutes prior to compound addition).
- After inspection of the response curves, export data from RTCA software at timepoints of interest, typically into a comma-separated-values (.csv) file or other Excel readable format.
- Compare Vmax and EC_{50} of different control compounds with respect to cell density and use Z' calculation to assess assay window and measurement variation from compound and vehicle treatment. Z' measurements will dictate screening assay suitability. Z' values between 0.5 – 1 are considered to be excellent, whereas measurements below 0.5 should be used with caution, as this indicates a narrow assay window and the potential for large data variation. Examples of curves and corresponding data are shown in Fig. (**2**).

a) $$Z' = 1 - \frac{3(\text{standard deviation}_{\text{positive control}} + \text{standard deviation}_{\text{negative control}})}{|\text{mean}_{\text{positive control}} - \text{mean}_{\text{negative control}}|}$$

Direct Assessment of the Degree of Cell Confluency at Different Plating Densities

A parallel assessment of cell density may be required in order to interpret changes observed in the impedance plates. Direct imaging in imaging plates can be challenging owing to the visual obstruction of cells by the electrodes, so the use of an alternative set of plates can provide additional insight.

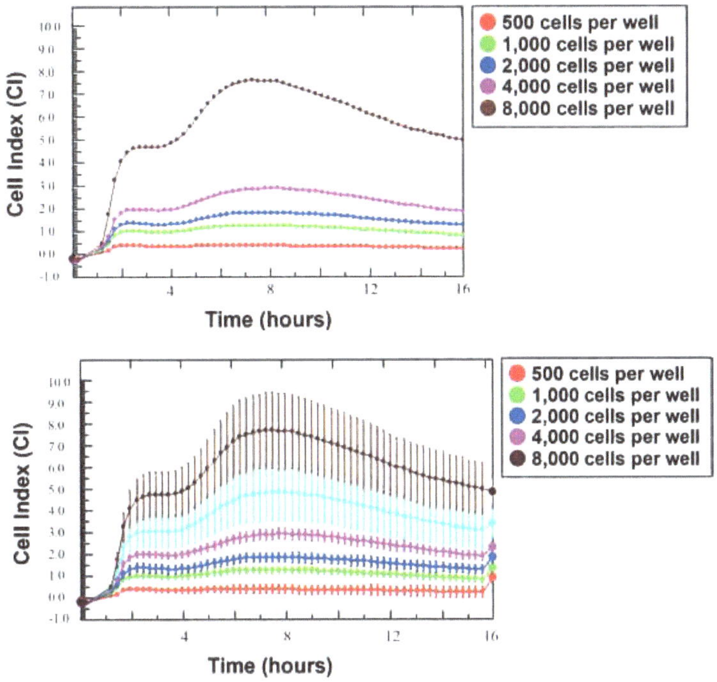

Fig. (1). – Raw impedance measurements at different seeding densities for NTM5 cells. Cell index (CI) measurements stabilize for each original plating density after 8 hours in the case of cells that exhibit contact inhibition. Top measurements are without standard deviation, whereas traces in the bottom panel show standard deviation under unoptimized conditions. Baseline impedance is higher with a greater number of cells.

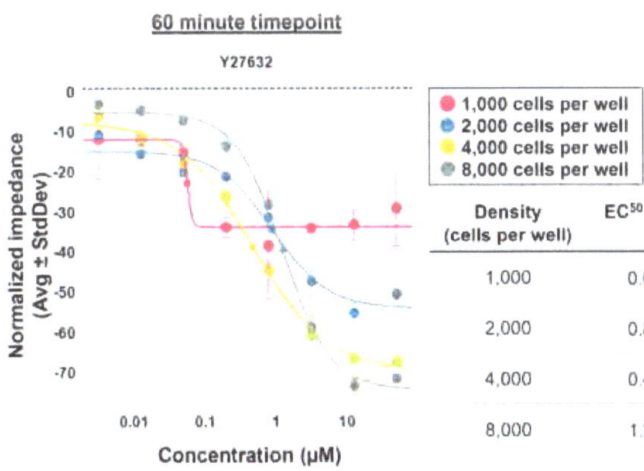

Density (cells per well)	EC50 (µM)	Z' at max concentration	Vmax
1,000	0.06	-2.39	-28.75%
2,000	0.88	0.84	-50.33%
4,000	0.47	0.82	-67.22%
8,000	1.23	0.85	-71.30%

Fig. (2). – Impedance magnitude of response and EC_{50} are dependent on cell density in NTM5 cells. Y27632, a ROCK inhibitor compound, causes a concentration-dependent decrease in impedance measurement (showing a 60-minute timepoint). Maximal response (Vmax, -67.22% relative to control), lowest EC_{50} (0.47 µM), and a good Z' (0.82) were observed at 4,000 cells per well, which could be selected as the appropriate plating density. We recommend using between 8 to 16 wells for control and test conditions to calculate Z'. Note that a combination of factors should be used to select the plating density; *e.g.* 8,000 cells/well of a 384-well plate provides a similar Vmax and Z' but a less sensitive EC_{50}.

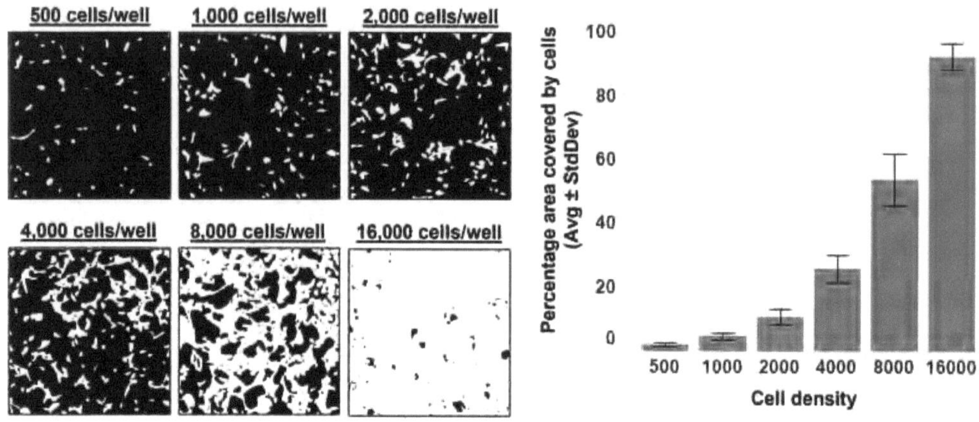

Fig. (3). – Assessment of NTM5 confluency at different cell densities. (A) Fluorescent images of CellMask stain at different densities are presented here following thresholding to demonstrate the relative level of confluence; black space is unoccupied, whereas white space is thresholded cell body (thresholded images generated with CellProfiler software). (B) The percentage area was calculated using a CellProfiler quantification algorithm. This information can be helpful in assessing cell behavior and factors contributing to Cell Index changes. For example, junctional changes may contribute more to Cell Index with increasing cell density. Cell confluency also varies depending on cell type.

- Detach cells from the culture flask using appropriate detachment media. Count cells using an automated counter (*e.g.*, ViCell, Beckman Coulter, California, USA).
- Calculate the volume of cells needed to seed different cell densities per well.
- Dispense cells in complete media to a 384-well clear-bottom, black-walled imaging plate (*e.g.*, Greiner μClear plates (Greiner BioOne, Germany)) using a multichannel pipettor or an automated dispenser (set at a low-speed setting to prevent cell shearing).
- Allow cells to settle for 10 to 15 minutes at room temperature before returning to the incubator to prevent uneven plating caused by convection at 37 °C.
- Place plates into the incubator and allow them to adhere. Keep cells in culture for an equivalent amount of time as used for the impedance assay (~32 hours).
- Fix cells by adding paraformaldehyde (PFA) to a final concentration of 4% in the wells, using either a multichannel pipettor or liquid handler. Incubate for 15 minutes – ensure that the addition of PFA is carried out in a chemical hood.
- Wash cells three times with buffer (*i.e.*, Tris-buffered saline, phosphate-buffered saline, *etc.*) to remove PFA. If available, an automated plate-washer can be used (*e.g.* EL406 plate-washer (BioTek/Agilent, California, USA)). Multi-channel pipettors are an acceptable alternative. Ensure PFA waste is appropriately handled per your organization's environmental health and safety regulations.
- After fixation, stain cells with a general dye that will capture bulk morphology (*e.g.*, CellMask) and nuclei (Hoechst) (ThermoFisher Scientific, Massachusetts). Permeabilization of cells will interfere with CellMask staining, so avoid the use

of reagents like Triton X-100 – both stains are naturally cell-permeable. Incubate at room temperature for 1 – 4 hours.

- Wash plates with buffer as described above.
- Obtain fluorescent images (using a 10X – 20X objective) of CellMask and Hoechst channels using a high-content imager (*e.g.*, InCell 2200, Cytiva, Massachusetts) or a microscope with a well plate holder. We recommend capturing multiple areas per well and use of a minimum of 2 wells in order to avoid local variation in cell density.
- CellMask staining is typically strong, and approximate confluency can be estimated by eye. For a more accurate assessment, images can be quantified using an image quantification application such as CellProfiler (Stirling *et al.*, 2021) or ImageJ, FIJI, *etc.* We have developed quantification algorithms using CellProfiler, where CellMask images are thresholded and classified as objects, which can then be measured for their area. Object/cell area is then divided by the total image area to calculate the percent area coverage for each density.

ASSESSING THE EFFECTS OF SERUM STARVATION ON ASSAY PERFORMANCE

Many complete growth media are supplemented with serum, which contains the known contractile agents sphingosine-1-phosphate (S1P) and lysophosphatidic acid (LPA) (Chrisman *et al.*, 2003). To reduce pro-contractile contributions from standard culture media, different low-serum or serum-starvation conditions can be evaluated for their effect on cell viability and assay quality from positive control compounds. Parameters to vary can include testing different concentrations of FBS or alternative supplements that support cell survival, such as insulin-transferrin-selenium (ITS) (ThermoFisher Scientific, Massachusetts).

Serum-starvation Optimization

- Prepare plates and cells as described in steps 1.1.2 through 1.1.10.
- The following day, wash cells three times into the desired different media conditions, *e.g.* serum-free media, 1% ITS, 0.5% FBS, or 10% FBS. We typically recommend using an EL405 plate washer (BioTek/Agilent, California, USA) located in a sterile biosafety cabinet and suggest automating these steps if possible to ensure accurate/consistent volume exchange between wells. Alternatively, if a plate-washer is unavailable, we suggest the use of a multichannel pipette. A typical final volume after washing is 30 µL per well of a 384-well plate.
- Return the plate to an RTCA electrode and monitor for at least 6 hours while recording impedance measurements every 15 minutes. We encourage running serum-starvation duration optimization experiments.

- Prepare compound treatments at X-fold greater concentrations such that the final delivered concentration will be 1X. For example, in the current experiment, our post-wash volume is 30 µL, so we can deliver 10 µL of 4X final concentration. Dilution series should be conducted as previously described.
- Add diluted compounds as previously described.
- In impedance software, set impedance measurements to record at 1-minute intervals for 4 hours, after which measurements can be recorded every 15 minutes for the subsequent 16 – 18 hours or another desired length of time. Time course and measurement recordings may be application-dependent and require empirical evaluation.
- Within RTCA software, normalize impedance measurements by dividing them into a pre-compound addition time-point measurement. Export data from RTCA software at timepoints of interest.
- Compare Vmax and AC_{50} of different compounds with respect to serum conditions. Z' measurements can also be assessed. Typical data and effects on response, EC50, and Z' are shown in Fig. (**4**).

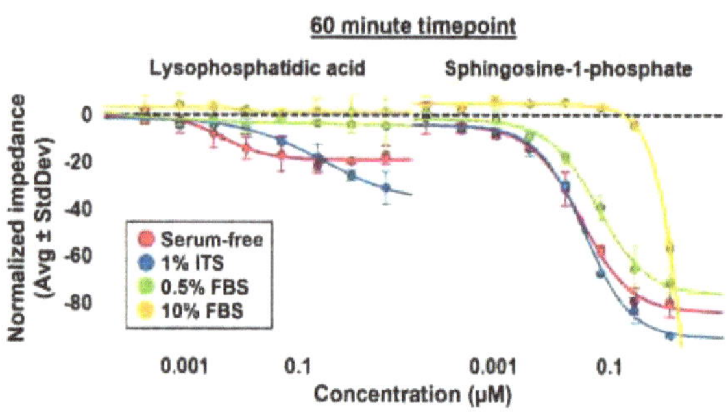

Treatment	Serum Condition	EC^{50} (µM)	Z' at max concentration	Vmax
LPA	Serum-free	0.001	-0.34	-15.9%
	1% ITS	0.1	0.03	-30.1%
	0.5% FBS	>3	-8.30	-3.8%
	10% FBS	>3	-22.40	2.32%
S1P	Serum-free	0.03	0.51	-78.4%
	1% ITS	0.03	0.94	-92.6%
	0.5% FBS	0.05	0.78	-70.3%
	10% FBS	2.31	0.72	-55.1%

Fig. (4). – Responsiveness of NTM5 cells to stimuli in different serum conditions. Serum content can influence impedance measurements (60-minute time point). In this assay setup, compounds have the best $EC_{50,}$ Vmax, and response in serum-free or 1% ITS conditions. Lysophosphatidic acid (LPA) and Sphingosine-1-phosphate (S1P) yielded minimal impedance change in the presence of 10% FBS. S1P shows some response with 0.5% FBS, but no response is observed with LPA.

ASSESSMENT OF CELL ADHERENCE FOLLOWING SERUM STARVATION AND WASHING

Cell types have different substrate adhesion properties, which can be influenced by altering growth conditions. Further, cell loss during wash steps can impact the interpretation of impedance results, leading to false positives or negatives. Assessment of the effect of cell washing under the desired assay conditions can assist in assay optimization and reduce the risk of data misinterpretation. This section describes a parallel imaging approach to evaluate this parameter.

Imaging Assessment of Cell Adherence

- Prepare and dispense cells as previously described above.
- Place plates into an incubator and allow them to adhere overnight (approximately 16 hours)
- The following morning, wash each individual plate 0 – 5 times. For example, subject plate 1 to 1 wash cycle and set aside, subject plate 2 to 2 wash cycles and set aside, and so on (reserve a plate for no wash control).
- Fix cells using 4% PFA for 15 minutes. Wash cells with buffer to remove PFA. Ensure PFA waste is appropriately handled per your organization's environmental health and safety regulations.
- After fixation, stain nuclei with Hoechst dye (Thermo Fisher Scientific, Massachusetts). Incubate at room temperature for 1 hour.
- Wash plates into the imaging buffer as described above.
- Obtain fluorescent images (10X – 20X objective) of the Hoechst channel using any high-content imager or microscope with a well plate holder.
- Use image quantification software (*i.e.* CellProfiler, ImageJ, FIJI, *etc.*) to develop a quantification algorithm that will count the number of nuclei. Normalize data relative to average counts for 0 wash plates – set this value to 100. A minimal loss of cells (~5%) post-washing is acceptable.

ASSESSMENT OF CELL TOLERANCE TO VEHICLES AND SOLVENTS

Low-molecular-weight compounds are often dissolved in dimethylsulfoxide (DMSO), ethanol, or other solvents, all of which have the potential to be cytotoxic or alter assay performance at high concentrations. Some compounds are poorly soluble at high stock concentrations, which requires a higher administration of DMSO volume to achieve activity; other compounds simply require higher concentrations to elicit activity, which can increase the final DMSO concentration. Different cell types have varying degrees of DMSO sensitivity, and RTCA instrument measurements are highly sensitive to cell density, so we advise assessing vehicle tolerability by measuring cell viability and/or baseline impedance. Cell Titer Glo reagents (CTG, Promega, Wisconsin, USA) measure cellular ATP content, which can often be a good proxy for cell viability. The approach may also be used to assess false positives from a screen – *e.g.*, to identify compounds or treatments that appear to cause an effect but instead lower Cell Index by killing cells.

Vehicle-tolerability Assessment and Viability Counter-Screen for False-Positives

- Prepare plates and cells as described above.
- The following morning, wash cells into serum-free media as previously

described. Return the E-plate to the RTCA electrode and serum-starve for 6 hours while recording impedance measurements every 15 minutes.

- Prepare DMSO treatments (or other vehicle/solvent) at X-fold greater concentrations such that the final delivered concentration would be 1X. For example, in the current experiment, our post-wash volume is 30 µL, so in order to administer 1% DMSO, we would need to prepare a 4% DMSO solution (4X final concentration) with 10 µL delivered. DMSO is typically administered at a final concentration of 0.1 – 0.5%, so we recommend starting in this range and evaluating higher and lower concentrations to establish boundaries (*e.g.*, 0.005% to 10% DMSO).
- Add DMSO to E-plates, return to RTCA electrode, and record impedance measurements at 1-minute intervals for 4 hours, after which measurements can be recorded every 15 minutes for the subsequent 16 – 18 hours.
- Thaw and prepare CTG reagents according to the manufacturer's instructions.
- Dispense CTG reagent to E-plates.
- Incubate sample plates for 5 minutes at room temperature.
- Transfer lysates to a 384-well white-walled plate for absorbance measurement using a suitable plate reader (*e.g.*, Envision, Perkin Elmer)
- Process CTG data and normalize the measurement from no DMSO treatment (set to 100). Typical data obtained are shown in Fig. (**5**).
- As an alternative to running a CTG assay, a parallel imaging experiment can be run on an imaging plate using the time parameters described in this section. See Fig. (**6**).

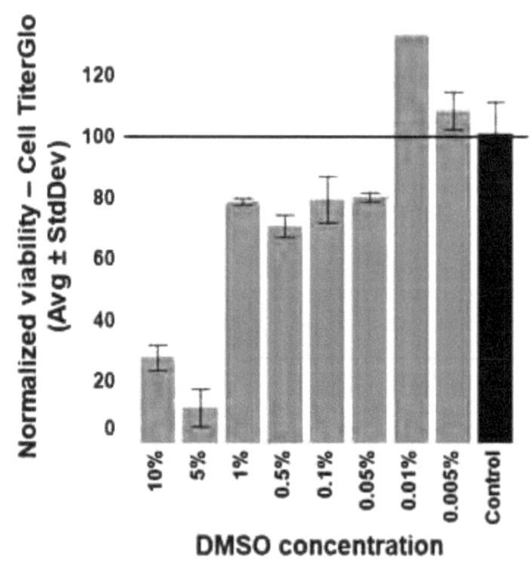

Fig. (5). – Increasing DMSO concentration impacts cell viability in NTM5 cells. ATP content was measured in NTM5 cells following treatment with a range of DMSO concentrations (0.005 to 10%) for 48 hours. Low concentrations of DMSO (0.005% - 0.01%) had little to no impact on viability, with a subtle (~20%) decrease in viability observed from the range of 0.05% to 1% DMSO. Significant ATP reduction was observed with 5 – 10% DMSO. In this example, final DMSO concentrations should be 1% or less to avoid significant effects on viability.

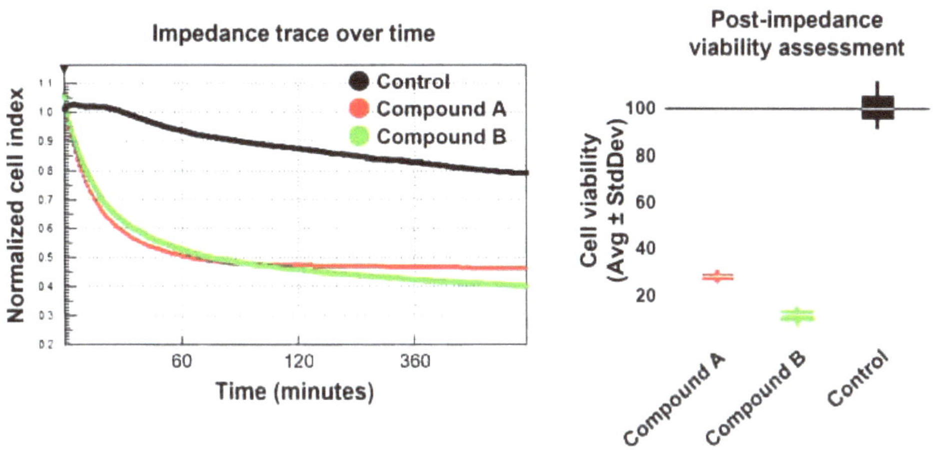

Fig. (6). –Viability counterscreens identify false positive hits. Manual inspection of impedance traces for Compounds A and B suggests a rapid response that could be indicative of changes in the cytoskeleton. Counterscreening for viability confirms that a decrease in impedance measurement correlates with compound-associated toxicity.

DATA EXTRACTION AND ANALYSIS

Impedance measurements on the RTCA instrument are reported by Cell Index (CI), which is calculated by taking the impedance measurement at time point X and subtracting the cell-free impedance measurement recorded at baseline. Data can be further normalized within the impedance software by dividing each CI measurement by a pre-treatment impedance baseline measurement.

Impedance measurements on an RTCA instrument can be set to record at any desired interval and for any number of measurements. Data from all recorded measurements is available for export in a list or matrix format. Depending on the interval duration and frequency of measurements, an individual experiment can have hundreds of timepoints. When assessing effects on cellular contractility, responses to compound treatment are often in the order of minutes, and so extraction of data from earlier timepoints (*e.g.* 5-240 minutes) is typically warranted. Depending on the responsiveness of cells to different compound types, a focus on later timepoints may be considered. Careful and manual inspection of the amplitude and timing of the responses in an experiment are needed to determine the appropriate normalization timepoints and times to extract data. Data can also be exported in a comma-delimited, Excel-readable format, which allows further data visualization by programs such as Excel or Spotfire (TIBCO, California, USA). An example of this would be plotting normalized impedance changes (as a percentage) against different compound concentrations, as exemplified in Figs. (**2** and **4**).

CORROBORATING IMPEDANCE CHANGES WITH ACTIN CYTOSKELETAL CHANGES BY IMMUNOFLUORESCENCE

It is important to corroborate impedance assays with a more focused investigation of phenotypes/functional changes that can be observed. Compounds that elicit changes in impedance assay can be orthogonally validated to understand the cytoskeletal implications of the impedance measurement. Phalloidin dye (Thermo Fisher Scientific, Massachusetts) will stain filamentous actin and is available conjugated to multiple fluorescent dyes (*i.e.*, AlexaFluor488, 568, 657, *etc.*). Clear resolution of actin dynamics can suffer as a consequence of tight cell-cell proximity/packing, so evaluating multiple cell densities may be required to create an opportunity for interpreting images. Impedance trace kinetics should be used to select timepoint(s) for analysis.

Actin staining with phalloidin

- Prepare, plate, and fix cells according to steps described above. In cell preparation, the addition of benchmark compounds such as Rho kinase inhibitors, latrunculin A, and endothelin-1 should be considered to provide relevant benchmarks for actin depolymerization and stress fiber formation, respectively. Other types of compounds can also be used to verify/validate the system (Fig. 7).
- After fixation, stain cells with phalloidin and Hoechst (nuclei) and any other dyes or antibodies as desired. Methanol fixation will depolymerize actin, so we encourage the use of PFA. Incubate at room temperature for 1 – 4 hours.
- Wash plates with buffer as previously described
- Obtain fluorescent images (10X – 20X objective) of phalloidin and Hoechst channels using a high-content imager or a fluorescent microscope with a well plate holder. We recommend capturing multiple areas per well to avoid local variation in cell density.
- Visually inspect images for differences in cell size, shape, actin stress fibers, cortical actin, *etc.* For a more accurate assessment, images can be quantified using an image-quantification software such as CellProfiler (Stirling *et al.*, 2021) or ImageJ, FIJI, *etc.* We have developed quantification algorithms using CellProfiler, where F-actin images are thresholded, classified as objects, and measured for intensity. Object/intensity is then divided by total image area to calculate the percent area coverage for each density.

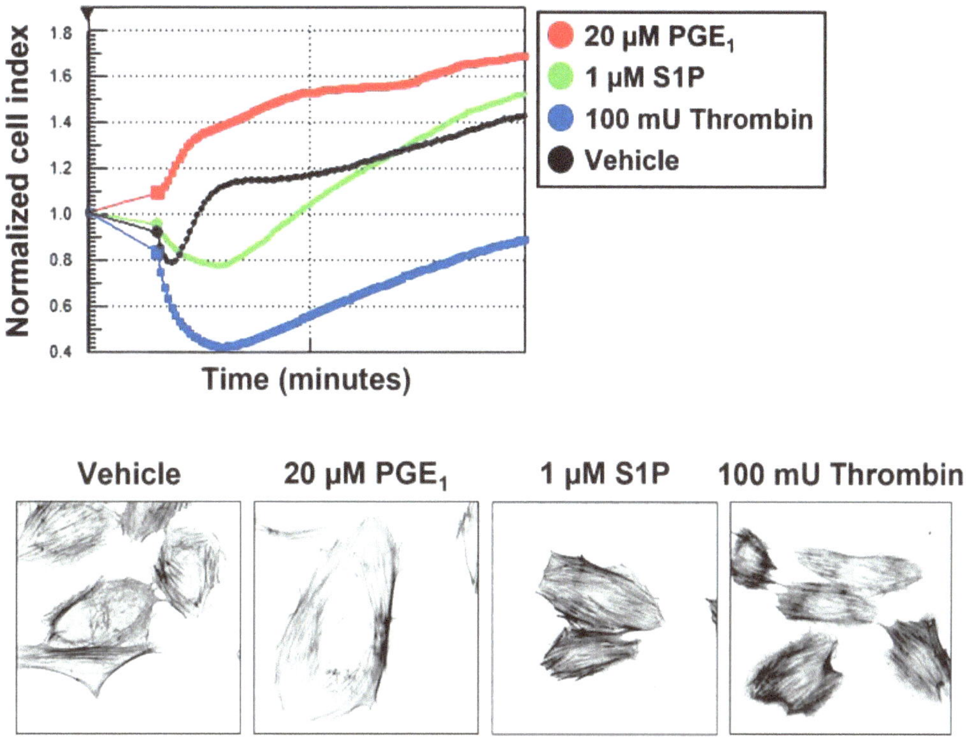

Fig. (7). – Assessment of the actin cytoskeleton is essential for interpretation of results. Single-donor human umbilical vein endothelial cells (HUVEC) (Promocell, Heidelberg, Germany) were treated with various contractile or relaxing agents and assessed for impedance response and F-actin staining. (11α,13E,15S)-11,15-Dihydroxy-9-oxoprost-13-enoic acid (alprostadil, labeled as PGE1), a cell relaxing agent, leads to increased cell size and decreases in filamentous actin staining, whereas S1P and thrombin, known contractile agents, lead to decreased cell size and increases in filamentous and cortical actin staining.

CONSIDERATIONS FOR HIGH-THROUGHPUT SCREENING WORKFLOWS

Screening of compound libraries is typically conducted at a single or limited number of high compound concentrations (*i.e.*, 10 uM and 2 uM in 2-3 replicate plates). In this format, many compounds are tested, hits are rescreened for confirmation of false hits, false positives are removed, and true hits are confirmed by assessing the cellular response to differing concentrations of the compound. Mechanistic studies can then be performed in order to confirm that the observed impedance changes correlate with changes in the actin cytoskeleton or other relevant biology. It should also be noted that relaxation or contraction of the cytoskeleton is not consistently associated with the same direction of impedance change. For instance, both PGE1 and Y27632, known relaxing agents, show opposite effects on Cell Index. This should be considered when interpreting data and is another reason to orthogonally validate interpretations by cytoskeletal staining.

One limitation of high-throughput screening in the RTCA system is the maximum capacity of 4 plates per instrument at any one time. The implication of this is that testing hundreds to thousands of compounds cannot be accomplished over a few days. Nonetheless, it is possible to do so if attention is paid to cell performance over time, ensuring that Vmax, EC_{50}, and Z' values of control compounds do not change significantly after passaging. Further, the same assay controls should be included on every assay plate. These assay controls can be used to calculate Z' for every plate, and plates that show a diminished assay window (*e.g.* Z' < 0.5) should be discarded from further analysis.

CONCLUSION

Impedance measurements are highly sensitive to alterations in cell contractility, relaxation, migration, and barrier function and can provide a useful, label-free approach to monitoring cellular behavior. There are numerous caveats and considerations to enable the careful interpretation of data and to ensure that the responses in impedance change are associated with a particular behavior. We hope that the protocols and factors outlined here provide a framework for the community to incorporate this platform and approach into their assessments of cellular behavior.

ACKNOWLEDGEMENTS

We thank Ernie Hixon, Enhua Zhou, Michael Twarog, YongYao Xu, and Dennis Rice for their support and contributions to impedance-based assays at our institution and Vijay Raghunathan for critically reading the manuscript in preparation.

REFERENCES

Benson, K, Cramer, S & Galla, HJ (2013) Impedance-based cell monitoring: barrier properties and beyond. *Fluids Barriers CNS,* 10, 5.
[http://dx.doi.org/10.1186/2045-8118-10-5] [PMID: 23305242]

Cavet, ME, Vollmer, TR, Harrington, KL, VanDerMeid, K & Richardson, ME (2015) Regulation of Endothelin-1–Induced Trabecular Meshwork Cell Contractility by Latanoprostene Bunod. *Invest Ophthalmol Vis Sci,* 56, 4108-16.
[http://dx.doi.org/10.1167/iovs.14-16015] [PMID: 26114488]

Chrisman, TD, Perkins, DT & Garbers, DL (2003) Identification of a potent serum factor that causes desensitization of the receptor for C-Type natriuretic peptide. *Cell Commun Signal,* 1, 4.
[http://dx.doi.org/10.1186/1478-811X-1-4] [PMID: 14627441]

Doijen, J, Van Loy, T, Landuyt, B, Luyten, W, Schols, D & Schoofs, L (2019) Advantages and shortcomings of cell-based electrical impedance measurements as a GPCR drug discovery tool. *Biosens Bioelectron,* 137, 33-44.

[http://dx.doi.org/10.1016/j.bios.2019.04.041] [PMID: 31077988]

Keller, KE, Bhattacharya, SK, Borrás, T, Brunner, TM, Chansangpetch, S, Clark, AF, Dismuke, WM, Du, Y, Elliott, MH, Ethier, CR, Faralli, JA, Freddo, TF, Fuchshofer, R, Giovingo, M, Gong, H, Gonzalez, P, Huang, A, Johnstone, MA, Kaufman, PL, Kelley, MJ, Knepper, PA, Kopczynski, CC, Kuchtey, JG, Kuchtey, RW, Kuehn, MH, Lieberman, RL, Lin, SC, Liton, P, Liu, Y, Lütjen-Drecoll, E, Mao, W, Masis-Solano, M, McDonnell, F, McDowell, CM, Overby, DR, Pattabiraman, PP, Raghunathan, VK, Rao, PV, Rhee, DJ, Chowdhury, UR, Russell, P, Samples, JR, Schwartz, D, Stubbs, EB, Tamm, ER, Tan, JC, Toris, CB, Torrejon, KY, Vranka, JA, Wirtz, MK, Yorio, T, Zhang, J, Zode, GS, Fautsch, MP, Peters, DM, Acott, TS & Stamer, WD (2018) Consensus recommendations for trabecular meshwork cell isolation, characterization and culture. *Exp Eye Res,* 171, 164-73.
[http://dx.doi.org/10.1016/j.exer.2018.03.001] [PMID: 29526795]

Perkumas, KM & Stamer, WD (2012) Protein markers and differentiation in culture for Schlemm's canal endothelial cells. *Exp Eye Res,* 96, 82-7.
[http://dx.doi.org/10.1016/j.exer.2011.12.017] [PMID: 22210126]

Ramachandran, C, Patil, RV, Combrink, K, Sharif, NA & Srinivas, SP (2011) Rho-Rho kinase pathway in the actomyosin contraction and cell-matrix adhesion in immortalized human trabecular meshwork cells. *Mol Vis,* 17, 1877-90. a
[PMID: 21850162]

Ramachandran, C, Patil, RV, Sharif, NA & Srinivas, SP (2011) Effect of elevated intracellular cAMP levels on actomyosin contraction in bovine trabecular meshwork cells. *Invest Ophthalmol Vis Sci,* 52, 1474-85. b
[http://dx.doi.org/10.1167/iovs.10-6241] [PMID: 21071747]

Scrace, S, O'Neill, E, Hammond, EM & Pires, IM (2013) Use of the xCELLigence system for real-time analysis of changes in cellular motility and adhesion in physiological conditions. *Methods Mol Biol,* 1046, 295-306.
[http://dx.doi.org/10.1007/978-1-62703-538-5_17] [PMID: 23868595]

Stamer, WD, Piwnica, D, Jolas, T, Carling, RW, Cornell, CL, Fliri, H, Martos, J, Pettit, SN, Wang, JW & Woodward, DF (2010) Cellular basis for bimatoprost effects on human conventional outflow. *Invest Ophthalmol Vis Sci,* 51, 5176-81.
[http://dx.doi.org/10.1167/iovs.09-4955] [PMID: 20435598]

Stirling, DR, Swain-Bowden, MJ, Lucas, AM, Carpenter, AE, Cimini, BA & Goodman, A (2021) CellProfiler 4: improvements in speed, utility and usability. *BMC Bioinformatics,* 22, 433.
[http://dx.doi.org/10.1186/s12859-021-04344-9] [PMID: 34507520]

Tamm, E, Flügel, C, Baur, A & Lütjen-Drecoll, E (1991) Cell cultures of human ciliary muscle: Growth, ultrastructural and immunocytochemical characteristics. *Exp Eye Res,* 53, 375-87.
[http://dx.doi.org/10.1016/0014-4835(91)90244-9] [PMID: 1936174]

Tanna, AP & Johnson, M (2018) Rho Kinase Inhibitors as a Novel Treatment for Glaucoma and Ocular Hypertension. *Ophthalmology,* 125, 1741-56.
[http://dx.doi.org/10.1016/j.ophtha.2018.04.040] [PMID: 30007591]

Thieulent, C, Hue, ES, Sutton, G, Fortier, C, Dallemagne, P, Zientara, S, Munier-Lehmann, H, Hans, A, Paillot, R, Vidalain, PO & Pronost, S (2020) Identification of antiviral compounds against equid herpesvirus-1 using real-time cell assay screening: Efficacy of decitabine and valganciclovir alone or in combination. *Antiviral Res,* 183, 104931.
[http://dx.doi.org/10.1016/j.antiviral.2020.104931] [PMID: 32926887]

Vollmer, TR, Zhou, EH, Rice, DS, Prasanna, G, Chen, A & Wilson, CW (2020) Application of Cell Impedance as a Screening Tool to Discover Modulators of Intraocular Pressure. *J Ocul Pharmacol Ther,* 36, 269-81.
[http://dx.doi.org/10.1089/jop.2019.0078] [PMID: 32176566]

Wang, JW, Woodward, DF & Stamer, WD (2013) Differential effects of prostaglandin E2-sensitive receptors on contractility of human ocular cells that regulate conventional outflow. *Invest Ophthalmol Vis Sci,* 54,

4782-90.
[http://dx.doi.org/10.1167/iovs.13-12363] [PMID: 23766471]

Webber, HC, Bermudez, JY, Millar, JC, Mao, W & Clark, AF (2018) The Role of Wnt/β-Catenin Signaling and K-Cadherin in the Regulation of Intraocular Pressure. *Invest Ophthalmol Vis Sci,* 59, 1454-66.
[http://dx.doi.org/10.1167/iovs.17-21964] [PMID: 29625468]

Xing, JZ, Zhu, L, Jackson, JA, Gabos, S, Sun, XJ, Wang, X & Xu, X (2005) Dynamic monitoring of cytotoxicity on microelectronic sensors. *Chem Res Toxicol,* 18, 154-61.
[http://dx.doi.org/10.1021/tx049721s] [PMID: 15720119]

Zhang, JH, Chung, TDY & Oldenburg, KR (1999) A Simple Statistical Parameter for Use in Evaluation and Validation of High Throughput Screening Assays. *SLAS Discov,* 4, 67-73.
[http://dx.doi.org/10.1177/108705719900400206] [PMID: 10838414]

CHAPTER 16

Protocols for Studying Ocular Cell Volume Changes in Aqueous Humor Outflow Regulating Cells *In Vitro*

Dorette Z. Ellis[1,*]

[1] *Department of Pharmaceutical Sciences, University of North Texas System College of Pharmacy, North Texas Eye Research Institute, University of North Texas Health Science Center, Fort Worth, Texas, USA*

Abstract: This chapter describes a protocol for measuring trabecular meshwork and Schlemm's cell volume with different experimental conditions over time, utilizing fluorescence and confocal microscopic methods. A fluorescence probe is applied to the cells, and a confocal microscope captures pixeled, z-stacked images with 8 bits of resolution. The images are converted from 8-bit to 1-bit or binary. Threshold values are determined using fluorescent latex beads of known diameter, and cell volume is analyzed. ImageJ software is used to calculate the number of voxels in the region of interest in the image stack. This methodology is of interest, as the outflow of aqueous humor is actively controlled by cellular and molecular mechanisms in the aqueous humor outflow pathway that includes the trabecular meshwork and Schlemm's canal. Several cellular mechanisms have been characterized by which changes in aqueous humor outflow can occur, including changes in the trabecular meshwork and Schlemm's canal cell volume.

Keywords: Cell volume, Fluorescence probe, Ocular hypertension, Schlemm's canal, Trabecular meshwork.

INTRODUCTION

Elevated intraocular pressure (IOP) places patients at an increased risk for developing visual field loss in the progressive blinding disease, glaucoma. IOP results from the balance between aqueous humor secretion by the ciliary processes and its outflow through the trabecular meshwork and Schlemm's canal (SC) within the anterior chamber of the eye. Major routes for the outflow of aqueous humor are the trabecular meshwork comprising of uveal and corneoscleral tra-

* **Corresponding author Dorette Z. Ellis:** Department of Pharmaceutical Sciences, University of North Texas System College of Pharmacy, North Texas Eye Research Institute, University of North Texas Health Science Center, Fort Worth, Texas, USA; Tel: (817) 735-2000; E-mail: dorette.ellis@unthsc.edu

Najam A. Sharif and Sunny E. Ohia (Eds.)

becular meshwork (TM) and the juxtacanalicular cells (JCT-trabecular meshwork), in conjunction with the Schlemm's canal (SC), and also the uveoscleral pathway that occurs across the ciliary muscle (CM) through small spaces between CM bundles (Lee *et al.*, 1982; Kaufman *et al.*, 1984; Krupin *et al.*, 1995). An imbalance of aqueous humor secretion and outflow will yield high pressures within the eye that can damage the retina and the optic nerve and thus cause loss of vision.

Once thought to be a passive process, the outflow of aqueous humor is now known to be actively controlled by the cells in the aqueous humor outflow pathways. Several cellular mechanisms have been characterized by which changes in aqueous humor outflow can occur. These include TM contractility and cell volume changes, CM contractility, alterations of the extracellular matrix in the TM, and formation of pores and vacuoles (Fig. **1**) in the inner wall of the SC (Banerjee *et al.*, 2017; Mitchell *et al.*, 2002; Soto *et al.*, 2004; O'Donnell *et al.*, 1995; Al-Aswad *et al.*, 1999; Stumpff *et al.*, 2000; Bradley *et al.*, 1998; Grierson *et al.*, 1998).

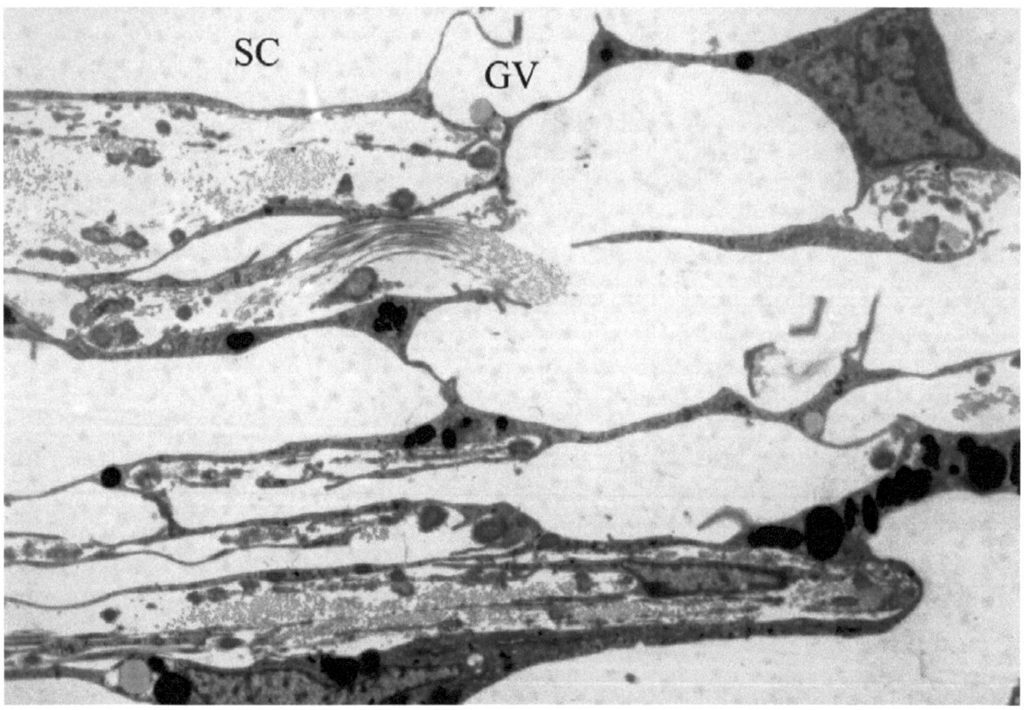

Fig. (1). Transmission electron micrograph of the aqueous humor pathway comprising the trabecular meshwork, JCT region, and Schlemm's canal (SC), showing giant vacuoles (GV) in the SC region. Image generated in the Ellis Lab.

Cell volume changes in the aqueous humor outflow pathway are of interest as they have been correlated with changes in the aqueous humor outflow facility. Studies demonstrate that a hypotonic or hypertonic challenge to a perfused eye anterior segment will decrease or increase the outflow facility respectively (Al-Aswad *et al*., 1999). To begin to understand mechanisms by which changes in TM and SC cell volume would affect aqueous humor drainage requires an understanding of the architecture of the aqueous humor outflow pathway (Fig. **1**). The TM is composed of interwoven collagen-covered elastin "beams". Trabecular endothelial cells (TM cells) line the outflow pathway and have been suggested to perform a number of functions, including phagocytosis (Polansky *et al*., 1984) and extracellular matrix (ECM) turnover (Alexander *et al*., 1991). As aqueous humor flows deeper into the TM towards the SC, the open spaces available for fluid to flow through decrease. As the spaces through which fluid flows narrow, the volume of the TM cells lining these openings would begin to exert more influence over the outflow facility. Increasing or decreasing the volume of these cells would, therefore, decrease or increase the rate by which fluid exits the eye, respectively.

Over the years of ocular cell volume regulation studies, several methodologies have been utilized to measure cell volumes. They include electronic cell sizing of suspended TM cells using a Coulter counter (O'Donnell *et al*., 1995; Li *et al*., 2011; Banerjee *et al*., 2017) and radioisotopes [^{14}C]urea and [^{14}C]sucrose as markers of cell volume of total intracellular and extracellular space(O'Donnell *et al*., 1995). While these are widely accepted methodologies, there are limitations on their uses. For example, electronic cell sizing utilizes non-adherent cells in suspension that have been treated with trypsin, a potential cell stressor and damaging enzyme. Additionally, the status of individual cells cannot be monitored during a given experimental run. This chapter describes a protocol that allows the measurement of cell volume of TM and SC cells that may be exposed to different experimental conditions over time using fluorescence and confocal microscopy (Mitchell *et al*., 2002; Bush *et al*., 2003 and 2005; Dismuke *et al*., 2008; Ellis *et al*., 2010)

EXPERIMENTAL PROTOCOLS

Cell Culture

Background

This section describes the protocol for the preparation of previously isolated and characterized primary cultured TM and SC cells for use in measuring cell volume (Fig. **2** and Table **1**) (Ellis *et al*., 2010).

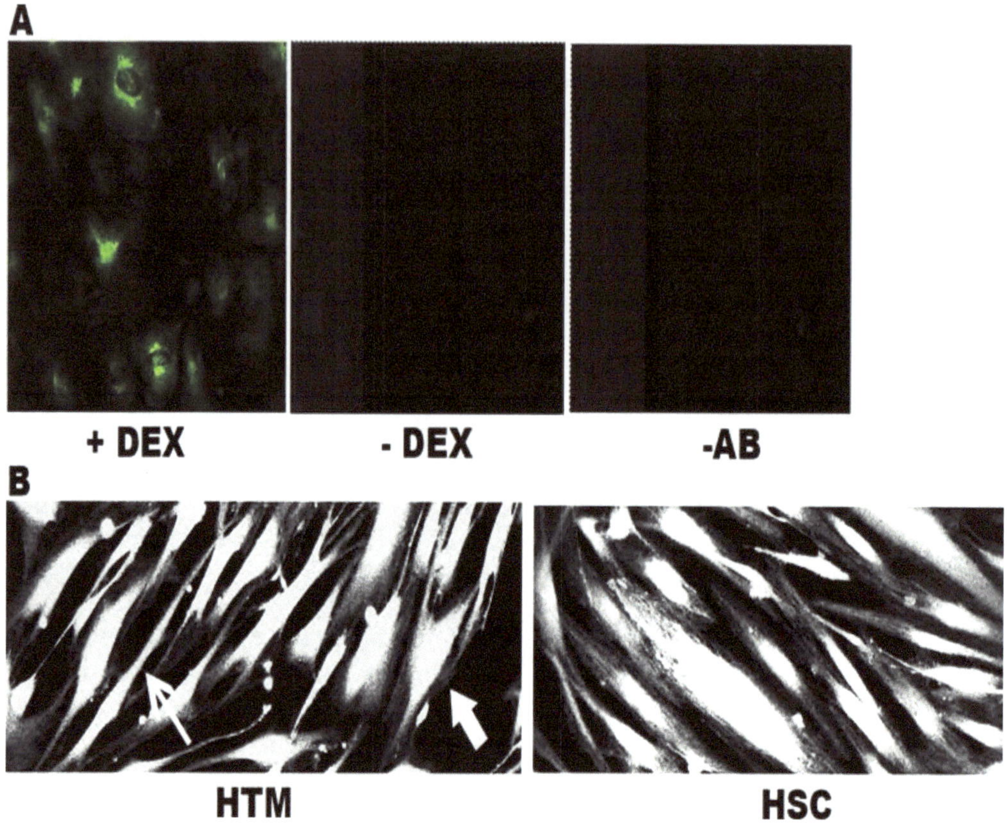

Fig. (2). Characterization of human trabecular meshwork and Schlemm's canal cells by dexamethasone treatment and morphological analysis. A. Dexamethasone treatment resulted in increased myocilin expression (+Dex) in trabecular meshwork cells but not in Schlemm's canal cells (data not shown). B. Trabecular meshwork cells contain a more heterogeneous cell population when compared with the Schlemm's canal cell population. Arrows point to morphologically different cells. Previously published in IOVS, Ellis *et al.*, 2010.

Table 1. Characterization of human trabecular meshwork cells and Schlemm's canal cells by their transendothelial electrical resistances. Schlemm's canal cells transendothelial electrical resistance measured ≥10 Ωcm2 after 1 week at confluence (Table 1). Human SC cells and TM cells (numbers represent the ages of the human donors) were grown on filters, as described below, and transendothelial resistance was measured using EVOM2 Voltometer. Data are expressed as Ωcm2 and represent the difference (Difference) between the resistance of the cells (Readings) and the resistance of the blank (Blank) filter. Previously published in IOVS, Ellis et al., 2010.

Cells	Readings(si)	Blank(S)	Difference(S)
SC 14	84	72	12
SC 25	91	70	21
SC 24	84	70	14
TM 84	77	72	5

Protocol

- Obtain well-characterized low-passage (2-5 passages) primary TM or SC (Fig. **2** and Table **1**). For the duration of the experiments, examine that cells are healthy and free from contamination by fibroblasts, bacteria, or fungus.
- For growth in 6-well plates, seed cells approximately $1x10^5$ cells/well.
- Add cell-growth medium containing low-glucose (1 g/l) DMEM, 10% FBS, 100 U/ml penicillin, and 100 µg/ml streptomycin to the cells. Allow cells to grow to 80-100% confluency in a cell-growth medium in a sterile incubator at 37°C in an atmosphere of 5% CO_2.
- Add trypsin (0.25% trypsin) to confluent cells as per the manufacturer's direction for the use of trypsin.
- Place re-suspended cells on either collagen-coated chambered cover-glass or collagen-coated 35mm petri dishes.
- Allow cells to grow to 80% confluency in the cell-growth medium in a sterile incubator at 37°C in an atmosphere of 5% CO_2.
- Carefully remove the media after the cells achieve 80% confluency.
- Add fresh culture medium without FBS (serum-free medium).

Note: TM cells can be incubated in serum-free media for 48 hrs. SC cells are more fragile and can be incubated in serum-free media for 24 hrs.

Measurement of Cell Volume Changes Using Fluorescent Indicators and Microscopy

Background

Prior to the use of fluorescent indicators and microscopy for the measurement of cell volume, changes in TM cell volume could not be measured in the same cells that were firmly attached to their substrate (*e.g.*, Petri dish and culture plate), which is the normal state for TM cells *in vitro*. The confocal microscopy instrumentation captures 1024 ×1024 or 512x512 pixel images with 8 bits of resolution. The confocal microscope captures images in z-stacks, which are a series of images captured at different equally spaced depths. For reference, a pixel represents a two-D area, whereas a voxel represents a three-D volume. The size of a voxel is determined for each image stack by the area of the pixel (for example, in μm^2, as given by the Leica confocal software) multiplied by the separation of the images in the stack (for example, in µm; z-section separation =1 µM). ImageJ software is then used to determine which images in the image stack represent the topmost and bottommost sections of the cell. The images are converted from 8-bit to 1-bit or binary configuration. A region of interest is selected, and the ImageJ software is used to calculate the number of voxels in the region of interest in the image stack. Cell volume is determined by multiplying the number of voxels by the size of 1 voxel. Threshold levels are determined using fluorescent latex beads of known diameter and volume that are imaged under conditions identical to those used for TM cells. Such calibration is important.

Fluorescent dye Preparation and Cell Loading

Background

Based on many literature reports, the cell-permeable fluorescent probe, calcein acetoxymethyl ester (calcein AM), is preferred for measuring cell volume in TM cells (Mitchell *et al.*, 2002; Dismuke *et al.*, 2008) and Schlemm's canal cells (Ellis *et al.*, 2010). Many other fluorescent probes exist (Oregon green, MQAE, fluorescein, and fura 2); however, the advantages of using calcein AM are that it is stable in TM and SC cells for up to 70 minutes and can easily enter the cells in the AM form. Additionally, calcein is an indicator of cell viability since calcein fluoresces only after hydrolysis of the acetoxymethyl ester by intracellular esterases, which are present in living cells.

Protocol

- Calcein AM needs to be reconstituted (dissolved) in high quality anhydrous dimethyl sulfoxide (DMSO) at 1 mg/mL and by following the manufacturer's instructions.
- Dilute calcein in serum-free medium containing low-glucose (1 g/l) DMEM, 100 U/ml penicillin, and 100 μg/ml streptomycin for a final working concentration of 1-2 μM.
- Load cells with 1-2 μM calcein-AM and incubate at 37°C in a 5% CO_2 incubator for 60 min to ensure a stable baseline.
- Aspirate out the medium containing the dye, add fresh medium, and image cells using a fluorescence microscope.

Note: Concentration-response experiments determined that 1-2 μM at 1 hr incubation time is optimum for our experiments. Optimization may require adjustments to incubation time and concentration of the dye. Note, in experiments, $\leq$ 0.1% DMSO in the medium had no effect on cell volume.

Confocal Microscopiv Imaging

Background

Proper use of a confocal microscope requires training, or utilizing the services of a trained microscopist is ideal. Optimize settings on the confocal microscope and use these settings throughout the entire experiment. The confocal images are captured with an intensity resolution of 8 bits or 256 (i.e., 2^8) shades from light to dark.

Cell Volume Measurement of Untreated Cells

- Place calcein AM-treated cells under the microscope
- Select an objective (20x) and select and focus on a region of interest in cells for imaging.
- Set spacing between images in the image stack. 1µm is optimum.
- Set scan speed at 400hz, and capture individual confocal images in an 8-bit, 1024x1024 or 512x512 pixel format.
- Set the upper and lower bounds of the area to be scanned, at least 1µm above and below where the cells' upper and lower portion appeared to be. This is done to ensure that both the upper and lower portions of the cells being imaged are included in the image stack.
- To capture images of the same cells over time, set the microscope to capture image stacks at desired intervals for a desired time period.

Cell Volume Measurement of Drug-Treated (Experimental) Cells

Background

To capture images of the same cells over time, the microscope can be set to capture image stacks at, for example, 5-minute intervals for 20 minutes. The first image stack is captured, and upon completion, the experimental compound is added to the dish containing the cells using the process described below. The microscope will then capture four additional image stacks 5, 10, 15, and 20 minutes following the addition of the test compound. For studies involving inhibitors or activators, the compounds may be added 5 minutes prior to capturing the initial image stack or for a time period determined to be optimum for a particular drug and /or experiment.

To image the same cells that are exposed to test compounds/ drugs, a technique was developed to deliver compounds to the cells on the coverslips to ensure that the slides did not shift during the imaging and that the images of the same cells were taken. The process was as follows:

- Drill several ports on the sides or covers of the glass chambers.
- Attach tubes to syringes and insert them into each port (allowing for the exchange of media and drugs at appropriate times)
- Mount slides containing calcein AM-treated cells onto the microscope and select the 20x objective.

- Select a region of interest on cells for imaging, and set the spacing between images in the image stack at 1μm.
- Set the upper and lower bounds of the area to be scanned, at least 1μm above and below where the cell's upper and lower portions appear to be (this is to ensure that both the upper and lower portions of the cells being imaged are included in the image stack).
- Select a scan speed of 400hz (a speed allowing measurements at 5-minute intervals for the duration of the calcein stability).
- Capture individual confocal images in an 8-bit, 1024x1024 or 512x512 pixel format.
- Capture images without drug treatment at (0) time point; this served as the experimental control.
- Add test agents to the cells through the ports without shifting the coverslip at the desired time period(s).
- Capture images at desired time intervals with the test agent present in the cells.

Cell Volume Measurement of Hypo- or Hypertonic Cells

Background

For experiments involving a hypo- or hypertonic challenge (fast-acting compounds or experimental treatments), modification of the above protocol may be needed. For example, 5-minute intervals for cell volume measurements may be too long a time period to capture the rapid volume changes induced by tonicity changes. The need to quickly capture image stacks for each time point may require a reduced resolution of 512x512 and an increased scan speed like 700hz. This necessitates a 1.7 ratio digital zoom, reducing the number of cells per treatment that can be imaged. By altering the protocol this way, a complete z-stack image with a 1μm z-spacing can be captured in less than 1 minute, allowing measurement of an initial resting cell volume. Then, the hypo- or hypertonic solution can be subjected to the cells, and cell volume can be measured at 1-minute intervals for the desired time period(s).

Protocol

- Grow cells in slides containing ports that may be used with syringes for the exchange of the medium and/or test compounds.
- Incubate cells in media-containing calcein AM as described above.
- Remove calcein-AM-containing media and replace with fresh isotonic medium.
- Place slides on a microscope and select 20x objective
- Select a region of interest on cells for imaging and set the spacing between images in the image stack at 1μm.

- Set the upper and lower bounds of the area to be scanned, at least 1μm above and below the cell's upper and lower portions.
- Select a scan speed of 700hz (a speed allowing measurements at 1-minute intervals).
- Capture individual confocal images in an 8-bit, 512x512 pixel format.
- Capture images in an isotonic medium.
- *Media preparation:* Hypertonic medium was made by the addition of 150 mM mannitol to DMEM (~469 mOsm/kg), and hypotonic medium was made by the addition of deionized water to DMEM for a final concentration of 30% water and 70% DMEM (~208 mOsm/kg).
  Hypertonic solution
    a. D-mannitol dissolved in DMEM, 300mM stock
  Hypotonic solution
    a. DMEM:deionized water (2:3, v:v)
- Using the syringe, aspirate isotonic media and replace it with either hypo- or hypertonic medium and scan for a desired period of time.

Image Analysis and Quantification of Cell Volume

Background

To quantify cell volume measurements from the confocal image stacks, NIH ImageJ software and a custom voxel counting macro can be used. First, a fluorescence intensity threshold value needs to be determined to allow demarcation of the boundaries between the intracellular and extracellular spaces. To accomplish this, image fluorescent microspheres of known diameter and volume that have similar fluorescence intensity as calcein. As previously stated, the confocal images are captured with an intensity resolution of 8 bits or 256 (i.e., 2^8) shades from light to dark. In defining a threshold value to use in cell volume analysis, a brightness between 0 and 255 is selected, which will thereafter define the intracellular (bright from calcein fluorescence) and extracellular (dark) space. To select this threshold value, the volume of a number of the fluorescent microspheres using all 256 possible threshold values is analyzed. The threshold value yielding the most accurate microsphere volume (known from the manufacturer) can then be used as the threshold value for further cell volume analyses. Image stacks from the experiment are then imported into ImageJ, and the outer, lateral boundary of each cell in the first image stack (the initial or "0" time point, without drug) is defined by hand (known as a "region of interest" [ROI]) and saved. The threshold value determined above is then applied to the image stack, yielding a black and white or binary image, and all thresholded pixels (black) within each ROI are counted for each image in the image stack. The resulting number is the voxel count, a number representing the volume of each cell in the image stack. This number is used as the initial resting cell volume prior to test agent addition. Similarly, the image stack from the next time point is imported, and the voxel counting macro is analyzed again using the saved RIOs from the initial (0-time point) image stack (Fig. **3**). By ensuring that the microscope stage did not shift during the experiment, the RIOs defined in the 0-time point image stack should also accurately define the outer boundary of each cell in the subsequent image stacks. The voxel counts for each cell at each time point are then imported into a spreadsheet.

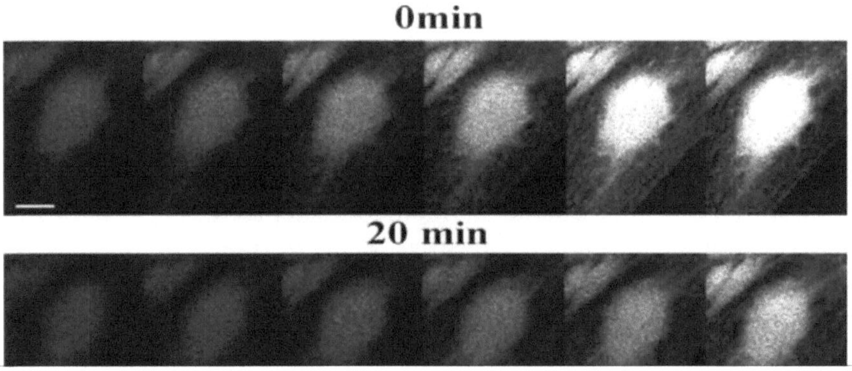

Fig. (3). Nitric oxide decreases Schlemm's canal cell volume. Threshold z-stack images of a single Schlemm's canal cell. At 0 minutes, the threshold voxels were qualitatively and quantitatively greater than at 20 minutes after DETA-NO (100 µM. Voxel count for cell: 0 minute: 11,606; 20 minutes: 7,435. Scale bar, 20 µm. Previously published in IOVS, Ellis *et al*., 2010.

To represent these data as a percentage change in cell volume, divide the voxel count for each cell at each time point by the voxel count of that cell at the 0-time point (Fig. **4**). For these experiments, statistical comparisons are performed by ANOVA followed by the Holm-Sidak or Fisher least significant difference method for the comparison among different means.

Protocol

- Determine threshold value: Measure the volume of a number of the fluorescent microspheres using all 256 possible threshold values. The threshold value yielding the most accurate microsphere volume will be used as the threshold value for further cell volume analyses.
- Import the image stacks into ImageJ software, and free-hand draw the outer lateral boundary (region of interest, ROI) of each cell in the first image stack and save.
- The resulting number is the voxel count, a number representing the volume of each cell in the image stack.
- Continue data analyses as described above.

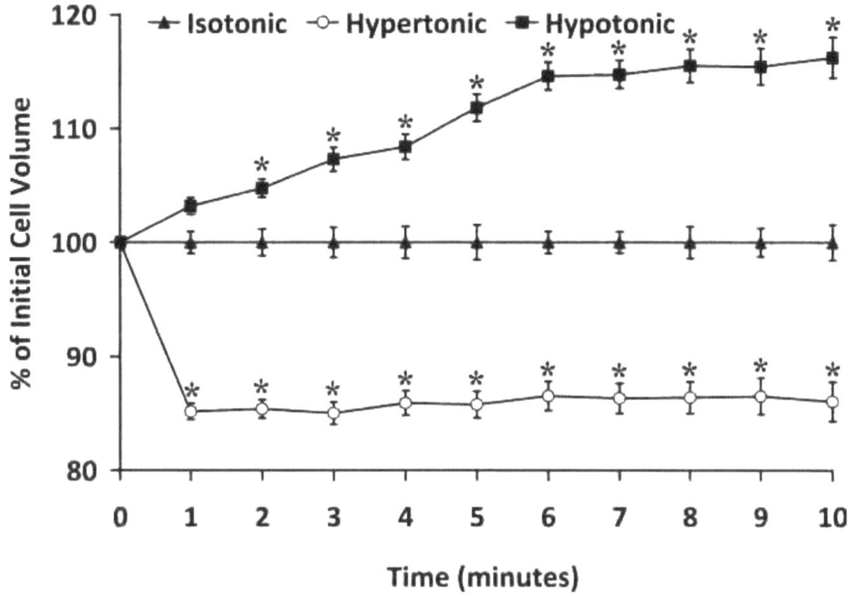

Fig. (4). Schlemm's canal cell volume is altered in response to changes in osmolarity. Hypotonic DMEM increased cell volume (mean ± SEM; n = 38 cells), whereas hypertonic DMEM decreased cell volume (mean ± SEM; n = 45 cells). There were no changes in cell volume in cells incubated in isotonic medium (mean + SEM; n = 59 cells, representing mean controls for hypotonic and hypertonic treatments). Data are expressed as percentage volume at the 0-minute time point; for hypotonic, hypertonic, and isotonic DMEM, they are 6994 ± 776, 3287 ± 245, and 5437 ± 279, respectively. *$P < 0.05$, significantly different from control (0-minute time point). Previously published, IOVS, Ellis *et al.*, 2010

CONCLUSION

Since aqueous humor fluid dynamics in the anterior chamber of the eye regulate the intraocular pressure, it is important to understand how cell volume in the major AQH outflow pathway can influence the IOP. This chapter provides fairly sensitive methods to determine the TM and SC cell volumes using fluorescence technology with and without the influence of ocular hypotensive drugs. When such drugs have been examined in either TM or SC cells, data reported in published papers (Dismuke *et al.*, 2009; Ellis *et al.*, 2010) can be successfully obtained to help make informed decisions about future experiments.

REFERENCES

Al-Aswad, LA, Gong, H, Lee, D, O'Donnell, ME, Brandt, JD, Ryan, WJ, Schroeder, A & Erickson, KA (1999) Effects of Na-K-2Cl cotransport regulators on outflow facility in calf and human eyes *in vitro*. *Invest Ophthalmol Vis Sci,* 40, 1695-701.
[PMID: 10393038]

Alexander, JP, Samples, JR, Van Buskirk, EM & Acott, TS (1991) Expression of matrix metalloproteinases and inhibitor by human trabecular meshwork. *Invest Ophthalmol Vis Sci,* 32, 172-80.
[PMID: 1846130]

Banerjee, J, Leung, CT, Li, A, Peterson-Yantorno, K, Ouyang, H, Stamer, WD & Civan, MM (2017)

Regulatory Roles of Anoctamin-6 in Human Trabecular Meshwork Cells. *Invest Ophthalmol Vis Sci,* 58, 492-501.
[http://dx.doi.org/10.1167/iovs.16-20188]

Bradley, JM, Vranka, J, Colvis, CM, Conger, DM, Alexander, JP, Fisk, AS, Samples, JR & Acott, TS (1998) Effect of matrix metalloproteinases activity on outflow in perfused human organ culture. *Invest Ophthalmol Vis Sci,* 39, 2649-58.
[PMID: 9856774]

Bush, PG & Hall, AC (2003) The volume and morphology of chondrocytes within non-degenerate and degenerate human articular cartilage. *OsteoarthritisCartilage,* 242-51.
[http://dx.doi.org/10.1016/S1063-4584(02)00369-2]

Bush, PG, Hodkinson, PD, Hamilton, GL & Hall, AC (2005) Viability and volume of *in situ* bovine articular chondrocytes—changes following a single impact and effects of medium osmolarity. *Osteoarthritis Cartilage,* 13, 54-65.
[http://dx.doi.org/10.1016/j.joca.2004.10.007] [PMID: 15639638]

Dismuke, WM & Ellis, DZ (2009) Human trabecular meshwork cell volume decrease by NO-independent soluble guanylate cyclase activators YC-1 and BAY-58-2667 involves the BKCa ion channel. *Invest Ophthalmol Vis Sci,* 50, 3353-9.
[http://dx.doi.org/10.1167/iovs.08-3127] [PMID: 19234350]

Dismuke, WM, Mbadugha, CC & Ellis, DZ (2008) NO-induced regulation of human trabecular meshwork cell volume and aqueous humor outflow facility involve the BK_{Ca} ion channel. *Am J Physiol Cell Physiol,* 294, C1378-86.
[http://dx.doi.org/10.1152/ajpcell.00363.2007] [PMID: 18385281]

Dismuke, WM & Ellis, DZ (2009) Activation of the BK(Ca) channel increases outflow facility and decreases trabecular meshwork cell volume. *J Ocul Pharmacol Ther,* 25, 309-14.
[PMID: 19552602]

Ellis, DZ, Sharif, NA & Dismuke, WM (2010) Endogenous regulation of human Schlemm's canal cell volume by nitric oxide signaling. *Invest Ophthalmol Vis Sci,* 51, 5817-24.
[http://dx.doi.org/10.1167/iovs.09-5072] [PMID: 20484594]

Ellis, DZ, Dismuke, WM & Chokshi, BM (2009) Characterization of soluble guanylate cyclase in NO-induced increases in aqueous humor outflow facility and in the trabecular meshwork Invest Ophthalmol. *Vis Sci,* 50, 1808-13.

Grierson, I & Johnson, NF (1981) The post-mortem vacuoles of Schlemm's canal. *Albrecht Von Graefes Arch Klin Exp Ophthalmol,* 215, 249-64.
[http://dx.doi.org/10.1007/BF00407664] [PMID: 6908820]

Kaufman, PL (1984) Aqueous humor outflow. *Curr Top Eye Res,* 4, 97-138.
[PMID: 6329604]

Krupin, T & Civan, MM (1995) The physiological basis of aqueous humor formation. In: Ritch, R., Shields, M.B., (Eds.), *The Glaucomas* Mosby, St. Louis 251-80.

Lee, WR, Grierson, P & McMenamin, PG (1982) The Morphological Response of the Primate Outflow System. In: Lutjen-Drecoll, E., (Ed.), *Basic Aspects of Glaucoma Research* F.K. Schattauer, Stuttgart 123-39.

Mitchell, CH, Fleischhauer, JC, Stamer, WD, Peterson-Yantorno, K & Civan, MM (2002) Human trabecular meshwork cell volume regulation. *Am J Physiol Cell Physiol,* 283, C315-26.
[http://dx.doi.org/10.1152/ajpcell.00544.2001] [PMID: 12055101]

O'Donnell, ME, Brandt, JD & Curry, FR (1995) Na-K-Cl cotransport regulates intracellular volume and monolayer permeability of trabecular meshwork cells. *Am J Physiol Cell Physiol,* 268, C1067-74.
[http://dx.doi.org/10.1152/ajpcell.1995.268.4.C1067] [PMID: 7733229]

Polansky, JR, Wood, IS, Maglio, MT & Alvarado, JA (1984) Trabecular meshwork cell culture in glaucoma

research: evaluation of biological activity and structural properties of human trabecular cells *in vitro*. *Ophthalmology,* 91, 580-95.
[http://dx.doi.org/10.1016/S0161-6420(84)34241-5] [PMID: 6540429]

Soto, D, Comes, N, Ferrer, E, Morales, M, Escalada, A, Pale´s, J, Solsona, C, Gual, A & Gasull, X (2004) Modulation of aqueous humor outflow by ionic mechanisms involved in trabecular meshwork cell volume regulation. *Invest Ophthalmol Vis Sci,* 45, 3650-61.
[http://dx.doi.org/10.1167/iovs.04-0060] [PMID: 15452073]

Stumpff, F & Wiederholt, M (2000) Regulation of trabecular meshwork contractility. *Ophthalmologica,* 214, 33-53.
[http://dx.doi.org/10.1159/000027471] [PMID: 10657743]

CHAPTER 17

Protocols for Studying Aquaporin Function Related to Ocular Hypertension *In Vitro*

Raj Patil[1,*]

[1] *OKYO Pharma Ltd, 420 Lexington Ave, Suite 1402, New York, NY-10170, USA*

Abstract: Aquaporins (AQPs) are a large family of membrane-bound water channels that facilitate water and small solute transport and have important physiological functions in all cells. At least thirteen types of aquaporins exist that exhibit a high level of phylogenetic homology, and many are present in ocular cells. Mouse knockout studies have demonstrated that AQPs play an important function in aqueous humor (AQH) dynamics in the anterior chamber cells and also have a role in retinal function. In contrast to the rich literature on aquaporin function, very little is known about how to assess water movement mediated by AQPs in their native environment, such as across ciliary epithelial cell membranes where AQH is manufactured. In part, the reason could be the lack of appropriate procedures for studying water movement across ciliary epithelial layers. This chapter describes methods to measure AQP function *in vitro* using ciliary epithelial cells, including a high-throughput screening assay method. In addition, a procedure to determine aquaporin function in its native environment is also presented.

Keywords: Aquaporins, Ciliary epithelium, Eye, Fluid transport, Glaucoma, Homeostasis, Intraocular pressure, Protocol, Retina.

INTRODUCTION

Aquaporins (AQPs) are a family of membrane channel proteins that transport water and small molecule solutes across cell membranes and possess important roles in physiological functions (Beitz and Schultz 1999; Agre, King *et al.* 2002; Verkman 2003, Patil; Wang *et al.* 2018,; Allegra, Cicero *et al.* 2022; Schey, Gletten *et al.* 2022; Ximenes-da-Silva, Capra *et al.* 2022; Bhend, Kempuraj *et al.* 2023; Bill 2023, Smith and Stroka 2023; Wang, Xu *et al.* 2023). Accordingly, AQPs play critical roles in a multitude of normal physiological and pathological functions and thus represent targets for drug discovery to modulate their activities. Selective inhibition of AQP can provide new approaches for treating many disor-

* **Corresponding author Raj Patil:** OKYO Pharma Ltd, 420 Lexington Ave, Suite 1402, New York, NY-10170, USA; Tel: +917-225-9692; E-mail: rpatil@okyopharma.com

Najam A. Sharif and Sunny E. Ohia (Eds.)

ders, including ocular hypertension/glaucoma, corneal and macular edema, brain swelling associated with a stroke, *etc.* At least 12 types of AQPs prevail in mammalian tissues (Table **1**), and several members are present in the eye. AQP1, which is a water-selective channel, is present in the cornea, ciliary body, trabecular meshwork, retina, and micro-vessels of the choroid, regulating fluid homeostasis (Patil, Saito *et al.* 1997; Verkman 2003). Genetic knockout studies on mice have shown that AQP1 plays important functions such as in AQH dynamics and thus in intraocular pressure (IOP) regulation and retinal angiogenesis (Li, Patil *et al.* 2002; Zhang, Vetrivel *et al.* 2002). Ciliary epithelium, which is composed of the proximal (or outer) pigmented epithelium (PE) and the distal (or inner) non-pigmented epithelium (NPE), produces and secretes AQH (Fig. (**1**). These ciliary epithelial cells have been isolated and cultured and characterized for the presence of several ion transporters and receptors (Wax and Patil 1994; Mukhopadhyay, Geoghegan *et al.* 1997; Ortego and Coca-Prados 1999). It is known that AQH secretion is driven by the transport of electrolytes from the plasma into the posterior chamber of the eye, followed by the rapid movement of water and key solutes. In contrast to the rich information available for electrolyte movements, less is known about water movement across ciliary epithelial cell membranes *in situ* or in isolated cells.

Table 1. Listing of mammalian aquaporins.

Aquaporin	Size	Permeability	Distribution
AQP0	26 kD	*Water (poor)*	Lens
AQP1	28 kD	Water (ions?)	RBCs, Kidney, eye, brain
AQP2	29 kD	Water	Kidney
AQP3	31 kD	Water, glycerol, urea	Kidney, red blood cells, eye
AQP4	32 & 34 kD	Water (Hg insensitive)	Brain, eye, kidney, lung, ear
AQP5	29 kD	Water	Salivary gland, eye, lung
AQP6	28-30 kD	*Water (poor)*	Kidney
AQP7	26 kD	Water, glycerol	Adipose tissue, testis, kidney
AQP8	27 kD	Water	Testis, pancreas, liver
AQP9	32 kD	Water, glycerol, urea	Liver, testis, brain
AQP10	28 kD	*Water (poor),* glycerol	Small intestine
AQP11	30 kD	Water?	Liver, testis, kidney
AQP12	31 kD	Water?	Pancreas

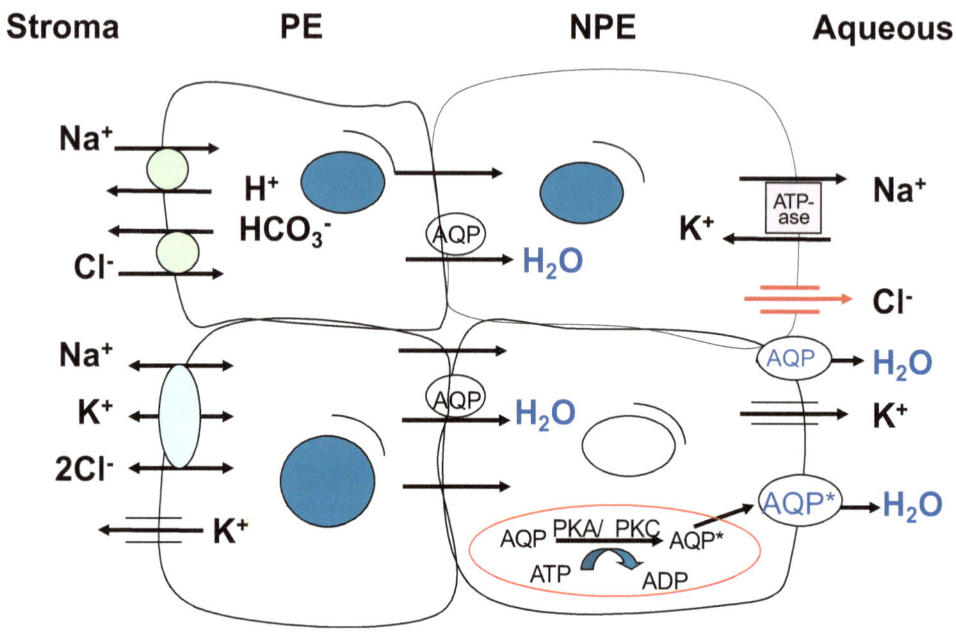

Fig. (1). Role of AQP1 in AQH production and secretion.

This chapter describes methods to measure AQP function *in vitro,* including a high-throughput screening assay, by capturing and analyzing the fluorescence dequenching of entrapped calcein in a confluent layer of AQP-expressing cells following exposure to a hypotonic shock. A high-throughput screening (HTS) assay method was successfully utilized to screen a library of novel compounds to identify potential AQP1 inhibitors/modulators (Patil, Xu *et al.* 2016). In addition, a procedure to assess AQP function in its native environment using proteoliposomes reconstituted with purified AQP1 is described below. These *in vitro* protocols represent valuable tools in defining the role of AQPs in normal physiological and pathological states. These methods can be used to find novel AQP1 inhibitors/modulators to treat many eye disorders, including ocular hypertension/glaucoma and edematous corneal and macular diseases.

Aquaporins Function in Native Cells Expressing AQP.

The *in vitro* method described below utilizes human non-pigmented ciliary epithelial (NPE) cells in culture to determine the function of aquaporin-1 in fluid transport by ciliary epithelium responsible for the secretion of aqueous humor into the posterior chamber of the eye.

Experimental Protocol

- Please refer to Patil, Han *et al.* (2001) for a detailed description of the chamber used for fluid flow measurements using cultured NPE cells.
- Grow SV40-transformed cultured human NPE cells (passage 8-10) on 24.5-m--diameter transparent, permeable, collagen-treated supports (Transwell, Costar) at a density of 1 X 10^6 per support in Dulbecco's modified Eagle's medium (DMEM) supplemented with 10% fetal bovine serum (FBS) in a 5% CO_2 atmosphere at 37°C.
- Experiments should be performed within 1–7 days after cells achieve confluence. Determine confluency by microscopy and ascertain by determining the resistance of each insert before the experiment. The electrical resistance of NPE layers should be determined using an Endohm chamber and a resistance meter (WPI, Sarasota, FL), but other similar devices should be fine.
- Now, assess the resistance of a control insert without any cells and subtract that value from that determined for an insert with a layer of cells.
- Calculate the specific resistance by multiplying the area of the insert (4.7 cm2 in this method). Typical values obtained for control inserts are ~56.4 $\Omega \cdot cm^2$. However, for a set of five NPE cell cultured layers, the corrected specific resistance should be ~73.32 ± 15.6 $\Omega \cdot cm^2$. Such numbers are similar to those noted for other cell types in these systems (*e.g.*, αTN4 cells: 130 ± 7.3 $\Omega \cdot cm^2$; bovine lens epithelial cells: 85.4 ± 5.9 $\Omega \cdot cm^2$).
- Two hours before and throughout the experiment, top-up the cell layers with DMEM containing FBS without antibiotics.
- The basal side of the NPE cell layer generated in this manner is close to the collagen support, whereas the apical side should face away from the support.
- The chamber typically used consists of two Lucite halves, with water jackets for temperature control, that are kept saturated with water when not being used (Fig. (**1**). Note that the chamber can be customized as needed from Harvard Apparatus (Holliston, MA).
- The top half of the chamber holds the Costar Transwell insert, while a rubber gasket separates the plastic bottom of the insert from a seat in the bottom chamber. In this manner, the clamping force to adequately seal the chamber is exerted on the plastic surfaces and not on the cells. The bottom chamber seat for the insert possesses a stainless-steel wire mesh to reduce/prevent sagging of the flexible permeable support. The bottom chamber is to be sealed with a plug and an O-ring and should be pierced by a 16-gauge stainless steel tube. The top chamber is also sealed with a plug and an O-ring and pierced by several tubes, and is gassed continuously with moist 95% air and 5% CO_2. The steel tube from the bottom plug should be connected to the automatic fluid level detector device (Fig. **2**).

- In this protocol, the signal from the detector can be used to provide negative feedback and to keep the volume of the bottom compartment constant. Fluid volume flow recordings represent the rate of injection (or removal) of fluid from the bottom chamber. The juxtapositions of the chamber and the detector should be such that the hydrostatic pressure difference applied to the apical side of the cultured cell layer in the top chamber is ~3 cm of H_2O. No gassing of the bottom chamber is necessary at this point.
- An example of fluid movement across the NPE cell layer in the expected direction, from the apical to the basal surface, and consistent with an absorptive epithelium activity is shown in Fig. (**3A**). As shown, the movement of fluid occurred continuously for many hours. It is not obvious whether AQH secretion *in vivo* requires the presence of both the PE and NPE cell layers transporting fluid in tandem or not.
- An example of the effect of an AQP1 antisense oligonucleotide on fluid movement across NPE cells is shown in Fig. (**3B**). As can be seen, the initial rates of fluid movement in both control (Fig. **3A**) and treated layers (Fig. **3B**) were quite similar. The overall steady-state rates of fluid movement measured over 6–8 h were different: control cell layers = $3.6 \pm 0.2\ \mu l \cdot h^{-1} \cdot cm^{-2}$($n$ = 3), and in cell layers exposed to the antisense oligonucleotide = $1.8 \pm 0.2\ \mu l \cdot h^{-1} \cdot cm^{-2}$ (n = 4). The decrease in fluid transport after AQP1 antisense treatment (~50%) was similar to the inhibition observed with mercuric chloride (Patil *et al.* 2001).
- The protocol described above was useful in confirming AQP1 function in fluid transportation by the cultured NPE cell layer. However, this procedure can be adapted to assess the function of this or other AQPs in different cell types.

Note: In the current experiments, the NPE cells (on the permeable support) were incubated with AQP1 antisense oligonucleotides at a final concentration of 5 μM for 16–18 h before measuring the fluid flow. Importantly, the nonsense oligonucleotides were inactive in this system. Here, AQP1 antisense oligonucleotides reduced AQP1mRNA levels in the NPE cells, whereas AQP1 nonsense oligonucleotide treatment failed to influence AQP1 protein and mRNA levels (Patil *et al.*, 2001).

AQP High Throughput Screening Method

The protocol described below is a high-throughput screening assay for AQP1. It relies on recording the fluorescence dequenching of entrapped Calcein-AM fluorescent dye (Dojindo, Rockville, MD, USA) due to rapid osmotic changes in a confluent layer of AQP1- -expressing cells following a hypotonic shock. This protocol can be adapted to any other members of the AQP family and can be run at a low or high throughput on the fluorescent reader used. As such, this procedure was successfully utilized to rapidly screen a library of compounds to identify potential inhibitors/modulators of AQP1 (Patil *et al.*, 2016).

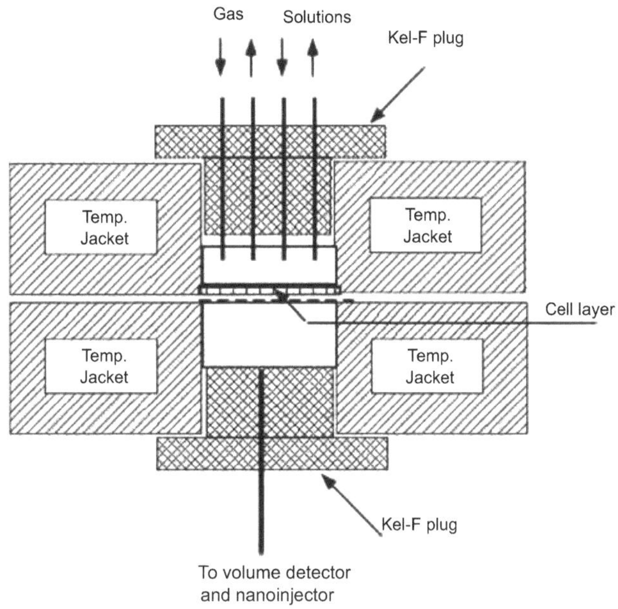

Fig. (2). Schematic representation of the chamber utilized in measuring fluid transport across ciliary epithelial cells.

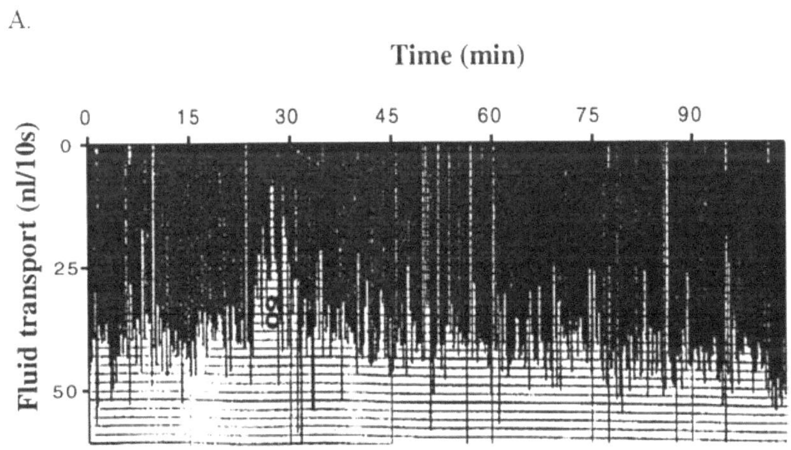

Fig. (3A). Chart recording of fluid movement by cultured non-pigmented ciliary epithelial layer (NPE). Recording began after a ~15-min stabilization period. Individual deflections represent fluid accumulating during a fixed time interval (10 s) in the downward direction, after which the accumulator is reset and the process restarts. The downward direction corresponds to fluid movement from the top chamber to the bottom chamber, *i.e.*, from the apical to the basal side of cells. The fluid level in the top chamber section was 3 cm above that of the detector communicating with the bottom chamber. The cultured monolayer transported fluid for several hours; the longest time monitored was 8 h (not shown). Similar results were obtained in 4 separate experiments with different batches of NPE cells.

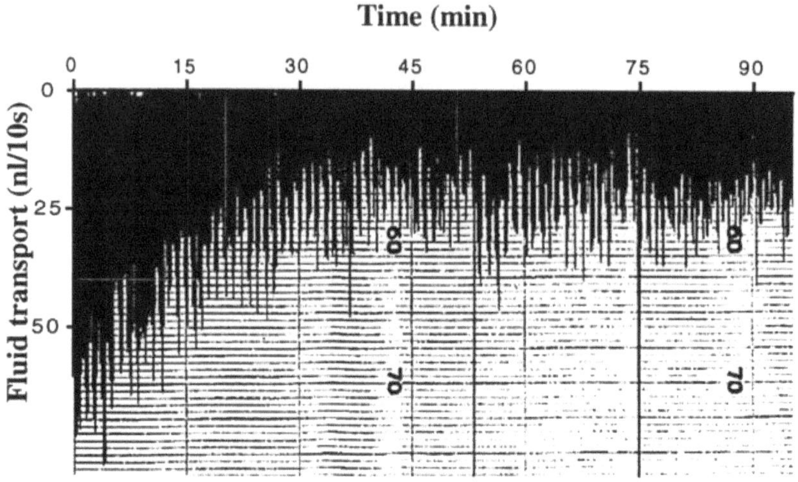

Fig. (3B). Effect of aquaporin-1 (AQP1) antisense oligonucleotides on fluid movement by NPE. A phosphorothioated antisense oligonucleotide targeted toward the region encompassing the ATG start codon of AQP1 mRNA was used. Cells were grown without oligos and incubated with an antisense oligonucleotide (5 μM) for 16–18 h before measurement of fluid movement. The initial transient change in the rate of fluid movement lasting 0.5 h represents the adjustment of the cell layer and support after the mounting procedure. The steady-state rate of fluid flow was much lower than in the control series exemplified in Fig. (**3A**). Similar results were obtained in 4 separate experiments with different batches of NPE cells.

Experimental Protocol

Transfection of the CHO-K1 Cells with the Human aqp1 Gene

- Although this procedure describes the transfection of CHO-K1 cells with the human *aqp1* gene, it can be used for any AQP analog to generate a stably transfected AQP-expressing cell line.
- Create a plasmid construct with the human *aqp1* gene utilizing the *aqp1* coding sequence from the I.M.A.G.E. consortium clone ID: CS0DA009YJ21 accession: AL518392 from Invitrogen (Invitrogen, Carlsbad, CA, USA) in the pcDNA3.1+ vector.
- The sequences of selected clones should be verified by a series of restriction analyses, colony polymerase chain reaction (PCR), and sequence analysis.
- Now, the isolation of the *aqp1* plasmid from verified clones and transfection into CHO-K1 cells (ATCC, Manassas, VA, USA) can proceed using Lipofectamine 2000 (Invitrogen) according to the manufacturer's guidelines.
- Selection of transfected cells can be accomplished after 48 h by adding 2 mg/mL of geneticin (Invitrogen) to the cell cultures.
- In parallel, a pcDNA3.1+ vector control-transfected cell line, with no insert in CHO-K1 cells, should be generated.
- Confirm the expression of AQP1 protein by Western blot analysis using cell extracts prepared from stably transfected cells utilizing an antibody directed

against the AQP1 protein's carboxyl-terminal tail (amino acid region 243–261; Millipore, Temecula, CA, USA).

- Next, assess many clones for AQP1 expression. Then, select the most preferred one based on the expression analysis data for further studies.
- In these procedures, the CHO-pcDNA3.1+ (no insert) clone should be used as a background control.

Measurement of AQP function in transfected cells

In the current studies, FlexStation II 384™ microplate reader for low throughput assays and FLIPR Tetra for high throughput assays (both from Molecular Devices (Sunnyvale, CA)) were utilized.

- CHO-AQP-1_9C8 expressing cells should be allowed to grow (80-90% confluent) once seeded at ~33×10^6 cells/T-150 cm^2 flask density in Dulbecco's modified Eagle's medium [DMEM] without pyruvate and L-glutamine containing 10% fetal bovine serum (FBS) from Invitrogen) in an incubator at 37 °C and under 5% CO_2 and 95% air.
- Incubate cells with 6 μM Calcein-AM for approximately 30 min at room temperature (RT; 24°C) in order for cells to absorb the Calcein-AM dye.
- Next, carefully and gently harvest the cells and sub-culture (10,000 cells/well) in 20 μL of assay media (DMEM without pyruvate and L- glutamine containing 10% FBS) into 384-well black clear-bottom assay plates (*e.g.*, Corning, Lowell, MA, USA) using a multidrop liquid dispenser (*e.g.*, Thermo Fisher Labsystems, Waltham, MA, USA).
- Incubate cells overnight at 37 °C in an atmosphere of 95% air and 5% CO_2 in a tissue culture incubator. If possible, allow cells to achieve 80-90% confluency.
- Gently wash the cell plates with 50 μL PBS twice using a plate washer (ELx405 BioTek; Winooski, VT, USA).
- Now, add 20 μL of PBS buffer per well to each assay plate and incubate cells at RT for 15 min.
- The test compounds (1-2 μL) can now be added to specified plate wells, ensuring that if dimethyl sulfoxide (DMSO) is used, its final concentration is less than 1% in the assay buffer in the well. When multiple compounds need to be tested, a liquid handling robotic system can be utilized (*e.g.*, Biomek FX (Beckman Coulter, Indianapolis, IN, USA).
- Incubate assay plates with test compounds for 10 min at room temperature. Then, the assay plates can be transferred to the FLIPR Tetra machine (Molecular Devices), and the baseline fluorescence reading can be recorded. Alternatively, the FlexStation II 384™ microplate reader can be used if the throughput of test agents is relatively small.

- After 15-20 seconds, add an equal volume of PBS without Ca^{2+} and Mg^{2+} (minimum response; Invitrogen) or H_2O (maximum response) automatically to the specified wells. The plate wells receiving H_2O represent the maximum cell volume change expected after the osmotic shock.
- The resultant fluorescence should be recorded in relative fluorescence units (RFU) at intervals of 0.5 seconds using an excitation (λex = 470–495 nm) and emission (λem = 515–575 nm, cutoff 515 nm) filter.
- The SOFTMAX PRO software (Molecular Devices) can be used to acquire the fluorescence values and then analyzed using Excel-fit software (Microsoft).
- An average of at least five consecutive points should be used to assess the rise time in fluorescence to yield the rate V (RFU/second). A typical fluorescence response depicting a rapid rise in fluorescence in the cells due to dequenching of entrapped calcein can be seen in Fig. (**4**).

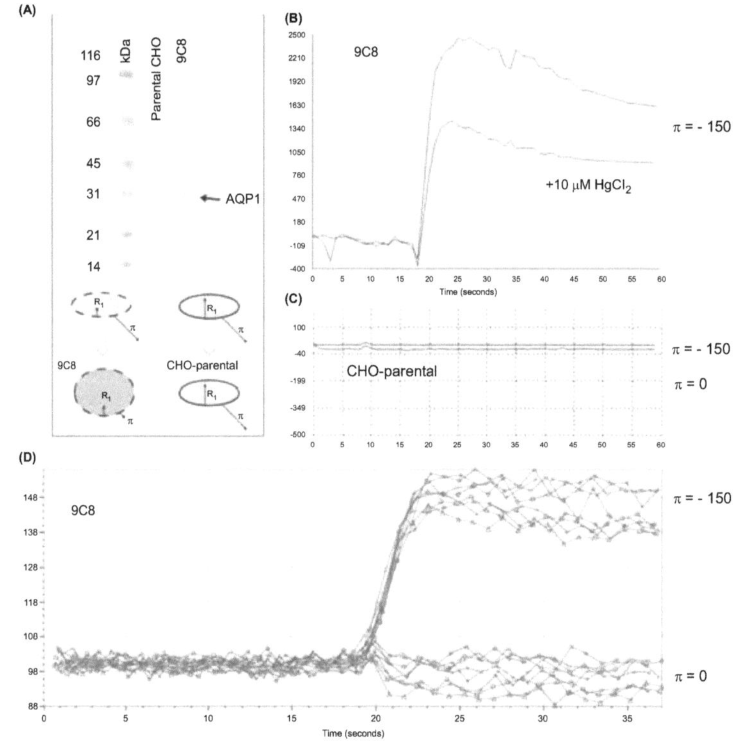

Fig. (4). Simultaneous calcein dequenching of confluent AQP1-expressing CHO cells using a robotic plate reader: (A) Western blot of CHO-K1 cells and CHO-9C8 AQP1-expressing cells (top), using an anti-AQP1 antibody (a.a. 243–261) (Millipore, Temecula, CA, USA). The cartoon (bottom) indicates the swelling of AQP1 cells by osmotic shock, while cells without AQP1 channels do not swell, notwithstanding the presence of the osmotic shock. (B) Characteristic fluorescence response showing a rapid rise in fluorescence as the result of dequenching of entrapped calcein. HgCl2 reduces the extent of the signal with a small effect in the rise time. (C) CHO cells without AQP1 do not respond to an osmotic pressure. (D) Representative data from a 96-well experiment showing responses of AQP1-expressing cells in the absence (bottom curves) and presence (top curves) of an osmotic gradient.

Xenopus Oocyte Assay to Measure Water Permeability of AQP1

It is important to eliminate any dequenching effect on calcein fluorescence independent of an AQP-mediated process, and thus, AQP activity determined by another procedure is desirable. One such alternative is to use a frog oocyte swelling assay without a fluorescent dye. The method described below provides guidelines to ascertain water permeability through AQP utilizing Xenopus oocytes.

- First, amplify the coding sequence of a desired AQP using polymerase chain reaction (PCR). For AQP1, wild-type human *aqp1* (WT-*aqp1*) use primers 5′ (atggccagcgagttcaagaag) and 3′ (ctatttgggcttcatctccac).
- Use pcDNA 3.1 myc-His vector (Invitrogen) carrying a T7 promoter for Xenopus oocyte to express the AQP1 in oocytes.
- Next, perform *in vitro* cRNA transcription using T7 RNA polymerase (mMESSAGE mMACHINE kit; Ambion®, ThermoFisher, WA, MA, USA) per manufacturer's guidance.
- Purify cRNA and then dissolve it in distilled water. This material needs to be stored at −80 °C until injection into the oocytes.
- Isolation of oocytes is achieved by surgically removing the ovarian lobes containing stage V and VI oocytes from the Xenopus laevis frog and defolliculation of the lobes using collagenase Type II enzyme (Sigma).
- After maintaining the oocytes at 18°C, inject 25 ng cRNA of the respective expression construct in a total volume of 25 nl/oocyte. For control oocytes, inject an equal volume of distilled water.
- Incubate injected oocytes in isotonic medium (200 mosmol modified Barth's buffer) at 18°C/24°C for 72 hrs to express the AQP.
- After this time, transfer oocytes from 200 mosmol modified Barth's buffer to the hypotonic medium (70 mosmol Barth's buffer diluted with distilled water).
- Record the osmotic volume increase due to water flux driven by an osmotic gradient *via* time-lapse video microscopy of the oocyte diameter.
- Acquire images of the oocyte silhouette every 2 s through a video camera attached to a stereomicroscope and analyze them using Optimas software version 5.2 (Media Cybernetics, Silver Spring, MD).
- Now, calculate the overall rate of oocyte volume change by linear regression of the first minute following exposure of the oocyte to the hypotonic medium.
- Calculate the water permeability (*P*f) of the oocyte membrane from the initial change in volume as per the equation shown below,

  where V (cm^3) is the oocyte volume calculated from the cross-sectional area, *S*m (cm^2) is the oocyte surface area calculated from the cross-sectional area, *V*w is the molar volume of water (18 cm^3/mol), and Δc is the change in bath osmolality (120 mOsm). The effect of AQP-1 modulators on water permeability in the oocyte assay is shown in Fig. (**5**).

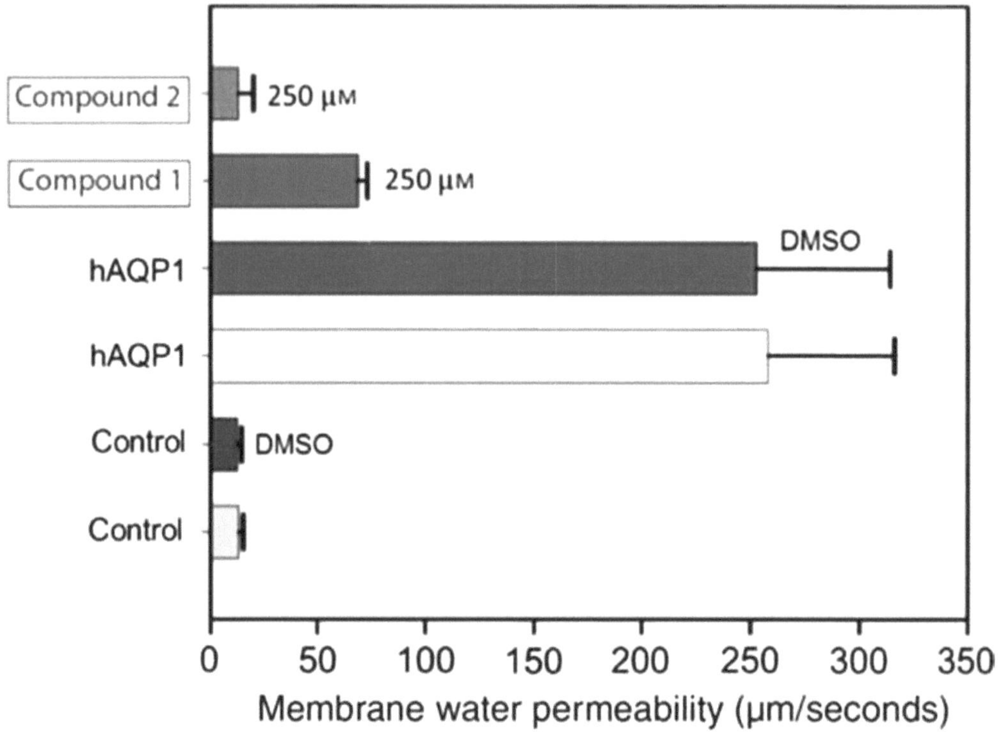

Fig. (5). Permeability of Xenopus laevis oocytes injected with distilled water (control) or 25 ng/ oocyte human AQP1 cRNA (experimental) is shown. Oocytes were incubated in a culture medium, DMSO (solvent used for dissolving the compound), or AQP1 inhibitor dissolved in DMSO, as represented in the figure. Membrane water permeability was determined as described in the Methods and Materials section. Each bar represents mean ± SD from 15 oocytes.

Measurement of AQP1 function in the native environment

In order to eliminate the possibility that cell swelling kinetics of CHO cells and Xenopus oocytes above could have arisen from non-AQP endogenous membrane proteins, it is deemed necessary to confirm AQP activity in another native environment. The method described below addresses this point.

An important prerequisite for the stop-flow method to be used is the availability of purified AQP1 protein before it can be incorporated into uncharged lipids that generate the native environment of AQP in cell membranes. For this purpose, outdated human red blood cells can be used to isolate and purify AQP1 using previously described procedures (van Hoek, *et al.* 1995) with some modifications. Please refer to Patil *et al.* (2016) for further details.

Preparation of AQP1 Proteoliposomes

- AQP1 proteoliposomes should be prepared using the synthetic lipid DOPC at a lipid-to-protein ratio of 10:1 (w:w).
- Remove the solvent of the DOPC stock (chloroform/ethanol) (4:1) by evaporating under nitrogen gas, and remove residual traces of the solvent using a SpeedVac at 24°C for 15–30 min.
- Now, add EDTA–phosphate buffer (pH 7.2), which contains 152 mM (4%) β-octyl-glucoside (βOG), to hydrate the lipid film by vortexing followed by a brief nitrogen purge and stirring for 2–3 hrs until clear.
- Now, add the purified AQP1 protein to lipid DOPC and incubate stirring overnight at 24°C.
- Remove βOG by adding biobeads (Biorad, 20 mg) to the AQP1: DOPC mixture and then incubate for an additional 2 hrs.
- Confirm the incorporation of AQP1 into proteoliposomes by SDS–PAGE of the reconstituted proteoliposome mixture/suspension.

Stopped-flow assay using AQP1 proteoliposomes

- Thirty minutes prior to the experiment, treat the proteoliposomes containing purified AQP1 with mercuric chloride (50–100 μM; positive control for inhibition) stored in ice.
- Osmotic water permeability of proteoliposomes should be determined at 24°C by monitoring 90° scattered light intensity at 520 nm wavelength using a PiStar 180 (Applied Photophysics, UK) or similar instrument with a dead time of 1–2 milliseconds.
- Create a hyperosmotic shock (inwardly directed osmotic gradient) by mixing the AQP1 proteoliposomes maintained in Buffer A (50 mM sodium phosphate buffer pH, 100 mM NaCl, 0.025% sodium azide, 1 mM EDTA) with an equal volume of 200 mM mannitol.
- In order to create an outwardly directed osmotic gradient/hypo-osmotic shock, preincubate AQP1 proteoliposomes with 200 mM mannitol and then mix with Buffer A.
- Now, measure the change in right-angle scattering light intensity for 1 or 2 seconds, as appropriate, and repeat each measurement at least three times to ensure reproducibility.
- An example of a light-scattering response using AQP1 reconstituted proteoliposomes is displayed in Fig. (**6**).

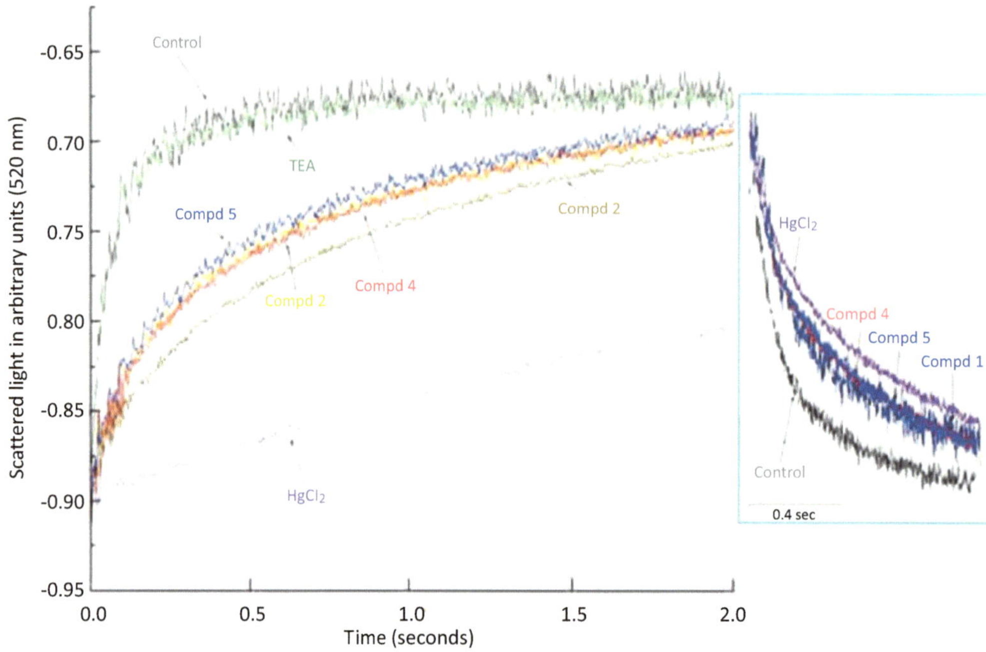

Fig. (6). Characterization of AQP1 inhibitors using vesicular assay. The plots represent swelling of NLS-treated AQP1-enriched erythrocyte ghosts under hypo-osmotic shock. Control is ghost only, without any compound. Inset shows a shrinkage assay for purified AQP1 reconstituted proteoliposomes exposed to hyper-osmotic shock. Control is AQP1 proteoliposome only, without any compound. In both sets of experiments, the compounds were at a final concentration of 75 μM while HgCl2 was at a concentration of 50 μM.

CONCLUSION

This chapter has provided experimental methods to measure AQP function *in vitro*, including a HTS assay method using a confluent layer of AQP-expressing cells. In addition, a method to determine AQP function in its native environment using proteoliposomes reconstituted with purified AQP1 is described. These *in vitro* procedures will be valuable tools in defining the role of AQPs in normal physiological and pathological conditions and will help discover suitable candidate drugs to treat eye diseases, in particular ocular hypertension, and other human diseases.

REFERENCES

Agre, P, King, LS, Yasui, M, Guggino, WB, Ottersen, OP, Fujiyoshi, Y, Engel, A & Nielsen, S (2002) Aquaporin water channels – from atomic structure to clinical medicine. *J Physiol,* 542, 3-16. [http://dx.doi.org/10.1113/jphysiol.2002.020818] [PMID: 12096044]

Allegra, A, Cicero, N, Mirabile, G, Cancemi, G, Tonacci, A, Musolino, C & Gangemi, S (2022) Critical Role of Aquaporins in Cancer: Focus on Hematological Malignancies. *Cancers (Basel),* 14, 4182. [http://dx.doi.org/10.3390/cancers14174182] [PMID: 36077720]

Beitz, E & Schultz, JE (1999) The mammalian aquaporin water channel family: A promising new drug target.

Curr Med Chem, 6, 457-67.
[http://dx.doi.org/10.2174/0929867306666220330183950] [PMID: 10213793]

Bhend, ME, Kempuraj, D, Sinha, NR, Gupta, S & Mohan, RR (2023) Role of aquaporins in corneal healing post chemical injury. *Exp Eye Res,* 228, 109390.
[http://dx.doi.org/10.1016/j.exer.2023.109390] [PMID: 36696947]

Bill, RM (2024) Drugging aquaporins. *Biochim Biophys Acta Biomembr,* 1866, 184164.
[http://dx.doi.org/10.1016/j.bbamem.2023.184164] [PMID: 37146744]

Li, J, Patil, RV & Verkman, AS (2002) Mildly abnormal retinal function in transgenic mice without Müller cell aquaporin-4 water channels. *Invest Ophthalmol Vis Sci,* 43, 573-9.
[PMID: 11818406]

Mukhopadhyay, P, Geoghegan, TE, Patil, RV, Bhattacherjee, P & Paterson, CA (1997) Detection of EP2, EP4, and FP receptors in human ciliary epithelial and ciliary muscle cells. *Biochem Pharmacol,* 53, 1249-55.
[http://dx.doi.org/10.1016/S0006-2952(97)00011-7] [PMID: 9214685]

Ortego, J & Coca-Prados, M (1999) Functional expression of components of the natriuretic peptide system in human ocular nonpigmented ciliary epithelial cells. *Biochem Biophys Res Commun,* 258, 21-8.
[http://dx.doi.org/10.1006/bbrc.1999.0573] [PMID: 10222228]

Patil, R, Wang, H, Sharif, NA & Mitra, A (2018) Aquaporins: Novel Targets for Age-Related Ocular Disorders. *J Ocul Pharmacol Ther,* 34, 177-87.
[http://dx.doi.org/10.1089/jop.2017.0024] [PMID: 28632458]

Patil, RV, Han, Z, Yiming, M, Yang, J, Iserovich, P, Wax, MB & Fischbarg, J (2001) Fluid transport by human nonpigmented ciliary epithelial layers in culture: a homeostatic role for aquaporin-1. *Am J Physiol Cell Physiol,* 281, C1139-45.
[http://dx.doi.org/10.1152/ajpcell.2001.281.4.C1139] [PMID: 11546649]

Patil, R, Saito, I, Yang, X & Wax, MB (1997) Expression of aquaporins in the rat ocular tissue. *Exp Eye Res,* 64, 203-9.
[http://dx.doi.org/10.1006/exer.1996.0196] [PMID: 9176054]

Patil, RV, Xu, S, van Hoek, AN, Rusinko, A, Feng, Z, May, J, Hellberg, M, Sharif, NA, Wax, MB, Irigoyen, M, Carr, G, Brittain, T, Brown, P, Colbert, D, Kumari, S, Varadaraj, K & Mitra, AK (2016) Rapid Identification of Novel Inhibitors of the Human Aquaporin-1 Water Channel. *Chem Biol Drug Des,* 87, 794-805.
[http://dx.doi.org/10.1111/cbdd.12713] [PMID: 26685080]

Schey, KL, Gletten, RB, O'Neale, CVT, Wang, Z, Petrova, RS & Donaldson, PJ (2022) Lens Aquaporins in Health and Disease: Location is Everything! *Front Physiol,* 13, 882550.
[http://dx.doi.org/10.3389/fphys.2022.882550] [PMID: 35514349]

Smith, IM & Stroka, KM (2023) The multifaceted role of aquaporins in physiological cell migration. *Am J Physiol Cell Physiol,* 325, C208-23.
[http://dx.doi.org/10.1152/ajpcell.00502.2022] [PMID: 37246634]

van Hoek, AN, Wiener, MC, Verbavatz, JM, Brown, D, Lipniunas, PH, Townsend, RR & Verkman, AS (1995) Purification and structure-function analysis of native, PNGase F-treated, and endo-beta-galactosidae-treated CHIP28 water channels. *Biochemistry,* 34, 2212-9.
[http://dx.doi.org/10.1021/bi00007a015] [PMID: 7532004]

Verkman, AS (2003) Role of aquaporin water channels in eye function. *Exp Eye Res,* 76, 137-43.
[http://dx.doi.org/10.1016/S0014-4835(02)00303-2] [PMID: 12565800]

Wang, F, Xu, W, Xu, C, Li, J & Lin, J (2023) Aquaporins and Neuropathic Pain. *Front Biosci (Landmark Ed),* 28, 35.
[http://dx.doi.org/10.31083/j.fbl2802035] [PMID: 36866545]

Wax, MB & Patil, RV (1994) Immunoprecipitation of A1 adenosine receptor-GTP-binding protein complexes in ciliary epithelial cells. *Invest Ophthalmol Vis Sci,* 35, 3057-63.

[PMID: 8206723]

Ximenes-da-Silva, A, Capra, D, Sanz, CK, Mendes, CB, de Mattos Coelho Aguiar, J, Moura-Neto, V & DosSantos, MF (2022) The role of aquaporins in hearing function and dysfunction. *Eur J Cell Biol,* 101, 151252.
[http://dx.doi.org/10.1016/j.ejcb.2022.151252] [PMID: 35779359]

Zhang, D, Vetrivel, L & Verkman, AS (2002) Aquaporin deletion in mice reduces intraocular pressure and aqueous fluid production. *J Gen Physiol,* 119, 561-9.
[http://dx.doi.org/10.1085/jgp.20028597] [PMID: 12034763]

CHAPTER 18

Measuring Elastic Moduli of Human Trabecular Meshwork Tissues, Cells, or Extracellular Matrices

VijayKrishna Raghunathan[1,*]

[1] *Department of Ophthalmology, Novartis Institutes for BioMedical Research, 22 Windsor St, Cambridge, MA 02139, USA*

Abstract: Exploration of the mechanical properties of biological tissues has sparked a growing interest in the mechanobiology of various ocular diseases. There is an increasing recognition that the change in mechanical attributes (of cells/tissues) may reflect disease states or may be a viable endpoint to assess cell/tissue function. As such, mechanobiological investigations often rely on developing substrates with properties mimicking the mechanical properties of the choice of cell/tissue, either in homeostasis or in disease. Variability in methods of mechanical characterization has resulted in confounding reports that subsequently impact reproducibility in science and the development of appropriate scientific hypotheses. Here, we describe a protocol for measuring the elastic moduli of cells, matrices, and tissues relevant to the outflow pathway. We discuss factors to be considered while selecting cantilevers and preparing samples for measurements and provide detailed instructions for calibration of cantilevers, collection of force-displacement curves, and a workflow for how to analyze the data and determine elastic modulus. Although the protocol is intended for the cells/tissues of the iridocorneal angle, readers may apply or adapt this protocol for other relevant tissues.

Keywords: Atomic force microscopy, Elastic modulus, Glaucoma, Indentation, Primary cells, Trabecular meshwork.

INTRODUCTION

Biophysical stimuli – whether mechanical (such as pressure, stretch, compression, or shear), topographical (ordered or random topology), or non-biochemical soluble and insoluble signals (oxygen-tension, pH, or electric field) – represent an integral part of the cellular microenvironment and tissue functionality. Indeed, a growing body of research has demonstrated the profound impact of biophysics on tissue development, homeostasis, and disease. All the while, it is important to place them in the larger context of tissue function, which includes biochemical

* **Corresponding author VijayKrishna Raghunathan:** Department of Ophthalmology, Novartis Institutes for BioMedical Research, 22 Windsor St, Cambridge, MA 02139, USA; E-mail: vijay.raghunathan@novartis.com

Najam A. Sharif and Sunny E. Ohia (Eds.)

and genetic factors. A fundamental characteristic exhibited by all biological materials is their innate biomechanical property that drives and partakes critically in their intrinsic structure-function relationship. Biomechanical properties of tissues are defined by their constitutive elements: cells and their extracellular matrix (ECM). Cellular biomechanics have become recognized as important contributors to cell and tissue (dys)function essentially due to the changes in cytoskeletal dynamics that may be governed by phenotypic processes such as migration and differentiation, as well as remodeling of the extracellular matrix or response to drugs. Cells themselves are intrinsically capable of both sensing and exerting physical forces in a context-dependent manner(Jahed *et al.* 2014; Kaminski *et al.* 2014; Martino *et al.* 2018). For example, forces exerted by cells on their microenvironment allow for matrix remodeling after injury or in response to wound repair. Similarly, changes in matrix stiffness can influence the amplitude of force transmitted across cell-adhesion sites and subsequently to the cytoskeleton and nucleus, thereby influencing nuclear shape and gene expression (Dahl *et al.* 2008; Jaalouk and Lammerding 2009). This bidirectional ability to sense and respond to physical forces helps maintain homeostasis. It is thus conceivable that if a cell misinterprets and misprocesses these biophysical stimuli, the consequences on cell fate decisions or transcriptional regulation of genes and subsequent post-translational modifications of proteins (including but not limited to ECM) may all contribute to pathology. Untangling causal relationships between microenvironment and cellular behavior requires experimentation that carefully matches both the biochemical and biophysical environment of normal and diseased tissues. Thus, there have been several attempts to quantify the biomechanical attributes of several tissues (liver, neural, musculoskeletal, dermal, ocular, *etc.*), cells, and ECM in homeostasis and pathology.

In the eye, approximately 75% of all aqueous humor flows through the trabecular meshwork (TM) and Schlemm's canal (SC) (Toris *et al.* 1999; Toris *et al.* 2002). The site of major resistance to this outflow is thought to reside within the cribriform region of the meshwork, the area around the juxtracanalicular region (JCT) of the meshwork, and the inner wall cells of the SC (Johnson *et al.* 1992; Tamm 2009; Tamm 2010; Tamm 2015; Tamm and Fuchshofer 2007). Whilst there have been several debates on ascertaining the relative contributions of JCT/TM and cells of the inner wall SC to outflow resistance, it is commonly accepted that ECM at the meshwork, particularly in the JCT, is a major contributor to the resistance. In addition to lending resistance to outflow, constituents of the JCT, trabecular lamellae, and ECM components act as load-bearing structures that contribute to innate mechanical properties of the tissue. Ascertaining the mechanical properties of tissues is inherently difficult due to tissue inaccessibility. A wide range of mechanical properties and methods available for measurement are largely context-dependent. Indeed, mechanical characterization of the TM has been performed either in isolation or in a combination of advanced optical imaging, indentation and tensile methods, acoustic force elastography, and finite element modeling (Ai *et al.* 2023; Camras *et al.* 2012; Camras *et al.* 2014; Gao *et al.* 2020; Huang *et al.* 2015; Johnson *et al.* 2015; Lee *et al.* 2021; Li *et al.* 2019; Li *et al.* 2013; Overby *et al.* 2014; Vahabikashi *et al.* 2019; Vargas-Pinto *et al.* 2013; Wang *et al.* 2018; Wang *et al.* 2017b; Yuan *et al.* 2011; Yuan *et al.* 2016; Zeng *et al.* 2010). Details regarding the merits or challenges of each individual method are out of the scope of this chapter, and we refer you to consult other reviews on this subject matter (Acott *et al.* 2021; Wang *et al.* 2017a). Nevertheless, our group has extensively reported the use of atomic force microscopy in characterizing TM cell/ECM/and tissue biomechanical properties (Chang *et al.* 2014; Dhamodaran *et al.* 2020; Last *et al.* 2011; Morgan *et al.* 2014; Morgan *et al.* 2015a; Morgan *et al.* 2015b; Peng *et al.* 2022a; Peng *et al.* 2022b; Raghunathan *et al.* 2017; Raghunathan *et al.* 2015a; Raghunathan *et al.* 2015b; Raghunathan *et al.* 2018; Vranka *et al.* 2018) from human, rabbit, and non-human primate models. In this chapter, we detail the salient steps required for such experiments.

EXPERIMENTAL DESIGN

Operating Principle

Atomic force microscopy is a form of scanning probe microscopy (SPM) whose operating principle (Fig. **1**) is defined by its ability to sense changes on a surface through deflections of a sharp tip (nanoscale) at the end of a cantilever beam (microscale). As the tip contacts the surface, its bends (known as *deflection*, **X**) as a function of force (**F**) exerted by the sample below. The bending of the cantilever is detected by a change in voltage using a laser diode and a split photodetector. Thus, the tip-sample interaction is inherently dependent on how much a cantilever may bend in response to the force (spring constant, **κ**). *i.e.* **F** = **κ . X**. The resulting output is known as a Force-Distance or Force-Displacement (F-D) curve.

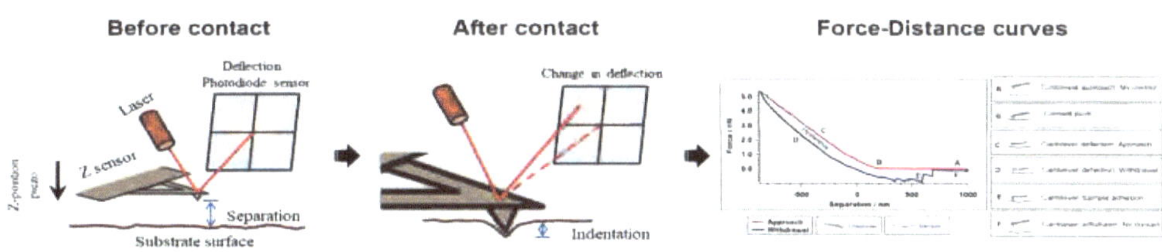

Fig. (1). Principle of operation of an atomic force microscope.

Factors Underlying Choice of AFM Equipment

There are several options now while considering the purchase of an AFM. For biological applications such as the measurement of mechanical properties of cells, tissues, *etc.*, ideally, your choice of AFM would include its utility in a hydrated environment. Depending on your budget constraints, you may want to consider a system that may be mounted on an inverted (epifluorescent, confocal, TIRF, *etc.*) or upright microscope with or without fluorescence capabilities. Coupling an AFM to a microscope allows us to gather complementary spatial information for image/mechanics layover and to visualize cells that may or may not have live cell staining/vector transduction. Further, it is essential to choose an AFM system with the ability to perform closed feedback loop measurements to allow for spatial positioning during imaging and mechanical characterization. The choice of AFM head depends on the intended application, *i.e.* long-range movement in the *z*-direction (up to 100 μm) may be required for highly adhesive samples or for single cell / single molecule force spectroscopy where the tip cantilever tip may be required to fully disengage following indentation. Standard *z*-length (up to 20 μm) would suffice for mechanical characterization (elasticity, viscoelasticity, force-map, *etc.*) and imaging of soft hydrated samples. Depending on the required speed and spatial precision, AFM heads may be mounted on manual or motorized stages. It is also advised to utilize a heated stage for the mechanical characterization of cells. Finally, it is strongly advised that the AFM-microscope system be mounted on an active anti-vibration table within an acoustic isolation system to minimize noise.

Important Considerations for using AFM to Assess TM Cell/Tissue Mechanics

Sample Preparation

One of the greatest strengths of the AFM is that it does not require expensive, tedious sample preparation methods that electron microscopes require. Many commercial AFMs employ a controlled environmental chamber. This is crucial as biological samples can be characterized in a biomimetic environment without the need for fixation or dehydration. The most common method to immobilize biological samples is by using cyanoacrylate or fibrin-based glues that can potentially introduce artifacts (Ebenstein and Pruitt 2006; Oyen 2013). For very small samples, Cell-Tak or poly-L-lysine may be used. While minimizing the amount of glue to minimize errors or discarding artifactual data is feasible, it is preferred that sample preparation is objective and controlled. This led us to develop a glue-free method for measuring TM moduli (Morgan *et al.* 2014).

Hydration Medium

Tissues are hydrated *in vivo* and thus must be adequately and appropriately hydrated while performing AFM. Physiological buffers like phosphate-buffered saline or Hank's balanced salt solution with divalent salts (Ca^{2+}/Mg^{2+}) will minimize electrostatic interactions and osmotic pressure and prevent potential swelling artifacts. Although useful to reduce tip-sample interactions, we recommend avoiding the use of agents such as pluronics or poly(ethylene glycol) as they may modulate osmolarity and affect cell function.

Cantilever Considerations

Since AFM is dependent on the deflection of a cantilever, the choice of appropriate cantilever stiffness (spring constant) should be matched with sample stiffness, *i.e.*, if a stiff cantilever is used to measure a sample by orders of magnitude, large deformations would not lead to detectable cantilever deflection. At the same time, the spring constant cannot be too small such that drag force due to motion through the buffer generates appreciable deflection. In addition, prior to every experiment, it is important to calibrate the spring constant and optical sensitivity of the cantilever (Table **1**). For example, for samples with moduli < 1 kPa, it is advisable to start with cantilevers with a spring constant of 0.01-0.08 N/m. For samples between 1-100 kPa, cantilevers with spring constant in the range 0.1 – 0.4 N/m are suggested. Finally, for rigid hydrogels whose moduli may exceed 100 kPa up to 1 MPa, cantilevers with a spring constant of 0.5-2 N/m are recommended. If the user intends to image samples in liquid, cantilevers of a short length are preferable as they help minimize drag forces in tapping mode. For all samples, optimal parameters for approach velocity and indentation depth have to be kept consistent. When using elastic approximations for viscoelastic tissues, the approach velocity of the cantilever must be carefully controlled.

Table 1. Cantilevers, their properties, and uses.

Cantilever	Vendor	Nominal Spring Constant (κ)	Borosilicate Bead (Diameter	Indenter Shape	Application
PNP-TR-TL (silicon nitride; Tipless)	Nano and More	0.32 N/m	Yes, 1-20 μm	Spherical	For bead modification & single-cell force spectroscopy
PNP-TR (silicon nitride)	Nano and More	0.32 N/m	Yes, 1 μm	Spherical	Tissue mechanics
PNP-TR (silicon nitride)	Nano and More	0.32 N/m	Yes, 1 or 5 μm	Spherical	Cell-derived matrices (CDM) mechanics

(Table 1) cont.....

Cantilever	Vendor	Nominal Spring Constant (κ)	Borosilicate Bead (Diameter	Indenter Shape	Application
PNP-TR (silicon nitride)	Nano and More	0.32 N/m	No	Pyramidal	Cells: Single indentation, Viscoelastic measurements
PF-QNM-LC	Bruker	0.01 N/m	No	Cone-sphere	Cells: Imaging, Force-volume
AC240TSR3	Asylum Research	2 N/m	No	Tetrahedral point	Imaging cells/CDM and single molecule force spectroscopy

Indenter Shape and Depth

This is a critical factor while obtaining force versus indentation curves for AFM analysis. The models used to fit force versus indentation curves are geometry-specific: rigid cone, sphere, or flat cylinder (Harding and Sneddon 1945; Love 1939). If cantilevers are modified with a sphere, the diameter of the sphere factors heavily in indentation depth and subsequent analysis of elastic modulus (Cheng *et al.* 2005; Cheng and Cheng 2005; Rodriguez *et al.* 2013; Rodriguez and Gutierrez 2003). For thin samples such as tissues or cell-derived matrices, it is essential to consider the influence of the underlying substrate, which is typically much stiffer. To mitigate substrate effects, the general rule is to limit the indentation depth to approximately 10% of the total sample thickness (Oliver and Pharr 1992; Pharr *et al.* 1992).

From our experience, we recommend the following types of cantilevers for the applications intended:

Once a cantilever is chosen, two key parameters are required: *deflection sensitivity* and the cantilever's *spring constant*. The *deflection sensitivity* is unique to each AFM system and needs to be measured before each experiment. The *deflection sensitivity* is a measure of how much a cantilever deflects (nm), resulting in a change in voltage (V) on the 4-quadrant photodiode. Variability is deflection sensitivity that can adversely impact moduli measurements, and special care must be taken to ensure clean surfaces, cantilever tips, *etc.*, during calibration. We recommend the use of a calibrating quartz chip or glass slide for determining deflection sensitivity. Once deflection sensitivity is measured, most commonly, we apply the thermal noise method to calculate the spring constant.

EXPERIMENTAL PROTOCOL

Modification of PNP-TR Cantilevers with Borosilicate Beads

- Clean surface contaminants off of PNT-TR cantilevers under UV-Ozone for 5 min prior to its utilization for experiments.
- On a fresh glass slide, add a few drops of UV-curable Norland electronic adhesive 123L (NOA123L) using a 10μl pipette tip, as shown in Fig. (**2**).
- Opposite the glue on the same side glass slide, add some borosilicate beads or the required diameter, as shown in Fig. (**2**).
- Mount the cantilever in the cantilever holder of the AFM head.
- Perform your laser alignment on the AFM software to obtain maximum sum and zero the horizontal and vertical measurements on the photodiode.
- Using the optical image on the camera of the microscope, position the cantilever tip over the glue by moving the sample holder and stage. Ensure glue is in focus.
- Lower the AFM head slowly by monitoring the change in amplitude (sum) on the photodiode and visualizing the *z*-level until it is close to the glue. Note that looking at the shadow of the cantilever tip on the camera would help position proximity.
- Once close to the surface, lower the head in increments of 1 – 5 μm steps until the tip makes contact with the small drop of glue (Fig. **3**). Contact is confirmed by monitoring a significant change in vertical deflection on the laser alignment window.
- Retract immediately (200-500 μm) and remove the tip from the glue. Ensure to use the smallest glue drop as possible to avoid contaminating the cantilever tip.
- Move the cantilever such that you are over a borosilicate bead and measure the bead diameter using the camera software.
- Lower the cantilever in large increments until you are close to the bead, and then in 1 μm increments.
- Make contact with the bead, which is confirmed by monitoring a significant change in vertical deflection on the laser alignment window.
- Pause for a second and retract (200-500 μm) and confirm that the bead is no longer present on the glass surface but is visible on the tip of the cantilever (Fig. **3**).
- Proper attachment of the bead to the cantilever is critical and requires patience and practice.
- Move the AFM head to its maximal height and remove the cantilever from the AFM head.
- UV the cantilever for 10 min to cure the glue.
- Confirm attachment of the bead under a stereomicroscope. For beginners, it is advised that you perform scanning electron microscopy to confirm proper bead attachment.

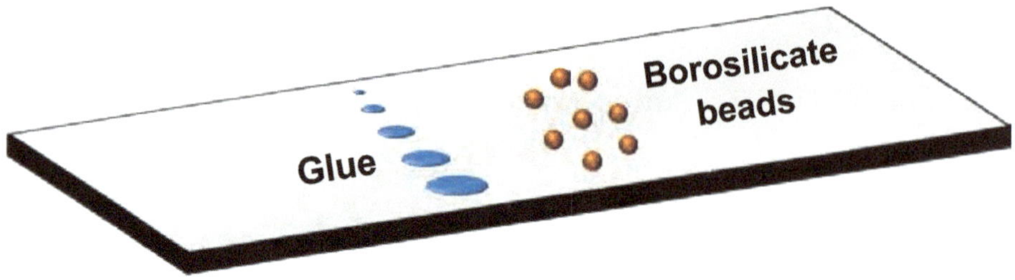

Fig. (2). Set up to modify cantilevers with borosilicate beads. To a clean glass slide, add NOA123L UV curable glue and borosilicate beads of the required diameter. Ensure separation between the beads and glue and good dispersion of beads.

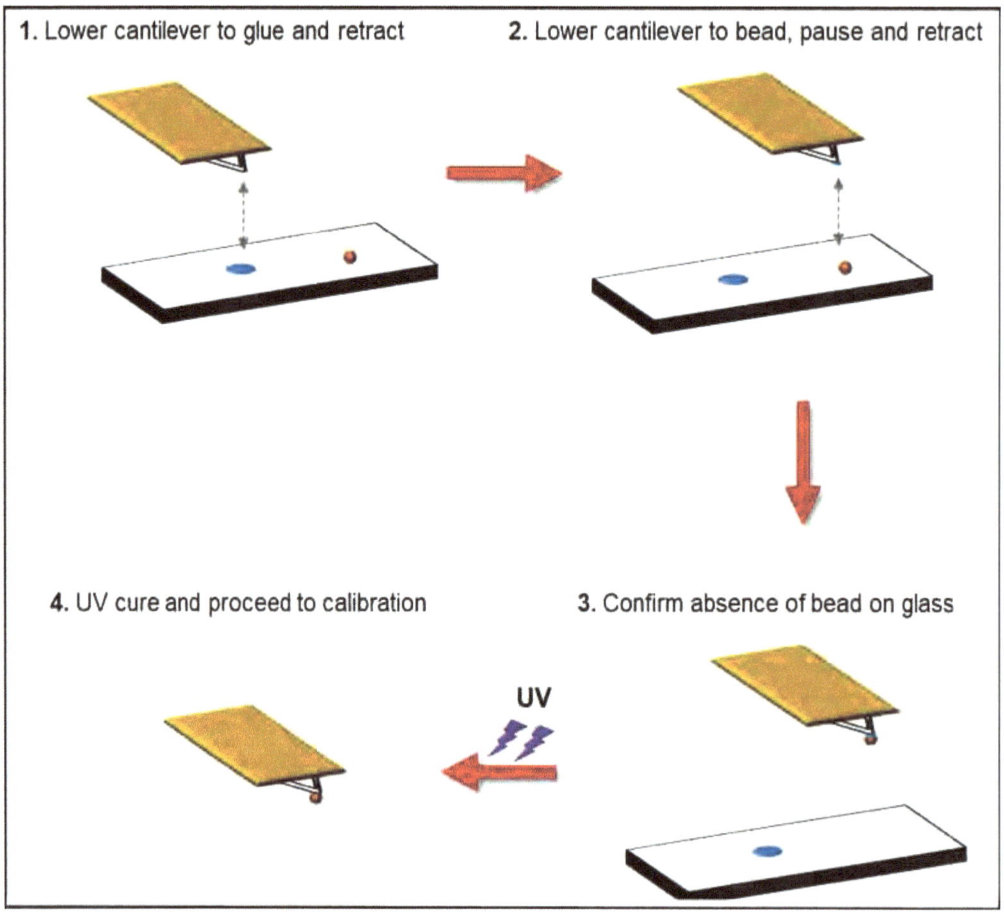

Fig. (3). Modification of cantilevers with borosilicate beads. First position the cantilever over a small drop of glue, lower it, and retract it immediately. Then move the cantilever over a single borosilicate bead, lower, pause, and retract. Remove cantilever from AFM head and cure using UV for 10 min. Confirm bead attachment to tip.

Calibration

- Mount the cantilever onto the AFM head, align the laser and photodiode to obtain maximum sum, zero the horizontal and vertical photodiodes, and center the laser.

Determining Deflection Sensitivity

- Using a *setpoint* of 0.8 V and a relative *setpoint* of 1.0 V, lower the cantilever towards a glass slide. Do not touch the surface of the slide.
- Once the tip is near the surface, *engage* the approach and lower the AFM head using the *Approach* function with constant velocity. Using the software's *approach/engage* function prevents the AFM head/cantilever from crashing into the glass slide.
- Once the cantilever is engaged with the surface, ensure that the deflection is stable by monitoring the laser alignment window.
- Collect one to five Force-Distance (F-D) curves with a *ramp distance* of 1 µm and 2 µm/s approach velocity.
- Open the software's calibration tab/manager, and by selecting the linear slope of the *extend* curve, adjust the deflection sensitivity (Fig. **4**).
- Accept the calculated deflection sensitivity and *withdraw* the cantilever from the surface.
- Repeat steps 2.2.4 through 2.2.6 at least three times and use the average deflection sensitivity across the measurements for your experiments.
- *Withdraw* and retract the AFM head by 200-500 µm from the surface

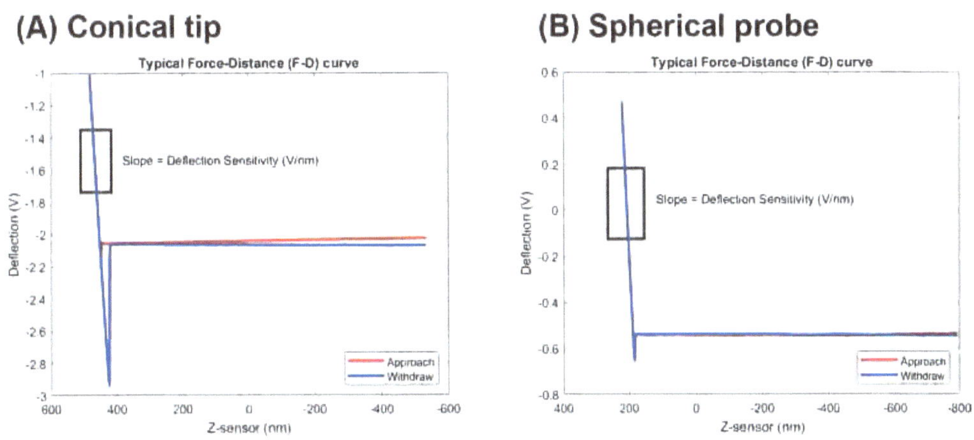

Fig. (4). Representative force-distance curve to determine deflection sensitivity for (A) conical tip or (B) spherical probe. Deflection and Z-sensor curve are used to determine the deflection sensitivity for the cantilevers used. Conical tip probes generally have stronger adhesion than probes modified with borosilicate beads (spherical).

Determining Spring Constant

- Ensure the cantilever is well above the surface of the glass slide.
- In the calibration manage/tab, select the thermal noise method for determining the spring constant.
- Remember to input the new/calculated *deflection sensitivity* for the cantilever on the day of the experiment.
- Based on the manufacturer's ratings for the cantilever, adjust the *thermal tune frequency* range.
- Acquire thermal sweep data and zoom in the region surrounding the peak.
- Select the *Lorentzian* function for calibration in *air* or the *simple harmonic oscillation* function for calibration in *fluid.*
- Fit data appropriately following the prompts on the software and record the calculated *spring constant.*
- The cantilever may be calibrated either pre- or post-bead attachment. The thermal noise method assumes that the mass of the tip is negligible compared with the mass of the cantilever. It is thus preferable to use beads of diameters < 20 μm for your experiments. The use of larger beads (*e.g.*, 50-200 μm) can impact the cantilever's resonance frequency and subsequent spring constant values. For this calibration, using the *weighted method* instead of thermal noise is advisable.
- For larger beads, use a tipless beam cantilever and calibrate prior to bead attachment. For smaller beads, confirm that the change in spring constant value is negligible prior to its usage.
- When doing AFM measurements in fluid, ensure laser and photodiode alignment and determination of deflection sensitivity and spring constant are all done in liquid. This is critical since changes in refractive indices from air to liquid will affect the photodiode sensitivity.

Sample Preparation

- We recommend the use of glass bottom AFM dishes such as the FluroDish (Catalog # FD5040-100, World Precision Instruments, Sarasota, FL) for cell culture and AFM. Alternatively, cells may be cultured on 12-13 mm Φ coverslips, which may be adhered to appropriate cell culture dishes prior to AFM measurements.
- Cell-derived matrices may be generated on glass bottom culture dishes or glass cover glasses modified with an amino silane. The detailed protocol to derive these is described in a prior chapter of this book.
- Care must be taken to ensure complete adhesion of cover glass to the substrate to minimize artifacts and noise.

- For tissues, most commonly, the TM is mounted onto substrates using cyanoacrylate glue. We, however, recommend a glue-free method that has been validated by our group (Morgan *et al.* 2014). Briefly,
  - Spin coat an AFM dish with a layer of silicone (Sylgard 527; Dow Corning, Midland, MI),
  - Cure at 65°C for 4 h and cool to room temperature. These may be stored at room temperature for up to 30 days prior to use.
  - Dissect out the TM from corneoscleral rims and cut into small 2-5 mm long samples.
  - Dab the sample briefly but quickly on a Kimwipe or Weck-Cel® cellulose eye spear to remove excess fluid.
  - Place the JCT side up of the TM on the center of the silicone-coated dish.
  - A Soft-Clamping Immobilizing Retainer of Tissue (SCIRT) is made by using a 1.25-4 mm biopsy punch to create a window in a 13 mm Thermanox coverslip (ThermoFisher Scientific, Waltham, MA), and small droplets of cyanoacrylate glue are placed around its periphery (Fig. **5**).
  - Utilizing a dissection microscope (Stemi V6, Carl Zeiss AG, Oberkochen, Germany), the SCIRT is then placed such that the tissue is accessible through the window, and it is monitored throughout the mounting to ensure the sample is not physically stretched or compressed by the SCIRT or contacts the glue.
  - Dulbecco's phosphate-buffered saline is immediately added to the dish to keep the tissue hydrated and cure the glue beneath the SCIRT (Fig. **5**).

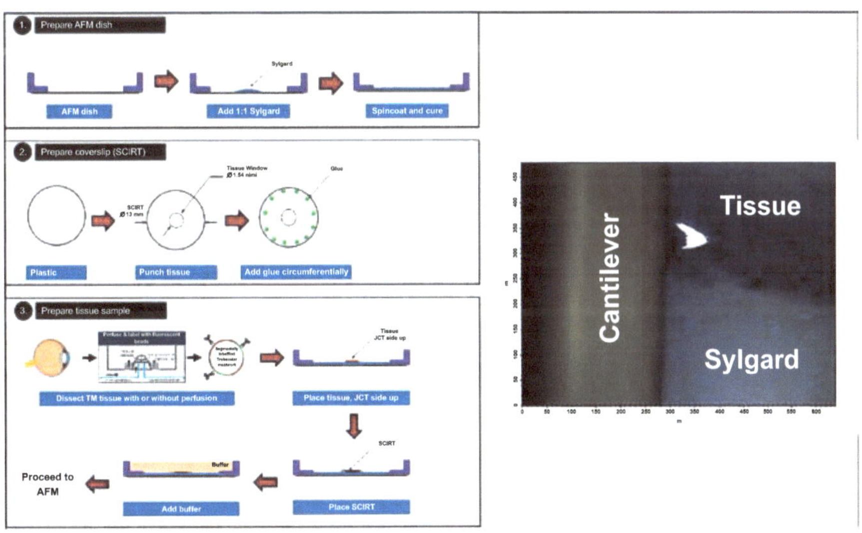

Fig. (5). Representation of a glue-free method to anchor TM tissue for AFM measurements. The cantilever here is in contact with the edge of the tissue, which must be avoided for elastic moduli measurements

Obtaining Force-Distance Curves

- F-D curves for elastic moduli measurements are routinely performed in contact mode AFM.
- Confirm that your calculated *deflection sensitivity* and *spring constant* are appropriately present/entered in the indentation parameters.
- Depending on sample stiffness, set your *relative setpoint* between 2-10 nN. It is our recommendation that you use a *relative setpoint* of 5 nN for TM cells, ECM, or tissues. It is good practice to empirically start with lower setpoints until satisfactory F-D curves are obtained. Higher *relative setpoints* may require greater indentation depths. It is also likely that a greater *relative setpoint* may be required if using large beads as indenters.
- For soft biological materials (*e.g.*, TM cell/ECM/tissue), we recommend setting the *ramp rate* at 2 µm/s. However, various groups use between 2-15 µm/s.
- Set your *ramp distance* as appropriate for the sample. For soft and adhesive samples (*e.g.*, tissues and ECM), you may need a longer *ramp distance* to ensure complete tip detachment from the sample. We recommend the following ramp distance for the following sample types:

Sample type	Ramp distance (µm)
Primary TM cells	1-3 µm
Human TM tissue	3-5 µm
Cell derived matrices	5-7 µm
Polyacrylamide hydrogels	
1-25 kPa	3 µm
>25 kPa	1 µm
Collagen gels	
Cell-free collagen gels	5-7 µm
Cell-laden collagen gels	3-5 µm

- Alter the *approach* parameters and *feedback control* depending on sample properties.
- Once your parameters have been set, you may proceed to obtain F-D curves. For tissues or cell-derived matrices, you may approach any location on your sample randomly. For cells, we recommend approaching the nucleus, which would be the highest point in the sample (Fig. **6**). It is encouraged that cells are single and not in contact with other cells for accurate cell mechanical characterization.
- Adjusting the focus and phase on your microscope enables viewing the nucleus of cells.

- Equilibrate your sample at 37°C using the heated stage for at least 30 min prior to measurements. Variations in temperature can impact reproducibility, so ensure that temperature is kept constant. Note that the tip temperature may differ from the sample temperature slightly.
- Confirm that the laser and photodiode are stable, and if there has been a discernable drift in the sum and photodiode, realign to obtain maximal sum and zero the horizontal and vertical photodiode.
- Lower the cantilever/AFM head towards the surface of the sample by following the shadow of the tip in the camera. Do not make contact with the sample yet.
- When close to the surface, engage and approach with constant velocity.
- Ensure the *autosave* function is enabled and collect F-D curves.
- Ensure that both *extend* and *retract* curves are saved for *height* and *deflection* channels.
- We recommend obtaining 3 to 5 F-D curves per location. Representative F-D curves for TM cell/ECM and tissue are illustrated in Fig. (**7**).
- If you are keen on determining viscoelasticity, utilize the hold function at either constant height or constant force to obtain stress relaxation or creep deformation curves, respectively.
- Force maps (*e.g.*, 100 μm x 100μm) may be obtained as required. Please note that force maps take time and generate a lot of force curves. Unless the user has the ability to automate AFM analysis, we recommend obtaining force maps at 16x16 points.
- Once a location has been completed, *withdraw*, *retract,* and move to the next location/cell for F-D measurements.
- We recommend users to obtain 3 to 5 F-D curves from at least 20 locations/cells.
- Avoid, when possible, measuring F-D curves close to the edges of samples, and keep the acoustic enclosure closed and the anti-vibration platform active.

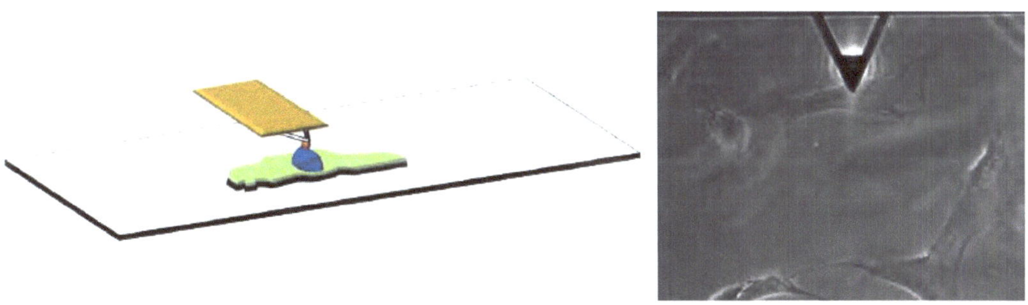

Fig. (6). Demonstration of tip position in relation to the nucleus.

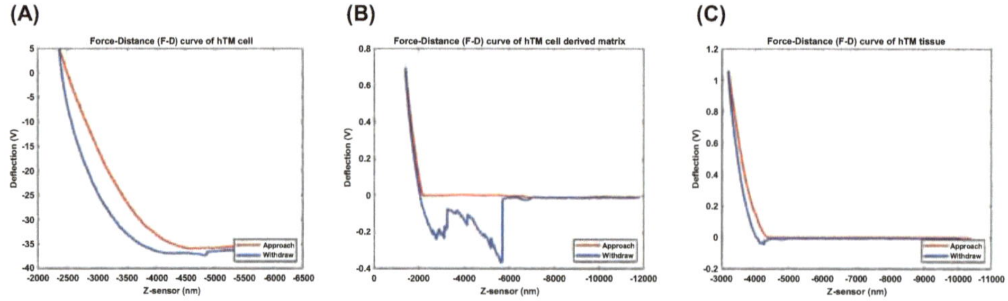

Fig. (7). Representative F-D curves for (**A**) hTM cell, (**B**) hTM cell derived matrix, (**C**) hTM tissue.

Analyzing F-D Curves

- We recommend exporting the F-D curves as ASCII files and proceeding with analysis using a custom script in MATLAB.
- A detailed description of automated custom analysis and accompanying MATLAB code is provided elsewhere (Chang *et al.* 2014).
- If limitations for such exist, one may use the built-in analysis tool. A general workflow for these may be as follows:
    - Confirm *deflection sensitivity* and *spring constant* for all F-D curves. Any discrepancies may need to be corrected appropriately.
    - Perform a *baseline offset* correction to correct for any tilt and offset.
    - Calculate *tip-sample* separation, which is critical to correct for any bending the cantilever may have undergone during measurements.
    - Check for the quality of F-D curves and discard those with abnormalities.
    - For each force curve, identify the appropriate contact point and determine the elastic modulus.
    - If utilizing the *extend* curves for analysis of *elastic moduli*, the use of the Sneddon model for conical tips and the Hertz model for spherical tips are recommended. Be sure to select and input the appropriate model and fit parameters (*e.g.*, tip radius). We assume a Poisson's ratio of 0.5 (incompressible material) for all samples (Anseth *et al.* 1996; Dimitriadis *et al.* 2002; Vinckier and Semenza 1998). A representative curve fit is demonstrated in Fig. (**8**).
    - Alternate models for analysis using the *retract* curve have been reported by various groups. Most commonly, the Oliver-Pharr model is utilized. Details of the analysis may be reviewed here (Oliver and Pharr 1992; Pharr *et al.* 1992).
    - Proceed toward statistical analysis and graphing.

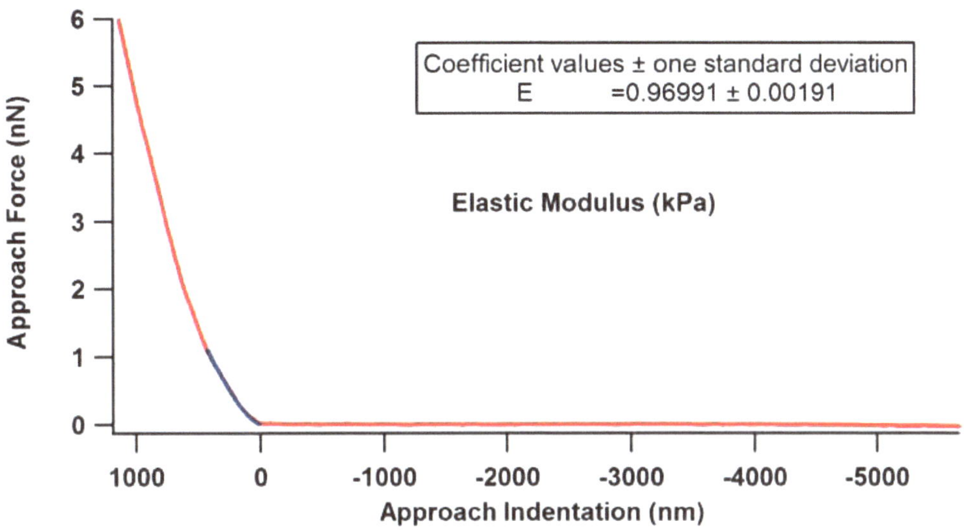

Fig. (8). Representative curve fit to determine elastic modulus from F-D curves. Red line is the extend curve. Using the Hertzian model for spherical indenter, based on contact point method, curve fitting was performed (blue line) and the elastic modulus was determined.

Generating data plots

It is feasible to assume that a large number of data points for elastic moduli would be obtained for these measurements. As such, different plot types may be employed. However, in our experience, we have observed a significant spread in data obtained from primary ocular cells and tissues. As such, we recommend demonstrating elastic moduli measurements in the form of SuperPlots (Kenny and Schoen 2021; Lord *et al.* 2020) that allow visualization of heterogeneity within and between samples. Further, we recommend the inclusion of data fit as supplementary information.

Troubleshooting

Since no experimental equipment and/or design can be trouble-free, we have listed a number of elements to check, as in Table **2**.

Table 2. Troubleshooting potential problems and suggested solutions.

Problem	Possible reason	Remedy
Laser and photodiode alignment	1. Improper cantilever mount 2. Defective or contaminated cantilever 3. Excessive glue during bead attachment	• Remove the cantilever and remount • Clean cantilever with UV-ozone treatment and remount • If excess glue is observed, replace it with a new cantilever

(Table 2) cont.....

Problem	Possible reason	Remedy
Calibration failure	1. Static interactions between the sample surface and cantilever tip	• Retract cantilever significantly. Increase *setpoint force* and modify *feedback* • Increase ramp (Z-length) • Decrease *approach height* • Change the glass surface or use a calibrating disk
	2. Spring constant value aberrant for choice of cantilever	• Measure the spring constant before attaching the bead • The bead may not have cured properly, or insufficient glue may have caused the displacement of the bead during thermal calibration
Unsuccessful *engage* and *approach*	1. Small Z-range 2. Inadequate *setpoint* 3. Feedback is slow	• Increase *setpoint* and *approach velocity*. • *Engage* closer to the sample
Noisy or non-standard F-D curves	1. Vibrations 2. High sample rate 3. Dirty cantilever/debris attached to tip 4. Glue leaching into the fluid medium	• Reduce sampling rate from 2048 points to 1024 points • Ensure the acoustic isolation chamber is closed and the anti-vibration table is active • The sample may not be adequately adhered to the substrate • Avoid measurements at the edges of samples • Ensure there are no contaminants in the sample and change fluid media • The cantilever may have become dirty from prior measurements
Inappropriate elastic modulus values	1. Poorly calibrated deflection sensitivity and/or spring constant 2. Damaged or dirty cantilever during measurements 3. Incorrect *contact point* 4. Incorrect model applied 5. Poor quality check on F-D curves	• Recalibrate the cantilever and ensure sensitivity and spring constant remain unaltered. It may require to be UV-ozone cleaned or changed • Ensure the extend curve is used for the analysis of elastic modulus. *Sneddon* model should be applied for conical tips and *Hertz* for spherical probes • Determine a contact point such that the region of elasticity is linear (McKee *et al.* 2011). • Reject F-D curves that are noisy or not smooth. Reject curves where tip/sample interactions are large and, especially when the tip is not completely retracted from the sample prior to the next measurement

CONCLUSION

In summary, we describe the various factors to be considered while choosing an AFM system, during the preparation of samples, and while selecting cantilevers.

Further, we provide a detailed protocol to modify cantilevers with beads to obtain spherical probes and use them to characterize the elastic moduli of biological samples (cells, tissues, or cell-derived matrices). In addition, we also provide details of a glueless technique that our group has used (and validated) to prepare hTM samples for AFM measurements. Lastly, we provide a general workflow for how to obtain F-D curves and analyze data using geometry relevant models. Where appropriate, we provide recommendations based on our user experience when using the AFM for vision science applications.

REFERENCES

Acott, TS, Vranka, JA, Keller, KE, Raghunathan, V & Kelley, MJ (2021) Normal and glaucomatous outflow regulation. *Prog Retin Eye Res,* 82, 100897.
[http://dx.doi.org/10.1016/j.preteyeres.2020.100897] [PMID: 32795516]

Ai, S, Zhang, Y, Shi, G, Wang, Y, Liu, G, Han, X, Zhao, Y, Yang, H & He, X (2023) Acoustic radiation force optical coherence elastography: A preliminary study on biomechanical properties of trabecular meshwork. *J Biophotonics,* e202200317.
[http://dx.doi.org/10.1002/jbio.202200317]

Anseth, KS, Bowman, CN & Brannon-Peppas, L (1996) Mechanical properties of hydrogels and their experimental determination. *Biomaterials,* 17, 1647-57.
[http://dx.doi.org/10.1016/0142-9612(96)87644-7] [PMID: 8866026]

Camras, LJ, Stamer, WD, Epstein, D, Gonzalez, P & Yuan, F (2012) Differential effects of trabecular meshwork stiffness on outflow facility in normal human and porcine eyes. *Invest Ophthalmol Vis Sci,* 53, 5242-50.
[http://dx.doi.org/10.1167/iovs.12-9825] [PMID: 22786899]

Camras, LJ, Stamer, WD, Epstein, D, Gonzalez, P & Yuan, F (2014) Circumferential tensile stiffness of glaucomatous trabecular meshwork. *Invest Ophthalmol Vis Sci,* 55, 814-23.
[http://dx.doi.org/10.1167/iovs.13-13091] [PMID: 24408980]

Chang, YR, Raghunathan, VK, Garland, SP, Morgan, JT, Russell, P & Murphy, CJ (2014) Automated AFM force curve analysis for determining elastic modulus of biomaterials and biological samples. *J Mech Behav Biomed Mater,* 37, 209-18.
[http://dx.doi.org/10.1016/j.jmbbm.2014.05.027] [PMID: 24951927]

Cheng, L, Xia, X, Scriven, LE & Gerberich, WW (2005) Spherical-tip indentation of viscoelastic material. *Mech Mater,* 37, 213-26.
[http://dx.doi.org/10.1016/j.mechmat.2004.03.002]

Cheng, YT & Cheng, CM (2005) Relationships between initial unloading slope, contact depth, and mechanical properties for spherical indentation in linear viscoelastic solids. *Mater Sci Eng A,* 409, 93-9.
[http://dx.doi.org/10.1016/j.msea.2005.05.118]

Dahl, KN, Ribeiro, AJS & Lammerding, J (2008) Nuclear shape, mechanics, and mechanotransduction. *Circ Res,* 102, 1307-18.
[http://dx.doi.org/10.1161/CIRCRESAHA.108.173989] [PMID: 18535268]

Dhamodaran, K, Baidouri, H, Sandoval, L & Raghunathan, V (2020) Wnt Activation After Inhibition Restores Trabecular Meshwork Cells Toward a Normal Phenotype. *Invest Ophthalmol Vis Sci,* 61, 30.
[http://dx.doi.org/10.1167/iovs.61.6.30] [PMID: 32539133]

Dimitriadis, EK, Horkay, F, Maresca, J, Kachar, B & Chadwick, RS (2002) Determination of elastic moduli of thin layers of soft material using the atomic force microscope. *Biophys J,* 82, 2798-810.
[http://dx.doi.org/10.1016/S0006-3495(02)75620-8] [PMID: 11964265]

Ebenstein, DM & Pruitt, LA (2006) Nanoindentation of biological materials. *Nano Today,* 1, 26-33. [http://dx.doi.org/10.1016/S1748-0132(06)70077-9]

Gao, K, Song, S, Johnstone, MA, Zhang, Q, Xu, J, Zhang, X, Wang, RK & Wen, JC (2020) Reduced Pulsatile Trabecular Meshwork Motion in Eyes With Primary Open Angle Glaucoma Using Phase-Sensitive Optical Coherence Tomography. *Invest Ophthalmol Vis Sci,* 61, 21. [http://dx.doi.org/10.1167/iovs.61.14.21] [PMID: 33326017]

Harding, J & Sneddon, I. (1945) The elastic stresses produced by the indentation of the plane surface of a semi-infinite elastic solid by a rigid punch, Cambridge Univ Press. 16-26.

Huang, J, Camras, LJ & Yuan, F (2015) Mechanical analysis of rat trabecular meshwork. *Soft Matter,* 11, 2857-65. [http://dx.doi.org/10.1039/C4SM01949K] [PMID: 25710888]

Jaalouk, DE & Lammerding, J (2009) Mechanotransduction gone awry. *Nat Rev Mol Cell Biol,* 10, 63-73. [http://dx.doi.org/10.1038/nrm2597] [PMID: 19197333]

Jahed, Z, Shams, H, Mehrbod, M & Mofrad, MRK (2014) Chapter Five - Mechanotransduction Pathways Linking the Extracellular Matrix to the Nucleus. In: Kwang, W.J., (Ed.), *International Review of Cell and Molecular Biology* Academic Press 171-220.

Johnson, M, Schuman, JS & Kagemann, L (2015) Trabecular Meshwork Stiffness in the Living Human Eye. *Invest Ophthalmol Vis Sci,* 56, 3541-1.

Johnson, M, Shapiro, A, Ethier, CR & Kamm, RD (1992) Modulation of outflow resistance by the pores of the inner wall endothelium. *Invest Ophthalmol Vis Sci,* 33, 1670-5. [PMID: 1559767]

Kaminski, A, Fedorchak, GR & Lammerding, J (2014) The cellular mastermind(?)-mechanotransduction and the nucleus. *Prog Mol Biol Transl Sci,* 126, 157-203. [http://dx.doi.org/10.1016/B978-0-12-394624-9.00007-5] [PMID: 25081618]

Kenny, M & Schoen, I (2021) Violin SuperPlots: visualizing replicate heterogeneity in large data sets. *Mol Biol Cell,* 32, 1333-4. [http://dx.doi.org/10.1091/mbc.E21-03-0130] [PMID: 34264756]

Last, JA, Pan, T, Ding, Y, Reilly, CM, Keller, K, Acott, TS, Fautsch, MP, Murphy, CJ & Russell, P (2011) Elastic modulus determination of normal and glaucomatous human trabecular meshwork. *Invest Ophthalmol Vis Sci,* 52, 2147-52. [http://dx.doi.org/10.1167/iovs.10-6342] [PMID: 21220561]

Lee, C, Li, G, Stamer, WD & Ethier, CR (2021) In vivo estimation of murine iris stiffness using finite element modeling. *Exp Eye Res,* 202, 108374. [http://dx.doi.org/10.1016/j.exer.2020.108374] [PMID: 33253706]

Li, G, Lee, C, Agrahari, V, Wang, K, Navarro, I, Sherwood, JM, Crews, K, Farsiu, S, Gonzalez, P, Lin, CW, Mitra, AK, Ethier, CR & Stamer, WD (2019) In vivo measurement of trabecular meshwork stiffness in a corticosteroid-induced ocular hypertensive mouse model. *Proc Natl Acad Sci USA,* 116, 1714-22. [http://dx.doi.org/10.1073/pnas.1814889116] [PMID: 30651311]

Li, P, Shen, TT, Johnstone, M & Wang, RK (2013) Pulsatile motion of the trabecular meshwork in healthy human subjects quantified by phase-sensitive optical coherence tomography. *Biomed Opt Express,* 4, 2051-65. [http://dx.doi.org/10.1364/BOE.4.002051] [PMID: 24156063]

Lord, SJ, Velle, KB, Mullins, RD & Fritz-Laylin, LK (2020) SuperPlots: Communicating reproducibility and variability in cell biology. *J Cell Biol,* 219, e202001064. [http://dx.doi.org/10.1083/jcb.202001064] [PMID: 32346721]

Love, AEH (1939) Boussingesq's problem for a rigid cone. *Q J Math,* os-10, 161-75. [http://dx.doi.org/10.1093/qmath/os-10.1.161]

Martino, F, Perestrelo, AR, Vinarský, V, Pagliari, S & Forte, G (2018) Cellular Mechanotransduction: From Tension to Function. *Front Physiol,* 9, 824.
[http://dx.doi.org/10.3389/fphys.2018.00824] [PMID: 30026699]

McKee, CT, Last, JA, Russell, P & Murphy, CJ (2011) Indentation versus tensile measurements of Young's modulus for soft biological tissues. *Tissue Eng Part B Rev,* 17, 155-64.
[http://dx.doi.org/10.1089/ten.teb.2010.0520] [PMID: 21303220]

Morgan, JT, Raghunathan, VK, Thomasy, SM, Murphy, CJ & Russell, P (2014) Robust and artifact-free mounting of tissue samples for atomic force microscopy. *Biotechniques,* 56, 40-2.
[http://dx.doi.org/10.2144/000114126] [PMID: 24447138]

Morgan, JT, Raghunathan, VK, Chang, YR, Murphy, CJ & Russell, P (2015) Wnt inhibition induces persistent increases in intrinsic stiffness of human trabecular meshwork cells. *Exp Eye Res,* 132, 174-8. a
[http://dx.doi.org/10.1016/j.exer.2015.01.025] [PMID: 25639201]

Morgan, JT, Raghunathan, VK, Chang, Y-R, Murphy, CJ & Russell, P (2015) The intrinsic stiffness of human trabecular meshwork cells increases with senescence. *Impact Journals.*
[http://dx.doi.org/10.18632/oncotarget.3798]

Oliver, WC & Pharr, GM (1992) An improved technique for determining hardness and elastic modulus using load and displacement sensing indentation experiments. *J Mater Res,* 7, 1564-83.
[http://dx.doi.org/10.1557/JMR.1992.1564]

Overby, DR, Zhou, EH, Vargas-Pinto, R, Pedrigi, RM, Fuchshofer, R, Braakman, ST, Gupta, R, Perkumas, KM, Sherwood, JM, Vahabikashi, A, Dang, Q, Kim, JH, Ethier, CR, Stamer, WD, Fredberg, JJ & Johnson, M (2014) Altered mechanobiology of Schlemm's canal endothelial cells in glaucoma. *Proc Natl Acad Sci USA,* 111, 13876-81.
[http://dx.doi.org/10.1073/pnas.1410602111] [PMID: 25201985]

Oyen, ML (2013) Nanoindentation of Biological and Biomimetic Materials. *Exp Tech,* 37, 73-87.
[http://dx.doi.org/10.1111/j.1747-1567.2011.00716.x]

Peng, M, Rayana, NP, Dai, J, Sugali, CK, Baidouri, H, Suresh, A, Raghunathan, VK & Mao, W (2022) Cross-linked actin networks (CLANs) affect stiffness and/or actin dynamics in transgenic transformed and primary human trabecular meshwork cells. *Exp Eye Res,* 220, 109097. a
[http://dx.doi.org/10.1016/j.exer.2022.109097] [PMID: 35569518]

Peng, M, Margetts, TJ, Sugali, CK, Rayana, NP, Dai, J, Sharma, TP, Raghunathan, VK & Mao, W (2022) An ex vivo model of human corneal rim perfusion organ culture. *Exp Eye Res,* 214, 108891. b
[http://dx.doi.org/10.1016/j.exer.2021.108891] [PMID: 34896309]

Pharr, GM, Oliver, WC & Brotzen, FR (1992) On the generality of the relationship among contact stiffness, contact area, and elastic modulus during indentation. *J Mater Res,* 7, 613-7.
[http://dx.doi.org/10.1557/JMR.1992.0613]

Raghunathan, V, Eaton, JS, Christian, BJ, Morgan, JT, Ver Hoeve, JN, Yang, CYC, Gong, H, Rasmussen, CA, Miller, PE, Russell, P, Nork, TM & Murphy, CJ (2017) Biomechanical, ultrastructural, and electrophysiological characterization of the non-human primate experimental glaucoma model. *Sci Rep,* 7, 14329.
[http://dx.doi.org/10.1038/s41598-017-14720-2] [PMID: 29085025]

Raghunathan, VK, Morgan, JT, Chang, YR, Weber, D, Phinney, B, Murphy, CJ & Russell, P (2015) Transforming Growth Factor Beta 3 Modifies Mechanics and Composition of Extracellular Matrix Deposited by Human Trabecular Meshwork Cells. *ACS Biomater Sci Eng,* 1, 110-8. a
[http://dx.doi.org/10.1021/ab500060r] [PMID: 30882039]

Raghunathan, VK, Morgan, JT, Park, SA, Weber, D, Phinney, BS, Murphy, CJ & Russell, P (2015) Dexamethasone Stiffens Trabecular Meshwork, Trabecular Meshwork Cells, and Matrix. *Invest Ophthalmol Vis Sci,* 56, 4447-59. b
[http://dx.doi.org/10.1167/iovs.15-16739] [PMID: 26193921]

Raghunathan, VK, Benoit, J, Kasetti, R, Zode, G, Salemi, M, Phinney, BS, Keller, KE, Staverosky, JA, Murphy, CJ, Acott, T & Vranka, J (2018) Glaucomatous cell derived matrices differentially modulate non-glaucomatous trabecular meshwork cellular behavior. *Acta Biomater,* 71, 444-59. [http://dx.doi.org/10.1016/j.actbio.2018.02.037] [PMID: 29524673]

Rodriguez, ML, McGarry, PJ & Sniadecki, NJ (2013) Review on Cell Mechanics: Experimental and Modeling Approaches. *Appl Mech Rev,* 65, 060801. [http://dx.doi.org/10.1115/1.4025355]

Rodriguez, R & Gutierrez, I (2003) Correlation between nanoindentation and tensile propertiesInfluence of the indentation size effect. *Mater Sci Eng A,* 361, 377-84. [http://dx.doi.org/10.1016/S0921-5093(03)00563-X]

Tamm, ER (2009) The trabecular meshwork outflow pathways: Structural and functional aspects. *Exp Eye Res,* 88, 648-55. [http://dx.doi.org/10.1016/j.exer.2009.02.007] [PMID: 19239914]

Tamm, ER (2010) Functional Morphology of the Trabecular Meshwork. In: Dartt, D.A., (Ed.), *Encyclopedia of the Eye* Academic Press, Oxford 157-63. [http://dx.doi.org/10.1016/B978-0-12-374203-2.00092-0]

Tamm, ER (2015) 5 - Functional Morphology of the Trabecular Meshwork Outflow Pathways. In: Crowston, T.M.S.B.S.A.H.G., (Ed.), *Glaucoma* W.B. Saunders 40-6. [http://dx.doi.org/10.1016/B978-0-7020-5193-7.00005-4]

Tamm, ER & Fuchshofer, R (2007) What increases outflow resistance in primary open-angle glaucoma? *Surv Ophthalmol,* 52 (Suppl. 2), S101-4. [http://dx.doi.org/10.1016/j.survophthal.2007.08.002] [PMID: 17998032]

Toris, CB, Yablonski, ME, Wang, YL & Camras, CB (1999) Aqueous humor dynamics in the aging human eye. *Am J Ophthalmol,* 127, 407-12. [http://dx.doi.org/10.1016/S0002-9394(98)00436-X] [PMID: 10218693]

Toris, CB, Koepsell, SA, Yablonski, ME & Camras, CB (2002) Aqueous humor dynamics in ocular hypertensive patients. *J Glaucoma,* 11, 253-8. [http://dx.doi.org/10.1097/00061198-200206000-00015] [PMID: 12140404]

Vahabikashi, A, Gelman, A, Dong, B, Gong, L, Cha, EDK, Schimmel, M, Tamm, ER, Perkumas, K, Stamer, WD, Sun, C, Zhang, HF, Gong, H & Johnson, M (2019) Increased stiffness and flow resistance of the inner wall of Schlemm's canal in glaucomatous human eyes. *Proc Natl Acad Sci USA,* 116, 26555-63. [http://dx.doi.org/10.1073/pnas.1911837116] [PMID: 31806762]

Vargas-Pinto, R, Gong, H, Vahabikashi, A & Johnson, M (2013) The effect of the endothelial cell cortex on atomic force microscopy measurements. *Biophys J,* 105, 300-9. [http://dx.doi.org/10.1016/j.bpj.2013.05.034] [PMID: 23870251]

Vinckier, A & Semenza, G (1998) Measuring elasticity of biological materials by atomic force microscopy. *FEBS Lett,* 430, 12-6. [http://dx.doi.org/10.1016/S0014-5793(98)00592-4] [PMID: 9678586]

Vranka, JA, Staverosky, JA, Reddy, AP, Wilmarth, PA, David, LL, Acott, TS, Russell, P & Raghunathan, VK (2018) Biomechanical Rigidity and Quantitative Proteomics Analysis of Segmental Regions of the Trabecular Meshwork at Physiologic and Elevated Pressures. *Invest Ophthalmol Vis Sci,* 59, 246-59. [http://dx.doi.org/10.1167/iovs.17-22759] [PMID: 29340639]

Wang, K, Read, AT, Sulchek, T & Ethier, CR (2017) Trabecular meshwork stiffness in glaucoma. *Exp Eye Res,* 158, 3-12. a [http://dx.doi.org/10.1016/j.exer.2016.07.011] [PMID: 27448987]

Wang, K, Li, G, Read, AT, Navarro, I, Mitra, AK, Stamer, WD, Sulchek, T & Ethier, CR (2018) The relationship between outflow resistance and trabecular meshwork stiffness in mice. *Sci Rep,* 8, 5848.

[http://dx.doi.org/10.1038/s41598-018-24165-w] [PMID: 29643342]

Wang, K, Johnstone, MA, Xin, C, Song, S, Padilla, S, Vranka, JA, Acott, TS, Zhou, K, Schwaner, SA, Wang, RK, Sulchek, T & Ethier, CR (2017) Estimating Human Trabecular Meshwork Stiffness by Numerical Modeling and Advanced OCT Imaging. *Invest Ophthalmol Vis Sci,* 58, 4809-17. b [http://dx.doi.org/10.1167/iovs.17-22175] [PMID: 28973327]

Yuan, F, Camras, LJ & Gonzalez, P (2011) Trabecular Meshwork Stiffness in Ex Vivo Perfused Porcine Eyes. *Invest Ophthalmol Vis Sci,* 52, 6693-3.

Yuan, F, Schieber, AT, Camras, LJ, Harasymowycz, PJ, Herndon, LW & Allingham, RR (2016) Mathematical Modeling of Outflow Facility Increase With Trabecular Meshwork Bypass and Schlemm Canal Dilation. *J Glaucoma,* 25, 355-64. [http://dx.doi.org/10.1097/IJG.0000000000000248] [PMID: 25836658]

Zeng, D, Juzkiw, T, Read, AT, Chan, DWH, Glucksberg, MR, Ethier, CR & Johnson, M (2010) Young's modulus of elasticity of Schlemm's canal endothelial cells. *Biomech Model Mechanobiol,* 9, 19-33. [http://dx.doi.org/10.1007/s10237-009-0156-3] [PMID: 19387710]

CHAPTER 19

Derivation of Primary Human Trabecular Meshwork Cell-Derived Matrices

VijayKrishna Raghunathan[1,*]

[1] *Department of Ophthalmology, Novartis Institutes for BioMedical Research, 22 Windsor St, Cambridge, MA 02139, USA*

Abstract: Ocular hypertension (OHT) partly results from increased resistance to aqueous humor (AQH) outflow from the anterior chamber of the eye as a result of changes in the extracellular matrix (ECM) of trabecular meshwork (TM). Even though *in vivo* animal models of OHT often rely upon singular gene knockout systems, these do not reveal the complexities in matrix changes (structure and composition) in the disease. Also, *in vitro* systems mimic the native topography, mechanics, or biochemistry of native ECM exist but often fail to mimic the multifaceted environment around the cells. There is, thus, a paucity of physiologically relevant assays/models to perform non-clinical mechanism-based research. Cell-derived matrices (CDMs) represent a 3D microenvironment derived from a cell type of interest that partially simulates the matrix similar to conditions *in vivo*. To mimic homeostasis under normal conditions or pathological states, the CDM content can be altered by the addition of various classes of compounds. A protocol for generating CDMs from isolated and cultured primary TM cells is described in this chapter.

Keywords: Decellularization, Extracellular matrix, Glaucoma, Matrices, Primary cells, Trabecular meshwork.

INTRODUCTION

Primary open-angle glaucoma (POAG) is a common multifactorial age-associated ocular disease worldwide, which causes irreversible vision loss if left untreated. Elevated intraocular pressure (IOP) is intimately linked to the etiology and progression of POAG. However, IOP-lowering treatments can partially address this risk factor. The trabecular meshwork (TM) is the primary route of egress for aqueous humor (AQH) from the anterior chamber of the eye (Stamer and Acott, 2012). However, abnormally accumulated extracellular matrix (ECM) in and around the TM obstructs the AQH drainage and is the main contributor to the de-

* **Corresponding author VijayKrishna Raghunathan:** Department of Ophthalmology, Novartis Institutes for BioMedical Research, 22 Windsor St, Cambridge, MA 02139, USA; E-mail: vijay.raghunathan@novartis.com

Najam A. Sharif and Sunny E. Ohia (Eds.)

velopment of ocular hypertension (OHT) (Vranka *et al.*, 2015; Acott and Kelley, 2008). Existing experimental systems of OHT have often focused on studying the role of individual components of ECM *via* genetic manipulations or exogenous treatments (*e.g.*, the addition of tissue growth factor-beta (TGFβ) or corticosteroids such as dexamethasone). However, the ECM is a mixture of proteins, lipids, biochemical ligands (Dhamodaran *et al.*, 2022), and other structural elements that are linked and interact in a complex manner. Thus, in addition to contributing towards structure and physical resistance to AQH flow, ECM regulates cell fate and cellular identity (Humphries *et al.*, 2018; Keung *et al.*, 2010; Sart *et al.*, 2020; Schwartz, 2010; Sima, 2017; Sun *et al.*, 2012; Trappmann *et al.*, 2012; Tschumperlin *et al.*, 2013; Urbanczyk *et al.*, 2020; Vining and Mooney, 2017; Vogel and Sheetz, 2009; Wen *et al.*, 2014; Wolfenson *et al.*, 2019). Consequently, no single ECM component can sufficiently cause a diminution of AQH drainage. Instead, complex interactions among matricellular proteins, growth factors, glycoproteins, and fibrillary and non-fibrillary structural proteins most likely influence the rate of ECM aggregation and digestion and thereby increase the overall stiffness of the TM and the surrounding environment. These events and factors are thus responsible for the raised resistance to AQH efflux from the anterior chamber.

CDMs are composed of a mixture of ECM biomolecules that can potentially recapitulate highly complex extracellular milieu encountered *in vivo* at the level of the TM and offer means to elucidate the relationship between the ECM turnover and cellular functions (Cukierman *et al.*, 2001). Described below is a reproducible method to generate primary human TM CDMs that can be utilized to study cellular mechanics and responses to exogenous growth factors and dissect molecular signaling pathways (Raghunathan *et al.*, 2015a,b; 2018; Yemanyi *et al.*, 2019, 2020a-d). It must be mentioned here that the creation and harvesting of CDMs is a labor-intensive and tedious process that requires patience in order to obtain a cell-free product. Even though ECMs derived from different tissue sources tend to contain a similar core of constituents, each ECM does possess a unique 'matrisomal' signature (Naba *et al.*, 2012, 2016; Taha and Naba, 2019; Bingham *et al.*, 2020; Nerger *et al.*, 2022). Consequently, it is imperative that specific procedures and conditions for cell isolation, propagation, and decellularization are delineated to reproducibly and successfully generate the desired CDMs from any particular cell type.

EXPERIMENTAL PROTOCOLS

Reagents and Supplies Required

- Since the current topic is matrices derived from human TM (hTM) cells, the latter cells must first be isolated and cultured from post-mortem human donor eye TM tissue as previously described (Keller *et al.*, 2018). Various reagents are needed for this and future purposes and are listed below, including the vendors and their locations.
- Tissue culture-treated dishes, 60 mm diameter (Corning Life Sciences, Corning, NY)
- Fine-tipped sterile plastic transfer pipettes (VWR International, Radnor, PA)
- Round glass coverslips, 12 mm diameter (Ted Pella, Inc., Redding, CA)
- Dulbecco's modified Eagle Medium/Nutrient mixture F-12 (DME/F-12, 1:1); (GE Healthcare Life Sciences, Logan, UT).
- Fetal bovine serum (FBS) (Atlanta Biologicals, Flowery, GA).
- Penicillin/streptomycin/amphotericin-B (Life Technologies, Carlsbad, CA, USA).
- Phosphate buffered saline (PBS, without calcium and magnesium) (GE Healthcare Life Sciences, Logan, UT).
- Versene (EDTA), 0.02%; 0.2 g/L ethylenediaminetetraacetic acid (0.53 mM) in DPBS, without calcium and magnesium (BioWhittaker® Reagents, Lonza, Walkersville, MD)
- 0.05% Trypsin-EDTA (ThermoFisher Scientific, Waltham, MA).
- Ammonium hydroxide (EMD Millipore Corporation, Darmstadt, Germany).
- 3-aminopropyl trimethoxysilane (281778-100ML, Sigma-Aldrich, St. Louis, MO) or 3-aminopropyl triethoxysilane (APTES; Sigma-Aldrich, St. Louis, MO).
- Triton X-100 (VWR International, Solon, OH).
- DNase I (Spectrum Chemical, Gardena, CA).

Reagent Setup

- <u>*Complete growth medium:*</u> In order to culture and propagate primary hTM cells, prepare the growth medium by supplementing DME/F-12 with 2.5mM L-glutamine, 10% FBS, and 1% penicillin/streptomycin/amphotericin-B. Then, refrigerate this culture medium.
- <u>*Decellularization / Extraction buffer:*</u> Prepare the decellularization buffer under aseptic conditions as follows: to 498.5 mL of deionized sterile water, add 1.25 mL of ammonium hydroxide and 250 μL of Triton X-100 detergent and then keep it at the bench.
- <u>*DNase I solution:*</u> Now prepare DNase-I to 50 U/mL. This will be utilized to eliminate DNA from decellularized cell-derived matrices.

- Silanization:
  - Place parafilm across a Petridish and place coverslips on top of the parafilm. Dispense 1 ml of 0.1M NaOH onto each coverslip, and after 3 mins, aspirate this off.
  - Pipette 500 μl of APTES or APTMS on coverslips and aspirate the silane after 3 mins. Do not exceed this incubation time.
  - Rinse coverslips with 20 mL sterile deionized water for 5 min on a rocker three times, and carefully pour off the solution into an appropriate organic solution waste vessel.
  - Using 100% ethanol, carefully rinse the coverslips two times, and then dry them at 65°C for 45 mins.
  - Sterilize the silanized dishes by exposing them to UV light (30 mins) in a laminar flow hood at room temperature.

Cell Culture and Decellularization

- Perform all the steps under a laminar flow biosafety cabinet to maintain sterility. For experiments pertaining to RNA/protein isolation, use 60mm Petri dishes. For immunocytochemistry or atomic force microscopy, use 12 mm round glass coverslips.
- Isolate and characterize hTM cells from post-mortem donor eye TM tissue using previously reported methods and consensus guidelines (Keller *et al*., 2018).
- Culture the isolated hTM cells in T75-flasks using 10 mL of the previously prepared culture medium in a humidified atmosphere of 5% CO_2 at 37°C and allow to attain 80-90% confluency. These cells should be utilized only between 2-5 passages.
- After this time, aspirate growth media, wash with 5 mL of Versene containing EDTA, aspirate, and incubate cells using 3 mL of 0.05% Trypsin-EDTA for 5 min in the incubator at 37°C.
- Ensure neutralization of the trypsin by adding fresh growth culture medium (~7 ml) containing serum and gently swirling the fluid inside the flask. Centrifuge the contents of the flask using conical centrifuge tubes (15 ml) on a bench-top centrifuge (1440 rotations /min for 5 mins).
- Following careful aspiration of the supernatant, gently but thoroughly mix and resuspend the hTM cell pellet using a growth culture medium (~5ml) until a homogeneous single-cell suspension is obtained. Determine the cell count either manually or using an automated cell counter.
- Carefully place 10,000 hTM/ cm^2 in 4 mL of complete growth media cells in sterile 60 mm tissue culture-treated plastic dishes or on 12 mm salinized round cover glass pieces in 24-well dishes with 1 mL medium. Now, if ECM from steroid-treated cells is required, replace the complete growth medium with a medium containing 100 nM dexamethasone.

- Ensure cells are confluent prior to initiating treatments (if any; Fig. **1A**).
- Maintain cells in a humidity-controlled 37°C, 5% CO_2 incubator with growth media changes every 2 days for 4 weeks. This process will allow the deposition of a robust ECM (6-10 µm thick).
- After this period, very gently remove 3ml of medium and leave about 1ml medium in the dish ensuring not to disturb the ECM. After about 15s, gently add 3 mL of decellularization buffer along the inner sides of the dish.
- Repeat the above steps 7-10 times to ensure a complete exchange of growth medium with decellularization buffer. Subsequently, observe under a phase contrast microscope to ensure complete decellularization. At the end of each of the decellularization procedures, gently remove much of the buffer (~3 mL) so that the dish contains about 1 ml of the decellularization buffer.
- Now, wait for 10 s, and then slowly and carefully add sterile PBS (3ml; without calcium/magnesium), pointing the dispensing tip of the pipette at the inner wall of the dish.
- Repeat the above procedures 7-10 times so that fresh PBS completely replaces the decellularization buffer. Again, observe under a phase-contrast microscope and ensure the decellularized ECM is intact (Fig. **1B**).
- If, for some reason, cellular debris is observed or there is incomplete decellularization, repeat gentle additional decellularization buffer incubations with gentle PBS washes to ensure complete cellular debris removal.
- Finally, gently remove 2 mL of PBS, replace it with 2 ml DNase-I to achieve 50 U/mL final concentration of DNase-I, and incubate it at 37°C for 1 hr to remove nuclear materials.
- After gently removing the DNase-I buffer, rinse the dish with sterile PBS (3ml).
- Now, fix extra samples in 4% paraformaldehyde before and after decellularization for secondary confirmation by immunostaining for the presence of collagen IV and fibronectin and for the absence of DAPI (nuclear stain) and F-actin (cytoskeletal remnants).
- Next, add 2-3 mL of serum-free culture medium in order to prime the ECM by incubating for 1 hr at 37°C.
- In order to study cell-ECM interactions, plate out about 8000-10,000 cells/cm^2 onto the matrices utilizing a serum-free growth medium (Fig. **1C**).
- Now, maintain the cells in an incubator in a humid atmosphere of 5% CO_2 / 95% air at 37°C. A time course of cell-ECM interaction can thus be studied using a number of similarly processed dishes or plates.

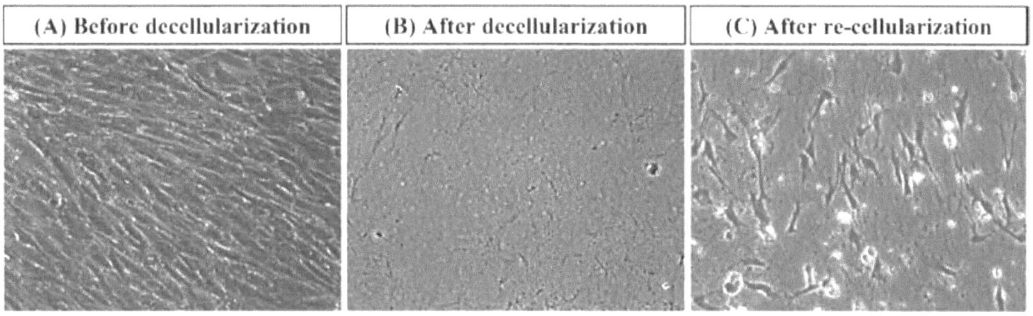

Fig. (1). Decellularization of chronically cultured primary hTM cells yield robust extracellular matrices. Representative images of (**A**) confluent culture of hTM cells prior to decellularization, (**B**) cell-derived matrices (CDMs) immediately after decellularization, and (**C**) CDMs reseeded with primary hTM cells and allowed to attach to substratum overnight.

Troubleshooting

- **Possible Problem:** Incomplete decellularization from matrices observed as dark patches on the ECM.
  Solution: Increase the volume of the decellularization buffer, incubation duration, and number of DNase I/PBS changes.
- **Possible Problem:** The demise of the hTM cells occurs during the month-ling CDM deposition process. **Solution**: Increase the number of medium changes and/or add a more complete growth culture medium.
- **Possible Problem:** The hTM cells detach from the plastic/glass substrates.
  - Solution:
    - Use early passage cells
    - Ensure cells are confluent prior to initiating any treatments
    - Reduce agitation of exchange buffer
    - Reduce the amount of suction force and avoid vacuum pump for aspiration
    - Decrease the number of buffer exchanges
    - Add solutions along the circumference of the Petri dish's inner walls instead of focusing on a single spot, and perform the additions in a circular, gentle manner
    - Utilize plasticware that has been treated to enhance CDM accumulation/deposition including for instance, "Easy-Grip" plasticware, Corning Life Sciences, Corning, NY
    - Alternatives include glass-bottom culture dishes and salinized slides in 4-well-format plates that offer good substrates for the CDMs

CONCLUSION

A comprehensive and detailed set of procedures has been described in this chapter that should yield hTM cell-derived CDMs. Some common troubleshooting steps have also been provided that should ensure success. Regardless, these matrices need to be further robustly evaluated to determine their test-retest variability, consistency in composition and morphology, and potential differences between postmortem human donors. Even though CDM utility is in its early phase, the promise of its application in future compound/drug screening, mechanism of action studies, and cell/tissue engineering approaches to help restore TM function *via* cell therapy remains high. Using bioengineering procedures to scale up CDM production and/or for the generation of customized TM-derived CDMs with homeostasis or disease relevance can enable the creation of bio-links (biological or polymer-conjugated). The latter can potentially be utilized to generate specific biomimetic microenvironment niches towards organ-on-chip devices and/or for 3D-bioprinting applications that have an enormous potential for discovering and developing future drugs directed at modulating ECM turnover and for mechanistic studies.

ACKNOWLEDGEMENTS

I would like to thank Dr. Ganesh Prasanna for the scientific discussions and for proofreading the manuscript. I would also like to thank Lions VisionGift (Portland, OR) and SavingSight (Kansas City, MO) for procuring all human donor eyes used in this work. Most importantly, I would like to thank the families of the organ donors, without whose consent these experiments would be impossible.

REFERENCES

Acott, TS & Kelley, MJ (2008) Extracellular matrix in the trabecular meshwork. *Exp Eye Res,* 86, 543-61. [http://dx.doi.org/10.1016/j.exer.2008.01.013] [PMID: 18313051]

Bingham, GC, Lee, F, Naba, A & Barker, TH (2020) Spatial-omics: Novel approaches to probe cell heterogeneity and extracellular matrix biology. *Matrix Biol,* 91-92, 152-66. [http://dx.doi.org/10.1016/j.matbio.2020.04.004] [PMID: 32416243]

Cukierman, E, Pankov, R, Stevens, DR & Yamada, KM (2001) Taking cell-matrix adhesions to the third dimension. *Science,* 294, 1708-12. [http://dx.doi.org/10.1126/science.1064829] [PMID: 11721053]

Dhamodaran, K, Baidouri, H, Nartey, A, Staverosky, J, Keller, K, Acott, T, Vranka, JA & Raghunathan, VK (2022) Endogenous expression of Notch pathway molecules in human trabecular meshwork cells. *Exp Eye Res,* 216, 108935. [http://dx.doi.org/10.1016/j.exer.2022.108935] [PMID: 35033558]

Humphries, JD, Chastney, MR, Askari, JA & Humphries, MJ (2019) Signal transduction *via* integrin adhesion complexes. *Curr Opin Cell Biol,* 56, 14-21. [http://dx.doi.org/10.1016/j.ceb.2018.08.004] [PMID: 30195153]

Keller, KE, Bhattacharya, SK, Borrás, T, Brunner, TM, Chansangpetch, S, Clark, AF, Dismuke, WM, Du, Y,

Elliott, MH, Ethier, CR, Faralli, JA, Freddo, TF, Fuchshofer, R, Giovingo, M, Gong, H, Gonzalez, P, Huang, A, Johnstone, MA, Kaufman, PL, Kelley, MJ, Knepper, PA, Kopczynski, CC, Kuchtey, JG, Kuchtey, RW, Kuehn, MH, Lieberman, RL, Lin, SC, Liton, P, Liu, Y, Lütjen-Drecoll, E, Mao, W, Masis-Solano, M, McDonnell, F, McDowell, CM, Overby, DR, Pattabiraman, PP, Raghunathan, VK, Rao, PV, Rhee, DJ, Chowdhury, UR, Russell, P, Samples, JR, Schwartz, D, Stubbs, EB, Tamm, ER, Tan, JC, Toris, CB, Torrejon, KY, Vranka, JA, Wirtz, MK, Yorio, T, Zhang, J, Zode, GS, Fautsch, MP, Peters, DM, Acott, TS & Stamer, WD (2018) Consensus recommendations for trabecular meshwork cell isolation, characterization and culture. *Exp Eye Res,* 171, 164-73.
[http://dx.doi.org/10.1016/j.exer.2018.03.001] [PMID: 29526795]

Keung, AJ, Healy, KE, Kumar, S & Schaffer, DV (2010) Biophysics and dynamics of natural and engineered stem cell microenvironments. *Wiley Interdiscip Rev Syst Biol Med,* 2, 49-64.
[http://dx.doi.org/10.1002/wsbm.46] [PMID: 20836010]

Naba, A, Clauser, KR, Ding, H, Whittaker, CA, Carr, SA & Hynes, RO (2016) The extracellular matrix: Tools and insights for the "omics" era. *Matrix Biol,* 49, 10-24.
[http://dx.doi.org/10.1016/j.matbio.2015.06.003] [PMID: 26163349]

Naba, A, Clauser, K R, Hoersch, S, Liu, H, Carr, S A & Hynes, R O (2012) The matrisome: *in silico* definition and *in vivo* characterization by proteomics of normal and tumor extracellular matrices. *Mol Cell Proteomics,* 11, 014647.
[http://dx.doi.org/10.1074/mcp.M111.014647]

Nerger, BA, Jones, TM, Rose, KWJ, Barqué, A, Weinbaum, JS, Petrie, RJ, Chang, J, Vanhoutte, D, LaDuca, K, Hubmacher, D & Naba, A (2022) The matrix in focus: new directions in extracellular matrix research from the 2021 ASMB hybrid meeting. *Biol Open,* 11, bio059156.
[http://dx.doi.org/10.1242/bio.059156] [PMID: 34994383]

Raghunathan, VK, Benoit, J, Kasetti, R, Zode, G, Salemi, M, Phinney, BS, Keller, KE, Staverosky, JA, Murphy, CJ, Acott, T & Vranka, J (2018) Glaucomatous cell derived matrices differentially modulate non-glaucomatous trabecular meshwork cellular behavior. *Acta Biomater,* 71, 444-59.
[http://dx.doi.org/10.1016/j.actbio.2018.02.037] [PMID: 29524673]

Raghunathan, VK, Morgan, JT, Chang, YR, Weber, D, Phinney, B, Murphy, CJ & Russell, P (2015) Transforming Growth Factor Beta 3 Modifies Mechanics and Composition of Extracellular Matrix Deposited by Human Trabecular Meshwork Cells. *ACS Biomater Sci Eng,* 1, 110-8. a
[http://dx.doi.org/10.1021/ab500060r] [PMID: 30882039]

Raghunathan, VK, Morgan, JT, Park, SA, Weber, D, Phinney, BS, Murphy, CJ & Russell, P (2015) Dexamethasone Stiffens Trabecular Meshwork, Trabecular Meshwork Cells, and Matrix. *Invest Ophthalmol Vis Sci,* 56, 4447-59. b
[http://dx.doi.org/10.1167/iovs.15-16739] [PMID: 26193921]

Sart, S, Jeske, R, Chen, X, Ma, T & Li, Y (2020) Engineering Stem Cell-Derived Extracellular Matrices: Decellularization, Characterization, and Biological Function. *Tissue Eng Part B Rev,* 26, 402-22.
[http://dx.doi.org/10.1089/ten.teb.2019.0349] [PMID: 32220216]

Schwartz, MA (2010) Integrins and extracellular matrix in mechanotransduction. *Cold Spring Harb Perspect Biol,* 2, a005066.
[http://dx.doi.org/10.1101/cshperspect.a005066] [PMID: 21084386]

Elena Sima, L (2016) Extracellular Signals for Guiding Mesenchymal Stem Cells Osteogenic Fate. *Curr Stem Cell Res Ther,* 12, 139-44.
[http://dx.doi.org/10.2174/1574888X10666151026114411] [PMID: 26496887]

Stamer, WD & Acott, TS (2012) Current understanding of conventional outflow dysfunction in glaucoma. *Curr Opin Ophthalmol,* 23, 135-43.
[http://dx.doi.org/10.1097/ICU.0b013e32834ff23e] [PMID: 22262082]

Sun, Y, Chen, CS & Fu, J (2012) Forcing stem cells to behave: a biophysical perspective of the cellular microenvironment. *Annu Rev Biophys,* 41, 519-42.

[http://dx.doi.org/10.1146/annurev-biophys-042910-155306] [PMID: 22404680]

Taha, IN & Naba, A (2019) Exploring the extracellular matrix in health and disease using proteomics. *Essays Biochem,* 63, 417-32.
[http://dx.doi.org/10.1042/EBC20190001] [PMID: 31462529]

Trappmann, B, Gautrot, JE, Connelly, JT, Strange, DGT, Li, Y, Oyen, ML, Cohen Stuart, MA, Boehm, H, Li, B, Vogel, V, Spatz, JP, Watt, FM & Huck, WTS (2012) Extracellular-matrix tethering regulates stem-cell fate. *Nat Mater,* 11, 642-9.
[http://dx.doi.org/10.1038/nmat3339] [PMID: 22635042]

Tschumperlin, DJ, Liu, F & Tager, AM (2013) Biomechanical regulation of mesenchymal cell function. *Curr Opin Rheumatol,* 25, 92-100.
[http://dx.doi.org/10.1097/BOR.0b013e32835b13cd] [PMID: 23114589]

Urbanczyk, M, Layland, SL & Schenke-Layland, K (2020) The role of extracellular matrix in biomechanics and its impact on bioengineering of cells and 3D tissues. *Matrix Biol,* 85-86, 1-14.
[http://dx.doi.org/10.1016/j.matbio.2019.11.005] [PMID: 31805360]

Vining, KH & Mooney, DJ (2017) Mechanical forces direct stem cell behaviour in development and regeneration. *Nat Rev Mol Cell Biol,* 18, 728-42.
[http://dx.doi.org/10.1038/nrm.2017.108] [PMID: 29115301]

Vogel, V & Sheetz, MP (2009) Cell fate regulation by coupling mechanical cycles to biochemical signaling pathways. *Curr Opin Cell Biol,* 21, 38-46.
[http://dx.doi.org/10.1016/j.ceb.2009.01.002] [PMID: 19217273]

Vranka, JA, Kelley, MJ, Acott, TS & Keller, KE (2015) Extracellular matrix in the trabecular meshwork: Intraocular pressure regulation and dysregulation in glaucoma. *Exp Eye Res,* 133, 112-25.
[http://dx.doi.org/10.1016/j.exer.2014.07.014] [PMID: 25819459]

Wen, JH, Vincent, LG, Fuhrmann, A, Choi, YS, Hribar, KC, Taylor-Weiner, H, Chen, S & Engler, AJ (2014) Interplay of matrix stiffness and protein tethering in stem cell differentiation. *Nat Mater,* 13, 979-87.
[http://dx.doi.org/10.1038/nmat4051] [PMID: 25108614]

Wolfenson, H, Yang, B & Sheetz, MP (2019) Steps in Mechanotransduction Pathways that Control Cell Morphology. *Annu Rev Physiol,* 81, 585-605.
[http://dx.doi.org/10.1146/annurev-physiol-021317-121245] [PMID: 30403543]

Yemanyi, F, Baidouri, H, Burns, AR & Raghunathan, V (2020) Dexamethasone and Glucocorticoid-Induced Matrix Temporally Modulate Key Integrins, Caveolins, Contractility, and Stiffness in Human Trabecular Meshwork Cells. *Invest Ophthalmol Vis Sci,* 61, 16. a
[http://dx.doi.org/10.1167/iovs.61.13.16] [PMID: 33170205]

Yemanyi, F, Vranka, J & Raghunathan, VK (2020) Crosslinked Extracellular Matrix Stiffens Human Trabecular Meshwork Cells *Via* Dysregulating β-catenin and YAP/TAZ Signaling Pathways. *Invest Ophthalmol Vis Sci,* 61, 41. b
[http://dx.doi.org/10.1167/iovs.61.10.41] [PMID: 32832971]

Yemanyi, F, Vranka, JA & Raghunathan, V (2019) Cell derived matrices modulate TGFβ2 signaling in human trabecular meshwork cells. *Invest Ophthalmol Vis Sci,* 60, 5146-6.

Yemanyi, F, Vranka, JA & Raghunathan, V (2020) Crosslinked ECM modulates β-Catenin and YAP/TAZ pathways in human trabecular meshwork cells. *Invest Ophthalmol Vis Sci,* 61, 1434-4. c

Yemanyi, F, Vranka, J & Raghunathan, V (2020) Generating cell-derived matrices from human trabecular meshwork cell cultures for mechanistic studies. *Methods Cell Biol,* 156, 271-307. d
[http://dx.doi.org/10.1016/bs.mcb.2019.10.008] [PMID: 32222223]

CHAPTER 20

Protocol for Studying TM Cell Function in a 3-D Matrix

Karen Y. Torrejon[1,*], **Andrea M. Unser**[1] and **Pujhitha Ramesh**[1]

[1] *Colleges of Nanoscale Science and Engineering, SUNY Polytechnic Institute, 257 Fuller Road, Albany 12203, New York, USA*

Abstract: This chapter describes the protocols to bioengineer a 3D human trabecular meshwork tissue model using Glauconix Biosciences' patented 3D-HTM™ system. These protocols combine species-relevant tissue with nanoengineering techniques in order to produce a 3D matrix to mimic the conventional outflow pathway, which is responsible for the majority of the aqueous humor drainage and intraocular pressure regulation in the eye. Currently, there is a lack of translation between glaucoma in the human eye and animal models, which fails to provide a sufficient platform for compound screening and intraocular pressure (IOP) assessment. To address this unmet need, a 3D-HTM™, which can be co-cultured with human Schlemm's canal cells and induced to a glaucomatous-like state, was developed to provide a more applicable model for the evaluation of IOP-lowering therapeutics. The included protocols address the engineering of this 3D tissue model, as well as the examination of key biological markers of diseased tissue using traditional biological techniques with a few modifications. Additionally, a methodology for indirectly measuring IOP within the bioengineered 3D tissue is described. Overall, these protocols provide an *in vitro* alternative for studying glaucoma at the anterior segment, which can propel the development of glaucoma therapeutics.

Keywords: 3D tissue, Conventional outflow, Eye, Fibrosis, Glaucoma, Intraocular pressure, Ocular hypertension, Schlemm's canal cells, Trabecular meshwork.

INTRODUCTION

The study of the anterior chamber of the eye, as it relates to the understanding of glaucoma and fibrosis, prompted the development of relevant 3D human glaucomatous tissue models for physiological and species-relevant research. The human trabecular meshwork (HTM) plays a critical role in maintaining intraocular pressure (IOP) and contributes to the maintenance of vision (Lütjen-

* **Corresponding author Karen Y. Torrejon:** Colleges of Nanoscale Science and Engineering, SUNY Polytechnic Institute, 257 Fuller Road, Albany 12203, New York, USA; Tel: +631-559-2727; E-mail:ktorrejon@glauconix-biosciences.com

Najam A. Sharif and Sunny E. Ohia (Eds.)

Drecoll, 1999; Zhou, Li and Yue, 1999; Llobet, Gasull and Gual, 2003). It is a sieve-like filtering structure that regulates the flow of aqueous humor to maintain IOP (Llobet, Gasull and Gual, 2003; Abu-Hassan, Acott and Kelley, 2014). The HTM is comprised of distinctive regions: uveal meshwork, corneoscleral, juxtacanalicular, inner wall of Schlemm's canal, and Schlemm's canal (Lütjen-Drecoll, 1999; Zhou, Li and Yue, 1999; Llobet, Gasull and Gual, 2003). The region believed to provide the most resistance to aqueous humor and hence linked to the regulation of intraocular pressure is the Juxtanacanlicular region and the inner wall of the Schlemm's canal. This area is comprised of human trabecular meshwork cells sitting on a basement membrane and interacting with Schlemm canal cells (Llobet, Gasull and Gual, 2003; Abu-Hassan, Acott and Kelley, 2014). The critical role of each of these components of the trabecular meshwork has been discussed in chapter 2 of this book. Bioengineering this structure enables studying key HTM and Schlemm's canal markers that may lead to novel targets for the treatment of ocular hypertension. In this chapter, we detail protocols to enable the monoculture of HTM cells on a basement membrane-like structure, coculture with Schlemm's canal cells for a more physiologically relevant representation of the anterior region, and creation of a disease-like state to mimic fibrosis and glaucoma. Finally, we discuss methods to evaluate IOP *in vitro.*

EXPERIMENTAL PROTOCOLS

Preparation of the Basement Membrane-Like Scaffold for the Culture of HTM and Schlemm Canal Cells

- Porous SU8 scaffolds are fabricated using established photolithography techniques, as seen in Fig. (**1**) below.
- Aluminum tape rings are made using a Cricut machine to the desired diameter of interest. Scaffolds are affixed to the rings in the biosafety cabinet by gently picking up the scaffold with tweezers and placing it onto the sticky side of an aluminum ring (see Fig. **2** below).
- The mounted scaffolds are sterilized by using 70% ethanol and allowed to dry for at least 20 minutes, followed by UV exposure for 1 hour.
- The sterile scaffolds are gelatin-coated by allowing them to be in direct contact with 1% gelatin and air-dried for 20 minutes overnight in the biosafety cabinet. These scaffolds can then be placed in 24 well plates, covered with Parafilm™, and stored at 4 °C until ready for cell culture.

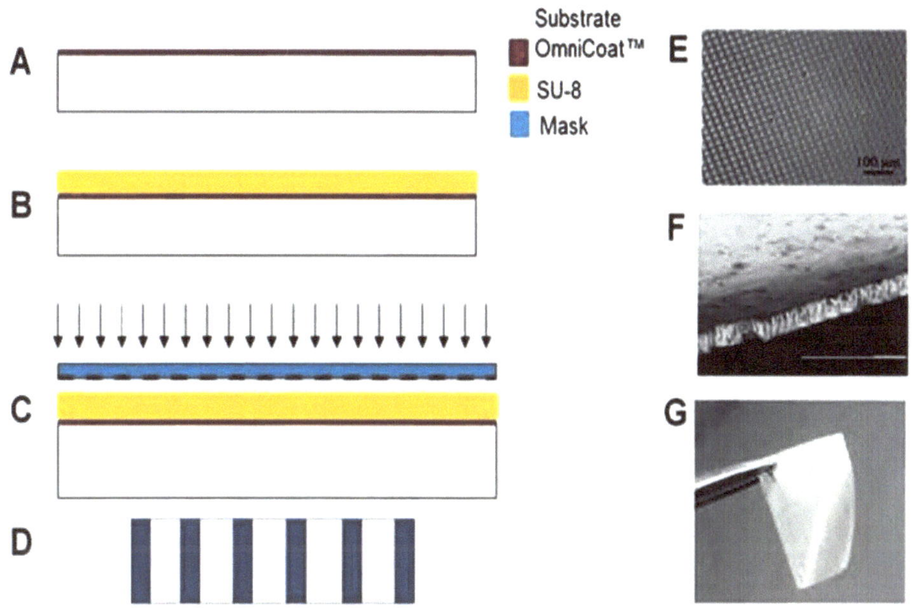

Fig. (1). Schematics of the fabrication of the micropatterned, porous SU-8 scaffold using photolithograpy. A: OmnicoatTM treatment on previously cleaned silica wafer for the release layer. B: SU-8 2010 coating. C: Exposure and post-exposure bake. D: Development. Representative scanning electron micrographs of top view (E) and cross-section (F), and optical image (G) of the freestanding scaffold. (E and F) Scale bar = 100 µm. (Torrejon *et al.*, 2013).

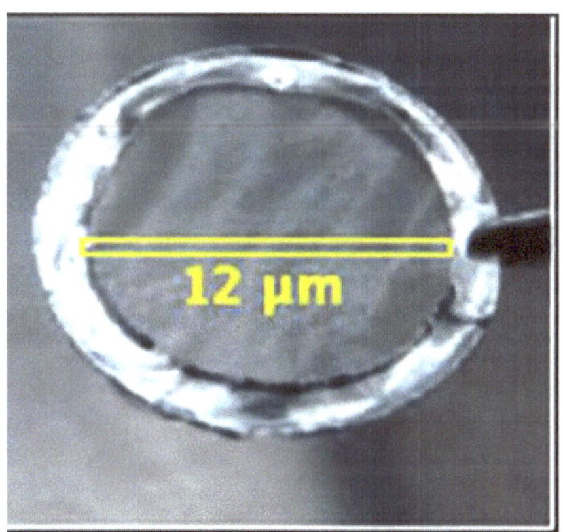

Fig. (2). Image of Glauconix Biosciences' patented SU-8 scaffold affixed to an aluminum ring. Diameter =12 µm.

Culture of Primary HTM Cells on Gelatin-coated SU8 Porous Scaffolds

- Primary HTM cells, isolated from the juxtacanalicular and corneoscleral regions of healthy human eyes, are plated in a T75 flask coated with 1% gelatin and supplemented with a 10% heat-inactivated FBS-IMEM medium. The medium is replaced every other day until the cell reaches confluency.

- When the primary HTM cells (up to passage 4) are confluent in the flask (see Fig. **3** below), the medium is removed and gently washed with sterile DPBS at room temperature.
- For a T75 flask, 3 mL of 0.25% cold trypsin EDTA are pipetted and placed into a 37 °C incubator for 7-10 minutes until cells are fully detached.
- Add 7 mL of pre-warmed 10% HI FBS-IMEM medium to the flask, and swirl and transfer it to a 15 mL conical tube. Repeat this step with 3 mL of medium to ensure all of the cells have been collected.
- Mix the entire cell suspension gently and thoroughly by pipetting and count the total number of cells in the suspension using traditional methods.
- Centrifuge the cell suspension at 1100 RPM for 7 minutes.
- Remove the supernatant and suspend the cells in pre-warmed 10% HI FBS-IMEM at a desired concentration. Seed 50,000 cells/150 µL per well.
- The samples are incubated at 37 °C undisturbed for two hours to facilitate attachment of the majority of the cells to the scaffold.
- Add 850 µL of media gently along the edges of the well. Incubate at 37 °C.
- Maintain in culture until confluent (anywhere from 5-10 days) with media changes every other day.

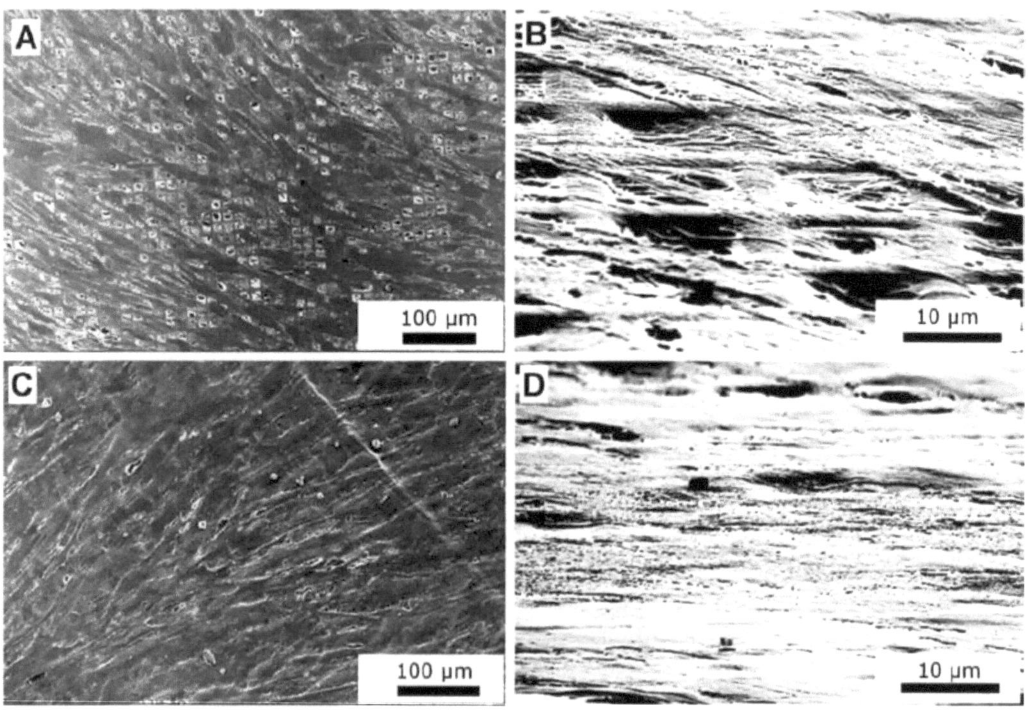

Fig. (3). SEM micrographs of HTM cells grown on su-8 scaffolds with a pore size of 12 um pore size for 7 days (A and B) and 14 days (C and D). (A) and (C) Scale bar = 100 µm.. (B) and (D) Scale bar = 10 µm. (Torrejon *et al.*, 2013).

Culture of Primary Human Schlemm's Canal Cells (HSCs) on Extracel® Coated SU8 Dcaffolds

Primary HSCs are isolated from the anterior chamber of human cadaveric eyes, as described previously by Stamer *et al.*, 1998. HSCs that are grown by themselves on scaffolds (not cocultured with HTM) need to be put on a surface with Extracel coating as determined by previous work (Fig. **4**) (Dautriche *et al.*, 2015).

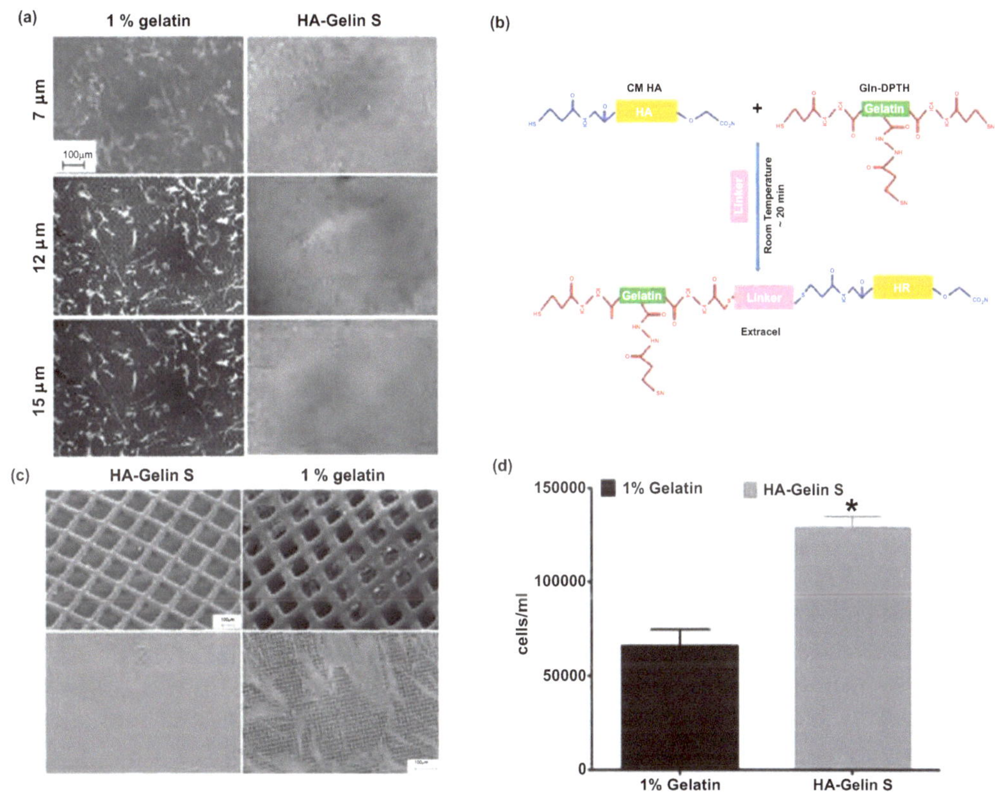

Fig. (4). Evaluation of human Schlemm's canal cell growth on well defined, microfabricated, porous SU-8 scaffolds. (a) Scanning electron microscopy (SEM) images showing that HSC cell growth on SU-8 scaffolds depended on the coating for biochemical signals and was independent of the pore size. Scale bar. 100 mm. (b) Schematic of the polymerization scheme for Extracel (HA-GelinS). (c) SEM images of SU-8 scaffolds (12-mm pores) coated with 1% gelatin or Extracel (ESU-8) (top panel). SEM images revealing establishment of a continuous HSC monolayer on the Extracel-coated SU-8 scaffold (bottom panel). Scale bar. 100 mm. (d) Live cell count demonstrating over 2-fold increase in HSC cell growth on ESU-8 scaffolds compared to gelatin-coated scaffolds. * (P 0.001, Extracel vs 1% gelatin) Mean ± SD with N-4. (Dautriche *et al.*, 2015).

Extracel (Hystem-c Hydrogel Kit) Coating Protocol

- Warm up 1 vial of gelin-s, 1 vial of degassed water, 1 vial of glycosil, and Extralink™ at 37 °C in the incubator for at least 30 mins.

- Using a syringe, add 1 mL of degassed water to the gelin-s vial. Swirl the vial to mix.
- Using a new syringe, add 1 mL of degassed water to the glycosil vial. Swirl the vial.
- Place both the glycosil and gelin-s back into the incubator for at least 20 mins. Do not vortex.
- Once ready to coat the scaffolds, add 0.5 mL of degassed water to the Extralink™ vial using a syringe. Swirl the vial to mix.
- Mix the following solutions together using their respective syringes and do not let the needle touch any of the liquid in the tube between mixings. Once completed, pipet up and down to mix well.
    a. 1 volume of gelin-s
    b. 1 volume of glycosil
    c. ½ volume of Extralink™
- Place half of the solution in a Petri dish and submerge both sides of the scaffold.
- Allow coated scaffolds to dry at room temperature for several minutes. Scaffolds should not dry while in direct contact with the Petri dish; instead, be sure that the scaffold dries while standing sideways and no part of the scaffold is touching the plate. For transwell-scaffold inserts, flip them upside down onto a Petri dish to dry.
- Once dry, place the scaffolds and transwell-scaffold inserts in the well plates and then seed cells on the scaffolds.

Coculture of HSC with HTM Cells

- After the HTM cells have become confluent, Schlemm's canal cells (HSCs) can be seeded on the other side of the scaffolds.
- When the primary human HSCs are confluent in the flask, remove the medium, gently wash the flask with sterile DPBS at room temperature, and immediately remove them.
- For a T75 flask, add 3 mL of 0.25% cold trypsin EDTA and place it into a 37 °C incubator for 7-10 minutes. After 10 minutes, inspect the cells under a brightfield microscope to ensure cells have detached. Trypsinize longer if needed.
- Add 7 mL of pre-warmed 10% pFBS-DMEM medium to the flask and pipet up and down to mix. Transfer this 7 mL to a 15 mL conical tube. Repeat this with 3 mL of medium to ensure that all of the cells have been removed for a total volume of 10 mL.
- Mix the entire cell suspension gently and thoroughly by pipetting. Count the cells using traditional cell-counting methods.
- Centrifuge the cells at 1100 RPM for 7 minutes.

- Remove the supernatant and resuspend the cells in pre-warmed 10% pFBS-DMEM at a desired concentration.
- Invert the scaffolds and seed the HSCs at 50,000 cells/150 µL/well on the inverted side of the scaffold.
- Incubate the samples at 37 °C undisturbed for two hours to facilitate attachment of the majority of the cells to the scaffold.
- Add 850 µL of media gently along the edges of the well. Incubate at 37 °C.
- Maintain in culture until confluent (~ 7-12 days) with media changes every other day (Fig. **5**).

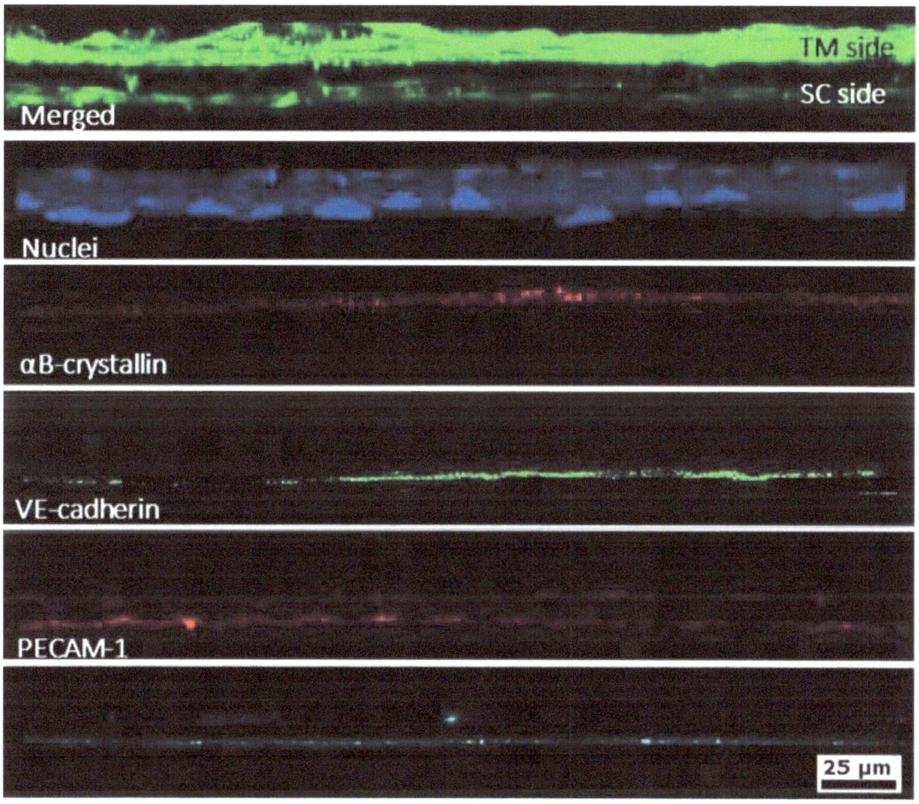

Fig. (5A). Confocal images of 3D HTM cocultured with HSC cells (side view). Images of phalloidin and DAPI staining (F-actin), immunocytochemistry of HTM marker alpha B crystallin, and HSC markers: VE-cadherin, PECAM-1 (CD31) and Fibulin-2.

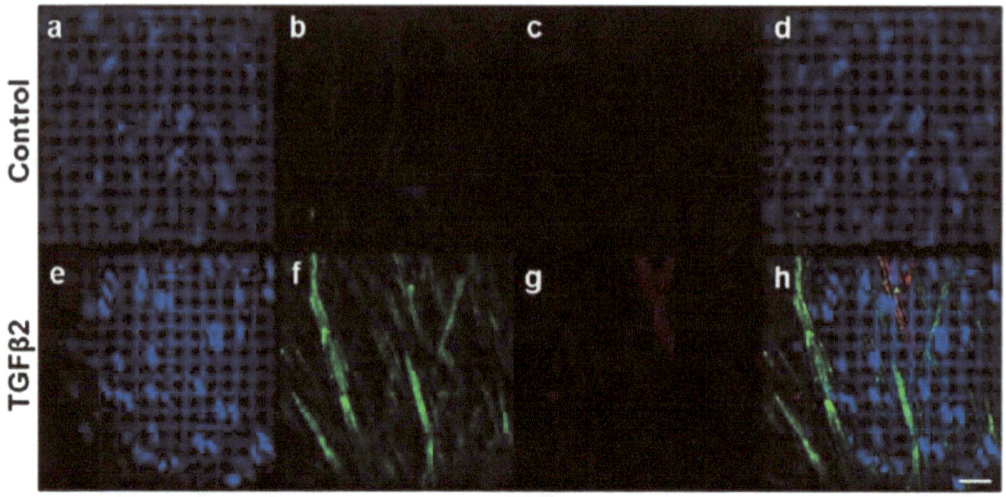

Fig. (5B). Confocal images of F-actin expression and a- SMA localization in 3D HTM cultures after TGFß2 treatment for 9 days. (a-d) Vehicle-treated controls. (e-h) TGFß 2 treatment. (a,e) DAPI-stained nuclei in blue. (b,f) Phalloidin-stained F-actin in green. (c,g) Immunocytochemistry of a -SMA in red. (d,h) Merged images. Scale bar = 30 μm. (Torrejon *et al.*, 2013).

Diseasing the Bioengineered 3D HTM and HTM/HSC Tissue

The 3D HTM and 3D HTM/HSC can be induced into a "glaucomatous state" (hypertensive) using either glucocorticoids (dexamethasone or prednisolone) or transforming growth factor-beta 2 (TGFβ2). Glucocorticoids have long been linked to primary open-angle glaucoma (POAG), given that in susceptible patients, they can induce ocular hypertension (Torrejon *et al.*, 2015). Similarly, TGFβ2 has been involved in the pathogenesis of certain glaucomas (Picht *et al.*, 2001); in fact, organ-culture perfusion studies have shown reduced outflow of cytokines, leading to an elevation in IOP (Gottanka *et al.*, 2004).

- Once the tissue is confluent, all medium is removed from the wells and is replaced with a 1% starvation medium (1% HI FBS in IMEM for HTM only and 1% pFBS in DMEM for HTM/HSC) and incubated at 37 °C overnight.
- The next day, the tissues are treated with the desired disease-causing agent of interest as well as its corresponding vehicle, with 500 μL treatment media per well in 24-well plates (see Table **1** below).
- Maintain in culture for 6-9 days with treatment media changes every 3 days and then assay for markers associated with a glaucomatous state including but not limited to an increase in α-smooth muscle actin (α-SMA), F-actin, myocilin, collagen IV, and fibronectin (see Figs. **5** and **6** below).

Table 1. Treatment of diesese-causing agent and their corresponding vehicle.

-	TGFβ	Dexamethasone	Prednisolne
Final Concentration	5ng/mL	250-500nM	300nM
Vehicle	Sterile 4mM HCl	Sterile DMSO	Ethanol or DMSO

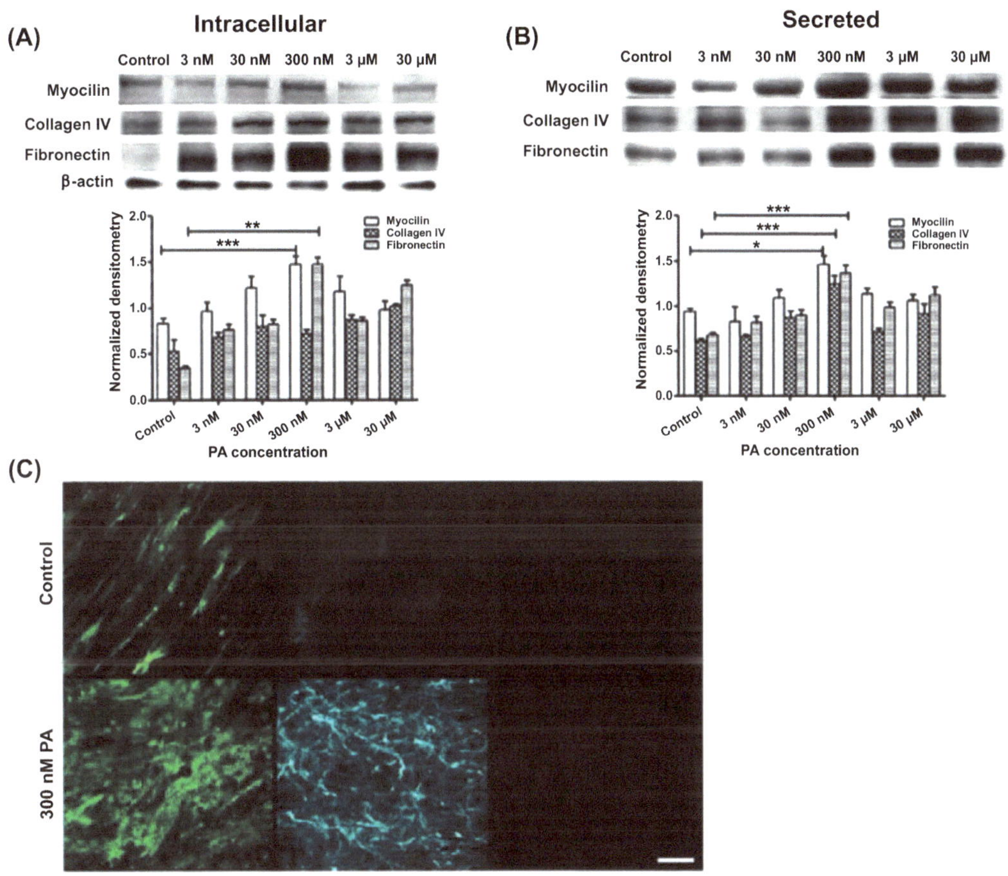

Fig. (6). Effects of glucocorticoid treatment on expression of myocilin and ECM proteins in 3D HTM cultures. Western blot analysis of dose-response to prednisolone acetate (PA) on (A) intracellular expression and (B) secretion of myocilin, collagen IV, and fibronectin. (C) Confocal images of immunocytochemistry of myocilin (left), collagen IV (middle) and fibronectin (right) in 3D HTM after perfusion with vehicle control (top panel) or 300nM PA (lower panel) for 9 days. Scale bar- 40 um. (Torrejon *et al.*, 2015).

Modified Protocols for Protein and Gene Analysis

- Immunocytochemistry (ICC): Protocols are followed as usual with the following difference in mounting the samples:
  - Clean up the glass slide and label the samples you will mount.
  - Carefully lift the scaffold out of wells by the aluminum ring with fine

forceps, and dip the sample in diH_2O.

- Remove the aluminum ring by holding one spot of the aluminum ring with forceps and then carefully take another pair of forceps, puncture an edge of the scaffold near the aluminum ring, and circle around the entire ring to release the scaffold.
- Place a drop of mounting media on the glass slide and a small coverslip, ensuring there are no bubbles. Carefully using tweezers, place the scaffold (cells facing up) on the drop of mounting media on a glass slide, then place the small coverslip with mounting media directly on the scaffold and push down lightly to get rid of any potential bubbles that could form.
- Store mounted samples in the dark overnight at room temperature so the mounting media can harden.
- The next day, paint the edges of the coverslip with clear nail polish and allow it to harden for 10 min, then place samples in the slide book and store at 4 °C or image.

- Western Blot/ELISA: Protocols followed as usual with the following difference in lysing the scaffolds are as follows:
    - Prepare the lysis buffer by combining RIPA buffer with 2% HALT protease-phosphatase inhibitor. Maintain on ice.
    - Remove media from all wells and wash with cold 1X-PBS; leave plate on ice.
    - Add 200 µL of lysis buffer to the first well of interest per condition, mix up and down 10 times, and repeat for all the scaffolds in the same sample/treatment set.
    - Ensure to remove bubbles and lysates from each well and collect them in a 1.5 mL labeled Eppendorf tube. Keep on ice.
    - Vortex each lysate for 10 seconds. Spin samples at maximum speed for 5 minutes and transfer the supernatant to new labeled tubes.
    - Store lysates at -80 °C.
- Quantitative Polymerase Chain Reaction (qPCR): Qiagen RNeasy Protocol is followed as described by the manufacturer, with the following difference in the RNA extraction step:
    - Remove media from all wells and rinse them with 1X-PBS.
    - Add 350 µl of Buffer RLT to the first well for each treatment group. Pipette up and down and move to the next well for the treatment group.
    - On the last well, use a 20G needle pipette up and down 5 times.
    - Add 350 µl 70% ethanol to the well and mix.
    - Add 700 µl of sample in the RNeasy spin column (pink tube) placed in a 2 mL collection tube (clear tube) and centrifuge for 30 seconds at 9000xg (RCF). Discard the flow through in the clear collection tube.
    - Add 700 µl buffer RW1 and centrifuge as in step 7.

- Add 500 µl buffer RPE and centrifuge as in step 7.
- Add 500 µl buffer RPE and centrifuge for 2 minutes at 9000 RCF.
- Move the RNeasy spin column into a clean 1.5 mL tubes and add 30 µl RNase-free water directly to the spin column. Centrifuge for 1 minute at 9000 RCF and put back on ice.
- Store extracted RNA at -80°C or keep it on ice and move onto quantitation.

Assaying Intraocular Pressure *In Vitro* (Hydraulic Conductivity)

The following procedure is to be followed when performing perfusion studies. All the assembly of samples is performed in the biosafety cabinet, and the perfusion is conducted in incubators kept at 34 °C. A schematic representation is shown in Fig. (**7**).

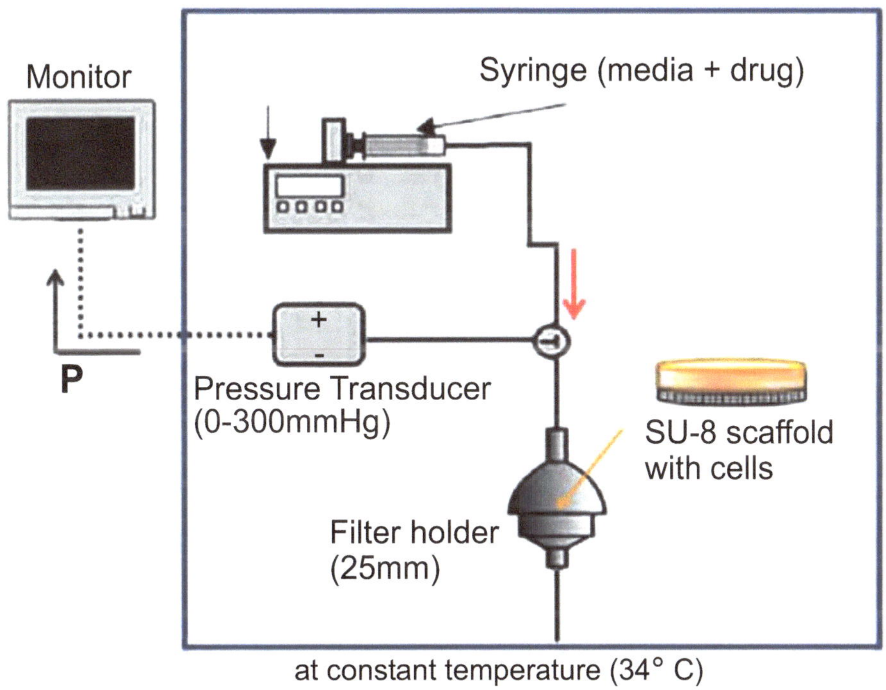

Fig. (7). Schematic of Glauconix Biosciences' perfusion system.

- Prepare perfusion medium and warm up in the incubator for at least 3 hrs.
- Thoroughly rinse sample holders, syringes, and clamps with 70% ethanol/30% water solution and place them in a biosafety cabinet. Assemble the sample holders using clamps.
- Thaw any treatments that need to be added to the perfusion media

- Place two (2) 50 mL tubes of the medium in the biosafety cabinet, but shake the tubes vigorously for 20 – 25 seconds outside the biosafety cabinet prior to use.
- Add the treatment group to the medium if needed and shake vigorously for 5 – 10 seconds.
- Prime 12 sample holders with medium.
- Place the perfusion samples (24-well plate) in the biosafety cabinet and place 6 samples on 6 of the sample holders, then return the 24-well plate to the incubator.
- Set up 6 perfusion samples, fill 6 syringes with perfusion media, and place the samples and syringes in the incubators.
- Place the perfusion samples (24-well plates) in the biosafety cabinet and place the next 6 samples onto 6 of the sample holders, then return the 24-well plate to the incubator.
- Set up the next 6 perfusion samples and 6 syringes with perfusion media and place the samples and tubes in the incubator.
- Fill 12 beakers up to the 200 mL mark with deionized water.
- Set up syringes and samples one incubator at a time.
- Set up the software and begin the perfusion experiment in all 3 incubators.
- Analyze data using the outflow facility (C) formula (change in the flow rate of fluid (f) divided by change in pressure (p))

$$C = \frac{f}{p}$$

CONCLUSION

The protocols described above have attempted to provide sufficient experimental details for the development of 3D conventional outflow tract tissues on micro-/nano-fabricated scaffolds and their applicability for glaucoma modeling. However, readers are encouraged to refer to the original publications where such methods are described. Additional literature searches may also be beneficial in order to find suitable modifications or refinements to the procedures described herein.

CONFLICT OF INTEREST STATEMENT

The authors declare the following financial interests/personal relationships: Drs. Torrejon, Unser, and Ramesh are employees of Glauconix, a company that developed this 3D tissue model. The authors have shared their knowledge on this technology in hopes that it may propel glaucoma research. The ultimate goal of this technology is to explore the mechanism of action of new and improved glaucoma therapies.

ACKNOWLEDGEMENTS

The authors would like to thank Dr. Feryan Ahmed, Dr. Vandhana Chari, and Hira Afzaal for their contribution to protocol development.

REFERENCES

Abu-Hassan, DW, Acott, TS & Kelley, MJ (2014) The Trabecular Meshwork: A Basic Review of Form and Function. *J Ocul Biol,* 2. http://fulltextarticles.avensonline.org/JOCB-2334-2838-02-0017.html [http://dx.doi.org/10.13188/2334-2838.1000017] [PMID: 25356439]

Dautriche, CN, Szymanski, D, Kerr, M, Torrejon, KY, Bergkvist, M, Xie, Y, Danias, J, Stamer, WD & Sharfstein, ST (2015) A biomimetic Schlemm's canal inner wall: A model to study outflow physiology, glaucoma pathology and high-throughput drug screening. *Biomaterials,* 65, 86-92. [http://dx.doi.org/10.1016/j.biomaterials.2015.06.034] [PMID: 26142779]

Gottanka, J, Chan, D, Eichhorn, M, Lütjen-Drecoll, E & Ethier, CR (2004) Effects of TGF-β2 in perfused human eyes. *Invest Ophthalmol Vis Sci,* 45, 153-8. [http://dx.doi.org/10.1167/iovs.03-0796] [PMID: 14691167]

Llobet, A, Gasull, X & Gual, A (2003) Understanding trabecular meshwork physiology: a key to the control of intraocular pressure? *Physiology (Bethesda),* 18, 205-9. [http://dx.doi.org/10.1152/nips.01443.2003] [PMID: 14500801]

Lütjen-Drecoll, E (1999) Functional morphology of the trabecular meshwork in primate eyes. *Prog Retin Eye Res,* 18, 91-119. [http://dx.doi.org/10.1016/S1350-9462(98)00011-1] [PMID: 9920500]

Picht, G, Welge-Luessen, U, Grehn, F & Lütjen-Drecoll, E (2001) Transforming growth factor β2 levels in the aqueous humor in different types of glaucoma and the relation to filtering bleb development. *Graefes Arch Clin Exp Ophthalmol,* 239, 199-207. [http://dx.doi.org/10.1007/s004170000252] [PMID: 11405069]

Stamer, WD, Roberts, BC, Howell, DN & Epstein, DL (1998) Isolation, culture, and characterization of endothelial cells from Schlemm's canal. *Invest Ophthalmol Vis Sci,* 39, 1804-12. [PMID: 9727403]

Torrejon, KY, Papke, EL, Halman, JR, Stolwijk, J, Dautriche, CN, Bergkvist, M, Danias, J, Sharfstein, ST & Xie, Y (2016) Bioengineered glaucomatous 3D human trabecular meshwork as an *in vitro* disease model. *Biotechnol Bioeng,* 113, 1357-68. [http://dx.doi.org/10.1002/bit.25899] [PMID: 26615056]

Zhou, L, Li, Y & Yue, BYJT (1999) Oxidative stress affects cytoskeletal structure and cell-matrix interactions in cells from an ocular tissue: The trabecular meshwork. *J Cell Physiol,* 180, 182-9. [http://dx.doi.org/10.1002/(SICI)1097-4652(199908)180:2<182::AID-JCP6>3.0.CO;2-X] [PMID: 10395288]

CHAPTER 21

Protocols for Studying Neurotransmitter Release from Isolated Ocular Tissues

Sunny E. Ohia[1,*], **Catherine A. Opere**[2], **Anthonia Okolie**[1], **Fatima Muili**[1], **Pratik Bhankele**[2] and **Ya Fatou Njie-Mbye**[1]

[1] *Department of Pharmaceutical Sciences, College of Pharmacy and Health Sciences, Texas Southern University, Houston, Texas, USA*

[2] *Department of Pharmacy Sciences, School of Pharmacy and Health Professions, Creighton University, Omaha, Nebraska, USA*

Abstract: Neurotransmitters mediate signals from nerve terminals to the postsynaptic receptors within central and peripheral nervous systems. The release of the transmitters depends on the action potential within the cognate nerves. Herein, protocols are described for measuring the release of neurotransmitters (such as norepinephrine) from isolated anterior uveal tissues (such as the iris/ciliary bodies), which influence the production and secretion of aqueous humor (AQH). The production and drainage of AQH and the ultimate volume within the anterior segment of the eye determine the intraocular pressure (IOP). Isolated neural retinal tissues can also be used to study neurotransmitter release under conditions where there is a need to assess the ability of compounds to offer neuroprotection in the eye. For instance, compounds that can prevent the release of glutamate from the retinal slices or whole tissue may prove to be neuroprotective by preventing neurodegeneration. The use of radiolabeled neurotransmitters to mimic the physiological actions of their endogenous counterparts and the release of the tritiated transmitter, for example, can be triggered using an electrical field stimulus, a potassium-depolarizing pulse, and hypoxia and glucose-deprivation, for instance, can emulate ischemic conditions *in vivo*. Protocols for measuring the release of radiolabeled norepinephrine and serotonin from iris/ciliary bodies of various species will be described in this chapter. Additionally, protocols for measuring radiolabeled D-aspartate release from the neural retina of these species will also be discussed.

Keywords: Ciliary body, Iris-ciliary body, Release mechanism, Retina, Transmitter.

[*] **Corresponding author Sunny E. Ohia:** Department of Pharmaceutical Sciences, College of Pharmacy and Health Sciences, Texas Southern University, Houston, Texas, USA; E-mail: Sunny.ohia@tsu.edu

Najam A. Sharif and Sunny E. Ohia (Eds.)

INTRODUCTION

Communication between nerves and effector cells is often mediated *via* neurotransmitters that are released by depolarization of the nerve terminal evoked by the arrival of action potentials in the peripheral and central nervous system (CNS). This process depends on the membrane potential at the nerve terminal and on the availability of stored neurotransmitters. Transmitter release parameters can be studied both *in vitro* and *in vivo,* and the effect of drugs and exogenous agents on such processes can be measured and quantified. A major focus of pharmacological studies using drugs that interfere with the release of neurotransmitters is their ability to alter the activity of presynaptic and/or postsynaptic receptors, thereby influencing the final biological response, whether it be hormone release, tissue contraction, or induction of sleep.

Presynaptic receptors act as a homeostatic control switch where they can either inhibit or enhance the release process. The depolarizing stimulus, whether electrical or chemical, may be employed continuously or intermittently, and the process of neurotransmitter release is measured in a super-fusion or a static system. The measurement of neurotransmitter release requires the rapid dissection of tissues from appropriate organs and immediate transfer to oxygenated buffer solutions. For the static system, it is important to gently agitate the incubation medium to enable adequate oxygenation and diffusion of endogenous materials/chemicals into the bathing medium. With the super-fusion system, flow rates of 0.25 to 2 ml/min are used to allow an adequately oxygenated and stable environment for the tissues. In order to enable adequate equilibration and stabilization of tissues under study in either of the static or super-fusion systems, it is highly recommended that tissues undergo a 20-60 minute preincubation at room temperature. The tissues should then be gently washed by a series of gentle centrifugation/filtration steps to remove endogenous transmitter substances before the actual experiments begin. In a static system, the measurement of neurotransmitter release is performed in test tubes or beakers. For the super-fusion system, a custom-made chamber to place the washed tissues is utilized with appropriate connections to a peristaltic pump using flexible tubing. Studies on the *in vitro* release of neurotransmitters from static and super-fusion systems have utilized the radiolabeled form of a transmitter of interest to enable their uptake and storage *via* selective and high-affinity carriers within the tissue nerve terminals or cells. Quantification of release of endogenous pools of neurotransmitters can be determined using selective and sensitive analytical tools such as high-pressure liquid chromatography (HPLC) or liquid chromatography with tandem mass spectrometry (LC-MS-MS).

OVERALL GENERAL EXPERIMENTAL PROCEDURES

Studies on neurotransmitter release from isolated ocular tissues involve the use of iris-ciliary bodies and/or the neural retina. All experiments using animals should be in accordance with the Statement for the Use of Animals in Ophthalmic and Vision Research from the Association for Research in Vision and Ophthalmology. Approval of protocol for the use of human tissue should be obtained from the Institutional Review Board prior to the acquisition and use of postmortem human eyes.

Experiments Using Electrical Stimulus to Induce the Release of Radiolabeled Neurotransmitters from Isolated Iris/Ciliary Bodies

Tissue Preparation

Eyeballs from freshly sacrificed cows, pigs, or rabbits should be kept on ice until ready for dissection. Human eyeballs should be obtained within 6-8 hours post-mortem and can be stored in sealed vials containing oxygenated Krebs buffer solution at 2-4°C for up to 12 hours. While the whole iris/ciliary bodies from rabbit, pig, and human eyes can be mounted in specially designed perfusion chambers for neurotransmitter release studies, iris/ciliary bodies from cows can be divided into 4 quadrants for ease of fit into the chambers. [^{3}H]- 5-hydroxytryptamine ([^{3}H]-5HT, 1.6 μM) and [^{3}H]-norepinephrine ([^{3}H]NE, 2.5 μCi/ml) can be used for neurotransmitter uptake and release studies using the iris/ciliary bodies.

Protocol for Measuring [^{3}H]NE release from Anterior Uveal Tissues

The procedures used in studies on [^{3}H]NE secretion from the iris/ciliary bodies have been previously described by several investigators (Ohia and Jumblatt, 1990; Ohia and Jumblatt, 1991; Salvi *et al.*, 2016). Briefly, freshly isolated bovine, porcine, rabbit, or human iris-ciliary bodies (ICB) are incubated with 4 ml of well-oxygenated Krebs buffer solution containing 0.1-1 μM [^{3}H]-NE at 37°C for 1 hour. The Krebs buffer solution is composed of (mM) NaCl 118, KCl 4.8, $CaCl_2$ 1.3, KH_2PO_4 1.2, $NaHCO_3$ 25, $MgSO_4$ 2.0, and dextrose 10 (pH 7.4). Ascorbic acid (56.7mM) is added to Kreb's buffer solution, and in some experiments, flurbiprofen (FBF 3 μM), a cyclooxygenase (COX) inhibitor, is added to the buffer to reduce the contribution of endogenously produced prostaglandins to the study. After this incubation, tissues are gently rinsed twice with fresh Krebs buffer for 5 minutes each, mounted between nylon mesh cloth, and placed in thermostatically controlled superfusion chambers (Warner Instrument Corp., CT). Tissues are then super-fused with oxygenated Krebs buffer solution at a rate of 2 ml/min, with effluent buffer being collected at 4-minute intervals.

Tissues are super-fused with the buffer for at least 1-2 hrs to set the baseline of the unstimulated release of the radiolabeled neurotransmitter. [^{3}H]-NE release is then electrically evoked using 300 d.c. electrical pulses (5 Hz, 2 msec pulse width, 12V/cm, 60 sec, supramaximal voltage), which are applied at 13 min (S_1) and 45/53 min (S_2) following the start of the super-fusion. Collected [^{3}H-NE--containing perfusate samples are then analyzed by liquid scintillation spectrometry. The electrically stimulated [^{3}H]-NE release is estimated by subtracting the extrapolated basal tritium efflux from the total tritium released in the 28-minute period after electrical stimulation. The basal tritium efflux is assumed to decline linearly between pre-stimulation and post-stimulation fractions. To examine the effect of test compounds on [^{3}H]-NE release, each agent should be applied 29 minutes after the onset of super-fusion. To determine the effect of receptor antagonists on the activity of test compounds, the antagonists should be added to the super-fusion buffer 20 minutes prior to S_1 and during S_2. Stimulation-evoked [^{3}H]-NE release during S_1 and S_2 is then graphically determined, and the ratio (S_2/S_1) is calculated and compared with those obtained for untreated controls.

Data Analysis

Results are expressed as the absolute S_2/S_1 ratios and/or as percentage inhibition of [^{3}H]-NE outflow relative to control conditions. The calculated IC_{50} value represents the concentration of a compound that causes 50% inhibition of the total field-stimulated [^{3}H]-NE release. Conversely, if the compounds further stimulate [^{3}H]-NE outflow, the concentration-response curves can be used to derive the concentration that produces 50% of the maximal stimulation (EC_{50}). Reproducibility of data should be confirmed by repeating the experiments in separate and fresh new ICB preparations, and the data must be pooled to derive the mean ± standard error of the mean (SEM) of the stimulatory or inhibitory parameters. Analysis of variance (ANOVA) followed by Tukey's post-test analysis can then be used to determine the statistical significance between different experimental conditions and for various agonists and antagonists, with p-values < 0.05 being statistically significant.

Protocol for Measuring [^{3}H]-5HT Release from Anterior Uveal Tissues

The procedures used for the studies on [^{3}H]-serotonin (5-hydroxytryptamine, 5-HT) release have been previously described in detail by Harris *et al.* (2001) and Kawasaki *et al.* (1989). Briefly, isolated ICB tissue should be incubated in well oxygenated Krebs buffer solution containing 1.6 μM [^{3}H]-5-HT, the monoamine oxidase inhibitor pargyline (10 μM), and the cyclooxygenase inhibitor flurbiprofen (3 μM) at 37°C. Following tissue loading with [^{3}H]-5-HT, the ICBs are thoroughly rinsed in excess fresh Krebs buffer to remove any adsorbed radioisotope on the surface of the tissues and then loaded into the super-fusion chambers as described above. Using fresh Krebs buffer containing clomipramine (10 μM), a 5-HT uptake inhibitor, ICBs can be perfused (2ml/min), and samples of the perfusates are collected every 4 mins. These samples can then be added to 12 ml of aqueous-accepting scintillation cocktail (Ecolume; ICN Radiochemicals, CA) and thoroughly mixed, and the $[^3H]$-5-HT can be ascertained on a β-radioactivity counter.

After an initial 1-3 hours of perfusion of tissues to establish a stable baseline of spontaneous tritium efflux, the release of $[^3H]$-5-HT should be elicited by consecutive trains of 300 d.c. pulses (5 Hz, 2 msec p.d., supramaximal voltage) delivered to platinum chamber electrodes using a Grass S48 stimulator. Stimulation-induced release can be determined by subtracting the extrapolated basal efflux from the total released $[^3H]$-5-HT during the 20-minute period following the stimulation. Basal (unstimulated) $[^3H]$-5-HT efflux is assumed to decrease linearly between pre-stimulation and post-stimulation. All tissues should receive two stimulations 30 minutes apart. Stimulation-induced $[^3H]$-5-HT release during S_1 and S_2 are determined graphically, and the ratio of the two peaks (S_2/S_1) should be calculated and compared with untreated control preparations. Data are analyzed as described above for $[^3H]$-NE release.

Studies on the Release of Radiolabeled Neurotransmitters from Isolated Neural Retina

$[^3H]$D-aspartate is taken up into pre-synaptic terminals of neurons that use glutamate as a neurotransmitter and has been validated as a useful biomarker of the glutamatergic activity or release from the retinae of many species (Lopez-Colome and Roberts,1987; Santos *et al.*,1996; Storm-Mathisen,1981).

Tissue Preparation

Enucleated eyeballs from freshly sacrificed animals obtained from local abattoirs for study should be kept on ice and brought to the laboratory. Donor human eyes should be acquired as soon as possible post-mortem and kept in a freshly prepared, ice-cold, well-oxygenated medium. Protocol approval for the use of human tissue should be obtained from an Institutional Review Board prior to the acquisition of human eyes, and all due precautions should be taken when handling human tissues. It is preferred that when conducting experiments on human retinae, the assays be conducted in a laminar flow hood where sterility and operations can be safely conducted. Even though whole retinae of pigs, rabbits, and humans can be mounted in specially designed perfusion chambers for $[^3H]$-neurotransmitter release studies, tissues from cows may be divided into 4 quadrants for ease of fit into the study chambers.

Protocol for Measuring Potassium-Depolarization-Induced Release of [^{3}H]D-Aspartate

The methodology employed for studies on [^{3}H]D-aspartate release is essentially the same as described by Lopez-Colome and Roberts (1987) in chick retina with some modifications by Opere *et al.* (2009) and Ohia *et al.* (2000). Freshly isolated neural retinae from different species should be placed in freshly prepared and well-oxygenated Krebs buffer, which contains 0.2 μM [^{3}H]D-aspartate and flurbiprofen (300 μM) at 37°C for 60 mins. After this pre-incubation, the retinal tissue should be placed in a small beaker containing room temperature Krebs buffer (25 mL) for 5 minutes to remove adsorbed radioisotope and then gently placed between nylon mesh cloths loaded into the super-fusion chambers. The retinae can now be super-fused (1.5 ml/min), and perfusate samples must be collected every 6 mins. The released radioisotope can be determined on a β-counter as described above. Now, [^{3}H]D-aspartate release should be determined by using 50 mM KCl as a stimulus applied at 80–88 minutes (S_1) and at 114–124 minutes (S_2) after the perfusion begins to set the baseline efflux. [^{3}H]D-aspartate secretion caused by the K^+-stimulus is then estimated by subtraction of the extrapolated basal [^{3}H]D-aspartate efflux from total [^{3}H]D-aspartate release during 20 minutes following the onset of the KCl challenge. In order to determine the effects of test drugs on K^+-stimulated [^{3}H]D-aspartate secretion, the retinae should be exposed to the test compound 12 minutes before S_2 (*i.e.*, 126 minutes after the start of super-fusion). Any inhibitor or antagonist to the receptor-activated [^{3}H]D-aspartate secretion should be added to the superfusion buffer at least 30 minutes prior to the S_1 phase (*i.e.*, 60 min after super-fusion) and during the S_2 phase. Then, the K^+-induced [^{3}H]D-aspartate release during S_1 and S_2 should be graphically determined. The comparative sizes of the peaks (S_2/S_1 ratios) should be ascertained and compared with the appropriate controls. The [^{3}H]D-aspartate is released into perfusates, and the data obtained from such studies is analyzed as described above.

Protocol for Measuring Hypoxia-Induced [^{3}H]D-Aspartate Release

For this section, the assays and data analysis used for studies on [^{3}H]D-aspartate release from retinae of different species are essentially performed as described above. The only difference is that Krebs buffer used during the K^+- or drug-induced [^{3}H]D-aspartate release should have been deprived of oxygen by pre-gassing the normal buffer with 95% N_2: 5% CO_2 for at least one hour (Hankins and Ikeda, 1993). Both K^+- and hypoxia-stimulated [^{3}H]D-aspartate release can be determined by subtracting the extrapolated basal [^{3}H]D-aspartate egress from total [^{3}H]D-aspartate secreted in the 24-minute period following the onset of stimulation. In these assays, the K^+ (50 mM, S_1)-induced release should be taken as a control response, and the drug effects must be measured relative to the latter. Once again, the addition of inhibitors or antagonists of the test compound effect should be perfused in the hypoxic buffer half an hour prior to the S_1 and be present during the S_2 phase.

Protocol for Measuring Glucose-Deprivation-Induced Release of [^{3}H]D-Aspartate

The procedures for conducting assays to determine the effect of glucose/dextrose-deprivation upon release of [^{3}H]D-aspartate from retinae of various species is essentially the same as described above except that the Krebs buffer perfused through the retinae during the course of the KCl- or drug stimulation lacks glucose or dextrose.

CONCLUSION

In conclusion, the use of isolated ocular tissues to study the release of various radiolabeled neurotransmitters is an effective technique to study the effects of various physiological and pathological conditions on tissue responses. Transmitter release from tissues from normal or ocular hypertensive animals may shed light on possible defects in transmitter uptake or release. Likewise, retinal neurotransmitter release studied under aglycemic, hypoxic, or neurotrophic factor withdrawal may provide insights into and possible linkage to glaucomatous optic neuropathy disease. As discussed above, the use of an appropriate stimulus (electrical, depolarizing agent, hypoxia, glucose deprivation, *etc.*) is critical for the successful execution of experiments using the aforementioned techniques. The additional benefit of utilizing [^{3}H]-neurotransmitter release as a biomarker is the ability to evaluate selective agonists and antagonists to pharmacologically define the presence or malfunction of active receptors and their sub-types involved in the transmitter release process (Ohia and Jumblatt, 1990; Ohia *et al.*, 2000; Harris *et al.*, 2001; Salvi *et al.*, 2016)

REFERENCES

Harris, LC, Awe, SO, Opere, CA, LeDay, AM, Ohia, SE & Sharif, NA (2001) [(^{3})H]-serotonin release from bovine iris-ciliary body: pharmacology of prejunctional serotonin (5-HT(7)) autoreceptors. *Exp Eye Res,* 73, 59-67.
[http://dx.doi.org/10.1006/exer.2001.1012] [PMID: 11428863]

Kawasaki, H, Urabe, M & Takasaki, K (1989) Presynaptic α2-adrenoceptor modulation of 5-hydroxytryptamine and noradrenaline release from vascular adrenergic nerves. *Eur J Pharmacol,* 164, 35-43.
[http://dx.doi.org/10.1016/0014-2999(89)90228-8] [PMID: 2546786]

López-Colomé, AM & Roberts, PJ (1987) Effect of excitatory amino acid analogues on the release of

D-[^{3}H]aspartate from chick retina. *Eur J Pharmacol,* 142, 409-17.
[http://dx.doi.org/10.1016/0014-2999(87)90080-X] [PMID: 3428354]

Ohia, SE & Jumblatt, JE (1990) Prejunctional inhibitory effects of prostanoids on sympathetic neurotransmission in the rabbit iris-ciliary body. *J Pharmacol Exp Ther,* 255, 11-6.
[PMID: 2170622]

Ohia, SE & Jumblatt, JE (1991) Prejunctional prostaglandin receptors in the human iris-ciliary body. *Curr Eye Res,* 10, 967-75.
[http://dx.doi.org/10.3109/02713689109020333] [PMID: 1659973]

Ohia, SE, Opere, CA, Awe, SO, Adams, L & Sharif, NA (2000) Human, bovine, and rabbit retinal glutamate-induced [^{3}H]D-aspartate release: role in excitotoxicity. *Neurochem Res,* 25, 853-60.
[http://dx.doi.org/10.1023/A:1007525725996] [PMID: 10944004]

Opere, CA, Monjok, EM, Kulkarni, KH, Njie, YF & Ohia, SE (2009) Regulation of [^{3}H] D-aspartate release from mammalian isolated retinae by hydrogen sulfide. *Neurochem Res,* 34, 1962-8.
[http://dx.doi.org/10.1007/s11064-009-9984-x] [PMID: 19760175]

Salvi, A, Bankhele, P, Jamil, JM, Kulkarni-Chitnis, M, Njie-Mbye, YF, Ohia, SE & Opere, CA (2016) Pharmacological actions of hydrogen sulfide donors on sympathetic neurotransmission in the bovine anterior uvea, *in vitro*. *Neurochem Res,* 41, 1020-8.
[http://dx.doi.org/10.1007/s11064-015-1784-x] [PMID: 26700431]

Santos, PF, Duarte, CB & Carvalho, AP (1996) Glutamate receptor agonists evoked Ca2+-dependent and Ca2+-independent release of [3H]d-Aspartate from cultured chick retina cells. *Neurochem Res,* 21, 361-8.
[http://dx.doi.org/10.1007/BF02531653] [PMID: 9139243]

Storm-Mathisen, J & Ottersen, OP (1987) Tracing of neurons with glutamate or γ -aminobutyrate as putative transmitters. *Biochem Soc Trans,* 15, 210-3.
[http://dx.doi.org/10.1042/bst0150210] [PMID: 2884148]

CHAPTER 22

Protocols for Studying Contraction/Relaxation of Ocular Tissues *In Vitro*

Kalu K. Ngele[1], **Sunny E. Ohia**[1], **Catherine A. Opere**[2], **Anthonia Okolie**[1], **Fatima Muili**[1], **Pratik Bhankele**[1] and **Ya Fatou Njie-Mbye**[1,*]

[1] *Department of Pharmaceutical Sciences, College of Pharmacy and Health Sciences, Texas Southern University, Houston, Texas, USA*

[2] *Department of Pharmacy Sciences, School of Pharmacy and Health Professions, Creighton University, Omaha, Nebraska, USA*

Abstract: Tissues isolated from organs have been extensively used in pharmacology or toxicology to study the effects of chemicals and drugs. A major advantage of using isolated tissues (instead of studying responses *in vivo*) is the exclusion of connective tissues, hormonal influences, or homeostatic mechanisms that may interfere with responses expected of the tissue under experimentation. The use of isolated tissues from the eye for physiological/pharmacological studies can yield significant amounts of information that is pertinent to the identification of new pathways or processes. Indeed, the ability to use various isolated ocular smooth muscles (iris, ciliary, vascular), skeletal muscle (rectus), and the TM to study contractions/relaxations to a wide range of drugs and chemicals provides a unique opportunity to identify potential new drugs for the treatment of diseases of the anterior segment such as glaucoma.

Keywords: Connective tissues, Glaucoma, Homeostatic mechanisms, Hormonal influences, Ocular smooth muscles, Ocular tissues, Skeletal muscles.

INTRODUCTION

Tissues isolated from organs have been extensively used in pharmacology or toxicology to study the effects of chemicals and drugs. A major advantage of using isolated tissues (instead of studying responses *in vivo*) is the exclusion of connective tissues, hormonal influences, or homeostatic mechanisms that may interfere with responses expected of the tissue under experimentation. In the eye, muscles (smooth and striated) have been isolated for use in studying the responses to chemicals or drugs. Strips of the trabecular meshwork have also been used for the measurement of contractile responses initiated by the activation of pharmacological receptors. Both contraction and relaxation of ocular tissues can be assessed using transducers that can detect changes in isometric tension developed or changes in the length of tissues in response to force (isotonic ten-

* **Corresponding author Ya Fatou Njie-Mbye:** Department of Pharmaceutical Sciences, College of Pharmacy and Health Sciences, Texas Southern University, Houston, Texas, USA; E-mail: YaFatou.Mbye@tsu.edu

Najam A. Sharif and Sunny E. Ohia (Eds.)

sion). Isolated ocular tissues should be placed immediately in a physiological salt solution with a composition that closely mimics the internal environment. For instance, Krebs buffer solution is used for most isolated smooth muscle preparations, while Ringer's solution is used for isolated trabecular meshwork strips. Typically, isolated tissues placed in physiological salt solutions should be maintained at a temperature that closely mimics the internal one (depending on the tissue) and gassed with appropriate gas (such as oxygen, carbon dioxide, or air). When used under the appropriate conditions, isolated ocular tissues can remain viable for more than six hours.

GENERAL EXPERIMENTAL PROTOCOLS

Experiments using isolated ocular tissues such as iris/ciliary muscles, trabecular meshwork, and blood vessels from rabbits, pigs, cows, and humans can be performed using specialized tissue/organ baths. After procurement from the slaughterhouse or Eye Banks, the eyeballs should be transported to the laboratory on ice. Careful dissection of tissues should lead to the isolation of the iris/ciliary muscles, trabecular meshwork, and blood vessels from an eyeball. All experiments using animals should be in accordance with the Statement for the Use of Animals in Ophthalmic and Vision Research from the Association for Research in Vision and Ophthalmology. Approval of protocol for the use of human tissue should be obtained from the Institutional Review Board prior to the acquisition of human eyes.

MEASUREMENT OF CONTRACTION/RELAXATION OF ISOLATED OCULAR SMOOTH MUSCLES

Tissue Preparation

Eyeballs from freshly sacrificed cows, pigs, or rabbits are transported to the laboratory on ice. When used, human eyeballs should be procured within six hours post-mortem and can be stored in sealed vials containing oxygenated Krebs buffer solution at 2°C for up to 12 hours. Approval of protocol for the use of human tissue should be obtained from the Institutional Review Board prior to the acquisition of human eyes. The iris smooth muscle/ciliary muscle can be dissected out of eyeballs from different species; whole irises/ciliary muscles from pigs, humans, or rabbits can be used, while each whole irise from cows can be cut into half for experiments. All dissected tissues should be placed in Krebs buffer solution in preparation for the experiment.

Protocol for Measuring Contraction/Relaxation of Iris/Ciliary Smooth Muscles

The methodology used for studies on the contraction/relaxation of isolated iris of pigs and ciliary muscle of cows are described by us and other investigators (Ohia *et al.*, 2010; Romano and Lograno, 2013; Ohia *et al.*, 2018.). For pigs, whole irises are isolated, placed in a Krebs buffer solution, and prepared for contraction/relaxation studies. For cows, ciliary muscle from each eyeball is quickly dissected under a binocular microscope, and 4-5 mm length is placed in Krebs buffer solution, which is then prepared for contraction/relaxation studies. After the setup of tissues in a thermostatically maintained (37°C) organ bath containing oxygenated (95% O_2: 5% CO_2) Krebs solution (pH 7.4). The Krebs solution should have the following composition (mM): potassium chloride, 4.8; sodium chloride, 118; calcium chloride, 2.3; potassium dihydrogen phosphate, 1.2; sodium bicarbonate, 25; magnesium sulfate, 2.0; and dextrose, 10. The muscle preparation in the organ bath is then connected to a force-displacement transducer (Ugo Basile, Stoelting Co., Wood Dale, IL 60191, USA) under resting tensions of 150 mg (for porcine tissues) and 300 mg (for bovine tissues). The tissues are then allowed to equilibrate in the oxygenated Kreb buffer solution in the organ bath for 60 minutes (with bath fluid replaced every 15 minutes). Changes in isometric tension of the tissues are captured using the computer software Digital Recorder DataCapsule-Evo, Stoelting Co., Wood Dale, IL 60191, USA). Before the addition of any drug, all muscle strips should be given a submaximal concentration of the muscarinic receptor agonist, carbachol, to check for the functionality of the tissues. After equilibration, contraction of the muscles can be elicited using different concentrations of muscarinic receptor agonists such as carbachol. To study the relaxant response of tissues, tone can be induced with a contractile agent that can maintain sustained tone (*e.g.*, carbachol), enabling the study of responses of different concentrations of an inhibitory agent (*e.g.*, β-adrenoceptor agonist such as isoproterenol) on the induced tone. For pharmacological studies, both contractile concentration-response and relaxant concentration-response curves can bc constructed in this system. After analysis of the data obtained under control and test conditions, relevant pharmacological information (such as the EC_{50} or IC_{50} values) can be obtained.

MEASUREMENT OF CONTRACTION/RELAXATION OF ISOLATED OCULAR VASCULAR SMOOTH MUSCLES

Tissue Preparation

Posterior ciliary arteries can be dissected from cows, rabbits, and human eyeballs (Kulkarni-Chitnis *et al.*, 2015; Chuman *et al.*, 2017.). For all species, the entire globe with an attached optic nerve is needed for the isolation of the posterior ciliary arteries (PCA). Rings of 1-2 mm in length of PCAs are dissected and immediately placed in oxygenated (95% O2; 5% CO2) Krebs buffer solution maintained at 37oC (pH 7.4). The Krebs solution should have the following composition (mM): potassium chloride, 4.8; sodium chloride, 118; calcium chloride, 2.3; potassium dihydrogen phosphate, 1.2; sodium bicarbonate, 25; magnesium sulfate, 2.0; and dextrose, 10.

Protocol for Measuring The Contraction/Relaxation of Isolated Posterior Ciliary Arteries

The protocol for measuring the contraction/relaxation of PCAs from cows, rabbits, and humans is essentially the same as described by us (Kulkarni-Chitnis *et al*., 2015) and others (Chuman *et al*., 2017.). For cows, PCA rings (2 mm long) are prepared for contraction/relaxation studies using 25 ml organ baths containing oxygenated Krebs solution (pH 7.4) at 37oC. The rings are mounted on two tungsten wires (with one immobilized and the other connected to a force-displacement transducer, Ugo Basile, Stoelting Co., Wood Dale, IL 60191, USA) for measurement of isometric tension using the computer software Digital Recorder DataCapsule-Evo, Stoelting Co., Wood Dale, IL 60191, USA). Due to the small size of PCAs in humans and rabbits, a wire myograph system can be used for measuring isometric tension (Puckrin Z, 2023. In Drug Discovery. https://www.reprocell.com/blog/biopta/myograph). For cows, each PCA preparation is mechanically stretched to achieve a basal tension of 5.0 g and then allowed to equilibrate for 60 mins before the start of the experiment. After equilibration, contractile responses can be obtained to an α-adrenoceptor agonist such as phenylephrine or to high potassium (30 – 50 mM, iso-osmotic solutions). A cumulative concentration-response curve is an experimental protocol suitable for use with isolated PCAs since increasing concentrations of compounds can be added to the organ bath or myograph system without washes between the addition of each compound. It allows the potency and magnitude of responses to be readily observed and for the calculation of useful pharmacological parameters such as the EC_{50} value. For measuring the relaxation of PCAs, compounds can be tested on basal tone or in the presence of induced tone using a contractile agent. After the attainment of a stable induced tone (using a concentration of the contractile agent producing about 70% of the maximum response of the tissue under study), a cumulative concentration-response curve can be constructed using an increasing concentration of a relaxant compound such as isoproterenol. Under this experimental condition, pharmacological parameters such as potency (assessed as IC_{50}) or the magnitude of the relaxation can be assessed.

MEASUREMENT OF CONTRACTION/RELAXATION OF THE ISOLATED TRABECULAR MESHWORK

Tissue Preparation

Isolated strips of the trabecular meshwork (TM) from cow eyeballs can be used to study the effect of pharmacological agents on the contraction/relaxation of this tissue. Freshly isolated cow eyeballs are bisected 10 mm behind the limbus. The anterior chamber disc, including the whole ciliary body, is dissected, and the corneal epithelial side is placed downward. The iris is carefully removed leaving only the TM and ciliary muscle remaining on the corneal-scleral segment, distinguishable by structure and pigmentation. Two vertical incisions are then made in a circular direction, one in the black pigmented anterior meshwork and the other 0.5 mm anterior to the ciliary muscle insertion. Both circular cuts and the resulting TM strip are oriented parallel to the corneal insertion of the pectinate ligament. The tissue strip between these cuts is approximately 0.5 mm wide and 4 mm long and show the typical Velcro-like structure of the TM. The strip should be removed from the sclera with cuts made carefully in a circular strip and placed in a modified Ringer's buffer solution gassed with 5% CO_2 in air at 37°C (pH 7.4). The Ringers buffer solution should have the following composition (mM): Na^+, 151; K^+, 5; $Ca^{2+,}$ 1.7; Mg^{2+}, 0.9; Cl^-, 131; SO_4^{2-}, 0.9; $HCO3^-$, 28; H_2PO^{4-}, 1; and glucose 5.

Protocol for Measuring the Contraction/Relaxation of Isolated Trabecular Meshwork Strips

The methodology for setting up and measuring contractions/relaxations of isolated strips of TM is similar to that described by Lepple-Wienhues *et al.* (1991) and Thieme *et al.* (2006). Isolated TM strips 2-4 mm long should be mounted in a perfusion chamber containing aerated (5% CO2 in air) Ringer's buffer solution thermostatically maintained at 37°C for at least one hour. Tension developed in the TM strips is measured using an isotonic force-length transducer (Ugo Basile, Stoelting Co., Wood Dale, IL 60191, USA) with data captured by a computer software Digital Recorder DataCapsule-Evo, Stoelting Co., Wood Dale, IL 60191. Only TM strips showing a stable baseline contractile tone should be used for experiments. For pharmacological contractile studies in TM strips, drugs such as carbachol (muscarinic receptor agonist) can be used to elicit responses to individual or cumulative concentrations when added to the perfusion chamber. TM strips can also contract in the presence of high K^+ (120 mM iso-osmotic solutions), a response that can be blocked by the muscarinic receptor antagonist atropine. Both contractile and relaxant responses to TM strips can be assessed for the determination of pharmacological parameters such as potency (EC_{50} or IC_{50} values) or efficacy (magnitude of responses elicited in the tissue).

MEASUREMENT OF CONTRACTION/RELAXATION OF ISOLATED EXTRAOCULAR RECTUS MUSCLES

Tissue Preparation

Isolated extraocular rectus muscles of rabbits can be employed to investigate the pharmacological actions of drugs on this tissue. The dissection of eyeballs from the orbit of rabbits should be performed carefully to ensure the preservation of both superior and inferior rectus muscles. A suture is tied to the tendon of each muscle, and the tendon is cut at its insertion. The muscle is then freed from connective tissues and cut as far back towards the origin as possible by means of curved enucleation scissors. The dissected muscles are immediately placed in oxygenated (95% O_2; 5% CO_2) Krebs buffer solution maintained at 30°C (pH 7.4). The Krebs solution should have the following composition (mM): potassium chloride, 4.8; sodium chloride, 118; calcium chloride, 2.3; potassium dihydrogen phosphate, 1.2; sodium bicarbonate, 25; magnesium sulfate, 2.0; and dextrose, 10.

Protocol for measuring the contraction/relaxation of isolated extraocular rectus muscles

The methodology for measuring the contraction/relaxation of isolated extraocular rectus muscles is described by Van Pinxteren and Van Alphen (1985). Strips of isolated rectus muscles are set up in a 25 ml thermostatically maintained (30°C) organ bath containing Krebs buffer solution gassed with 95% O_2:5% CO_2 under a resting tension of 150 mg. Isometric tension developed by the muscles is measured *via* a force-displacement transducer (Ugo Basile, Stoelting Co., Wood Dale, IL 60191) with data captured by a computer software Digital Recorder DataCapsule-Evo, Stoelting Co., Wood Dale, IL 60191. After 60 mins of equilibration, tissues can be exposed to contractile agents such as muscarinic receptor agonist, acetylcholine, or the inhibitor of acetylcholinesterase, physostigmine. Contractile responses can also be obtained with adrenoceptor agonists but only in the presence of acetylcholine and physostigmine (Van Pinxteren and Van Alphen, 1985). Both contractile and relaxant responses of rectus muscles can be assessed for determination of pharmacological parameters such as potency (EC_{50} or IC_{50} values) or efficacy (magnitude of responses elicited in the tissue).

CONCLUSION

The use of isolated tissues from the eye for physiological/pharmacological studies can yield significant amounts of information that is pertinent to the identification of new therapeutic entities. Indeed, the ability to use various isolated ocular smooth muscles (iris, ciliary, vascular), skeletal muscle (rectus), and the TM to study contractions/relaxations to a wide range of drugs and chemicals provides a unique opportunity to identify potential new drugs for the treatment of diseases of the anterior segment such as ocular hypertension and glaucoma.

REFERENCES

Chuman, H, Sugimoto, T & Nao-I, N (2017) Vasodilatory effect of L-arginine on isolated rabbit and human posterior ciliary arteries *in vitro* and increased optic disc blood flow *in vivo*. *Graefes Arch Clin Exp Ophthalmol,* 255, 2381-8.
[http://dx.doi.org/10.1007/s00417-017-3824-5] [PMID: 29063193]

Kulkarni-Chitnis, M, Njie-Mbye, YF, Mitchell, L, Robinson, J, Whiteman, M, Wood, ME, Opere, CA & Ohia, SE (2015) Inhibitory action of novel hydrogen sulfide donors on bovine isolated posterior ciliary arteries. *Exp Eye Res,* 134, 73-9.
[http://dx.doi.org/10.1016/j.exer.2015.04.001] [PMID: 25845295]

Lepple-Wienhues, A, Stahl, F & Wiederholt, M (1991) Differential smooth muscle-like contractile properties of trabecular meshwork and ciliary muscle. *Exp Eye Res,* 53, 33-8.
[http://dx.doi.org/10.1016/0014-4835(91)90141-Z] [PMID: 1679018]

Ohia, SE, Opere, CA, Monjok, EM, Kouamou, G, Leday, AM & Njie-Mbye, YF (2010) Role of hydrogen sulfide production in inhibitory action of L-cysteine on isolated porcine irides. *Curr Eye Res,* 35, 402-7.
[http://dx.doi.org/10.3109/02713680903576716] [PMID: 20450253]

Ohia, SE, Njie-Mbye, YF, Robinson, J, Mitchell, L, Mckoy, M, Opere, CA & Sharif, NA (2018) Serotonin-2B/2C receptors mediate bovine ciliary muscle contraction: Role in intraocular pressure regulation. *J Ocul Pharmacol Ther,* 34, 70-5.
[http://dx.doi.org/10.1089/jop.2017.0123] [PMID: 29364761]

Puckrin, Z (2023) https://www.reprocell.com/blog/biopta/myograph

Romano, MR & Lograno, MD (2013) Signaling cross-talk between cannabinoid and muscarinic systems actives Rho-kinase and increases the contractile responses of the bovine ciliary muscle. *Eur J Pharmacol,* 702, 174-9.
[http://dx.doi.org/10.1016/j.ejphar.2013.01.053] [PMID: 23396229]

Thieme, H, Schimmat, C, Mu¨nzer, G, Boxberger, M, Fromm, M, Pfeiffer, N & Rosenthal, R (2006) Endothelin antagonism: effects of FP receptor agonists prostaglandin F2α and fluprostenol on trabecular meshwork contractility. *Invest Ophthalmol Vis Sci,* 47, 938-45.
[http://dx.doi.org/10.1167/iovs.05-0527] [PMID: 16505027]

Pinxteren, PCM & Alphen, GWHM (1985) Extraocular rectus muscles of the rabbit contain α_2 -and β_2 -adrenergic receptors. *Curr Eye Res,* 4, 989-94.
[http://dx.doi.org/10.3109/02713689509000006] [PMID: 2866066]

CHAPTER 23

Protocol for Studying Aqueous Outflow Facility from Anterior Eye Segments *In Vitro* as an Organ Culture Procedure

Najam A. Sharif[1,*] and **Saima Chaudhry**[2]

[1] *Vice President and Head of Research & Development Nanoscope Therapeutics Inc., 2777 N. Stemmons Fwy, Suite 1102, Dallas, TX-75207, USA*

[2] *Univ N. Texas at Arlington, 701 S Nedderman Dr, Arlington, TX-76019, USA*

Abstract: Open-angle glaucoma is a neurodegenerative eye disease that is associated with elevated intraocular pressure (IOP) and affects millions of people worldwide. Since the raised IOP is the only risk factor that can be treated, much effort is being expended in finding novel ways to promote the efflux of aqueous humor (AQH) from the anterior chamber (ANC) of the eye. This is important for lowering and controlling IOP in order to prevent the loss of retinal ganglion cells and their axons, thereby slowing down vision loss. Even though several animal models have been developed to study the efficacy of new compounds to reduce ocular hypertension (OHT), such studies are labor-intensive and expensive. An in vitro model to permit similar kinds of investigations has been created using ANC segments of animal and human postmortem eyes. This system capitulates the *in vivo* situation and is easier to use and less expensive than the animal models. An organ culture model system and techniques will be described in this chapter.

Keywords: Aqueous humor, Glaucoma, Intraocular pressure, Ocular hypertension, Perfused eye.

INTRODUCTION

Excessive accumulation of aqueous humor (AQH) in the anterior chamber of the eye is often associated with different forms of glaucoma, a constellation of neurodegenerative diseases with varied etiologies. The retention of AQH in the ANC results from pathological blockage of the main drainage system for the fluid, the trabecular meshwork (TM), by excessively deposited collagen, fibronectin, and myocilin proteins (Polansky *et al.*, 2000; Weinreb *et al.*, 2014). Over time, the

* **Corresponding author Najam A. Sharif:** Vice President and Head of Research & Development Nanoscope Therapeutics Inc., 2777 N. Stemmons Fwy, Suite 1102, Dallas, TX-75207, USA; Tel: +1(817)-565-7686; E-mail: nsharif@nanostherapeutics.com

Najam A. Sharif and Sunny E. Ohia (Eds.)

pressure in the ANC rises and is transmitted throughout the eye, leading to disturbances in the structure and function of retinal ganglion cells and their axons (which form the optic nerve), thereby resulting in visual impairment (Weinreb *et al.*, 2014; Bucolo *et al.*, 2018; Sharif, 2021). If left untreated, this ocular hypertension (OHT) can lead to irreversible loss of vision.

The mainstay treatment for OHT and such glaucomatous optic neuropathy is the lowering and controlling of the intraocular pressure (IOP) by pharmaceutical (*e.g.* topical instillation FP- and EP2-receptor agonist drugs or other ocular hypotensive agents) implantation of microshunts to remove the excess AQH and surgical means (Bucolo *et al.*, 2018; Sharif, 2021; Sharif *et al.*, 2023). Due to patient incompliance and side effects of existing treatments, new drugs to tackle OHT and glaucoma are needed. Screening of potential drug candidates for ocular hypotensive activity relies on animal models of OHT, which is an expensive and labor-intensive endeavor. To reduce animal use, increase the throughput, and lower the cost of testing compounds, the use of ANC segments of animal and human eyes postmortem can be a viable alternative (Johnson *et al.*, 1990; Clark *et al.*, 1995; Mao *et al.*, 2011). Such procedures can also provide mechanistic information about the test agents in these organ cultures of ANC segments (Webb *et al.*, 2006; Mao *et al.*, 2011).

Perfused Organ Culture Anterior Segments (POCAS) from human post-mortem or from a number of different animal species have been a standard model for examining the aqueous outflow pathway for over 30 years (Johnson *et al.*, 1990; Clark *et al.*, 1995). This ex-vivo model preserves the architecture of the aqueous outflow pathway and enables studies to be performed in a near physiologic state. Typically, POCAS are perfused in pairs from the same individual with one eye serving as control while the other as experimental control. This somewhat reduces the variability in the outflow facility measurements. For all perfused POCAS studies (irrespective of the species used), it is important to perform a histological examination of the outflow tissues after perfusion to ensure no gross disruption of the outflow pathways, which can dramatically affect the results occurred during the experimentation (Johnson *et al.*, 1990; Mao *et al.*, 2011). Histological examination should also be used to verify that the TM cellularity is within acceptable bounds, as loss of TM cells can lead to preparations that are not responsive to pharmacologic agents. It is also important to point out that perfused POCAS from many animal species (including those from primates) exhibit the "washout effect". This is an increase in outflow facility over time during the initial period of perfusion, which occurs in perfusion models and has been attributed to the removal of extracellular cells or ECM components in outflow pathway tissues. Whether washout is time- or volume-dependent is still not clear (Mao *et al.*, 2011). Although different animal species show varying amounts of this effect, the washout effect is absent in human and probably mouse eyes. The use of a POCAS-based organ culture system is described below.

Tissue Acquisition and Preparation

- Obtain enucleated animal or human eyeballs as fresh as possible from the appropriate source with due consent and related administrative paperwork and keep them on ice.
- Bisect the eye equatorially and carefully remove the vitreous, lens, and iris.
- Mount the anterior segment in a sterile Plexiglass culture dish and seal with a Plexiglass O-ring (Fig. **1**).
- Perfuse the eye segment with chemically defined media (Dulbecos's modified Eagle's medium; Sigma Chemical Co., St. Louis, MO) containing L-glutamine, penicillin, streptomycin, and gentamicin (Gibco/BRL, Grand Island, NY) at a fixed flow rate of 2 /xl/minute using a Harvard perfusion pump (Harvard Instruments, Cambridge, MA).
- Connect a pressure transducer (Stemtech, Houston, TX) connected to the second cannula and monitor the IOP within each eye. In this perfusion system, the perfusate exits the eye through the conventional aqueous humor outflow system. The TM cells of the outflow pathway remain viable for up to 4 weeks in the culture.
- After stabilization for 2-3 days, the test compound can be added to the culture media of one eye while the contralateral eye serves as the control, receiving an equivalent volume of the vehicle during the perfusion.
- Monitor and record the IOPs over several minutes/hours depending on when the peak and plateau phase is achieved.
- If mechanistic studies are undertaken, such as determining the role of matrix metalloproteinases (MMPs) in the molecular mechanism of action of a drug (Webb *et al.*, 2006), then inhibitors of MMPs can be added to the perfusion medium 20-30 minutes before the test compound is introduced. Appropriate controls for experimental arms would need to be designed and implemented. The MMPs can also be co-added with the drug and maintained in a perfused combination throughout the experiments. Here, samples of the perfusate are taken at various time points and later analyzed for Pro-MMPs before, during, and after the perfusion is commenced.
- Likewise, if the effect of corticosteroids on the IOP and outflow facility needs to be determined, then the dexamethasone (0.1-1 uM) would need to be added to the perfusion medium and the experiment continued (with appropriate controls) for 2 hours (Clark *et al.*, 1995; Mao *et al.*, 2011). The structural changes in the TM and adjoining tissues can then be morphologically determined, as outlined below.

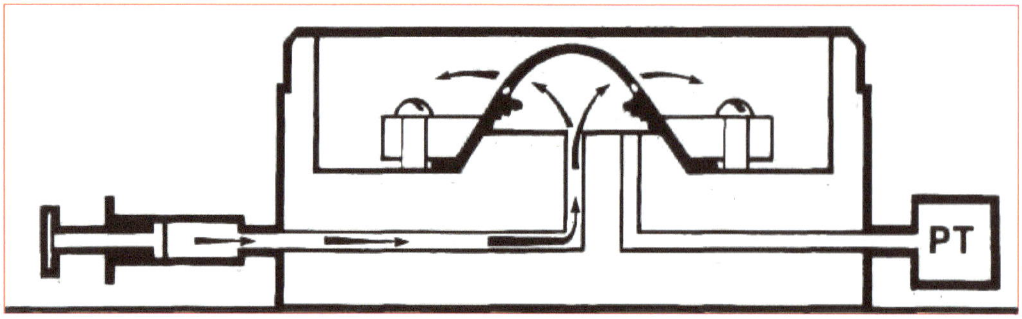

Fig. (1). Pictorial of a perfusion system for the ANC segment of the eye.
The anterior portion of the post-mortem human donor eye is clamped into the Plexiglas dish and perfused *via* a central cannula with chemically defined media using a perfusion pump. The media exits the eye through the conventional outflow pathway. A second cannula is connected to a pressure transducer (PT), which allows monitoring of intraocular pressure. (Clark *et al.*, 1995).

Determining the Morphological Changes in ANC Eye Segments

- The morphologic consequences of perfusion in the absence and presence of the test compound should be examined. The eye segments are fixed by perfusion at 15 mm Hg constant pressure with either 1) a fixative consisting of 4% paraformaldehyde in Sorenson's buffer, followed by immersion fixation in 2.5% glutaraldehyde and 2% paraformaldehyde in 0.1 M Sorenson's phosphate-buffered solution (pH 7.3) or 2) a fixative consisting of 1% paraformaldehyde, 1% glutaraldehyde, and 0.5% acroleiri in 0.1 M sodium cacodylate with pH 7.3.
- Wedge-shaped sections of the iridocorneal angle from four quadrants should be removed and processed for morphologic analysis by light microscopy. Samples of TM for immunohistochemical study should be taken immediately after constant pressure perfusion fixation in 4% paraformaldehyde. Frozen sections (20 um) need to be cut from segments of control and drug-treated ANC and labeled with a monoclonal antibody to human fibronectin (Cappel, West Chester, PA) followed by FITC-labeled rabbit anti-mouse IgG (Cappel, West Chester, PA) using standard immunohistochemical procedures.
- A standard confocal laser scanning microscope (BioRad Laboratories, Hercules, CA) can be used to obtain serial digital images of the inner wall of Schlemm's canal and juxtacanalicular tissue (JCT). Stacks of 0.5 um optical sections are then reconstituted three-dimensionally with BioRad software combined with the image restoration techniques of a Silicon Graphics 4D/240 GTX system (Silicon Graphics, Mountain View, CA).

CONCLUSION

The procedures described above have been successfully utilized to obtain important mechanistic information about the efficacy and mode of action of test compounds using animal and human ANC eye segments. Examples of data that can be garnered from such POCAS-based studies include those for cabergoline, a mixed serotonin-2 receptor and dopamine receptor agonist (Sharif *et al.*, 2009; Fig. **2**), and the effect of dexamethasone on IOP elevation (Clark *et al.*, 1995; Fig. **3**).

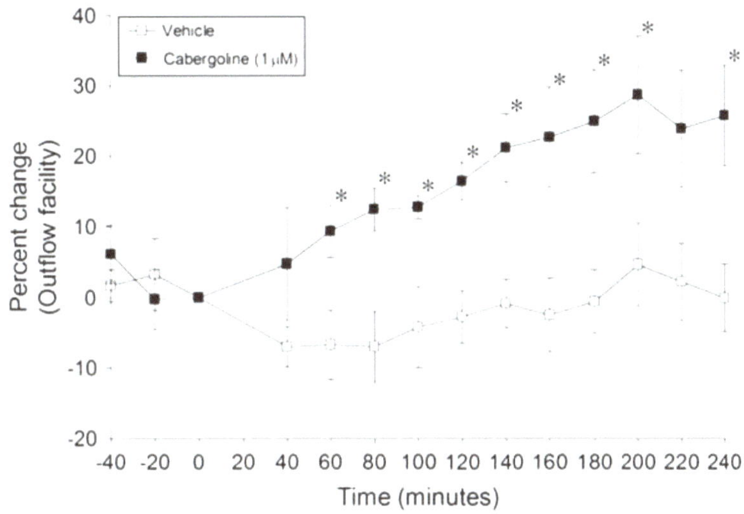

Fig. (2). Example of data showing TM-mediated aqueous fluid outflow enhancement by cabergoline, a mixed serotonin-2 receptor and dopamine receptor agonist, from perfused porcine ANC segments in vitro. The asterisks denote statistical significance relative to the vehicle controls. (Sharif *et al.*, 2009).

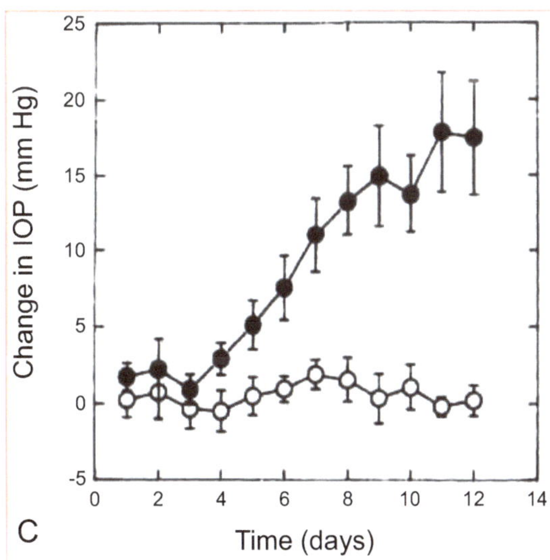

Fig. (3). The ability of corticosteroid and dexamethasone to elevate intraocular pressure (IOP) by suppressing the outflow of fluid from the anterior segment of the human eye in vitro is shown. Thirteen eyes developed a significant rise in IOP when exposed to 100 nM dexamethasone (•) compared to contralateral control eyes receiving media without dexamethasone (o). (Clark *et al.*, 1995).

REFERENCES

Bucolo, C, Platania, CBM, Drago, F, Bonfiglio, V, Reibaldi, M, Avitabile, T & Uva, M (2018) Novel therapeutics in glaucoma management. *Curr Neuropharmacol,* 16, 978-92.
[http://dx.doi.org/10.2174/1570159X15666170915142727] [PMID: 28925883]

Clark, AF, Wilson, K, de Kater, AW, Allingham, RR & McCartney, MD (1995) Dexamethasone-induced ocular hypertension in perfusion-cultured human eyes. *Invest Ophthalmol Vis Sci,* 36, 478-89.
[PMID: 7843916]

Johnson, DH, Bradley, JM & Acott, TS (1990) The effect of dexamethasone on glycosaminoglycans of human trabecular meshwork in perfusion organ culture. *Invest Ophthalmol Vis Sci,* 31, 2568-71.
[PMID: 2125032]

Mao, W, Tovar-Vidales, T, Yorio, T, Wordinger, RJ & Clark, AF (2011) Perfusion-cultured bovine anterior segments as an ex vivo model for studying glucocorticoid-induced ocular hypertension and glaucoma. *Invest Ophthalmol Vis Sci,* 52, 8068-75.
[http://dx.doi.org/10.1167/iovs.11-8133] [PMID: 21911581]

Polansky, JR, Fauss, DJ & Zimmerman, CC (2000) Regulation of TIGR/MYOC gene expression in human trabecular meshwork cells. *Eye (Lond),* 14, 503-14.
[http://dx.doi.org/10.1038/eye.2000.137] [PMID: 11026980]

Sharif, NA (2021) Therapeutic drugs and devices for tackling ocular hypertension and glaucoma, and need for neuroprotection and cytoprotective therapies. *Front Pharmacol,* 12, 729249.
[http://dx.doi.org/10.3389/fphar.2021.729249] [PMID: 34603044]

Sharif, NA, Odani-Kawabata, N, Lu, F & Pinchuk, L (2023) FP and EP2 prostanoid receptor agonist drugs and aqueous humor outflow devices for treating ocular hypertension and glaucoma. *Exp Eye Res,* 229, 109415.
[http://dx.doi.org/10.1016/j.exer.2023.109415] [PMID: 36803996]

Sharif, NA, McLaughlin, MA, Kelly, CR, Katoli, P, Drace, C, Husain, S, Crosson, C, Toris, C, Zhan, GL & Camras, C (2009) Cabergoline: Pharmacology, ocular hypotensive studies in multiple species, and aqueous humor dynamic modulation in the Cynomolgus monkey eyes. *Exp Eye Res,* 88, 386-97.
[http://dx.doi.org/10.1016/j.exer.2008.10.003] [PMID: 18992242]

Webb, JG, Husain, S, Yates, PW & Crosson, CE (2006) Kinin modulation of conventional outflow facility in the bovine eye. *J Ocul Pharmacol Ther,* 22, 310-6.
[http://dx.doi.org/10.1089/jop.2006.22.310] [PMID: 17076624]

Weinreb, RN, Aung, T & Medeiros, FA (2014) The pathophysiology and treatment of glaucoma: a review. *JAMA,* 311, 1901-11.
[http://dx.doi.org/10.1001/jama.2014.3192] [PMID: 24825645]

CHAPTER 24

Human TM Cells as Models for Pseudo-Exfoliation Glaucoma (PEXG)

Aparna Rao[1,*] and **Munmun Chakraborthy**[1]

[1] *Hyderabad Eye Research Foundation, LV Prasad Eye Institute, Patia, Bhubaneswar, MTC Campus, Bhubaneswar, Odisha, India*

Abstract: Exfoliation syndrome and exfoliation glaucoma (XFG; PEXG) remain an enigma with regard to their pathogenesis and cause of glaucoma. While several studies have characterized their clinical characteristics and different phenotypic variations, the mechanisms of formation for complex protein aggregates within ocular tissues like the trabecular meshwork (TM) in this disease entity are largely unknown. The risk factors for the onset of glaucoma in XFS remain a mystery, with only selected eyes developing glaucoma or raised intraocular pressure, IOP. Several molecular markers are known to be upregulated in XFS and XFG eyes, including oxidative stress markers, cytokines, and transforming growth factor (TGF-β1). Several studies have elucidated the differences between eyes with exfoliation and primary glaucoma. Yet, the molecular events that mark the onset of XFS or the development of glaucoma are under-investigated. This is largely because of the inability to sample ocular tissue like the TM or iris in early disease stages. The variable viability of cells from tissues obtained during surgery is a concern precluding easy understanding of the events involved specifically in this disease. In vitro human TM cell line models mimicking this disease allow us to study the temporal events that may mimic the disease's onset and progression over time. We herein present the protocols for establishing such an in vitro model for the study of exfoliation syndrome or XFG, which may be valuable for evaluating various molecular events responsible for the disease pathogenesis.

Keywords: Cell line model, Exfoliation syndrome, Exfoliation glaucoma, Human trabecular meshwork, Transforming growth factor.

INTRODUCTION

The trabecular meshwork (TM) is a tissue located in the eye that helps regulate the outflow of fluid from the eye and maintain normal intraocular pressure (IOP) (Fig. **1**). This is the primary site of injury in glaucoma caused by exfoliation syn-

* **Corresponding author Aparna Rao:** Hyderabad Eye Research Foundation, LV Prasad Eye Institute, Patia, Bhubaneswar, MTC Campus, Bhubaneswar, Odisha, India; Tel: +91 (674) 398 7999/7201; Fax: +91 (674) 398 7130; E-mail: vinodini10375@yahoo.com

Najam A. Sharif and Sunny E. Ohia (Eds.)

drome (Rao *et al.*, 2017; Rao *et al.*, 2014; Schlotzer-Schrehardt *et al.*, 1995; Sahay *et al.*, 2021; Garweg *et al.*, 2017). In glaucoma, elevated IOP can damage the optic nerve, leading to vision loss. As a result, the TM has been studied as a cellular model for understanding the pathophysiology of glaucoma and developing treatments for the disease (Schlotzer-Schrehardt *et al.*, 1995; Sahay *et al.*, 2021; Chakraborty *et al.*, 2021; Lee *et al.*, 2008; Evangelho *et al.*, 2019; Sahay *et al.*, 2017). The TM is composed of various types of cells, including extracellular matrix (ECM) proteins and various types of cells, such as fibroblasts, myofibroblasts, and inflammatory cells (Schlotzer-Schrehardt *et al.*, 1995; Chakraborty *et al.*, 2021). Studies using in vitro and ex vivo models of the TM have provided valuable insights into the cellular and molecular changes that occur in glaucoma and how they may contribute to the progression of the disease (Chakraborty *et al.*, 2021; Evangelho *et al.*, 2019). These models have also been used to test new therapies for glaucoma, such as drugs that target specific signaling pathways or ECM proteins involved in the regulation of IOP.

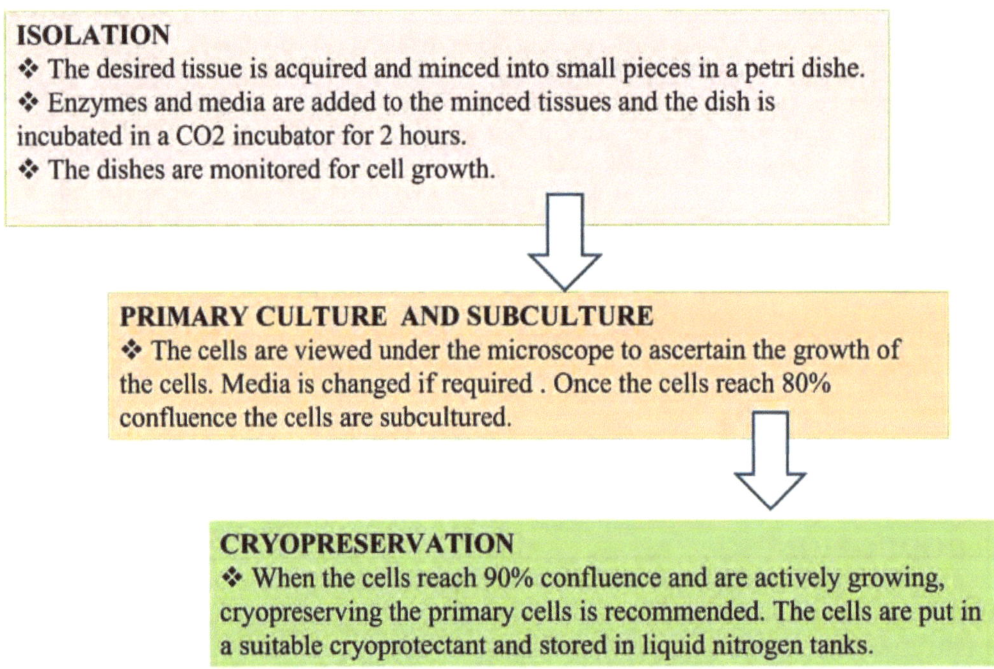

Fig. (1). Anatomy of the eye showing the trabecular meshwork and its relation to adjacent angle structures.

Exfoliation syndrome (XFS) or exfoliation glaucoma (XFG) represents a unique entity among all glaucoma types characterized by the presence of dandruff-like protein complex aggregates within the eye (Schlotzer-Schrehardt *et al.*, 1995; Sahay *et al.*, 2021; Chakraborty *et al.*, 2021; Lee *et al.*, 2008; Evangelho *et al.*,

2019; Sahay *et al*., 2017). These aggregates cause gradual obstruction of the TM and outflow channels that cause tissue dysfunction and TM cell death over time (Rao *et al*., 2017; Rao *et al*., 2014). This causes raised intraocular pressure and irreversible optic nerve damage, leading to blindness. This disease entity has evaded a clear explanation of its pathogenesis on how the aggregates form or what marks the onset of glaucoma. While the TM is the primary site of injury, sampling the TM in early disease stages is unethical, which makes the study of the molecular events causing tissue death impossible. This is precisely why in vitro models using HTM cell lines are important to studying specific temporal molecular events. Transforming growth factor (TGF β1; TGF) is known to be upregulated in XFS and XFG (Jampel *et al*., 1990; Zenkel *et al*., 2014; Hao *et al*., 2019; Rao *et al*., 2020; Chakraborty *et al*., 2022; Sahay *et al*., 2022). This is known to regulate key processes involved in TM cell repair and cell function, which get dysregulated by exfoliation deposits and result in TM dysfunction and glaucoma over time (Sahay *et al*., 2017; Chakraborty *et al*., 2022; Sahay *et al*., 2022). An in vitro model of exfoliation syndrome refers to a laboratory-based system for studying this disease outside of the human body (Chakraborty *et al*., 2021; Lee *et al*., 2008; Evangelho *et al*., 2019; Sahay *et al*., 2017). In vitro models are typically created using cell cultures or tissue samples obtained from healthy donors or patients with exfoliation syndrome. These models allow researchers to study the disease in a controlled environment, where various conditions and treatments can be precisely controlled and monitored. Though they may not simulate the actual disease that happens in vitro, they provide valuable insights into events that mark the onset of changes that cause cell dysfunction or cell death. They also give specific therapeutic targets to reverse these changes that may be used for preventing the onset of glaucoma or disease progression. The in vitro model of exfoliation syndrome has been used to study the cellular and molecular changes that occur in the disease and to test new treatments for exfoliation syndrome (Chakraborty *et al*., 2021; Lee *et al*., 2008; Sahay *et al*., 2017). For example, researchers may use the model to study the effects of drugs on the expression of specific genes or the accumulation of exfoliation material in the lens capsule. Advantages of using an in vitro model of exfoliation syndrome include the ability to precisely control and monitor various conditions, the availability of large amounts of tissue for analysis, and the ability to study the tissue over an extended period. In conclusion, the in vitro model of exfoliation syndrome is a valuable tool for studying the pathophysiology of the disease and developing new treatments for exfoliation syndrome. We present a simple method of harvesting, creating a primary human trabecular meshwork cell line model for exfoliation with specific treatments, and suggest experiments that may be required to validate the same.

METHODS

All experiments require a fully equipped cell culture lab with biosafety cabinets and a laminar hood where all cell-based experiments can be carried out.

We use a primary culture for human TM cell culture for our experiments for mimicking human disease in XFS or XFG. The advantage of using primary cultures is that they retain the characteristics of the tissue they originated from. They retain their normal morphology, cellular function, growth characteristics, cellular markers, signaling, and genetic integrity close to the *in vivo* conditions, which makes them most suited for preclinical or investigative trials. This is very crucial for experiments on XFS or XFG.

Primary Cell Culture of Human Trabecular Meshwork

For creating a primary cell culture, we need cadaver donor corneal buttons with the corneoscleral rims from healthy donors (Figs. **2**, **3**, and **4**). These cadaver eyes are preserved in any institutional eye banks in McCarey-Kaufman (MK). The process of harvesting the TM strip from donor corneas is as below-

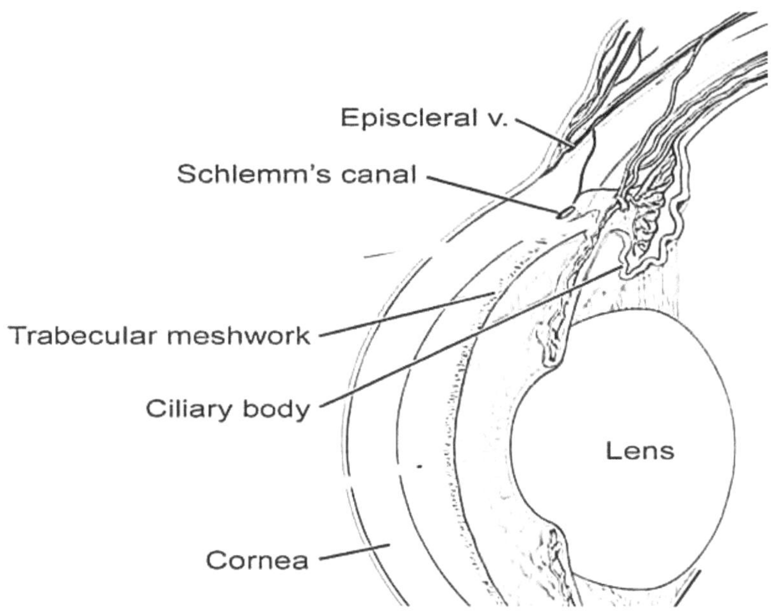

Fig. (2). Flowchart of basic processes involved in generating primary human trabecular meshwork cell culture.

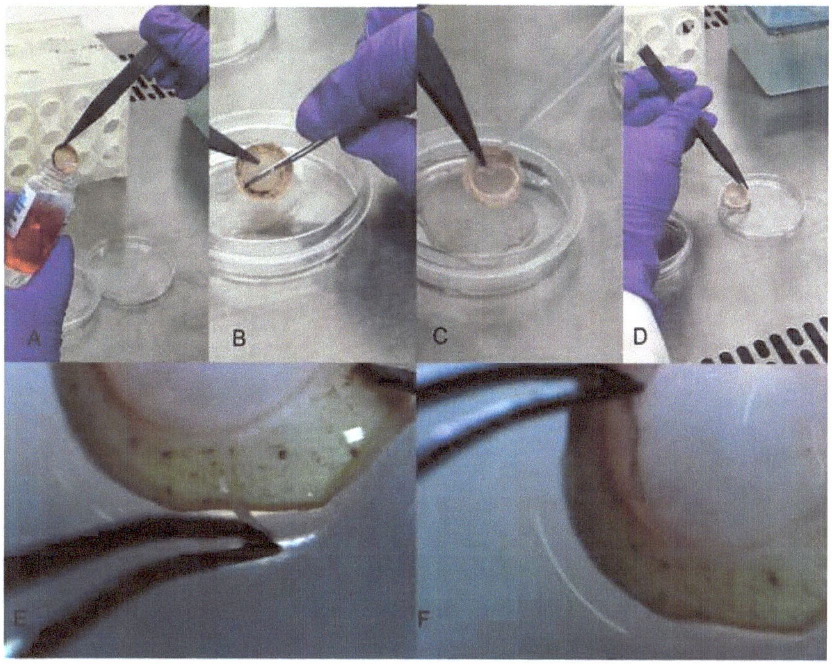

Fig. (3). Isolation of human trabecular meshwork from donor corneal buttons-see test for details.

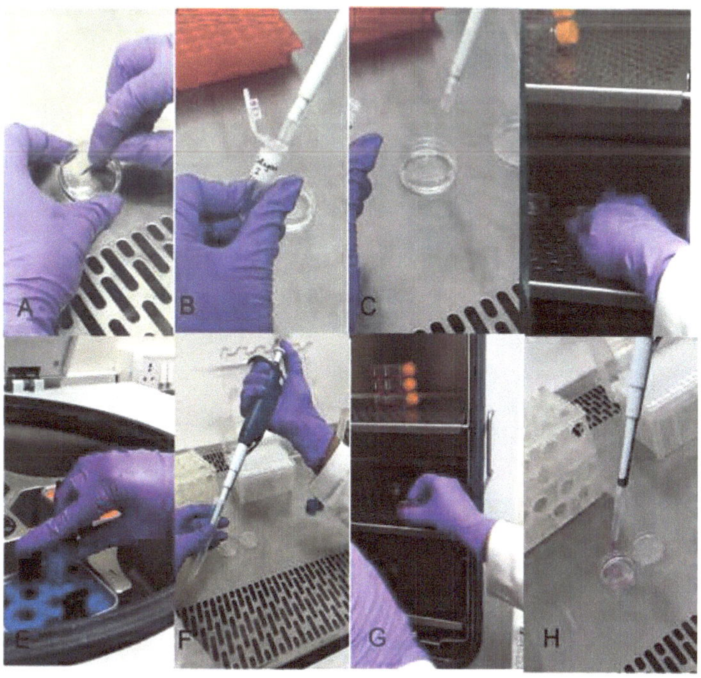

Fig. (4). Culture and sub-culture of harvesting human trabecular meshwork cells.

Isolation of TM Strip from Cadaver Eyes

- Cadaver corneas with intact corneoscleral rims are received in MK medium (Fig. **3**). Ensure the corneas retrieved from the institutional bank belong to young donors <30 years that have been retrieved within 4 hours of death. This is to ensure maximal retrieval of TM cells, preventing the requirement for multiple donor corneas for adequate primary cell culture from each donor. Aged corneas >30 years old have very less viable or healthy TM cells, which may not result in a successful primary culture, even from pooled samples.
- The cornea is first washed with Dulbecco Phosphate-buffered saline (PBS), ensuring the iris remnants on the rims are scraped off. It is washed again gently multiple times to remove the left-over iris tissue remnants and pigments. This step is very important to exclude iris contamination.
- Now, using Lim's forceps or any toothed microsurgical ophthalmic forceps, the TM tissue is carefully stripped off the angle and removed under the dissection microscope. If the tissue is to be stored for future use and not in culture immediately, it can be stored at this stage in any endothelial basal medium (like EBM™-2 medium) at 37°C incubator). This medium is essential for providing key vital growth factors that are essential for the growth of primary endothelial cells.
- If the tissues are put into culture immediately, 1ml of medium is added to a 35mm dish Petri dish, and the TM tissue is then minced into pieces (~0.5mm size) using a sterile surgical blade (Fig. **4**).
- Now, add around 30µL of 30 mg/ml collagenase to the minced tissues and incubate at 37°C for 2 hours in the incubator.

Culture and Sub-Culture of Harvested Primary HTM Cells

- The tissue is observed under the microscope regularly over periodic intervals. If cells are seen coming out of the tissue, the entire content of the Petri dish is transferred into a 15ml falcon and centrifuged at 1000 rpm/3min/25°C. The supernatant is discarded, and the pelleted cells/tissue are dissolved in 1ml trypsin (0.25% trypsin,5min).
- The cells/tissue are incubated at 37^0C for 5-7 min, followed by the addition of 1ml endothelial cell media to inhibit trypsin activity. Centrifugation is then done at 1000 rpm for 5 minutes to remove the excess trypsin.
- The cells are then resuspended in 2ml endothelial basal medium, plated on a 35mm dish, and left undisturbed for 2-3 days in the incubator at 37^0C and 5% CO2. The cells take 4-5 days to adhere and grow; they have to be handled with care during this period to avoid loss of the cells by frequent disturbances.
- The plate is then observed for cells that separate and move out of the minced pieces and assume the specific morphology of a TM cell (Fig. **5**).

- In the initial days, media can be changed every 3-4 days to prevent the loss of too many cells, which may not be so strongly adherent and, therefore, may be lost in the process of changing media.
- The TM cells also tend to float around in spheres, which should not be mistaken to be dead cells and removed. They would separate over time and assume adult TM cell morphology over time.
- Only flasks with 50-7-% confluence may be spilled and passaged using standard protocols. Only the third-fifth passage cells of 50-70% confluence are used for all study experiments.
- Check the morphology of the adult TM cells, which appear as regular elongated cells with intermittent connective tissue between them in a regular arrangement. Before using them for experiments, perform cell viability assays to ensure a viable cell population of each cell lineage. Validation of each TM cell lineage obtained from each donor must be confirmed by the upregulation of myocilin expression after dexamethasone treatment.

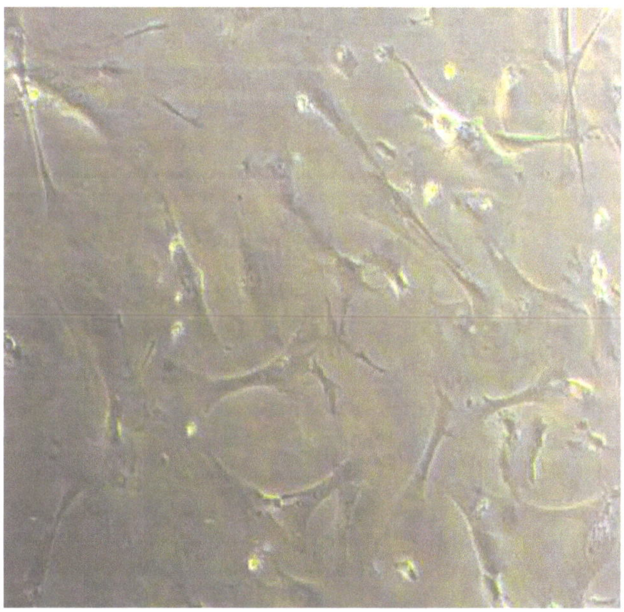

Fig. (5). Appearance of healthy primary human trabecular meshwork cells after culture.

Cryopreservation

- When the cells reach 90% confluence and are actively growing, cryopreserving the primary cells is recommended.
- The cells are put in a suitable cryoprotectant and stored in liquid nitrogen tanks.
- When required for experiments, the cells are thawed slowly and used for various experiments after validation and other assays, as detailed below.

Treatment of HTM Cells with TGF-β1

- Cultures that reach 50-70% confluence in flasks are serum starved for 24hrs, followed by treatment with TGF-β1.
- One set of cultures that is left untreated is used as control for all the experiments. Check the controls periodically to ensure the cells do not acquire senescent changes or become stressed.
- Check the viability and morphology of the cells after each treatment.
- Cell viability in control and treated cells is measured using the 3-(4,- -dimethylthiazol-2-yl)-2,5-diphenyltetrazolium bromide assay.
- Cells that are serum starved for 24hrs are now treated with or without TGF-β1(3ng/ml, 5ng/ml, 10ng/ml, 15ng/ml) for 24hrs, 36hrs, 48hrs, 72hrs, and 96hrs.
- After treatment, absorbance at 570 nm may be measured on an EPOCH microplate reader (BioTek, USA).
- Serum-starved and TGF-β1-treated (0ng/ml, 5ng/ml,10ng/ml, and 15ng/ml) HTM cells are analyzed for morphological changes in shape and structure at 24hrs, 48hrs, and 72hrs after treatment. Epithelial mesenchymal transformation (EMT), induced by TGF, is indicated when the cells become spindle-like and are more densely packed, losing the characteristic morphology of HTM cells. Rounded cells over time in clusters indicate stress that is removed on a periodic basis to avoid dead cells in the culture. Cell viability assays may be done to ensure cell viability changes with treatment over time.
- To confirm the recruitment of pro-fibrotic response after TGF treatment in treated cells, the expression of smooth muscle actin, α-SMA, and vimentin is determined, which are markers of mesenchymal cells.
- These treated cells can now be used for various experiments to evaluate molecular events after various periods of exposure to TGF that simulate changes seen in XFS/XFG.

CONCLUSION

The protocols described are for creating an in vitro model that may simulate exfoliation in a very controlled environment. However, readers are encouraged to check out the original publications where such methods were described and explore other models for studying glaucoma, including those inducing oxidative stress using hydrogen peroxide. An additional literature search is recommended for incorporating suitable modifications or refinements to the procedures described herein.

ACKNOWLEDGEMENTS

The authors would like to thank the Hyderabad Eye Research Foundation and DBT Wellcome Trust India Alliance for supporting the work on XFS/XFG.

REFERENCES

Chakraborty, M, Sahay, P & Rao, A (2021) Primary Human Trabecular Meshwork Model for Pseudoexfoliation. *Cells,* 10, 3448.
[http://dx.doi.org/10.3390/cells10123448] [PMID: 34943956]

Chakraborty, M & Rao, A (2022) Alternate Causes for Pathogenesis of Exfoliation Glaucoma, a Multifactorial Elastotic Disorder: A Literature Review. *Curr Issues Mol Biol,* 44, 1191-202.
[http://dx.doi.org/10.3390/cimb44030078] [PMID: 35723301]

Evangelho, K, Mastronardi, CA & de-la-Torre, A (2019) Experimental Models of Glaucoma: A Powerful Translational Tool for the Future Development of New Therapies for Glaucoma in Humans—A Review of the Literature. *Medicina (Kaunas),* 55, 280.
[http://dx.doi.org/10.3390/medicina55060280] [PMID: 31212881]

Garweg, JG, Zandi, S, Pfister, IB, Skowronska, M & Gerhardt, C (2017) Comparison of cytokine profiles in the aqueous humor of eyes with pseudoexfoliation syndrome and glaucoma. *PLoS One,* 12, e0182571.
[http://dx.doi.org/10.1371/journal.pone.0182571] [PMID: 28797085]

Hao, Y, Baker, D & ten Dijke, P (2019) TGF-β-Mediated Epithelial-Mesenchymal Transition and Cancer Metastasis. *Int J Mol Sci,* 20, 2767.
[http://dx.doi.org/10.3390/ijms20112767] [PMID: 31195692]

Hocevar, BA & Howe, PH (2000) Analysis of TGF-beta-mediated synthesis of extracellular matrix components. *Methods Mol Biol,* 142, 55-65.
[PMID: 10806613]

Jampel, HD, Roche, N, Stark, WJ & Roberts, AB (1990) Transforming growth factor-β in human aqueous humor. *Curr Eye Res,* 9, 963-9.
[http://dx.doi.org/10.3109/02713689009069932] [PMID: 2276273]

Lee, RK (2008) The molecular pathophysiology of pseudoexfoliation glaucoma. *Curr Opin Ophthalmol,* 19, 95-101.
[http://dx.doi.org/10.1097/ICU.0b013e3282f49cda] [PMID: 18301281]

Rao, A, Padhy, D, Sahay, P, Pradhan, A, Sarangi, S, Das, G & Raj, N (2017) Clinical spectrum of pseudoexfoliation syndrome—An electronic records audit. *PLoS One,* 12, e0185373.
[http://dx.doi.org/10.1371/journal.pone.0185373] [PMID: 29077713]

Rao, A & Padhy, D (2014) Pattern of pseudoexfoliation deposits on the lens and their clinical correlation--clinical study and review of literature. *PLoS One,* 9, e113329.
[http://dx.doi.org/10.1371/journal.pone.0113329] [PMID: 25478872]

Rao, A, Chakraborty, M, Roy, A, Sahay, P, Pradhan, A & Raj, N (2020) Differential miRNA Expression: Signature for Glaucoma in Pseudoexfoliation. *Clin Ophthalmol,* 14, 3025-38.
[http://dx.doi.org/10.2147/OPTH.S254504] [PMID: 33116354]

Sahay, P, Chakraborty, M & Rao, A (2022) Global and Comparative Proteome Signatures in the Lens Capsule, Trabecular Meshwork, and Iris of Patients With Pseudoexfoliation Glaucoma. *Front Mol Biosci,* 9, 877250-0.
[http://dx.doi.org/10.3389/fmolb.2022.877250] [PMID: 35517867]

Sahay, P, Rao, A, Padhy, D, Sarangi, S, Das, G, Reddy, MM & Modak, R (2017) Functional Activity of Matrix Metalloproteinases 2 and 9 in Tears of Patients With Glaucoma. *Invest Ophthalmol Vis Sci,* 58, BIO106-13.
[http://dx.doi.org/10.1167/iovs.17-21723] [PMID: 28586796]

Sahay, P, Reddy, S, Prusty, BK, Modak, R & Rao, A (2021) TGFβ1, MMPs and cytokines profiles in ocular surface: Possible tear biomarkers for pseudoexfoliation. *PLoS One,* 16, e0249759.
[http://dx.doi.org/10.1371/journal.pone.0249759] [PMID: 33914756]

Schlötzer-Schrehardt, U & Naumann, GO (1995) Trabecular meshwork in pseudoexfoliation syndrome with and without open-angle glaucoma. A morphometric, ultrastructural study. *Invest Ophthalmol Vis Sci,* 36,

1750-64.
[PMID: 7635652]

Zenkel, M & Schlötzer-Schrehardt, U (2014) The composition of exfoliation material and the cells involved in its production. *J Glaucoma,* 23 (Suppl. 1), S12-4.
[http://dx.doi.org/10.1097/IJG.0000000000000123] [PMID: 25275897]

ANIMAL MODELS OF OCULAR HYPERTENSION (OHT)/GLAUCOMA FOR DETERMINATION OF AQUEOUS HUMOR DYNAMICS

CHAPTER 25

Protocol for Inducing IOP-Elevation (OHT) Using Hypertonic Saline Injection into Episcleral Veins of Rats

Shahid Husain[1,*]

[1] *Department of Ophthalmology, Storm Eye Institute, Medical University of South Carolina, 167 Ashley Ave, Charleston, SC 29425, USA*

Abstract: This chapter provides a description of protocols utilized to develop ocular hypertension (OHT) in rats *via* episcleral/limbal veins occlusion using hypertonic saline injections. A procedure for measuring the elevated intraocular pressure (IOP) using a TonoLab rebound tonometer in these animals is also described. Furthermore, the impact of the raised IOP on retinal ganglion cell (RGC) function in this model of OHT/glaucoma, using pattern electroretinograms (Pattern ERG) as a measure of RGC function, is detailed.

Keywords: Episcleral veins, Glaucoma, Ontraocular pressure, Ocular hypertension, Pattern electroretinogram.

INTRODUCTION

It is now well-established that elevated intraocular pressure (IOP) is one of the major risk factors for developing open-angle, closed-angle, and many secondary forms of glaucoma (Weinreb *et al.*, 2014; Sharif, 2017, 2021). In order to decipher the cellular and molecular factors and events that cause ocular hypertension (OHT) due to abnormal accumulation of excess aqueous humor in the anterior chamber of the eye, a number of animal models of OHT/glaucoma have been generated. Some of these are described in other chapters in this book. The current chapter focuses on the classic method to induce elevated IOP, *i.e.*, by injecting hypertonic saline into the episcleral veins of lightly anesthetized rodents, especially in rats (Johnson *et al.*, 2005; Morrison, 2007; Pazos *et al.*, 2016; Morrison *et al.*, 2018). The author's own work in this arena of research where this rat model of OHT was developed in Brown Norway rats is described below and

* **Corresponding author Shahid Husain:** Department of Ophthalmology, Storm Eye Institute, Medical University of South Carolina, 167 Ashley Ave, Charleston, SC 29425, USA; Tel: 843-792-2792; Fax: 843-792-1155; E-mail: husain@musc.edu

Najam A. Sharif and Sunny E. Ohia (Eds.)

detailed in a number of publications (Husain, 2012, 2021; Abdul *et al*., 2013; Zaidi *et al*., 2020).

OHT/Glaucoma Model: Rat Episcleral/Limbal Vein Occlusion Model of IOP Elevation

The rat handling and housing were in accordance with the ARVO Statement for the Use of Animals in Ophthalmic & Vision Research, and the study protocol was approved by the Animal Care and Use Committee at MUSC. Brown Norway rats (~150–225 g body weight) were kept under a standard cycle of 12-hours:12-hours light/dark. The following procedure was used to raise IOP in rats.

Micro Injections Procedure

- First, we prepared a micro-injection assembly to inject hypertonic saline into the episcleral/limbal veins. The micro-injection apparatus consisted of 3 components: (1) a glass microneedle ~2-3 mm long with 50 micrometers in diameter, (2) a PE-50 polyethylene tubing (length can vary as needed), and (3) a 23-gauge needle attached to 2-5 ml syringe with a blunt tip. These components were assembled under a dissecting microscope using a 3-way stopcock. This microneedle assembly was attached with a 2 mL syringe, which was further attached with a 2-5 mL syringe with a 3-way stopcock to provide sufficient fluid pressure at the needle tip, as shown in Fig. (**1**).
- Prior to any intraocular pressure (IOP) elevation, a stable baseline IOP was determined.
- Once a stable IOP was determined, IOP was raised by injecting hypertonic saline injections. Rats were then anesthetized with ketamine (75 mg/kg) and xylazine (8 mg/kg), and their body temperature was maintained at 37°C using a heating pad. Next, a drop of topical proparacaine (0.5%) was applied to numb the cornea 5 minutes prior to the ocular injections.
- The microneedle was held by a pair of curved forceps and pointed toward the limbus. It was then carefully positioned parallel to the vessel wall and slowly inserted into a circumferential limbal vein close to the cornea.
- About 50 μL of 2.0 M hypertonic saline solution (NaCl) was then injected into the limbal venous system as described earlier (Husain, 2012, 2021; Abdul *et al*., 2013; Zaidi *et al*., 2020). For the saline injection, a gentle force was used to sufficiently blanch the limbal artery. The blanching of the circular limbal vein is an indication of proper infusion of hypertonic saline into the veins. Generally, when a greater force is used, it results in excessive IOP elevation, which is detrimental to the subsequent experimental paradigm.

- A little neomycin (an antibacterial ointment) was applied at the injection site of each animal to prevent infection. The rats were kept on the heating pad, monitored, and allowed to recover from anesthesia.
- To control potential pain, animals were given a recommended dose of buprenorphine after surgery, and we continued the analgesic injections for the next 24 hours at an interval of 6-8 hours.
- Animals were observed for general activity and weighed and their IOP was measured on a regular basis (*i.e.*, 3, 7 days, and weekly afterward).
- The anterior chamber was periodically examined to check for potential inflammation.
- In general, a significant elevation in IOP was seen on day 7 and onwards.
- If no changes in IOP were detected after 2 weeks, a second injection of hypertonic saline was performed in an episcleral vein as described above.
- The optic nerve head and retinal vasculature were also assessed by viewing the fundus with a direct ophthalmoscope through pupils dilated with 1% tropicamide and 2% phenylephrine hydrochloride.
- To measure changes in IOP and retinal ganglion cell (RGC) function, IOP and pattern electroretinograms (Pattern-ERG) were routinely measured at an interval of 1-2 weeks post-surgery.

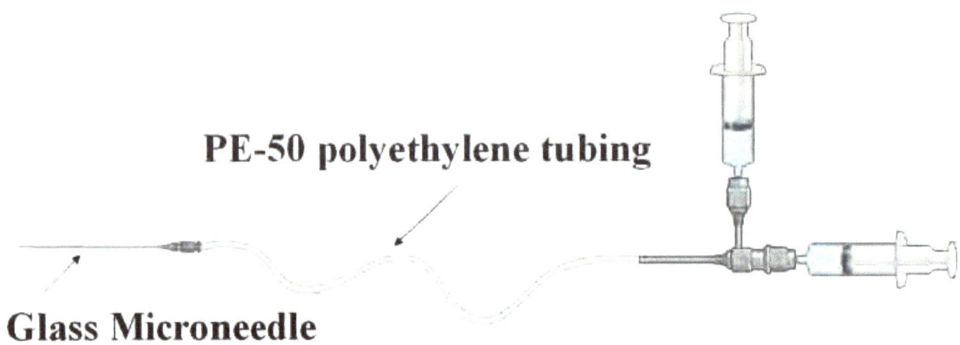

Fig. (1). Schematic showing microinjection assembly.

Measurement of Intraocular Pressure (IOP) in Rats

- IOP was measured in conscious animals in a masked fashion using the TonoLab rebound tonometer (Colonial Medical Supply Co. Inc., Franconia, NH).
- To minimize any discomfort to the animal during tonometry, corneas were lightly anesthetized by the topical application of 0.1% proparacaine (3 μl).
- Baseline IOP readings of both eyes were determined. To ensure the accuracy of the tonometer, the TonoLab read-outs were calibrated against the rat IOPs set by perfusing the rat anterior chamber using saline from a reservoir set at various heights.

- To raise the IOP, rats were anesthetized (ketamine, 33 mg/kg and xylazine, 6 mg/kg), and eyes were cannulated with a 35-gauge needle inserted through the limbus.
- This calibration procedure utilized the open stopcock method, where the IOP was measured with a pressure transducer (Model BLPR 5326, WPI, Sarasota, FL) connected in parallel between the eye and the saline reservoir.
- A calibration curve was established from 8-40 mmHg and used to correct readouts from the anesthetized rats.
- Once the Tonolab was calibrated, the IOPs in normal and ocular hypertensive rats were recorded as the average of 6-8 consecutive measurements before and after the surgery.
- Later on, IOPs were measured on a weekly basis in all groups of rats as previously described (Husain, Abdul *et al.* 2012; Abdul, Akhter *et al.* 2013; Zaidi, Guzman *et al.* 2020; Husain, Zaidi *et al.* 2021).
- Exposure to elevated IOPs for each rat was calculated by performing separate integration of the IOP over days of exposure for the control eyes and the drug-treated eyes. By subtracting the control eye integrated values from the drug-treated eye values, "IOP-integral difference" was obtained. The final values were then expressed as mm Hg-days.
- Only rats with elevated IOP, which was at least 25% above the baseline IOP (~18–20 mm Hg), were subsequently included in the experiments.

Pattern Electroretinogram (Pattern-ERGs)

- Rats were anesthetized with ketamine (75 mg/kg) and xylazine (8 mg/kg), and their body temperature was maintained at 37°C with a heating pad.
- Pattern-ERG recordings (without dark adaptation) were performed in both eyes (sequentially) 3 days before the IOP increase using the hypertonic saline injection as described above and then every 2 weeks following the surgery, as previously described (Husain, 2012, 2021; Abdul *et al.*, 2013; Zaidi *et al.*, 2020).
- Next, a micromanipulator was used to place the pattern-ERG electrode on the corneal surface, and the electrode was positioned to encircle the undilated pupil so that the field of view remained unobstructed.
- In order to keep the cornea and lens moist during each recording, a drop of sterile saline was applied to the cornea.
- Next, a visual stimulus created by black/white alternating contrast reversing bars (mean luminance, 50 cd/m2; spatial frequency, 0.033 cycle/deg; contrast, 100%; and temporal frequency, 1 Hz) was aligned with the projection of the undilated pupil of each rat at an 11 cm distance using the P-ERG machine (UTAS-2000 (LKC Technologies, Gaithersburg, MD).

- Each PERG was represented by an average of 300 sweeps at an interval of 1 second. In order to determine the pattern of ERG amplitudes, measurements were recorded between a peak and an adjacent trough of the waveform, as shown and previously described (Husain *et al.*, 2012).

CONCLUSION

Animal models of ocular hypertension and glaucoma have led to a better understanding of the disease processes and factors implicated in the causality of these eye diseases. Furthermore, testing of and comparative studies on potential novel IOP-lowering and/or neuroprotective compounds have been made possible using such animal models. One of the most well-characterized animal models to date is the episcleral vein hypertonic saline injection model described in the current chapter. Typical data gathered from such studies can be found in several publications listed in the references section below.

ACKNOWLEDGEMENTS

This study was supported by NIH/NEI grant EY-034514.

REFERENCES

Abdul, Y, Akhter, N & Husain, S (2013) Delta-opioid agonist SNC-121 protects retinal ganglion cell function in a chronic ocular hypertensive rat model. *Invest Ophthalmol Vis Sci,* 54, 1816-28.
[http://dx.doi.org/10.1167/iovs.12-10741] [PMID: 23404122]

Husain, S, Abdul, Y & Crosson, CE (2012) Preservation of retina ganglion cell function by morphine in a chronic ocular-hypertensive rat model. *Invest Ophthalmol Vis Sci,* 53, 4289-98.
[http://dx.doi.org/10.1167/iovs.12-9467] [PMID: 22661469]

Husain, S, Zaidi, SAH, Singh, S, Guzman, W & Mehrotra, S (2021) Reduction of Neuroinflammation by δ-Opioids *Via* STAT3-Dependent Pathway in Chronic Glaucoma Model. *Front Pharmacol,* 12, 601404.
[http://dx.doi.org/10.3389/fphar.2021.601404] [PMID: 33628191]

Johnson, EC, Jia, L, Cepurna, WO, Doser, TA & Morrison, JC (2007) Global changes in optic nerve head gene expression after exposure to elevated intraocular pressure in a rat glaucoma model. *Invest Ophthalmol Vis Sci,* 48, 3161-77.
[http://dx.doi.org/10.1167/iovs.06-1282] [PMID: 17591886]

Morrison, JC (2005) Elevated intraocular pressure and optic nerve injury models in the rat. *J Glaucoma,* 14, 315-7.
[http://dx.doi.org/10.1097/01.ijg.0000169410.09258.bf] [PMID: 15990616]

Morrison, JC, Johnson, EC & Cepurna, WO (2018) Hypertonic Saline Injection Model of Experimental Glaucoma in Rats. *Methods Mol Biol,* 1695, 11-21.
[http://dx.doi.org/10.1007/978-1-4939-7407-8_2] [PMID: 29190014]

Pazos, M, Yang, H, Gardiner, SK, Cepurna, WO, Johnson, EC, Morrison, JC & Burgoyne, CF (2016) Expansions of the neurovascular scleral canal and contained optic nerve occur early in the hypertonic saline rat experimental glaucoma model. *Exp Eye Res,* 145, 173-86.
[http://dx.doi.org/10.1016/j.exer.2015.10.014] [PMID: 26500195]

Sharif, NA (2017) Ocular hypertension and glaucoma: a review and current perspectives. *Int J Ophthalmol. Vis Sci,* 2, 22-36.

Sharif, NA (2021) Therapeutic drugs and devices for tackling ocular hypertension and glaucoma, and need for neuroprotection and cytoprotective therapies. *Front Pharmacol,* 12, 729249. [http://dx.doi.org/10.3389/fphar.2021.729249] [PMID: 34603044]

Weinreb, RN, Aung, T & Medeiros, FA (2014) The pathophysiology and treatment of glaucoma: a review. *JAMA,* 311, 1901-11. [http://dx.doi.org/10.1001/jama.2014.3192] [PMID: 24825645]

Zaidi, SAH, Guzman, W, Singh, S, Mehrotra, S & Husain, S (2020) Changes in Class I and IIb HDACs by δ-Opioid in Chronic Rat Glaucoma Model. *Invest Ophthalmol Vis Sci,* 61, 4. [http://dx.doi.org/10.1167/iovs.61.14.4] [PMID: 33263714]

CHAPTER 26

Protocol for Inducing Ocular Hypertension in Mice Using Magnetic Microbeads

Najam A. Sharif[1,*] and **Saima Chaudhry**[2]

[1] *Vice President and Head of Research & Development Nanoscope Therapeutics Inc., 2777 N. Stemmons Fwy, Suite 1102, Dallas, TX-75207, USA*

[2] *Univ N. Texas at Arlington, 701 S Nedderman Dr, Arlington, TX-76019, USA*

Abstract: In many types of glaucoma, a set of chronic neurodegenerative diseases of the retina and optic nerve, elevated intraocular pressure (IOP) is a major culprit. In order to study the disease mechanisms and help discover novel drugs and devices that lower and control IOP, several animal models of ocular hypertension (OHT) have been developed. This chapter focuses on and describes protocols to induce OHT in mice (or rats) using magnetic microbeads (MMBs). Intracameral injection of a suspension of MMBs occludes the trabecular meshwork and prevents or drastically reduces the outflow of aqueous humor (AQH). This gradually raises the IOP. If the IOP is not elevated by 2-fold from baseline and maintained for at least 4 weeks, additional microbeads may need to be injected. Many researchers have successfully created such animal models of OHT and shown them to be useful for drug screening for IOP-lowering efficacy and glaucomatous optic neuropathy studies aimed at finding suitable neuroprotective therapies to preserve vision.

Keywords: Anterior chamber, Eye, Glaucoma, Intraocular pressure, Magnetic microbeads, Ocular hypertension, Optic nerve, Protocol, Retina.

INTRODUCTION

Humans and animals suffer from numerous eye diseases and disorders. Animal models of ocular disease play a central role in defining the factors involved in the pathogenesis of human disease. They also provide a useful model to assess the *in vivo* efficacy of pharmacological agents that may be beneficial in treating the human condition. Accordingly, since glaucoma is a major ocular degenerative disease of concern and varying etiologies, and elevated intraocular pressure (IOP) is a leading cause of many forms of glaucoma (Weinreb *et al.*, 2014; Sharif, 2018, 2021), several animal models have been developed where ocular hypertension

* **Corresponding author Najam A. Sharif:** Vice President and Head of Research & Development Nanoscope Therapeutics Inc., 2777 N. Stemmons Fwy, Suite 1102, Dallas, TX-75207, USA; Tel: +1(817)-565-7686; E-mail: nsharif@nanostherapeutics.com

(OHT) has been induced acutely or on a more chronic basis (Urcola *et al.*, 2006; Morrison *et al.*, 2011; Bouhenni *et al.*, 2012). Many such animal models have been described, including those using latex microbeads to raise IOP (Weber and Zelenak, 2001; Cone *et al.*, 2010; Sappington *et al.*, 2010; Samsel *et al.*, 2011) and more recently utilizing magnetic microbeads (Samsel *et al.*, 2011; Bunker *et al.*, 2015; Ito *et al.*, 2016).

The purpose of this chapter is to describe the key elements of experimental protocols to induce and maintain OHT in mice using magnetic microbeads (Samsel *et al.*, 2011; Bunker *et al.*, 2015; Ito *et al.*, 2016) injected into the anterior chamber of the mouse eye and directing their accumulation into the trabecular meshwork to prevent aqueous humor (AQH) outflow. These procedures permit the raising and maintenance of elevated IOP for up to six weeks in order to investigate the effects of chronic OHT on the structure and function of the retina and optic nerve. Such mouse and rat models also provide platforms for testing the ability of pharmacological agents to reduce the IOP and/or protect the retinal ganglion cells (RGCs) and reduce damage to their axons that form the optic nerve. Some representative data obtained from this model of OHT/glaucoma are presented to illustrate the type of information that can be obtained from such studies with a focus on the methods described by Ito *et al.* (2016).

EXPERIMENTAL PROTOCOLS

The following procedures should be performed in compliance with the guidelines for the Use of Experimental Animals and the Statement for the Use of Animals in Ophthalmic and Visual Research from the Association for Research in Vision and Ophthalmology (ARVO). The majority of the procedures described herein are adapted from Ito *et al.* (2016). Alternative methods are also available (Bunker *et al.*, 2015).

Glass Microneedle Preparation for Intracameral Injection of the Microbeads

Whilst glass capillary-based microneedles are used in the current protocol (Ito *et al.*, 2061), it is possible to use sterile 33 G beveled metal needles (Bunker *et al.*, 2015).

- First, create borosilicate glass capillary microneedles using standard glass-pulling techniques
- At an angle under a microscope, use a sharp metal blade to carefully generate an elliptical opening (approx 190 µm and 70 µm) at microneedle tips. Using distilled water, the uniformly created microneedles are then beveled at a 20° angle (relative to the plate in the beveling system) for up to 10 min to ensure that

the final products are smooth and without rough edges or surfaces and, of course, still with sharp ends.

- An aerosol duster is then used to remove any debris on and in the microneedle tips.
- For quality control purposes, ensure that all beveled microneedles are clean and unfractured and then sterilized with ethanol and then with a sterile balanced salt solution (BSS). Allow the microneedles to air dry in a sterile cell culture hood.

Magnetic Microbead Suspension Preparation

Removal of Epoxy Groups from Magnetic Beads

- The epoxy groups coated on the magnetic microbeads need to be removed first before proceeding to the animal work.
- Suspend the magnetic microbeads (MMBs; 4.5 μm diameter, 4 x 10^8 beads/ml) in a solution of 0.02 M sodium hydroxide made up of 10x Tris buffer. Gently vortex the stock of MMBs suspension until the beads are uniformly dispersed and suspended in solution.
- Rapidly remove 1 ml of this suspension and add it to 50 ml of 0.02 M NaOH in 10x Tris buffer. Allow this tube to rotate for 1 day at room temperature in order to free the beads off the epoxy groups.
- Using a magnet, collect the beads at the bottom of the tube and gently remove the supernatant. Re-suspend the beads in fresh 50 ml of 0.02 M NaOH in 10x Tris buffer, gently disperse, and repeat the tube rotation for another 4 hrs as above.
- Using a magnet, collect the beads at the bottom of the tube and gently remove the supernatant without disturbing the "MMBs pellet".
- Gently vortex the pellet in 50 ml of 10x Tris-buffer until the beads are well suspended, and repeat steps 5 & 6 as above.

Concentration and Resuspension of MMBs in Sterile Balanced Salt Solution

- Now concentrate the MMBs in sterile BSS to obtain a final concentration of 1.6 x 10^6 beads/μl.
- Suspend the concentrated MMBs in 5 ml of ultra-pure laboratory-grade water by gently mixing for 2 min on a vortex. Then, concentrate them to the bottom of the tube with a magnet as before and remove the supernatant.
- Repeat the MMBs washing procedure described above an additional 3 times and obtain the washed MMB pellets.
- Under sterile conditions in a laminar flow hood, wash the beads with 0.5 ml of sterile BSS by gentle trituration (pipetting up and down a few times).

- With a magnet, collect/concentrate the washed MMBs to the bottom of the tube and gently remove the supernatant. Repeat the above sterile washing process 3 more times and end up with concentrated MMBs.
- Now resuspend the MMBs by trituration in 250 µl of sterile BSS until the beads are evenly dispersed/ suspended. The final concentration of the stock bead suspension should be 1.6 x 10^6 beads/µl.
- Now, rapidly aliquot 25 µl of this suspension into sterile 0.5 ml plastic tubes and store them at 4 °C until needed for the injections.

Ocular Hypertension in Mice

This procedure requires two skilled technicians, one to handle the animal and the other to perform the MMB injection. Animals used for studies of this type can range from normal C57BL/6 mice and gene-knockout mice to transgenic mice of either sex. Ideally, the former mice should be utilized to aid successful handling and OHT creation.

- In order to determine the baseline IOPs, inject one drop of proparacaine hydrochloride in the corneas of the eyes in conscious 3-4.5 months old C57BL/6 mice to numb the tissue.
- Carefully but gently restrain the mouse by holding the skin between the ears and positioning it on the benchtop so the eyes are easily accessible. Holding the tonometer perpendicular to the corneal surface, take at least 3-sets of ten consecutive readings per eye to obtain an average IOP. If mice are to be handled after anesthesia, then they are anesthetized using an intraperitoneal injection (1 µl/g of body weight) of a cocktail of 20 mg/ml ketamine, 2 mg/ml xylazine, and 0.4 mg/ml acepromazine.
- To minimize pain, administer 0.05 mg per kg body weight of buprenorphine subcutaneously.
- In order to induce pupil dilation to more easily perform the MMB injection, inject an eyedrop of tropicamide into the mouse eye that will receive the MMBs. Apply a small amount of topical ointment to the corneal surface of the contralateral eye (un-operated) to minimize tear evaporation and possible damage due to desiccation.
- To prepare for the MMB injection, attach a clean microneedle to the injection assembly of the microsyringe pump.
- Technician 1 should transfer the anesthetized mouse to the operating platform of the microscope and ensure that the pupil is fully dilated, ocular muscles are relaxed, and the mouse eye is perfectly still. The tropicamide is gently removed from the cornea with a sterile swab.
- Technician 2 mixes the MMB suspension by gentle trituration. Now, using the microsyringe pump, quickly load the microneedle with 1.5 µl of the mixed

MMBs to have 2.4 x 10^6 beads available for injection but without any air bubbles at the tip of the microneedle.

- The loaded microneedle is positioned at a 45° angle and placed anteriorly relative to the limbus. Technician 1 supports the eye using plastic forceps to allow the angle between the microneedle and the plastic forceps to be around 90°.
- Technician 2 should carefully and gently puncture the cornea so that the tip of the microneedle enters the anterior chamber of the eye, ensuring that the loaded microneedle remains at a 45° angle relative to the limbus during the puncture. Any and all contact of the microneedle with the lens or the iris should be completely avoided, and the microneedle should not enter the posterior chamber. During this procedure, Technician 1 continues to support the eye using plastic forceps.
- Technician 1 should place a magnet beside the eye opposite to the microneedle tip. This will draw the MMBs into the anterior chamber and minimize contact of the beads with the inner surface of the cornea. Technician 2 should now carefully and gently inject 1.5 μl of the MMB suspension into the anterior chamber. The MMBs should be injected slowly over the next 15 - 30 seconds while Technician 1 continues to hold the magnet opposite to the microneedle tip during the entire duration of the injection.
- Technician 2 should slowly withdraw the microneedle from the eye once the MMBs have been fully released into the eye. Technician 1 should continue to use the magnet to draw the MMBs into the anterior chamber over the next 1 min and thus prevent potential reflux of the MMBs and the liquid.
- Technician 1 should use the magnet to help disperse the MMBs within the iridocorneal angle and around the circumference of the anterior chamber. Due caution should be exercised to avoid moving the MMBs toward the inner cornea.
- Now, instill an eyedrop of an antibiotic to the corneal surface to reduce potential infection risk.
- For the next 3-4 hrs, place the mouse on a heated pad until fully awake. Ensure that the operated eye faces upwards to reduce the gravity-assisted MMBs accumulating on the inner corneal cells.
- IOP measurements should only be performed on the operated mice after at least 2 days of recovery. IOPs should be determined at least once a week or more frequently, as necessary, and at the same time of the day to reduce circadian rhythm-related spikes and other changes.
- The non-operated eye can be used to determine the normal (control) IOP. Additional IOP readings can be determined in sham-operated mice, which can serve as naïve controls.

Future IOP-related studies on operated mice can utilize the elevated IOP as a new baseline of OHT and permit testing of pharmacological compounds of different classes for their ability to lower and control IOPs in control and OHT mouse eyes over a period of time. Concentration- or dose-response studies of test agents can be performed on these mice when the peak IOPs have been attained. Similarly, AQH dynamics studies can be conducted on these mice with well-known and new ocular hypotensive compounds to determine the mechanism of action of IOP reduction by the compounds as previously described (Roy Chowdhury *et al.*, 2017).

Since the subsequent analysis of the retinas and optic nerves of the control mice and those with MMB-induced OHT is beyond the scope of this chapter, readers are encouraged to consult the original publications where the use of such techniques of raising IOPs and outcome measures determined have been reported (Bunker *et al.*, 2015; Ito *et al.*, 2016). A common feature of this MMB-induced OHT animal model is that raised IOP leads to a slow loss of RGCs during the first three weeks post-MMB injection. However, 3 weeks after the procedure, an accelerated and significant RGC loss and axon dropout can be expected. Thus, this means of OHT induction permits the determination of acutely and chronically (relatively speaking) elevated IOP (Fig. **1**) on the structure and function of retinal cells and the optic nerve.

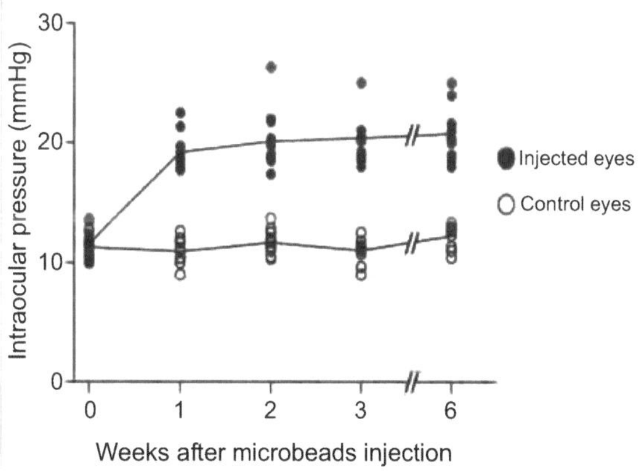

Fig. (1). Induction of OHT in mice using magnetic microbeads injected into the anterior chamber of the eye to block the AQH drainage *via* the trabecular meshwork and Schlemm's canal.

CONCLUSION

The procedures described above have endeavored to provide sufficient experimental details for researchers to conduct the studies to establish this animal model of OHT. However, readers are encouraged to check out the original publications where such methods were described, which are referenced below. Additional literature searches may also be beneficial in order to find suitable modifications or refinements to the procedures described herein. Additional modifications have included using hyaluronic acid to suspend and also deliver the microbeads to the anterior chamber of the eye.

CONFLICT OF INTEREST STATEMENT

The author declares that no conflict of interest exists. The sole aim of the chapter is to disseminate information and pass on knowledge to other researchers in the ocular field so that continuous progress can be made in finding suitable novel treatments for OHT and glaucoma.

ACKNOWLEDGEMENTS

The authors are grateful for having access to published and open-access material that permitted the writing of this set of protocols. The papers provided invaluable guidance and are appropriately acknowledged and cited herein.

REFERENCES

Bouhenni, RA, Dunmire, J, Sewell, A & Edward, DP (2012) Animal models of glaucoma. *J Biomed Biotechnol,* 2012, 692609.
[http://dx.doi.org/10.1155/2012/692609] [PMID: 22665989]

Bunker, S, Holeniewska, J, Vijay, S, Dahlmann-Noor, A, Khaw, P, Ng, YS, Shima, D & Foxton, R (2015) Experimental glaucoma induced by ocular injection of magnetic microspheres. *J Vis Exp,* 52400.
[http://dx.doi.org/10.3791/52400-v] [PMID: 25742031]

Cone, FE, Gelman, SE, Son, JL, Pease, ME & Quigley, HA (2010) Differential susceptibility to experimental glaucoma among 3 mouse strains using bead and viscoelastic injection. *Exp Eye Res,* 91, 415-24.
[http://dx.doi.org/10.1016/j.exer.2010.06.018] [PMID: 20599961]

Ito, YA, Belforte, N, Cueva Vargas, JL & Di Polo, A (2016) A magnetic microbead occlusion model to induce ocular hypertension-dependent glaucoma in mice. *J Vis Exp,* e53731, e53731.
[http://dx.doi.org/10.3791/53731-v] [PMID: 27077732]

Morrison, JC, Cepurna Ying Guo, WO & Johnson, EC (2011) Pathophysiology of human glaucomatous optic nerve damage: Insights from rodent models of glaucoma. *Exp Eye Res,* 93, 156-64.
[http://dx.doi.org/10.1016/j.exer.2010.08.005] [PMID: 20708000]

Roy Chowdhury, U, Rinkoski, TA, Bahler, CK, Millar, JC, Bertrand, JA, Holman, BH, Sherwood, JM, Overby, DR, Stoltz, KL, Dosa, PI & Fautsch, MP (2017) Effect of cromakalim prodrug 1 (CKLP1) on aqueous humor dynamics and feasibility of combination therapy with existing ocular hypotensive agents. *Invest Ophthalmol Vis Sci,* 58, 5731-42.
[http://dx.doi.org/10.1167/iovs.17-22538] [PMID: 29114841]

Samsel, PA, Kisiswa, L, Erichsen, JT, Cross, SD & Morgan, JE (2011) A novel method for the induction of experimental glaucoma using magnetic microspheres. *Invest Ophthalmol Vis Sci,* 52, 1671-5.
[http://dx.doi.org/10.1167/iovs.09-3921] [PMID: 20926815]

Sappington, RM, Carlson, BJ, Crish, SD & Calkins, DJ (2010) The microbead occlusion model: a paradigm for induced ocular hypertension in rats and mice. *Invest Ophthalmol Vis Sci,* 51, 207-16.
[http://dx.doi.org/10.1167/iovs.09-3947] [PMID: 19850836]

Sharif, NA (2018) iDrugs and iDevices discovery and development- preclinical assays, techniques and animal model studies for ocular hypotensives and neuroprotectants. *J Ocul Pharmacol Ther,* 34, 7-39.
[http://dx.doi.org/10.1089/jop.2017.0125] [PMID: 29323613]

Sharif, NA (2021) Therapeutic drugs and devices for tackling ocular hypertension and glaucoma, and need for neuroprotection and cytoprotective therapies. *Front Pharmacol,* 12, 729249. [http://dx.doi.org/10.3389/fphar.2021.729249] [PMID: 34603044]

Urcola, JH, Hernández, M & Vecino, E (2006) Three experimental glaucoma models in rats: Comparison of the effects of intraocular pressure elevation on retinal ganglion cell size and death. *Exp Eye Res,* 83, 429-37. [http://dx.doi.org/10.1016/j.exer.2006.01.025] [PMID: 16682027]

Weber, AJ & Zelenak, D (2001) Experimental glaucoma in the primate induced by latex microspheres. *J Neurosci Methods,* 111, 39-48. [http://dx.doi.org/10.1016/S0165-0270(01)00443-5] [PMID: 11574118]

CHAPTER 27

Protocol for the Rat Episcleral Vein Cauterization Model of OHT/Glaucoma

Anthonia Okolie[1], **Ya Fatou Njie Mbye**[1,*], **Fatima Muili**[1], **Catherine A. Opere**[2] and **Sunny E. Ohia**[1]

[1] *Department of Pharmaceutical Sciences, College of Pharmacy and Health Sciences, Texas Southern University, 3100 Cleburne Street, Houston, TX 77004, USA*

[2] *Department of Pharmacy Sciences, School of Pharmacy and Health Professions, Creighton University, Omaha, Nebraska, USA*

Abstract: Glaucoma caused by ocular hypertension (OHT) poses a grave health problem as our society's demographics tilt towards an ever-increasing aged population. In order to study this ocular disease, several different models of OHT involving a variety of different animal species have been developed over the years. In the current chapter, we will focus on a method to raise intraocular pressure (IOP) by cauterizing two or three trunks of episcleral veins in the eye of rats to induce OHT.

Keywords: Eye, Glaucoma, Intraocular pressure, Ocular hypertension, Protocol, Retina, Retinal ganglion cells, Tonometry, Uveitis.

INTRODUCTION

A rise in intraocular pressure (IOP) occurs when the balance between aqueous humor formation and outflow resistance is compromised, resulting in ocular hypertension (OHT). Long-term elevated eye pressure is a critical risk factor for glaucoma and the leading cause of blindness in the world (Jayanetti *et al.*, 2020). Glaucoma is a neurodegenerative disease that has hallmark features that involve loss of retinal ganglion cells (RGCs), thinning of the optic nerve, and the resultant visual field loss affecting mostly the peripheral vision at the beginning, which progressively worsens over time (Bai *et al.*, 2014). Over the last two decades, researchers have established and validated numerous animal models that mimic clinical features of OHT and glaucomatous optic neuropathy. Some examples include the hypertonic saline episcleral vein injection model (Mittag *et al.*, 2000),

* **Corresponding author Ya Fatou Njie Mbye:** Department of Pharmaceutical Sciences, College of Pharmacy and Health Sciences, Texas Southern University, 3100 Cleburne Street, Houston, TX 77004, USA;
E-mail: yafatou.mbye@tsu.edu

Najam A. Sharif and Sunny E. Ohia (Eds.)

the laser-induced OHT model (Fu *et al.*, 2010), the trabecular meshwork-occlusion with microspheres model (Sappington *et al.*, 2010), and spontaneous or genetically-created mouse glaucoma models (Harada *et al.*, 2019). The episcleral vein cauterization rat model of OHT involves obstructing two or three trunks of episcleral veins. This rat model of OHT is beginning to be utilized in OHT/glaucoma research since it is quite reproducible and relatively cheap. The purpose of this chapter is to provide a series of steps that can serve as a guide for researchers in the utilization of *in vivo* models of glaucoma in glaucoma research to help discover new etiological factors related to OHT/glaucoma development and for discovering new therapeutic modalities.

EXPERIMENTAL PROTOCOLS

The following procedure was adapted from methods similar to that of Shi *et al.* (2007) and Bai *et al.* (2014). The detailed protocol should be approved by and performed according to guidance provided by the Association for Research in Vision and Ophthalmology (ARVO) "Use of Animals in Ophthalmic and Vision Research" and the Institutional Animal Care and Use Committee (IACUC).

Preparation of the Animals

- Female Wistar Hannover rats (225-250 gm) should be kept in a 12-hour dark-light cycle paradigm and provided food and water ad libitum.
- Use a cocktail of ketamine, xylazine, and acepromazine (injected intraperitoneally at a dose ratio of 50/5/1 mg/kg) to deeply anesthetize the rats on the day of the surgery.

Induction of OHT / Glaucoma

- In the anesthetized rats, make an incision in the conjunctiva followed by isolation of extra-ocular muscles and identification of major limbal drainage veins.
- Cauterize two dorsal episcleral veins and one temporal episcleral vein using a 30″ cautery tip.
- Observe the morphology of the episcleral veins before and after cauterization to ensure no bleeding is present. Use a small amount of a broad topical antibiotic ointment to prevent any future infection.
- Use the contralateral eye with sham surgery as a control.

IOP Measurement

- For IOP measurement, anesthetize the treated rats using light anesthesia consisting of oxygen and a 3% isoflurane mixture (1 liter/min).

- Measure and record the IOPs using a Tono-Pen-XL Applanation tonometer per the manufacturer's instructions.
- Take baseline measurements immediately after cauterization and then every week after the surgery until the rats are sacrificed.
- Each measurement should be repeated at least 3 times, recorded, and later averaged for each time point. IOP readings should be performed at the same time every day or every week as deemed fit.
- The effect of test drugs topically applied to the eye can be determined when the IOP has reached maximum levels. Again, multiple readings should be taken post-drug application over time to determine the time course of IOP changes in the absence and presence of the test compound.

Retinal Thickness Measurements

- Under full anesthesia, apply a topical pupil dilation solution (atropine sulfate 1%, Alcon, USA) to the cornea/conjunctiva.
- Acquire images of retinas from experimental rats using a non-invasive prototype optical coherence tomography (OCT) system.
- Scan 2-4-volumes in each eye in different quadrants of the retina.
- For each volume, take six high-quality frames and take four measurements in one frame adjacent to 1 mm from the optic nerve head.
- Average the four recordings as the thickness of each frame.
- The OCT measurements need to be performed before and after the cauterization procedure to detect changes in the retinal thickness.

Retinal Function Determination

- Following 15 hours of adaptation following the vein cauterization surgery, rats should be anesthetized and kept under dim red illumination light ($\lambda > 600$ nm).
- Now, dilate the pupil using topical atropine treatment.
- Place the gold ring electrode of the electroretinogram (ERG) system over the central part of the corneal surface.
- Place a reference electrode and a ground electrode onto the ear and in the tail, respectively.
- Now, take ERG measurements simultaneously from both eyes. Later, using a photic stimulator (Ganzfeld Q400, USA), record at least 10 retinal responses to flashes of unattenuated white light (5 ms, 0.2 Hz).

CONCLUSION

The rat episcleral cauterization protocol described herein has been developed and validated in several studies. It is a fairly cheap, reproducible, and reliable animal model of OHT, which can be an asset for studying factors involved in

OHT/glaucoma and can be utilized to find and help develop new therapeutic drugs to lower and control IOP.

REFERENCES

Bai, Y, Zhu, Y, Chen, Q, Xu, J, Sarunic, MV, Saragovi, UH & Zhuo, Y (2014) Validation of glaucoma-like features in the rat episcleral vein cauterization model. *Chin Med J (Engl),* 127, 359-64.
[http://dx.doi.org/10.3760/cma.j.issn.0366-6999.20132398] [PMID: 24438629]

Fu, CT & Sretavan, D (2010) Laser-induced ocular hypertension in albino CD-1 mice. *Invest Ophthalmol Vis Sci,* 51, 980-90.
[http://dx.doi.org/10.1167/iovs.09-4324] [PMID: 19815738]

Harada, C, Kimura, A, Guo, X, Namekata, K & Harada, T (2019) Recent advances in genetically modified animal models of glaucoma and their roles in drug repositioning. *Br J Ophthalmol,* 103, 161-6.
[http://dx.doi.org/10.1136/bjophthalmol-2018-312724] [PMID: 30366949]

Jayanetti, V, Sandhu, S & Lusthaus, JA (2020) The latest drugs in development that reduce intraocular pressure in ocular hypertension and glaucoma. *J Exp Pharmacol,* 12, 539-48.
[http://dx.doi.org/10.2147/JEP.S281187] [PMID: 33244278]

Mittag, TW, Danias, J, Pohorenec, G, Yuan, HM, Burakgazi, E, Chalmers-Redman, R, Podos, SM & Tatton, WG (2000) Retinal damage after 3 to 4 months of elevated intraocular pressure in a rat glaucoma model. *Invest Ophthalmol Vis Sci,* 41, 3451-9.
[PMID: 11006238]

Sappington, RM, Carlson, BJ, Crish, SD & Calkins, DJ (2010) The microbead occlusion model: a paradigm for induced ocular hypertension in rats and mice. *Invest Ophthalmol Vis Sci,* 51, 207-16.
[http://dx.doi.org/10.1167/iovs.09-3947] [PMID: 19850836]

Shi, Z, Birman, E & Saragovi, HU (2007) Neurotrophic rationale in glaucoma: A TrkA agonist, but not NGF or a p75 antagonist, protects retinal ganglion cells *in vivo. Dev Neurobiol,* 67, 884-94.
[http://dx.doi.org/10.1002/dneu.20360] [PMID: 17506493]

CHAPTER 28

Protocol for Silicone Oil-Induced Ocular Hypertension

Alyssa Hostert[1], **Sunny E. Ohia**[2], **Ya Fatou Njie Mbye**[2] and **Catherine A. Opere**[1,*]

[1] *Department of Pharmacy Sciences, School of Pharmacy and Health Professions, Creighton University, Omaha, Nebraska, USA*

[2] *Department of Pharmaceutical Sciences, College of Pharmacy and Health Sciences, Texas Southern University, Houston, Texas, USA*

Abstract: This chapter describes the protocols to induce ocular hypertension in rabbits using silicone oil. This process consists of many steps and sub-steps, including preparation of the animal for anesthesia, preparation of materials, administration of anesthesia, preparation for silicone oil (SO) injection, intracameral injection of SO, and finally, postoperative care. Healthy animals free of ocular morphological abnormalities or disease states should be chosen for inclusion before beginning the protocol. Following these steps will allow for the simulation of ocular hypertension while also ensuring an aseptic environment.

Keywords: Eye, Glaucoma, Intraocular pressure, Ocular hypertension, Protocol, Retinal ganglion cells, Silicone oil.

INTRODUCTION

Changes to aqueous humor (AH) flow can have a significant impact on visual acuity in both humans and animals. In the normal function of the eye, AH must flow through the anterior chamber to drain through the trabecular meshwork (TM); however, if this pathway is altered, pressure differentials can occur (Zhang *et al.*, 2019). If AH outflow through the TM is excessive, this can cause intraocular pressure (IOP) to decrease, and uveitis may occur. Conversely, if AH outflow is obstructed, IOP may increase, potentially leading to glaucoma and damage to the retinal ganglion cells (RCGs) (Zhang *et al.*, 2019; Ofri, 2020).

* **Corresponding author Catherine A. Opere:** Department of Pharmacy Sciences, School of Pharmacy and Health Professions, Creighton University, Omaha, Nebraska, USA; Tel: +402-280-3726; Fax: 402-280-1883; E-mail: copere@creighton.edu

Najam A. Sharif and Sunny E. Ohia (Eds.)

Animal models can be useful not only for understanding the pathophysiology of naturally occurring ocular disease but also for presenting models of disease that may be modified by researchers to create targeted drug therapies. One such animal model is the rabbit. At a comfortable baseline, rabbits typically produce IOP values in the range of 15-23 mm Hg (Vareilles *et al.*, 1977). Instead of waiting years for the possible occurrence of natural glaucoma in these animals, it is possible to simulate glaucoma using an intracameral injection of silicone oil (SO) (Zhang *et al.*, 2019). The purpose of this chapter is to describe a veterinary protocol for the artificial induction of ocular hypertension in rabbits. This will allow researchers to simulate the glaucomatous disease state so that they may evaluate new drug therapies for those afflicted.

EXPERIMENTAL PROTOCOLS

The following procedure should be performed in accordance with the Statement for the Use of Animals in Ophthalmic and Vision Research from the Association for Research in Vision and Ophthalmology (ARVO).

All testing should be performed on healthy rabbits. Those with a history of prior ocular disorders or morphological changes to the cornea should be excluded from this study.

Preparation of the Animal for Anesthesia

NOTE: There is no need for the animals to be placed on a fast before surgery, as rabbits are unable to vomit (Horn *et al.*, 2013).

- Using a scale, obtain an accurate weight in kilograms for the rabbit.
- Place the rabbit gently on a heating pad on top of the examination table.
- Gently restrain the rabbit by wrapping it in a towel.
- Shave a small area on the back of the rabbit's neck to prepare for subcutaneous injection.

Preparation of Materials

- Attach a sterile 25 G needle to a sterile plastic 3 mL Luer Lock syringe. Ensure that the needle is screwed on tightly.
- Use a 70% alcohol wipe to sterilize the injection site of a vial of 100 mg/mL ketamine before withdrawing a dose of 10 mg/kg body weight using the syringe prepared.
- Use a 70% alcohol wipe to sterilize the injection site of a vial of 20 mg/mL xylazine before withdrawing a dose of 2 mg/kg body weight using the syringe prepared above.
- Attach a sterile 25 G, 0.5-inch needle to a plastic 1 mL Luer Lock syringe.

Ensure that the needle is screwed on tightly and that the plunger is fully depressed.

- Use a 70% alcohol wipe to sterilize the injection site of a vial of 1,000 centistokes silicone oil (SILIKON®) before using the syringe as above to withdraw 1 mL of silicone oil.
- Prepare a dilute solution (1:50 in sterile normal saline) of betadine (Povidone-Iodine 10%) for pre-surgical irrigation of the eye.

Administration of Anesthesia

- Apply lidocaine cream topically to the area to be injected and wait for a few minutes before administering the anesthetic injection.
- Use a 70% alcohol wipe to sterilize the shaved portion of the rabbit's neck. Allow the alcohol to dry before injection.
- Using the thumb and forefinger of one hand, pinch the shaved skin on the back of the rabbit's neck and pull it away from the body.
- Insert the needle of the syringe containing ketamine into the pinched skin at a 45-degree angle and depress the plunger completely.
- Discard the used syringe and needle in a Sharps container.
- Repeat steps for the xylazine syringe.
- As sedation sets in, place the animal on heat support and maintain ½" of padding/material between the animal and the heat source.
- About 7-10 minutes following injection of anesthetic agents, place a face mask on the rabbit to administer oxygen mixed with 1% isoflurane initially. Isoflurane concentration may be increased up to 5% to maintain sedation.
- Pinch the rabbit's toe to monitor for degree of sedation and to determine if an additional sedation is required. If no whisker or tail movement is noted, sedation is sufficient.

NOTE: Once anesthesia has been administered, monitor the rabbit's heart rate, respiratory rate, and temperature continuously or every 5 minutes as resources allow.

Preparation for SO Administration

- While on the heat support/padding, place the rabbit on one side, in a lateral recumbent position, with the desired eye facing upward.
- Use two fingers of one hand to hold open the eye planned for injection.
- Using the other hand, irrigate animal eyes with 1:50 betadine/sterile water or sterile saline solution.
- Then, with the same hand, instill one drop of 0.5% proparacaine hydrochloride into the eye to coat the cornea.
- Wait 1-2 minutes to allow for absorption of proparacaine.

SO Intracameral Injection

- Insert the syringe containing silicone oil into the supertemporal quadrant of the cornea, approximately 1-2 mm from the limbus.
- With the needle's bevel facing down, depress the plunger until the silicone oil appears to cover approximately 75% of the anterior chamber when looking at the iris (approximately 0.1 mL).

NOTE: If higher volumes of silicone oil are desired, a sterile 25 G to 30 G needle and 1 mL syringe may first be used to aspirate the quantity of AH from the anterior chamber, which corresponds to the amount of SO to be added (Zhang *et al.*, 2019).

- After injecting the desired volume of SO, keep the needle in the injection site for about 10 seconds before slowly removing it, using caution to not touch the lens or iris.
- Discard the used syringe and needle in a Sharps container.
- Gently press on the rabbit's upper eyelid to ensure proper closure of the injection site.
- Apply one drop of 0.3% ofloxacin ophthalmic solution to the eye. Wait approximately 5 minutes before the next antibiotic administration.
- Apply a ribbon of neomycin/polymyxin/bacitracin ointment to the cul de sac of the eye.
- Remove the face mask from the rabbit to discontinue isoflurane.

Postoperative Care

- Monitor heart rate, respiratory rate, and temperature every 5 minutes for 15 minutes after the discontinuation of anesthesia.
- After 15 minutes, monitor heart rate, respiratory rate, and temperature every 10 minutes until the animal is awake and grooming.
- Do not take IOP readings for at least 48 hours to allow the eye to recover from the injection. Continue to apply antibiotics and artificial tears for lubrication.

CONCLUSION

The protocol described here is written to be sufficient for anyone in possession of the proper resources to be able to perform this procedure to simulate OHT/ glaucoma in rabbits for research purposes. Reversal of SO-induced glaucoma, as well as an exhaustive list of animal-handling procedures, is outside the scope of this protocol, and additional research would be needed for these purposes.

REFERENCES

Greenfield, EA (2018) Administering Anesthesia to Rabbits. *Cold Spring Harb Protoc,* 2018, pdb.prot100206.
[http://dx.doi.org/10.1101/pdb.prot100206] [PMID: 30181226]

Greenfield, EA (2018) Routes of Antigen Injection in Rabbits. *Cold Spring Harb Protoc,* 2018, pdb.prot100222.
[http://dx.doi.org/10.1101/pdb.prot100222] [PMID: 30181227]

Henke, J, Astner, S, Brill, T, Eissner, B, Busch, R & Erhardt, W (2005) Comparative study of three intramuscular anaesthetic combinations (medetomidine/ketamine, medetomidine/fentanyl/midazolam and xylazine/ketamine) in rabbits. *Vet Anaesth Analg,* 32, 261-70.
[http://dx.doi.org/10.1111/j.1467-2995.2005.00242.x] [PMID: 16135207]

Horn, CC, Kimball, BA, Wang, H, Kaus, J, Dienel, S, Nagy, A, Gathright, GR, Yates, BJ & Andrews, PLR (2013) Why can't rodents vomit? A comparative behavioral, anatomical, and physiological study. *PLoS One,* 8, e60537.
[http://dx.doi.org/10.1371/journal.pone.0060537] [PMID: 23593236]

Kiliç, N (2004) A comparison between medetomidine-ketamine and xylazine-ketamine anaesthesia in rabbits. *Turk J Vet Anim Sci,* 28, 921-6.

Thomas, BS, Bhat, KM & Mapara, M (2012) Rabbit as an animal model for experimental research. *Dent Res J (Isfahan),* 9, 111-8.
[http://dx.doi.org/10.4103/1735-3327.92960] [PMID: 22363373]

Nakamura, K, Refojo, MF, Crabtree, DV, Pastor, J & Leong, FL (1991) Ocular toxicity of low-molecula--weight components of silicone and fluorosilicone oils. *Invest Ophthalmol Vis Sci,* 32, 3007-20.
[PMID: 1938278]

Norman, BC, Oliver, J, Cheeks, L, Hull, DS, Birnbaum, D & Green, K (1990) Corneal endothelial permeability after anterior chamber silicone oil. *Ophthalmology,* 97, 1671-7.
[http://dx.doi.org/10.1016/S0161-6420(90)32374-6] [PMID: 1708117]

Ofri, R (2020) An overview of canine glaucoma. *Dvm360,* 52.

Ohira, A, Chihara, E & Soji, T (1994) Egress route of emulsified 20 centistokes silicone oil from anterior chamber of rabbit. *Curr Eye Res,* 13, 489-95.
[http://dx.doi.org/10.3109/02713689408999880] [PMID: 7924413]

Papp, A, Kiss, EB, Tímár, Ö, Szabó, E, Berecki, Á, Tóth, J & Páli, J (2007) Long-term exposure of the rabbit eye to silicone oil causes optic nerve atrophy. *Brain Res Bull,* 74, 130-3.
[http://dx.doi.org/10.1016/j.brainresbull.2007.06.002] [PMID: 17683798]

Sternberg, P, Jr, Hatchell, DL, Foulks, GN & Landers, MB, III (1985) The effect of silicone oil on the cornea. *Arch Ophthalmol,* 103, 90-4.
[http://dx.doi.org/10.1001/archopht.1985.01050010096027] [PMID: 3977681]

Vareilles, P, Conquet, P & Le Douarec, JC (1977) A method for the routine intraocular pressure (IOP) measurement in the rabbit: Range of IOP variations in this species. *Exp Eye Res,* 24, 369-75.
[http://dx.doi.org/10.1016/0014-4835(77)90149-X] [PMID: 858319]

Zhang, J, Fang, F, Li, L, Huang, H, Webber, HC, Sun, Y, Mahajan, VB & Hu, Y (2019) A reversible silicon oil-induced ocular hypertension model in mice. *J Vis Exp,* e60409.
[http://dx.doi.org/10.3791/60409-v] [PMID: 31789319]

CHAPTER 29

Protocol for Inducing Ocular Hypertension in Rats and Mice Using Circumlimbal Sutures

Da Zhao[1], Zheng He[1], Pei Ying Lee[1], Brianna Caroline Afiat[1], Anna Van Koeverden[1], Vickie Hoi Ying Wong[1], Christine Tram Oanh Nguyen[1] and **Bang Viet Bui[1,*]**

[1] *Department of Optometry & Vision, 202 Berkeley St, Parkville, The University of Melbourne, Victoria 3010, Australia*

Abstract: The circumlimbal suture technique for inducing experimental ocular hypertension (OHT) in rodents can be utilized to achieve chronic intraocular pressure (IOP) elevation, however, it is fully reversible. This protocol provides guidance for the application and adjustments of the suturing approach for both rats and mice. In brief, by placing the animals under general anesthesia, a "purse-string" suture is threaded through and anchored to the conjunctiva around the equator, behind and parallel to the eyeball limbus. Using this procedure, moderate levels of IOP increases can be achieved over a 12-week time period. This protocol can induce retinal dysfunctions, specifically both structural and functional, commensurate with retinal ganglion cell demise and optic nerve damage. Removal of the suture and restoration of IOP back to baseline levels afford functional recovery when the intervention is early. This circumlimbal suture procedure is a minimally invasive and cost-effective means to induce OHT that reliably results in RGC and optic nerve injury in rodents. The effects of potential IOP-lowering and neuroprotectants can be assessed in this novel animal model of OHT.

Keywords: Circumlimbal suture, Eye, Glaucoma, Intraocular pressure, Ocular hypertension, Optic nerve, Protocol, Retinal ganglion cells.

INTRODUCTION

Development and validation of suitable animal models are important to study neurodegeneration due to ocular hypertension (OHT)/glaucoma. Many inducible models have been established to produce long-term increases in intraocular pressure (IOP), the most important risk factor for the development of glaucoma. These approaches induce OHT (Bunker *et al.* 2015; Chiu *et al.* 2007; Feng *et al.* 2013; Moreno *et al.* 2005; Morrison *et al.* 1997; Quigley and Addicks 1980;

* **Corresponding author Bang V Bui:** Department of Optometry & Vision, 202 Berkeley St, Parkville, The University of Melbourne, Victoria 3010, Australia; Tel: +61 3 83447006; E-mail: bvb@unimelb.edu.au

Najam A. Sharif and Sunny E. Ohia (Eds.)

Weber and Zelenack 2001), with the goal of recapitulating specific and progressive injury to retinal ganglion cells (RGCs), with minimal complications such as trauma and inflammation.

In this chapter, we describe a step-by-step protocol for inducing chronic IOP elevation in rats (Lakshmanan *et al.* 2020; Liu *et al.* 2015) and mice (Zhao *et al.* 2017a) using a circumlimbal suture, which increases episcleral venous pressure (Wong *et al.* 2021) resulting in sustained IOP elevation. One important feature of this model is the reversibility of the IOP to baseline by simply removing the suture. IOP normalization may be useful for studying the cellular and molecular correlates of reversible and irreversible RGC injury (Liu *et al.* 2017; Zhao *et al.* 2019).

EXPERIMENTAL PROTOCOLS

All experimental procedures were conducted according to the Australian Code of Practice for the Care and Use of Animals for Scientific Purposes, set by the National Health and Medical Research Council in Australia, as well as the Statement for the Use of Animals in Ophthalmic and Vision Research from the Association for Research in Vision and Ophthalmology (ARVO).

Intraocular Pressure Measurement in Conscious Rodents

Note: To obtain robust baseline IOP, measurements can be undertaken for several days (*e.g.*, 3 -5 days) prior to surgery to acclimatize animals to the procedure. Measurements can be taken using a calibrated rebound tonometer with or without a topical drop of proparacaine hydrochloride. For longitudinal monitoring, the IOP should be measured at about the same time of day and under the same lighting conditions for consistency (Aihara *et al.*, 2003; Jia *et al.*, 2000).

- Set the rebound tonometer to the correct calibration (rat or mice) as per the manufacturer's instructions.
- For ease of handling of rats, try to wrap the awake rat in a soft cloth and use gentle rocking motion to calm the animal. Gently expose the head and neck and carefully hold the torso in one hand, with the rat's back resting against the researcher's chest.
- For mice, hold the animal by the scruff of the neck and hold the tail between the ring finger and middle finger (or between the little finger and your palm). Avoid too much pressure on the skin so that little impact occurs on the eyes and potential suffocation is prevented.
- When using a rebound tonometer, use the other hand to align the tonometer so that the tip of the IOP probe is approximately 2 – 3 mm away from and perpen-

dicular to the corneal apex. Press the measurement button whilst ensuring that the tip of the probe contacts the corneal apex.

Note: A single beep of the tonometer confirms successful measurement, which can be read from the LCD screen. A measurement error is indicated by a dual beep. Such errors arise due to many factors, including excessive tilt, incorrect working distance, the probe striking the periphery of the cornea, and the touching of eyelashes or eyelids. Careful reading and executing the guidelines for the use of the rebound tonometer should reduce the potential measurement errors.

- Record individual reading for each of ten repeats, each at an interval of 1 – 2 seconds. Reset the tonometer after the 5th reading.

Note: If possible have another investigator take the IOP readings to ensure correct reproducible data are collected.

Induction of Intraocular Pressure Elevation in Anesthetized Rodents

- Autoclave all surgical equipment beforehand.
- Clean the surgical bench with disinfectant (*e.g.*, 0.5% chlorhexidine in 70% ethanol).
- Use sterile drapes to cover the bench.
- Appropriate personal protective equipment should be worn by all research staff (*e.g.*, sterilized gloves, gowns, and masks).
- Anaesthetize animals with 3 – 3.5% isoflurane with O_2 at a flow rate of 3 L/min (flow rate is usually the same as the size of the induction container) and then maintain using 1.5% isoflurane at 0.5 - 1 L/min. Place the animal on a heat pad to maintain body temperature during surgery. Adjust the isoflurane level to ensure sufficient surgical plane of anesthesia. Monitor and adjust the flow of the anesthetic to obtain about 60 breaths/min breathing rate.
- Now, select one eye and lightly numb the cornea with a drop of 0.5% proxymetacaine ophthalmic solution.
- Use sterile surgical drapes to cover the animal while leaving the treated eye exposed. To prevent desiccation of the other eye, place some lubricating gel on it.
- Under a microscope, weave a 7/0 nylon suture under (5 – 6 anchor points in rats; 4 – 5 anchor points in mice) and above the conjunctiva parallel and 2 mm posterior to the limbus (Fig. **1**). For mice, use a 10/0 nylon suture at 1 mm posterior to the limbus, avoiding penetration of the sclera. It is critical that compression of the major episcleral veins be avoided by threading the suture underneath the conjunctiva at the crossing of these veins. The episcleral veins are hard to distinguish/see in mice; thus, avoiding them may be somewhat difficult.

- Now, tie a slipknot followed by a second simple knot in order to fasten the purse-string suture (see Fig. **1**). In order to prevent a high post-surgical IOP spike, measure the IOP before completing the second knot. The tension of the slip knot at one end of the suture should be adjusted to achieve the desired IOP (see arrow in Fig. **1**A). When the needed IOP is obtained (30 – 40 mmHg in mice; 30 – 60 mmHg in rats), tying off the second knot can be performed while maintaining a continuous force on that end of the suture (see arrow in Fig. **1**A). The IOP should be measured again for confirmation. To prevent possible foreign body sensation, the ends of the suture should be trimmed and discarded after the second knot has been tightened.
- Treat the sutured eye with an antibiotic eye drop to minimize the risk of infection.
- Allow the animals to rest on the heat pad and periodically monitor them while they recover from the anesthetic.

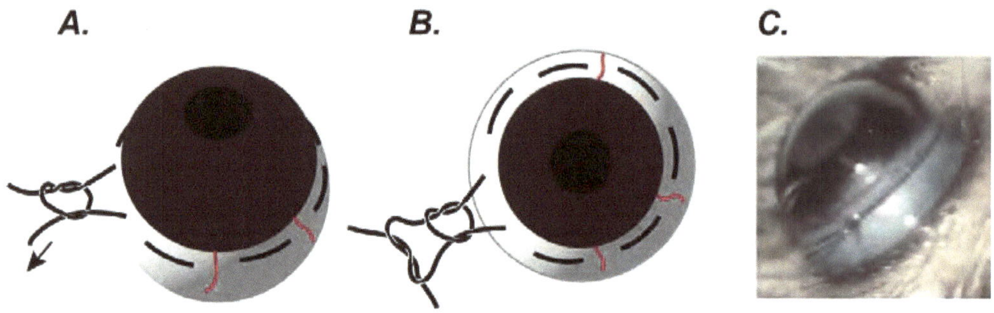

Fig. (1). Circumlimbal suture application to induce ocular hypertension. A: First, use a slipknot to gradually tighten the purse-string suture by pulling only one side (arrow) while ensuring adequate inward compression is maintained. IOP should be determined before fastening the second knot in order to achieve the desired target IOP. **B**: A second simple knot should be employed in order to lock the first knot. **C**: The final circumlimbal suture on a mouse eye is shown. (Schematic representation in **A** and **B** are re-used with permission from our previously published work, see references (Van Koeverden *et al.* 2018) and (Zhao *et al.* 2017b), respectively).

Monitoring IOP

- Measure the first IOP 2 minutes post-operatively. Monitor the IOP the next day and at least once a week or more frequently as deemed necessary. Randomize the IOP measurements in the treated and untreated contralateral eyes.

Restoring IOP Back to Baseline

- Use the procedure described above to anesthetize the animal and ensure that the body temperature is maintained using a heat pad.
- Numb the cornea with one drop of 0.5% proxymetacaine ophthalmic solution and use sterile saline to clean the eye if needed.

- Now, cut the suture, gently work through the conjunctiva, and draw away from the eye.

Note: In some cases, the knot of the suture will be embedded underneath the conjunctiva, especially when the suture is implanted for longer than 4 weeks. Make a small incision at the conjunctiva to allow suture removal.

- Treat the sutured eye with an antibiotic eye drop to minimize the risk of infection.
- Typical IOP data are shown in Fig. **2** below.

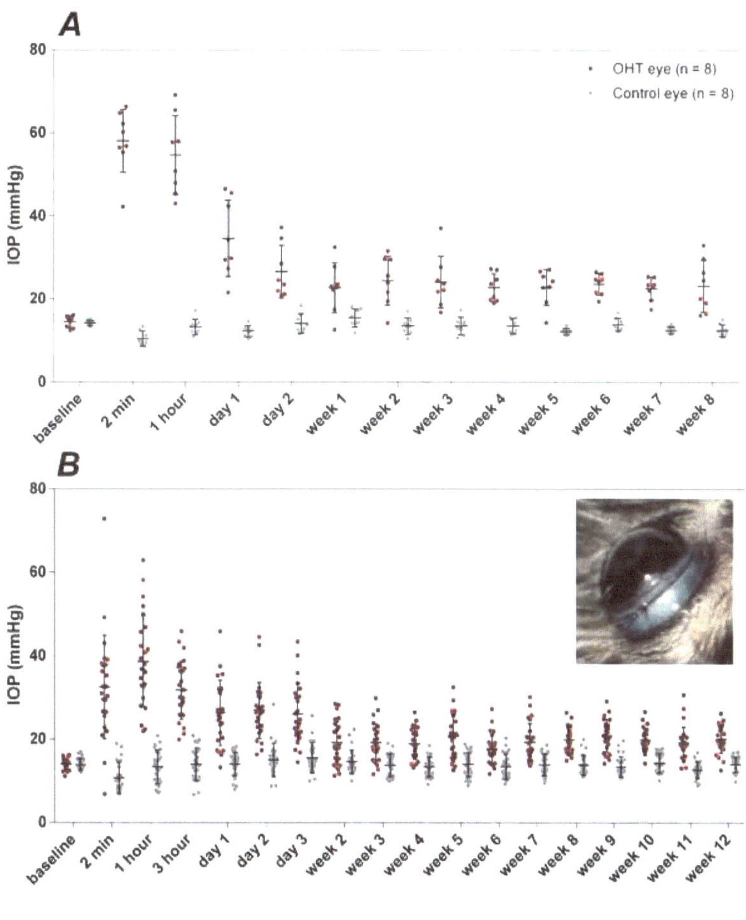

Fig. (2). Circumlimbal suture-induced IOP elevation over an 8-week period in rats (A, n = 8) and 12 weeks in mice (B, n = 23). IOP was elevated in OHT eyes [red] but remained unchanged in contralateral control eyes [grey]. Average and standard deviations are overlaid in black. Data are replotted with permission from our previous published work (Van Koeverden *et al.* 2018; Zhao *et al.* 2017b).

CONCLUSION

Whilst the protocol described above is known to work well in Long Evans rats and C57BL/6 mice, the effectiveness of the procedure may vary based on the strain of the animals. Researchers are encouraged to read additional literature (Kim *et al.* 2021; Lakshmanan *et al.* 2020; Lee *et al.* 2021; Lee *et al.* 2022) to find suitable modifications or refinements to the procedures described above that are suited to specific animal strain and study design. For example, to avoid the initial IOP spike over the first few days, a modification introduced by Mathew *et al.* (2021) can produce a more gradual level of IOP elevation.

REFERENCES

Aihara, M, Lindsey, JD & Weinreb, RN (2003) Twenty-four-hour pattern of mouse intraocular pressure. *Exp Eye Res,* 77, 681-6.
[http://dx.doi.org/10.1016/j.exer.2003.08.011] [PMID: 14609556]

Bunker, S, Holeniewska, J, Vijay, S, Dahlmann-Noor, A, Khaw, P, Ng, YS, Shima, D & Foxton, R (2015) Experimental glaucoma induced by ocular injection of magnetic microspheres. *J Vis Exp,* 52400.
[http://dx.doi.org/10.3791/52400-v] [PMID: 25742031]

Chiu, K, Chang, R & So, KF (2007) Laser-induced chronic ocular hypertension model on SD rats. *J Vis Exp,* 10, 549.
[http://dx.doi.org/10.3791/549-v] [PMID: 18989402]

Feng, L, Chen, H, Suyeoka, G & Liu, X (2013) A laser-induced mouse model of chronic ocular hypertension to characterize visual defects. *J Vis Exp,* 14, 50440.
[http://dx.doi.org/10.3791/50440-v] [PMID: 23979255]

He, Z, Zhao, D, van Koeverden, AK, Nguyen, CT, Lim, JKH, Wong, VHY, Vingrys, AJ & Bui, BV (2018) A Model of Glaucoma Induced by Circumlimbal Suture in Rats and Mice. *J Vis Exp,* 5, 58287.
[http://dx.doi.org/10.3791/58287-v] [PMID: 30346390]

Jia, L, Cepurna, WO, Johnson, EC & Morrison, JC (2000) Patterns of intraocular pressure elevation after aqueous humor outflow obstruction in rats. *Invest Ophthalmol Vis Sci,* 41, 1380-5.
[PMID: 10798653]

Kim, ML, Sung, K, Kwon, J, Choi, G & Shin, JA (2021) Neuroprotective Effect of Statins in a Rat Model of Chronic Ocular Hypertension. *Int J Mol Sci,* 22, 12500.
[http://dx.doi.org/10.3390/ijms222212500] [PMID: 34830387]

Lakshmanan, Y, Wong, FSY, Zuo, B, Bui, BV & Chan, HHL (2020) Longitudinal outcomes of circumlimbal suture model-induced chronic ocular hypertension in Sprague-Dawley albino rats. *Graefes Arch Clin Exp Ophthalmol,* 258, 2715-28.
[http://dx.doi.org/10.1007/s00417-020-04820-7] [PMID: 32623578]

Lee, KM, Song, DY & Kim, SH (2022) Effect of Strain on Rodent Glaucoma Models: Magnetic Bead Injection Versus Hydrogel Injection Versus Circumlimbal Suture. *Transl Vis Sci Technol,* 11, 31.
[http://dx.doi.org/10.1167/tvst.11.9.31] [PMID: 36173647]

Lee, SH, Shim, KS, Kim, CY & Park, TK (2021) Characterization of the role of autophagy in retinal ganglion cell survival over time using a rat model of chronic ocular hypertension. *Sci Rep,* 11, 5767.
[http://dx.doi.org/10.1038/s41598-021-85181-x] [PMID: 33707562]

Liu, HH, Bui, BV, Nguyen, CTO, Kezic, JM, Vingrys, AJ & He, Z (2015) Chronic ocular hypertension induced by circumlimbal suture in rats. *Invest Ophthalmol Vis Sci,* 56, 2811-20.
[http://dx.doi.org/10.1167/iovs.14-16009] [PMID: 25829414]

Liu, HH, He, Z, Nguyen, CTO, Vingrys, AJ & Bui, BV (2017) Reversal of functional loss in a rat model of chronic intraocular pressure elevation. *Ophthalmic Physiol Opt,* 37, 71-81.
[http://dx.doi.org/10.1111/opo.12331] [PMID: 27774623]

Mathew, DJ, Livne-Bar, I & Sivak, JM (2021) An inducible rodent glaucoma model that exhibits gradual sustained increase in intraocular pressure with distinct inner retina and optic nerve inflammation. *Sci Rep,* 11, 22880.
[http://dx.doi.org/10.1038/s41598-021-02057-w] [PMID: 34819548]

Moreno, MC, Marcos, HJA, Oscar Croxatto, J, Sande, PH, Campanelli, J, Jaliffa, CO, Benozzi, J & Rosenstein, RE (2005) A new experimental model of glaucoma in rats through intracameral injections of hyaluronic acid. *Exp Eye Res,* 81, 71-80.
[http://dx.doi.org/10.1016/j.exer.2005.01.008] [PMID: 15978257]

Morrison, JC, Moore, CG, Deppmeier, LMH, Gold, BG, Meshul, CK & Johnson, EC (1997) A rat model of chronic pressure-induced optic nerve damage. *Exp Eye Res,* 64, 85-96.
[http://dx.doi.org/10.1006/exer.1996.0184] [PMID: 9093024]

Quigley, HA & Addicks, EM (1980) Chronic experimental glaucoma in primates. I. Production of elevated intraocular pressure by anterior chamber injection of autologous ghost red blood cells. *Invest Ophthalmol Vis Sci,* 19, 126-36.
[PMID: 6766124]

Van Koeverden, AK, He, Z, Nguyen, CT, Vingrys, AJ & Bui, BV Systemic hypertension is not protective against chronic IOP elevation in a rodent model. *Sci Rep* In press

Weber, AJ & Zelenak, D (2001) Experimental glaucoma in the primate induced by latex microspheres. *J Neurosci Methods,* 111, 39-48.
[http://dx.doi.org/10.1016/S0165-0270(01)00443-5] [PMID: 11574118]

Wong, VHY, Zhao, D, Bui, BV, Millar, CJ & Nguyen, CTO (2021) Increased episcleral venous pressure in a mouse model of circumlimbal suture induced ocular hypertension. *Exp Eye Res,* 202, 108348.
[http://dx.doi.org/10.1016/j.exer.2020.108348] [PMID: 33166503]

Zhao, D, Nguyen, CTO, Wong, VHY, Lim, JKH, He, Z, Jobling, AI, Fletcher, EL, Chinnery, HR, Vingrys, AJ & Bui, BV (2017) Characterization of the Circumlimbal Suture Model of Chronic IOP Elevation in Mice and Assessment of Changes in Gene Expression of Stretch Sensitive Channels. *Front Neurosci,* 11, 41. a
[http://dx.doi.org/10.3389/fnins.2017.00041] [PMID: 28239332]

Zhao, D, Nguyen, CTO, Wong, VHY, Lim, JKH, He, Z, Jobling, AI, Fletcher, EL, Chinnery, HR, Vingrys, AJ & Bui, BV (2017) Characterization of the Circumlimbal Suture Model of Chronic IOP Elevation in Mice and Assessment of Changes in Gene Expression of Stretch Sensitive Channels. *Front Neurosci,* 11, 41. b
[http://dx.doi.org/10.3389/fnins.2017.00041] [PMID: 28239332]

Zhao, D, Wong, VHY, Nguyen, CTO, Jobling, AI, Fletcher, EL, Vingrys, AJ & Bui, BV (2019) Reversibility of Retinal Ganglion Cell Dysfunction From Chronic IOP Elevation. *Invest Ophthalmol Vis Sci,* 60, 3878-86.
[http://dx.doi.org/10.1167/iovs.19-27113] [PMID: 31529082]

CHAPTER 30

Protocol for Corticosteroid-Induced Ocular Hypertension and Glaucomatous Optic Neuropathy in Rodents

Najam A. Sharif[1,*] and **Saima Chaudhry**[2]

[1] *Vice President and Head of Research & Development Nanoscope Therapeutics Inc., 2777 N. Stemmons Fwy, Suite 1102, Dallas, TX-75207, USA*

[2] *Univ N. Texas at Arlington, 701 S Nedderman Dr, Arlington, TX-76019, USA*

Abstract: Many forms of glaucoma afflict patients around the world and rob them of their eyesight. Secondary glaucoma is induced by many factors, such as trauma to the eye, injury-induced inflammation, pathogen-induced inflammation, and drug-induced pathology of the major aqueous humor outflow system, the trabecular meshwork. When patients experience inflammation and irritation on the ocular surface or within the anterior chamber of the eye (*e.g.*, uveitis), they are prescribed topical ocular formulation of corticosteroid (*e.g.*, dexamethasone) and perhaps also oral anti-inflammatory steroids to reduce the symptoms and calm down the eye. However, a major side effect of such corticosteroid treatment is the development of secondary glaucoma in at least 30% of the population who are susceptible to steroids. In order to find suitable remedies for this condition, a variety of animal models of steroid-induced ocular hypertension (OHT) have been developed for testing drugs and other therapeutics. Some of these models and techniques will be described in this chapter.

Keywords: Animal model, Intraocular pressure, Ocular hypertension, Steroids, Secondary glaucoma.

INTRODUCTION

Ocular inflammation can be caused by many internal and external factors, including microbial infestation, blunt trauma to the eye, and irritation caused by drug eyedrop administration or airborne pollutants and allergens. A common treatment for such conditions is instillation of topical ocular and oral anti-inflammatory steroids such as dexamethasone (DEX). Unfortunately, steroid-induced elevation of intraocular pressure (IOP), ocular hypertension (OHT), and

* **Corresponding author Najam A. Sharif:** Vice President and Head of Research & Development Nanoscope Therapeutics Inc., 2777 N. Stemmons Fwy, Suite 1102, Dallas, TX-75207, USA; Tel: +1(817)-565-7686; E-mail: nsharif@nanostherapeutics.com

Najam A. Sharif and Sunny E. Ohia (Eds.)

glaucoma often result in 20-30% of patients who possess a gene that is switched on by corticosteroids (Stone *et al*., 1997). This gene overproduces a mutated form of an endogenous protein, mutant myocilin, which is released by cells within the major outflow pathway of aqueous humor (AQH) drainage from the anterior chamber of the eye, the trabecular meshwork (TM) (Clark *et al*., 1994, 1995). The chronic obstruction of the TM by accumulated extracellular matrix components such as collagen and fibronectin and the mutated myocilin reduces or halts the drainage of AQH, and this raises the IOP (Stone *et al*., 1995; Weinreb, 2005; Patel *et al*., 2017; Sharif, 2021, 2023). Over time, even acute OHT begins to damage the retinal ganglion cells and the optic nerve, and patients begin to experience visual impairment if the steroidal treatment is not curtailed and the steroid removed from the body. Corticosteroid-stimulated OHT develops within weeks in vulnerable patients. Its onset, severity, and final outcome (degree of vision loss) depend on the steroid potency, its ability to penetrate the cornea and conjunctiva (pharmacokinetics), duration of treatment, and route of administration, with topical ocular (or periocular injection, at least in animals) being the most rapid inducer of the OHT (Clark *et al*., 1995; Zhang *et al*., 2007; Whitlock *et al*., 2010; Zode *et al*., 2011, 2014; Maddineni *et al*., 2020).

In order to better understand the pathophysiology of steroid-induced IOP increase, a number of model systems have been developed that try to capitulate the human condition. These range from ex vivo cell and anterior eye segment organ cultures to *in vivo* animal models using rodents, cattle, and even non-human primates (Rybkin *et al*., 2017; Li *et al*., 2019). These model systems can then be utilized to investigate specific aspects of IOP elevation and to better understand the pathological sequelae involved in disease development and progression, as well as the means to find suitable remedies to overcome the symptoms of the disease and its consequences. Commonly used rodent models of steroid-induced glaucoma will be described in this chapter (Maddineni *et al*., 2020).

From a phylogenetic perspective, rodents are the lowest mammals where IOP increase with steroidal treatment has been reported. Even though rats offer a larger eye for manipulation and perhaps ease of handling, mice are cheaper, and they provide an animal platform that can be genetically altered. As such, three mouse models of steroid-induced OHT are currently available for utility in research. These include the following: 1). Topical ocular steroid treatment model. In this model, DEX eyedrops (0.1%) are instilled in the eyes of normal mice three times daily for 6 weeks (Zode *et al*., 2014). Here, the animals develop OHT starting at 2 weeks after steroid administration, and the IOP can be elevated by up to 7 mmHg from baseline. These mice develop glaucomatous optic neuropathy (GON), where the RGCs and their axons are significantly reduced (Zode *et al*., 2014). 2). Systemic corticosteroid treatment model. Here, mice are subjected to continuous systemic exposure to DEX, which is delivered *via* osmotic minipumps for up to 1 month (*e.g.*, 0.09 mg DEX/day) (Overby *et al.*, 2014; Whitlock *et al.*, 2010). Unfortunately, the systemic steroid treatment only elevates the IOP by 2-4 mmHg, and there is high mortality in the mice. 3). Periocular corticosteroid treatment model. Here, triamcinolone acetonide (40mg/ml – 20ul per eye) is given to the mice *via* the periocular route of administration (Maddineni *et al.*, 2020). This model shows an IOP increase with reduced TM outflow and GON (Maddineni *et al.*, 2020; Sharif *et al.*, 2024) and will be described below.

Periocular Administration of DEX to Raise IOP

Animal Preparation

- All experiments are to be performed after receiving and documenting written permission from the Institutional Animal Care and Use Committee (IACUC), and according to the guidelines provided by the Assoc. Research in Vision and Ophthalmology (ARV). At the conclusion of the experiments, mice should be sacrificed by CO_2 inhalation and then by cervical dislocation or as approved by institutional IACUC protocol.
- Use 3-month-old male C57BL/6 J mice (Jackson Laboratory; Bar Harbor, ME), feed rodent/mouse standard chow ad libitum, and maintain them on a 12 hrs light/dark cycle at 21°C-26 °C and with 40-70% humidity.

Periocular Administration of DEX and IOP Measurements

- Prepare DEX suspension by mixing 10 mg of micronized DEX-Acetate (Spectrum Chemicals, New Brunswick, NJ) in 1 mL of vehicle (Veh). A uniform suspension with a desired DEX particle size can be achieved by mixing the suspension along with two stainless steel 5-mm beads (Qiagen, Valencia, CA) in a Tissue Lyser LT (Qiagen) for 10 min at 50 oscillations/sec and further rotated overnight at 4°C.
- Anesthetize the mice with isoflurane (2.5%) and oxygen (0.8 L/min) and then peri-ocularly inject 200 μL/eye of either Veh or freshly made DEX (*i.e.*, 200 μg) using a 32-gauge needle attached to a Hamilton glass micro syringe. This procedure should be repeated on a weekly basis for up to 6-8 weeks to raise the IOP. For most experiments, both eyes should be injected with either vehicle alone or DEX (*i.e.*, bilaterally). To study axonal transport, one eye should be injected with the vehicle while the contralateral eye should receive the DEX.
- Anesthetize mice as above to measure their IOPs using a TonoLab rebound tonometer (Colonial Medical Supply, Franconia, NH). Day and night-time IOPs should be recorded once a week throughout the treatment period. IOP measurements should be obtained in a masked manner, and an average of six IOP readouts should be taken at each time point. Additionally, dark-adapted

night-time IOP recordings should also be taken.

- Ideally, complete the IOP measurements within 4 minutes to limit the effect of anesthetic on the IOP. Using a constant-flow infusion technique, AQH outflow facilities can be determined in vehicle-injected and DEX-injected mice. Using the aforementioned procedures, the IOP should remain elevated at 8-9 weeks after DEX-dosing as compared to vehicle-injected mice (Fig. **1a**).

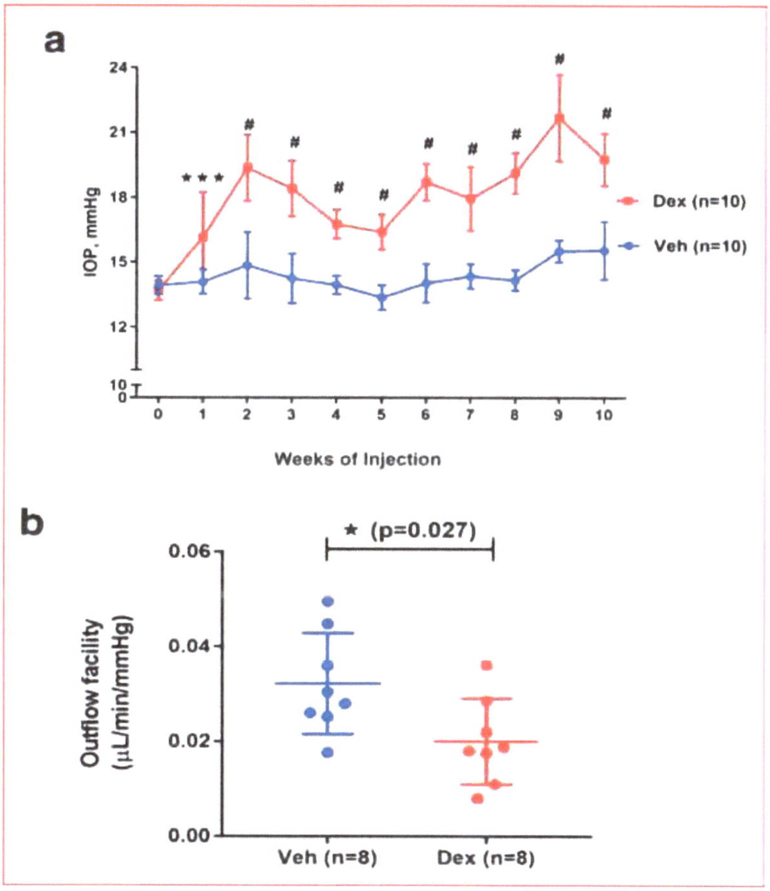

Fig. (1). Periocular DEX-induced OHT in mice (a) and reduction in AQH outflow facility (b) are shown. (Adapted from Maddineni *et al.*, 2020).

Outflow of AQH Measurements

- Using ketamine/xylazine solution (100/10 mg/kg), anesthetize the mice and place them on a 37 °C heating pad to maintain their body temperature.
- Apply one drop of topical ocular proparacaine HCl (0.5%) per eye to numb the cornea. Cannulate the anterior chambers using a 30-gauge needle through the cornea. Ensure that the needle does not touch the corneal endothelium, iris, or

anterior lens capsule. A pre-calibrated flow-through BLPR-2 pressure transducer should be connected to the needle and a continuous pressure should be maintained within the perfusion system. Connect the opposing end of the transducer to a 1 mL syringe placed into a microdialysis infusion pump. The entire perfusion system should be filled with sterile phosphate buffer solution (PBS). The cannulated eye should now be infused at a flow rate of 0.1-0.5 μL/min (in 0.1 μL/min increments), and 3 stabilize pressures must be recorded at 5 min intervals for each flow rate. Mean stabilized pressure is derived from averaging the 3-stabilized pressures.

- The AQH outflow facility value can be obtained from the reciprocal of the slope of a plot of mean stabilized pressure as the Y-axis ordinate and flow rate as the X-axis abscissa. Such corticosteroid injection procedures elevate the IOP and significantly decrease the AQH outflow from the anterior chamber of the eye (Fig. **1b**) (Millar *et al.*, 2011; Maddineni *et al.*, 2020).

Mouse Slit-lamp Examination

Use slit-lamp microscopy (SL-D7; Topcon) to check for any ocular abnormalities and inflammation in the vehicle- and DEX-injected eyes, and take digital photos as deemed necessary.

Fixing of Ocular and Extra-Ocular Tissues

- To fix the ocular and/or extra-ocular tissues of the anesthetized mice, perform an intracardiac perfusion of PBS followed by 4% paraformaldehyde (PFA) (see below).
- Mice should be weighed and then anesthetized using an injectable anesthetic cocktail (ketamine 100 mg/kg; xylazine 10 mg/ kg; acepromazine 3 mg/kg (intraperitoneally administered, 1 mL/100 g)). The intracardiac perfusion should be performed when there is no sign of flexor withdrawal response upon a tail pinch and in the absence of a blink reflex. After the intracardiac perfusion, confirm the animal is not breathing and a heartbeat is undetectable. Now perform a unilateral thoracotomy, after which ocular and/or extra-ocular tissues can be carefully dissected out and placed in 4% PFA for 12 h at 4 °C to fix the tissues.

Immunostaining of Tissues

- The fixed tissues should be sectioned once embedded in paraffin and cut and collected on microscope slides. Remove the paraffin from the sections by rinsing the slides in xylene and rehydrate gradually by rinsing in 100%, 95%, 70%, and 50% ethanol for 5 min in each solvent. Antigen retrieval should now be achieved by incubating the tissue section-bearing slides in citrate buffer (pH 6.0) for 13 minutes at 100°C and then another incubation in citrate buffer (pH 6.0) at room temperature for 30 minutes.

- When using OCT-embedded cryosections, dip the slides directly in the blocking buffer (PBS containing + 10% goat serum + 0.2% Triton X100) for 2 hrs in a dark and humidified container at room temperature. However, the concentration of Triton X-100 may be changed from 0.2 to 2% final, depending on the type of tissue under study. Tissue sections should then be briefly washed and then incubated with specific primary antibodies at 4°C overnight. After 3 washes in PBS, sections should be incubated with the appropriate secondary antibodies for 2 hrs at room temperature.
- Now wash the tissue sections in PBS and then mount them with mounting-medium containing DAPI nuclear stain (Vector Labs, Inc., Burlingame, CA, USA). After this, the images of the stained sections can be captured on a fluorescence microscope (Itasca, IL, USA) and processed with the ImageJ software/hardware system or another suitable image analysis program (Rueden *et al.*, 2017).
- To ensure that appropriate controls are run and accounted for, tissue sections that are incubated without the primary antibody and should be used as negative controls, and the relative signal intensities should be subtracted with averaged background intensity.

Pattern Electroretinography

- To study the functional activity of RGCs, pattern electroretinography (PERG) should be performed, and the ERG wave amplitudes and latency should be determined as previously described by Chou *et al.* (2014). The mice should be anesthetized with ketamine/xylazine solution (100/ 10 mg/kg) and maintained on a heated stage during the whole procedure. The PERG measurements should be conducted using the Miami PERG system (Jorvec, Miami, Fl) as per the manufacturer's guidelines or using another similar system.

Whole-mount Retinal Staining

In order to determine the number of surviving RGCs in vehicle and DEX-injected mice, retinal staining with RBPMS antibody needs to be performed as described below.

- Enucleate the eyes from the sacrificed mice and fix them in 4% PFA at 4 °C for 12 hrs. Rinse the eyeballs with PBS, remove the anterior chamber, and carefully separate the retina from the posterior eyeball cup.
- Incubate the isolated retinae in blocking buffer (PBS containing 10% goat serum and 0.2% Triton X-100) at 4°C for 12 hrs. Then, incubate the retinae with the RBPMS antibody at 4 °C for 3 days, and then rinse in PBS buffer for 2 h. After

this time, incubate the retinae with the appropriate secondary antibody (goat anti-rabbit 568, 1:500; from Invitrogen) for 2 hrs at 4°C, rinse them for 1 h in PBS, and then mount them with the mounting medium containing the DAPI nuclear stain.

- In order to determine the number of RBPMS-positive RGCs, capture at least 16 non-overlapping images from the entire retina (at 200x magnification) using a fluorescence microscope (*e.g.*, Keyence [Itasca, IL, USA]) and ascertain the number of cells with ImageJ or similar software.
- In order to determine the presence of reactive astrocytes in the isolated retinae, the whole-mounted retinae should be incubated with the GFAP antibody along with the RBPMS antibody, and the tissues must be processed accordingly as described above.
- For determining axonal anterograde transport in the mice, cholera toxin B (CTB) labelling should be utilized. After 5-, 8- or 10- weeks post injections of vehicle or DEX, mice should be anesthetized and injected intravitreally (using a Hamilton syringe with a 33-gauge needle) with 3 µL of 0.1% CTB (reconstituted in PBS), which is conjugated with either Alexa fluor 555 or Alexa fluor 480 fluorescence dyes (*e.g.*, Invitrogen, Life Technologies, Grand Island, NY, USA).
- After two days, euthanize the mice, remove the eyes and brains, and fix in 4% PFA 4 °C for 12 hrs. The fixed eyes and brains should now be rinsed in PBS, incubated in graded concentrations of sucrose solution (10-30%) for an additional 3 days, and then embedded in OCT compound followed by cryosectioning of the tissues (10 µm thick sections).
- For visualizing the axonal anterograde transport of CTB in the superior colliculus, cut and collect serial frontal 30 µm thick sections of the brain and collect them on microscope slides previously coated in gelatin. Wash the sections in PBS and mount them with a mounting medium containing DAPI nuclear stain. Image sections on a Keyence fluorescence microscope and capture digital photos of the images.

Assessment of Optic Nerve Damage

Paraphenylenediamine (PPD) stains fatty tissue. Hence, PPD lightly stains the myelin sheath of all healthy axons of the optic nerve, while the axoplasm of damaged or dying axons is darkly stained. For these studies, the optic nerve needs to be separated from the eyeball and fixed in phosphate-buffer 3% glutaraldehyde/paraformaldehyde mixture overnight at 4 °C. After an overnight treatment in 1% osmium tetroxide at 4 °C, rinse the optic nerves in 0.1 M phosphate buffer and 0.1 M sodium-acetate buffer, then dehydrate in graded ethanol concentrations as described above. Now embed the nerves in resin (Eponate-12; Ted Pella) and then cut 1 µm thick sections and stain in 1% PPD for 10 min at room temperature. Optic nerve axons can now be counted under a microscope. Thus, take 10 non-overlapping images of the optic nerve sections at 1630x magnification, and count the axons in an area equal to ~10% of the overall optic nerve cross-sectional area. The number of axons in the optic nerves derived from the corticosteroid-treated mice should be significantly lower than vehicle-treated animals (Maddineni *et al.*, 2020).

CONCLUSION

Many animal models of steroid-induced OHT are available to researchers. The most robust and reliable procedure appears to be using periocular injection of corticosteroids such as DEX in normal mice. This protocol reliably induces a 7-8 mmHg increase in IOP relative to baseline IOP (Maddineni *et al.*, 2020). The consequential damage to the retinal and optic nerve structure and function can also be studied using this model (Maddineni *et al.*, 2020). Recent examples of data that can be obtained from such animal models of OHT are illustrated in Fig. (**1**) (Maddineni *et al.*, 2020) and Fig. (**2**) (Sharif *et al.*, 2024).

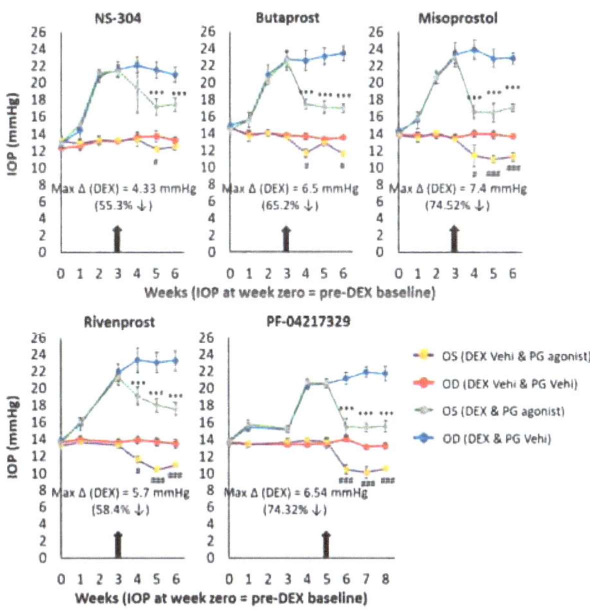

Fig. (2). Periocular DEX-induced IOP-elevation and its reduction by various topical ocularly delivered prostanoid receptor-selective agonist drugs. *** $p < 0.001$; the significance of the difference between PG agonist and corresponding PG vehicle groups in DEX-injected eyes; # $p < 0.05$; ### $p < 0.001$; the significance of the difference between PG agonist and corresponding PG vehicle groups in DEX Vehi injected eyes, as indicated by 2-Factor ANOVA followed by the Holm-Sidak post-hoc test. Vertical arrow (↓) indicates the maximum % reduction in IOP in the DEX-treatment group following topical ocular drug treatment. NS-304 is an IP-selective agonist; Butaprost and PF-04217328 are EP2-selective agonists; Misoprostol has affinity for EP3 and EP2 receptors; and Rivenoprost is an EP4-selective agonist. (Adapted from Sharif *et al.*, 2024) Vehi, vehicle.

REFERENCES

Chou, TH, Bohorquez, J, Toft-Nielsen, J, Ozdamar, O & Porciatti, V (2014) Robust mouse pattern electroretinograms derived simultaneously from each eye using a common snout electrode. *Invest Ophthalmol Vis Sci,* 55, 2469-75.
[http://dx.doi.org/10.1167/iovs.14-13943] [PMID: 24667861]

Clark, AF, Wilson, K, de Kater, AW, Allingham, RR & McCartney, MD (1995) Dexamethasone-induced ocular hypertension in perfusion-cultured human eyes. *Invest Ophthalmol Vis Sci,* 36, 478-89.
[PMID: 7843916]

Clark, AF, Wilson, K, McCartney, MD, Miggans, ST, Kunkle, M & Howe, W (1994) Glucocorticoid-induced formation of cross-linked actin networks in cultured human trabecular meshwork cells. *Invest Ophthalmol Vis Sci,* 35, 281-94.
[PMID: 8300356]

Li, G, Lee, C, Agrahari, V, Wang, K, Navarro, I, Sherwood, JM, Crews, K, Farsiu, S, Gonzalez, P, Lin, CW, Mitra, AK, Ethier, CR & Stamer, WD (2019) In vivo measurement of trabecular meshwork stiffness in a corticosteroid-induced ocular hypertensive mouse model. *Proc Natl Acad Sci USA,* 116, 1714-22.
[http://dx.doi.org/10.1073/pnas.1814889116] [PMID: 30651311]

Maddineni, P, Kasetti, RB, Patel, PD, Millar, JC, Kiehlbauch, C, Clark, AF & Zode, GS (2020) CNS axonal degeneration and transport deficits at the optic nerve head precede structural and functional loss of retinal ganglion cells in a mouse model of glaucoma. *Mol Neurodegener,* 15, 48.
[http://dx.doi.org/10.1186/s13024-020-00400-9] [PMID: 32854767]

Millar, JC, Clark, AF & Pang, IH (2011) Assessment of aqueous humor dynamics in the mouse by a novel method of constant-flow infusion. *Invest Ophthalmol Vis Sci,* 52, 685-94.
[http://dx.doi.org/10.1167/iovs.10-6069] [PMID: 20861483]

Overby, DR, Bertrand, J, Tektas, OY, Boussommier-Calleja, A, Schicht, M, Ethier, CR, Woodward, DF, Stamer, WD & Lütjen-Drecoll, E (2014) Ultrastructural changes associated with dexamethasone-induced ocular hypertension in mice. *Invest Ophthalmol Vis Sci,* 55, 4922-33.
[http://dx.doi.org/10.1167/iovs.14-14429] [PMID: 25028360]

Patel, GC, Phan, TN, Maddineni, P, Kasetti, RB, Millar, JC, Clark, AF & Zode, GS (2017) Dexamethasone-induced ocular hypertension in mice: effects of Myocilin and route of administration. *Am J Pathol,* 187, 713-23.
[http://dx.doi.org/10.1016/j.ajpath.2016.12.003] [PMID: 28167045]

Rueden, CT, Schindelin, J, Hiner, MC, DeZonia, BE, Walter, AE, Arena, ET & Eliceiri, KW (2017) ImageJ2: ImageJ for the next generation of scientific image data. *BMC Bioinformatics,* 18, 529.
[http://dx.doi.org/10.1186/s12859-017-1934-z] [PMID: 29187165]

Rybkin, I, Gerometta, R, Fridman, G, Candia, O & Danias, J (2017) Model systems for the study of steroid-induced IOP elevation. *Exp Eye Res,* 158, 51-8.
[http://dx.doi.org/10.1016/j.exer.2016.07.013] [PMID: 27450911]

Sharif, NA (2021) Therapeutic drugs and devices for tackling ocular hypertension and glaucoma, and need for neuroprotection and cytoprotective therapies. *Front Pharmacol,* 12, 729249.
[http://dx.doi.org/10.3389/fphar.2021.729249] [PMID: 34603044]

Sharif, NA (2023) Identifying new drugs and targets to treat rapidly elevated intraocular pressure for angle closure and secondary glaucomas to curb visual impairment and prevent blindness. *Exp Eye Res,* 232, 109444.
[http://dx.doi.org/10.1016/j.exer.2023.109444] [PMID: 36958427]

Sharif, NA, Millar, JC, Zode, G & Ota, T (2024) Steroid-induced ocular hypertension in mice is differentially reduced by selective EP2-, EP3-, EP4- and IP-prostanoid receptor agonists. *Int J Mol Sci,* 25, 3328.
[http://dx.doi.org/10.3390/ijms25063328] [PMID: 38542305]

Stone, EM, Fingert, JH, Alward, WLM, Nguyen, TD, Polansky, JR, Sunden, SLF, Nishimura, D, Clark, AF,

Nystuen, A, Nichols, BE, Mackey, DA, Ritch, R, Kalenak, JW, Craven, ER & Sheffield, VC (1997) Identification of a gene that causes primary open angle glaucoma. *Science,* 275, 668-70.
[http://dx.doi.org/10.1126/science.275.5300.668] [PMID: 9005853]

Weinreb, RN (2005) IOP and the risk of progression to glaucoma. *Graefes Arch Clin Exp Ophthalmol,* 243, 511-2.
[http://dx.doi.org/10.1007/s00417-005-1195-9] [PMID: 15909156]

Whitlock, NA, McKnight, B, Corcoran, KN, Rodriguez, LA & Rice, DS (2010) Increased intraocular pressure in mice treated with dexamethasone. *Invest Ophthalmol Vis Sci,* 51, 6496-503.
[http://dx.doi.org/10.1167/iovs.10-5430] [PMID: 20671272]

Zhang, X, Ognibene, CM, Clark, AF & Yorio, T (2007) Dexamethasone inhibition of trabecular meshwork cell phagocytosis and its modulation by glucocorticoid receptor β. *Exp Eye Res,* 84, 275-84.
[http://dx.doi.org/10.1016/j.exer.2006.09.022] [PMID: 17126833]

Zode, GS, Kuehn, MH, Nishimura, DY, Searby, CC, Mohan, K, Grozdanic, SD, Bugge, K, Anderson, MG, Clark, AF, Stone, EM & Sheffield, VC (2011) Reduction of ER stress *via* a chemical chaperone prevents disease phenotypes in a mouse model of primary open angle glaucoma. *J Clin Invest,* 121, 3542-53.
[http://dx.doi.org/10.1172/JCI58183] [PMID: 21821918]

Zode, GS, Sharma, AB, Lin, X, Searby, CC, Bugge, K, Kim, GH, Clark, AF & Sheffield, VC (2014) Ocular-specific ER stress reduction rescues glaucoma in murine glucocorticoid-induced glaucoma. *J Clin Invest,* 124, 1956-65.
[http://dx.doi.org/10.1172/JCI69774] [PMID: 24691439]

CHAPTER 31

Protocol for Measuring Intraocular Pressure in Guinea Pigs

Alyssa Hostert[1] and **Catherine A. Opere**[1,*]

[1] *Department of Pharmacy Sciences, School of Pharmacy and Health Professions, Creighton University, Omaha, Nebraska, USA*

Abstract: This chapter describes the protocols to measure intraocular pressure (IOP) in guinea pigs. The process consists of many steps and sub-steps, including the preparation of the animal, the preparation of the TonoVet-Plus® rebound tonometer, and finally, the measurement of IOP itself. Healthy animals free of ocular morphological abnormalities or disease states should be chosen for inclusion before beginning the protocol. Following this series of steps will ensure that IOP readings are taken accurately and with precision.

Keywords: Eye, Glaucoma, Intraocular pressure, Protocol, Retina, Retinal ganglion cells, Tonometry, Uveitis.

INTRODUCTION

Ocular disorders can have a significant impact on visual acuity in both human and animal populations. Changes in intraocular pressure (IOP) can cause lasting damage to the retina and adjoining tissues of the eye. In guinea pigs, for example, there is a wide range of normal IOP values; however, previous studies on normal, healthy guinea pigs found average IOP values ranging anywhere from 9 to 23 mm Hg, concentrating primarily around 15-19 mm Hg (Coster *et al.*, 2008; Di *et al.*, 2017; Wu *et al.*, 2020). IOP readings higher than the typically observed range of values indicate an increased risk for glaucoma, in which aqueous humor (AH) outflow is obstructed, leading to lasting damage to the retinal ganglion cells (RGCs) (Ofri, 2021; Gelatt, 2008). Lower than expected IOP values may indicate excess AH outflow, putting the patient at risk for uveitis (Ofri, 2021). For these reasons, careful monitoring and screening protocols are needed to ensure that these disease states are caught early so that they can be managed appropriately.

* **Corresponding author Catherine A. Opere:** Department of Pharmacy Sciences, School of Pharmacy and Health Professions, Creighton University, Omaha, Nebraska, USA; Tel: +402-280-3726;
Fax: 402-280-1883; E-mail: copere@creighton.edu

Najam A. Sharif and Sunny E. Ohia (Eds.)

The purpose of this chapter is to describe a veterinary protocol for the evaluation of IOP in guinea pigs. This will provide useful insight into the applicability of animal models for research into new drug therapies that may one day be used in human patients. It will allow for further establishment of baseline expected IOP values for these animals to detect any deviations from the norm, which may be targeted by drug therapies.

EXPERIMENTAL PROTOCOLS

The following procedure was performed in accordance with the Statement for the Use of Animals in Ophthalmic and Vision Research from the Association for Research in Vision and Ophthalmology (ARVO).

All testing should be performed on healthy guinea pigs. Those with a history of prior ocular disorders or morphological changes to the cornea should be excluded from this study.

Preparation of the Animal for Evaluation

- Gently place the guinea pig in a comfortable sternal recumbent position.
- Allow the guinea pig about five minutes to acclimate to this position. Do not begin testing if the animal is in distress or if excess force is needed to secure the animal in this position.

Preparation of the TonoVet-Plus®

Note: TonoVet-Plus® rebound tonometer has been shown to be more accurate than TonoVet® at measuring IOP when values exceed 14 mm Hg; however, if all values are expected to be below this threshold, TonoVet-Plus® or TonoVet® may be used interchangeably (Shim *et al*., 2020).

- Press the Select or Measure button on the tonometer to turn it on.
- Remove the red cap from the probe base.
- Remove the cap from the tube holding the probe and use the tube to insert the probe into the probe base. Do not touch the probe itself.
- A “play” symbol and species setting should appear on the tonometer’s display, indicating that it is ready for use.

Species Selection

Note: Previous IOP studies have been done on guinea pigs using the TonoVet-Plus® in the “Rabbit” setting due to the animals’ similarity in size (Wu *et al*., 2020). Normal IOPs for rabbits range from 15-23 mm Hg, which encompasses the range of expected values for guinea pigs (Vareilles *et al.* 1977). The TonoVet-

Plus® may be further calibrated in the "p" setting if IOP values are expected to differ from species pre-sets (Icare, 2015). Refer to the manufacturer's website for more information (tonovet.com).

- Press the select button on the tonometer.
- Use the Navigation buttons to find Setting, and then press Select again.
- Use the Navigation buttons to toggle through species until "Rabbit" appears, and then press Select.

IOP Measurement

Note: A study using the TonoVet® to measure differences in IOP based on probe distance from the eye found that the farther the probe was from the eye, the slower the probe speed and the higher the observed IOPs. The newer model tonometer is purported to have a faster probe speed to minimize this concern. As such, the manufacturer recommends holding the probe at 4-8 mm from the eye, with the range in distance accounting for human error (Rodrigues, 2021; Icare, 2015).

- Instill one drop of proparacaine hydrochloride (0.5%) into each animal's eye.
- Position one hand with fingers both above and below the left eye to hold the eyelids open.
- With the other hand, position the TonoVet-Plus® so that the probe tip is horizontal and perpendicular to the cornea, at a distance of 4-8 mm from the corneal surface. A green probe light indicates that the horizontal positioning is correct. If this light is red, the machine is being tilted vertically, and placement should be adjusted. If this light is blinking, press the Measure button to clear this error signal.
- Hold down the Measure button to initiate the collection of six consecutive measurements. The TonoVet-Plus® will automatically discard the highest and lowest readings and project an average of the remaining four IOP readings onto the display.
- If the ring surrounding the final IOP reading is yellow or red, repeat the sequence, as this will indicate that the standard deviation is greater than the accepted 5% (Gloe *et al.* 2019).
- Record the resulting IOP measurement.
- Repeat steps for the right eye.
- Discard the probe after use. The same probe may be used for both eyes in a single guinea pig as long as neither eye is infected.
- To turn off the tonometer, press and hold the Select button until the power sign appears. The device will also turn off automatically after three minutes of use.

CONCLUSION

The protocol described here is written to be sufficient that anyone in possession of a TonoVet-Plus® rebound tonometer might be able to repeat this procedure to measure IOP in guinea pig subjects. It does not contain an exhaustive report of all error messages that may be encountered. For that reason, readers are encouraged to visit the manufacturer's website (tonovet.com) for any additional inquiries.

REFERENCES

Coster, ME, Stiles, J, Krohne, SG & Raskin, RE (2008) Results of diagnostic ophthalmic testing in healthy guinea pigs. *J Am Vet Med Assoc,* 232, 1825-33.
[http://dx.doi.org/10.2460/javma.232.12.1825] [PMID: 18598151]

Di, Y, Luo, XM, Qiao, T & Lu, N (2017) Intraocular pressure with rebound tonometry and effects of topical intraocular pressure reducing medications in guinea pigs. *Int J Ophthalmol,* 10, 186-90.
[PMID: 28251075]

Gelatt, KN, Brooks, DE & Kallberg, ME (2008) The canine glaucomas. *Essentials of veterinary ophthalmology,* 2, 155-87.

Gloe, S, Rothering, A, Kiland, JA & McLellan, GJ (2019) Validation of the Icare® TONOVET plus rebound tonometer in normal rabbit eyes. *Exp Eye Res,* 185, 107698.
[http://dx.doi.org/10.1016/j.exer.2019.107698] [PMID: 31201805]

Icare (2015). TonoVet Plus®. Icare Veterinary Tonometer

Ofri R. (2020). An overview of canine glaucoma. *Dvm360.* 52

Rodrigues, BD, Montiani-Ferreira, F, Bortolini, M, Somma, AT, Komáromy, AM & Dornbusch, PT (2021) Intraocular pressure measurements using the TONOVET ® rebound tonometer: Influence of the probe-cornea distance. *Vet Ophthalmol,* 24 (Suppl. 1), 175-85.
[http://dx.doi.org/10.1111/vop.12832] [PMID: 33070466]

Shim, J, Kang, S, Park, Y, Kim, S, Go, S, Lee, E & Seo, K (2021) Comparative intraocular pressure measurements using three different rebound tonometers through in an ex vivo analysis and clinical trials in canine eyes. *Vet Ophthalmol,* 24 (Suppl. 1), 186-93.
[http://dx.doi.org/10.1111/vop.12771] [PMID: 32501651]

Vareilles, P, Conquet, P & Le Douarec, JC (1977) A method for the routine intraocular pressure (IOP) measurement in the rabbit: Range of IOP variations in this species. *Exp Eye Res,* 24, 369-75.
[http://dx.doi.org/10.1016/0014-4835(77)90149-X] [PMID: 858319]

Wu, D, de Linde Henriksen, M, Grant, K, Lyakhova, T, Sharp, JL & Daniels, JB (2020) Ocular findings and selected ophthalmic diagnostic tests in a group of young commercially available Guinea and Skinny pigs (*Cavia porcellus*). *Vet Ophthalmol,* 23, 234-44.
[http://dx.doi.org/10.1111/vop.12709] [PMID: 31562703]

CHAPTER 32

Protocol for Measuring Intraocular Pressure in Dogs

Pratik Bankhele[1], **Alyssa Hostert**[1] and **Catherine A. Opere**[1,*]

[1] *Department of Pharmacy Sciences, School of Pharmacy and Health Professions, Creighton University, Omaha, Nebraska, USA*

Abstract: This chapter describe the protocols to measure intraocular pressure (IOP) in canines. The process consists of many steps and sub-steps, including the preparation of the animal, the preparation of the TonoVet-Plus® rebound tonometer, and finally, the measurement of IOP itself. Healthy animals free of ocular morphological abnormalities or disease states should be chosen for inclusion before beginning the protocol. Following this series of steps will ensure that IOP readings are taken accurately and with precision.

Keywords: Eye, Glaucoma, Intraocular pressure, Protocol, Retina, Retinal ganglion cells, Tonometry, Uveitis.

INTRODUCTION

Like humans, ocular disorders are prevalent in the canine population. Changes in intraocular pressure (IOP) cause etiologies, which can lead to lasting damage to the retina. In dogs, for example, there is a wide range of normal IOP values, which may vary based on breed; however, 15 to 25 mm Hg is standard (Kulualp *et al.*, 2017; Ofri, 2021). IOP readings higher than the accepted range of values put the animal at risk for the development of glaucoma, in which the increased pressure contributes to the obstruction of aqueous humor (AH) outflow. This, in turn, can cause permanent damage to retinal ganglion cells (RCGs) (Ofri, 2021; Gelatt, 2008). Conversely, IOP values that are lower than expected are often associated with uveitis and can be attributed to excess AH outflow. When screening for these disease states, both eyes should have similar pressures within 10 mm Hg of each other. Any larger deviations may be suspicious for the development of glaucoma (Ofri, 2021).

[*] **Corresponding author Catherine A. Opere:** Department of Pharmacy Sciences, School of Pharmacy and Health Professions, Creighton University, Omaha, Nebraska, USA; Tel: +402-280-3726; Fax: 402-280-1883; E-mail: copere@creighton.edu

Najam A. Sharif and Sunny E. Ohia (Eds.)

The purpose of this chapter is to describe a veterinary protocol for the evaluation of IOP in canines. Animal models of eye disease provide valuable insight into identifying the potential factors underlying ocular disorders. Additionally, animal models present a useful tool for the evaluation of the *in vivo* pharmacological efficacy of drugs that may help treat eye conditions in both humans and animals. This protocol allows for the detection of any deviation from standard IOP values and, by extension, allows screening for potential ocular disease states, which may then be targeted by drug therapies.

EXPERIMENTAL PROTOCOLS

The following procedure should be performed in accordance with the Statement for the Use of Animals in Ophthalmic and Vision Research from the Association for Research in Vision and Ophthalmology (ARVO).

All testing should be performed on healthy, conscious dogs. Those with a history of prior ocular disorders or morphological changes to the cornea should be excluded from this study.

Preparation of the Animal for Evaluation

- Gently place the dog in a comfortable sternal recumbent position.
- Allow the dog about five minutes to acclimate to this position. Do not begin testing if the animal is in distress or if excess force is needed to secure the animal in this position.

Preparation of the TonoVet-Plus®

Note: TonoVet-Plus® rebound tonometer has been shown to be more accurate than TonoVet® at measuring IOP when values exceed 14 mm Hg; however, if all values are expected to be below this threshold, TonoVet-Plus® or TonoVet® may be used interchangeably (Shim *et al*., 2020).

- Press the Select or Measure button on the tonometer to turn it on.
- Remove the red cap from the probe base.
- Remove the cap from the tube holding the probe and use the tube to insert the probe into the probe base. Do not touch the probe itself.
- A “play” symbol and species setting should appear on the tonometer’s display, indicating that it is ready for use.

Species Selection

- If the species shown on the display is incorrect, press the Select button.
- Use the Navigation buttons to find Setting, and then press Select again.

- Use the Navigation buttons to toggle through species until "Canine" appears, and then press Select.

IOP Measurement

Note: A study using the TonoVet® to measure differences in IOP based on probe distance from the eye found that the farther the probe was from the eye, the slower the probe speed and the higher the observed IOPs. The newer model tonometer is purported to have a faster probe speed to minimize this concern. As such, the manufacturer recommends holding the probe at 4-8 mm from the eye, with the range in distance accounting for human error (Rodrigues, 2021; Icare, 2015).

- Instill one drop of proparacaine hydrochloride (0.5%) into each animal's eye.
- Position one hand with fingers both above and below the left eye to hold the eyelids open.
- With the other hand, position the TonoVet-Plus® so that the probe tip is horizontal and perpendicular to the cornea, at 4-8 mm from the corneal surface. A green probe light indicates that the horizontal positioning is correct. If this light is red, the machine is tilted vertically, and placement should be adjusted. If this light blinks, press the Measure button to clear this error signal.
- Hold down the Measure button to initiate the collection of six consecutive measurements. The TonoVet-Plus® will automatically discard the highest and lowest readings and project an average of the remaining four IOP readings onto the display.
- If the ring surrounding the final IOP reading is yellow or red, repeat the sequence, as this will indicate that the standard deviation is greater than the accepted 5% (Gloe *et al.* 2019).
- Record the resulting IOP measurement.
- Repeat steps 3.1-3.5 for the right eye.
- Discard the probe after use. The same probe may be used for both eyes in a single dog as long as neither eye is infected.
- To turn off the tonometer, press and hold the Select button until the power sign appears. The device will also turn off automatically after three minutes of use.

CONCLUSION

The protocol described here is sufficient for anyone in possession of a TonoVet-Plus® rebound tonometer who can repeat this procedure to measure IOP in canine subjects. It does not contain an exhaustive report of all error messages that may be encountered. For this reason, readers are encouraged to visit the manufacturer's website (tonovet.com) for any additional inquiries.

REFERENCES

Gelatt, KN, Brooks, DE & Kallberg, ME (2008) The canine glaucomas. *Exp Eye Res,* 2, 155-87.

Gloe, S, Rothering, A, Kiland, JA & McLellan, GJ (2019) Validation of the Icare® TONOVET plus rebound tonometer in normal rabbit eyes. *Exp Eye Res,* 185, 107698. [http://dx.doi.org/10.1016/j.exer.2019.107698] [PMID: 31201805]

Icare (2015). TonoVet Plus®. Icare Veterinary Tonometer

Kulualp, K, Yurdakul, I, Erol, H, Atalan, G & Kilic, S (2017) Measurement of intraocular pressure in clinically normal Turkish Shepherd Dogswith the rebound tonometer (TonoVet®) and the applanation tonometer (Tono-Pen Vet®). *Med Weter,* 1-6.

Ofri, R (2020) An overview of canine glaucoma. *Dvm360,* 52.

Rodrigues, BD, Montiani-Ferreira, F, Bortolini, M, Somma, AT, Komáromy, AM & Dornbusch, PT (2021) Intraocular pressure measurements using the TONOVET ® rebound tonometer: Influence of the probe-cornea distance. *Vet Ophthalmol,* 24 (Suppl. 1), 175-85. [http://dx.doi.org/10.1111/vop.12832] [PMID: 33070466]

Shim, J, Kang, S, Park, Y, Kim, S, Go, S, Lee, E & Seo, K (2021) Comparative intraocular pressure measurements using three different rebound tonometers through in an ex vivo analysis and clinical trials in canine eyes. *Vet Ophthalmol,* 24 (Suppl. 1), 186-93. [http://dx.doi.org/10.1111/vop.12771] [PMID: 32501651]

CHAPTER 33

Laser Model of Ocular Hypertension in Nonhuman Primates

Carol B. Toris[1,*] and **Shan Fan**[2]

[1] *Havener Eye Institute, Department of Ophthalmology and Visual Sciences, The Ohio State University Wexner Medical Center, Columbus, OH 43212, USA*

[2] *Department of Ophthalmology and Visual Sciences, University of Nebraska Medical Center, Omaha, Nebraska, USA*

Abstract: This chapter describes a protocol to generate a chronic model of elevated intraocular pressure in nonhuman primates. The main piece of equipment is a good laser designed for use in humans but dedicated exclusively for NHP use. The preoperative procedures include anesthesia, which should be done by certified trained personnel. The actual laser procedure only takes a few minutes, preferably by an ophthalmologist. Forty spots are administered to one eye around 8 clock hours of the trabecular meshwork (80 spots). The fellow eye remains untouched. The animal is allowed to recover for one month, during which time it is monitored daily. Intraocular pressures (IOPs) are taken every few days. The laser procedure is repeated at one month (30 spots) and possibly two months (15 spots) depending on the rise in pressure. The contralateral eye is never lasered. Recovery from the last laser procedure requires three to six months, after which time the animal is ready for study. The IOPs of the lasered eye will be more variable than the contralateral eye. A successful procedure yields unilateral ocular hypertension that persists for years.

Keywords: Argon laser, Glaucoma, Intraocular pressure, Ocular hypertension, Trabecular meshwork, YAG laser.

INTRODUCTION

The nonhuman primate (NHP) is a valuable model used to study glaucoma because of its similarity to humans in its anatomy, physiology, and response to intraocular pressure (IOP)-lowering treatments. Laser treatment to the trabecular meshwork can cause a chronic elevation in IOP that becomes glaucoma. The model was developed in the 1980s (Quigley and Hohman, 1983) and has been

* **Corresponding author Carol B. Toris:** Havener Eye Institute, Department of Ophthalmology and Visual Sciences, The Ohio State University Wexner Medical Center, Columbus, OH 43212, USA; Tel: +614-688-9573; E-mail: carol.toris@osumc.edu

Najam A. Sharif and Sunny E. Ohia (Eds.)

used over the past four decades in studies on IOP effects on aqueous humor dynamics (Toris *et al.*, 2000), optic nerve head ischemia (Bellezza *et al.*, 2003), electroretinograms (Marx *et al.*, 1986), progression of cupping (Pederson and Gaasterland, 1984), changes in visual fields (Sasaoka *et al.*, 2008), morphological changes in outflow pathways (Sasaoka *et al.*, 2008, Zhang *et al.*, 2009), prescribed IOP lowering drugs (Lee *et al.*, 1985, Podos *et al.*, 1989), and IOP lowering drugs in preclinical studies (Bastia *et al.*, 2021a, Bastia *et al.*, 2021b, Fuwa *et al.*, 2018a, May *et al* ., 2003, Toris *et al.*, 2005, Toris *et al.*, 2006).

The protocols used today in our lab are modifications of the original procedures from the 1980s. Three main changes have been incorporated. First, the laser procedure is less aggressive than the original method. Laser is done over two to three sessions with a month's recovery between treatments. Second, 10-15 degrees of the trabecular meshwork are always left untouched. This avoids excessive and painful extremes in IOP that reduce the usefulness of the model. Third, the laser treatment avoids the iris root so as not to cause a permanently dilated and asymmetric pupil. Below are details of our protocol for treating chronic glaucoma in NHPs.

EXPERIMENTAL PROTOCOLS

The following procedures were performed with the approval of the University of Nebraska Medical Center Institutional Animal Care and Use Committee and conformed to the Statement for the Use of Animals in Ophthalmic and Visual Research from the Association for Research in Vision and Ophthalmology (ARVO).

Outline of Procedures

Animals

i. Species most often used
    - *Macaca fascicularis* (cynomolgus macaques)
    - *Macaca mulatta* (Rhesus macaques)
ii. Number of animals
    - For IOP studies, 6 to 8 animals per group
    - For studies of aqueous humor dynamics, 12-16 animals per group
    - For morphological studies, 3-5 animals per group

Equipment

i. Neodymium-doped YAG diode laser or Argon Ophthalmic laser with adjustable table and slit lamp (Alcon, Ft. Worth, TX). The laser should be dedicated to animal use only. It should not be shared with humans.

Supplies

i. Personal Protective Equipment (PPEs); a set for each person handling or near animals
   - Kevlar gloves for handling awake animals
   - Surgical gloves for all other procedures
   - Coveralls
   - Mask
   - Face shield
   - Shoe covers
   - Hair net

ii. Prep area
   - Absorbent pads to cover surfaces that animals could contaminate
   - Sterile drapes to cover areas near the eye
   - Heating pad
   - Disinfectant
   - Soft tissue wipes

iii. Anesthesia
   - Isoflurane anesthesia delivery system
   - Isotec (isoflurane) gas canister
   - O_2 tank
   - Respirator
   - Laryngoscope
   - Endotracheal tube
   - Gauze tie
   - Syringe for inflating balloon
   - Surgical tape
   - Needles
   - Syringes
   - Scissors

iv. Drugs
   - Ketamine, for the safe handling of animals
   - Cetacaine for gag reflex suppression
   - Banamine (flunixin meglumine) or other pain reliever
   - Proparacaine hydrochloride, 0.5%, to anesthetize the cornea
   - Artificial tears, such as EyeStream (Alcon) to keep the cornea hydrated

v. Record keeping
   - Report Forms (one for each animal) to record all experimental procedures and data
   - Log book
   - Anesthesia record form
   - Pen
   - Timer and clock

vi. Laser procedure
   - Infant eye speculum
   - Forceps
   - Goniolens (child size)
   - Goniosol (Gonak, 2.5% hydroxy-propyl methylcellulose ophthalmic demulcent solution)
   - Safety goggles (one pair for each person involved in the laser procedure)

Preparation

i. Measure IOPs weekly for a month. IOP methods are described elsewhere in this book (Aqueous Humor Dynamic Measurements in Nonhuman Primates).

ii. Laser setup
   - Turn on the laser and allow it to warm up for several minutes.
   - Set the laser beam to all colors.
   - Set Power to 0.8 W.
   - Set Duration to 0.5 seconds.
   - On the slit lamp, set the Spot Size to 50 µm.

iii. Anesthesia. This is done by a veterinarian or vet tech in the pre-op room.
   - Administer an intramuscular injection of ketamine (10 mg/kg).
   - When sedated, place the anesthesia cone over the nose and mouth and infuse isoflurane gas (5%).
   - When lightly anesthetized, intubate the animal.
   - Continue administering isoflurane gas (3%) until deep anesthesia is obtained.

iv. Positioning of animal
   - Cover surfaces with absorbent pads and/or sterile drapes.
   - Place the animal on a water-circulating heating pad on an adjustable table in front of the slit lamp connected to the laser instrument. Reduce the isoflurane flow rate to 1% and monitor the animal's vitals constantly during the laser.
   - Place the animal's chin on the slit lamp chin rest, which is covered in a drape and gauze sponges.

Procedure

i. IMPORTANT: All personnel near the laser must wear safety goggles. All personnel handling animals must wear personal protective equipment (PPE).

ii. Up to three treatments are needed, separated by one month (Fig. **1**).
iii. Choose one eye for the laser procedure. The fellow eye is not lasered and remains normotensive.
iv. Place one drop of proparacaine on the cornea.
v. Place a generous drop of goniosol on goniolens.
vi. Place goniolens on the cornea.
vii. If you are lasering the left eye, hold the goniolens with the left hand and control the joystick with the right.
viii. Focus on the trabecular meshwork by moving the animal's head, the slit lamp's joystick, and the lens itself. Move the lens until glare is eliminated. Point the nose down and the eye looking directly ahead. Position the lens to view the superior aspect of the eye. This provides a view of the inferior trabecular meshwork.
ix. Do not apply pressure to the goniolens, which wrinkles the cornea and deforms the view. The goniolens should be pulled ever so slightly away from the cornea to keep the globe in proper shape.
x. Locate the outer edge of the trabecular meshwork (away from the iris).
xi. Laser evenly from 6:00 to 10:00 with 40 spots.
xii. Rotate the lens and laser evenly from 12:00 to 4:00 with 40 spots for a total of 80 spots.
   - Know exactly where you are looking and what you are lasering at all times. Remember that the image through the goniolens is a mirror image of the eye (up is down, and left is right).
   - Bubbles should appear beneath the spot, and the tissue should blanch.
   - Record the number of spots and draw a figure of where the spots were applied (Fig. **2**). You will need this for the next laser session in a month. Take careful notes on the individual animal's report form.

Recovery and Follow-up

i. The ventilator is unhooked, and the animal is moved to a recovery station.
ii. The animal is hooked up to another ventilator that is not dispensing isoflurane. When the animal begins to stir, the endotracheal tube is withdrawn.
iii. Banamine 0.5 mg/kg i.m. or other approved analgesia is given.
iv. When an animal can sit up on its own, place it in a darkened housing room. If possible, maintain dim room lighting for a week. The animals will be photosensitive, and a darkened room is more comfortable for them. If they are housed in cages stacked top and bottom, put the lasered animal in the bottom cage where it can avoid ceiling lighting.
v. Administer pain meds for a minimum of three days or as approved by the veterinarian and IACUC.
vi. Monitor animals daily and IOPs weekly

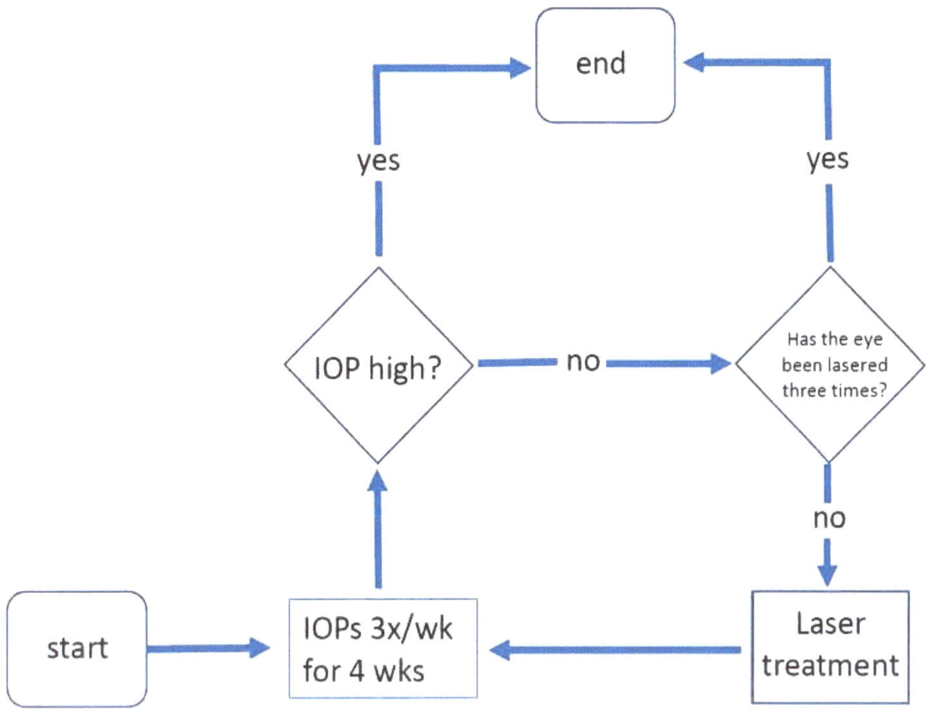

Fig. (1). Flowchart of IOP and laser procedures described in the protocol.

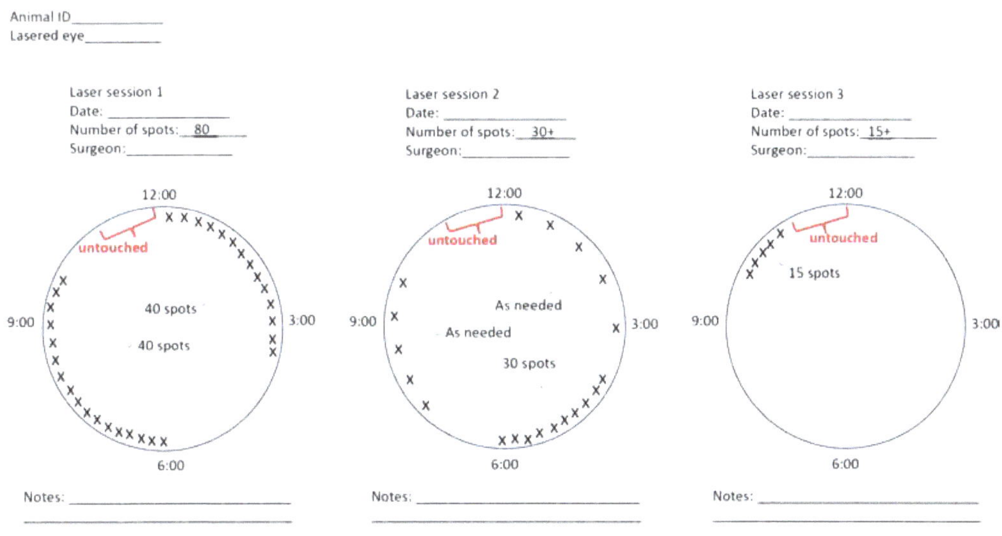

Fig. (2). Example of **Report Form** of the location of laser spots. Superior is at 12:00.

Repeat Laser Treatments

i. The second laser treatment is 4 weeks after the first laser treatment. Laser from 4:00 to 6:00 for a total of 30 or more spots. Re-laser unlasered tissue from 6:00 to 10:00 and 12:00 to 4:00 if needed, showing no set number of spots (**Figure 2**). Usually, two sessions are sufficient to achieve a consistently elevated IOP.
ii. From week 2 to 4 post laser, take IOPs 4 to 5 days/week.
iii. If IOP is not consistently >5 mmHg higher than the untreated eye or baseline, a third treatment is done 4 weeks after the second treatment. Laser from 10:00 to 11:00 (**Figure 2**).
iv. Take IOPs 4 to 5 days/week.
v. If IOP is consistently elevated more than 5 mmHg above baseline or contralateral eye, no more lasering is needed.
vi. A fourth laser session should not be done because it does not increase IOP.

CONCLUSION

The following are some important points to consider before choosing this model.

- Some animals never exhibit an IOP elevation with this treatment. They can be used as sham controls, or once completely recovered from the procedure, the fellow eye can be lasered and serve as the hypertensive eye.
- The IOPs of lasered eyes are more variable than unlasered eyes. Standard deviations can be large.
- Over time (years), the IOP may drift downward. Relasering at this point is not effective at elevating IOP. In this case, the animals are no longer useful for IOP studies.
- This is an injury model of glaucoma, a condition rare in humans. Because the trabecular meshwork is damaged, the effect of some outflow drugs may not be predictive of the human response. Nevertheless, if the laser is done carefully enough and sufficient time is given to recovery, the model can detect changes in the outflow facility (Fuwa *et al.*, 2018b; Toris *et al.*, 2016).
- If the laser is too aggressive and flow through the trabecular meshwork becomes severely limited or blocked entirely, then the model will fail because the IOP will be greatly increased and will not respond to drugs in a predictable manner. In these eyes, uveoscleral outflow will increase greatly to compensate for the lack of flow through the trabecular meshwork. This happens in patients on maximally tolerated medical therapy (Yablonski *et al.*, 1985). Extreme elevations in IOP become an ethical issue as the animal may experience severe and chronic discomfort and may need to be euthanized.
- For IOP studies, the best results occur when tonometry is done on unanesthetized animals. Take the time to train them to accept the measurements

while awake and unstressed. Sometimes, sedation can mask the IOP effect of an ocular hypotensive treatment.

Patience is the key factor in the success of this model. The best results occur when the animal is given sufficient time for recovery from each laser session. Repeated laser procedures cannot be rushed, and recovery cannot be shortened. Training of the animals to accept IOP measurements is time-consuming but worthwhile in the end.

Once the IOP is chronically elevated, the model is useful for years. Longitudinal information can be collected, and a detailed history of responses to certain treatments can be obtained. The model is often used in preclinical studies of new IOP-lowering treatments. No better model for these purposes exists.

REFERENCES

Bastia, E, Toris, C, Bukowski, JM, Brambilla, S, Galli, C, Almirante, N, Bergamini, MVW, Lucarini, L, Navratil, T & Impagnatiello, F (2021) NCX 1741, a Novel Nitric Oxide-Donating Phosphodiesterase-5 Inhibitor, Exerts Rapid and Long-Lasting Intraocular Pressure-Lowering in Cynomolgus Monkeys. *J Ocul Pharmacol Ther,* 37, 215-22.
[http://dx.doi.org/10.1089/jop.2020.0126] [PMID: 33595367]

Bastia, E, Toris, CB, Brambilla, S, Galli, C, Almirante, N, Bergamini, MVW, Masini, E, Sgambellone, S, Unser, AM, Ahmed, F, Torrejon, KY, Navratil, T & Impagnatiello, F (2021) NCX 667, a Novel Nitric Oxide Donor, Lowers Intraocular Pressure in Rabbits, Dogs, and Non-Human Primates and Enhances TGFβ2-Induced Outflow in HTM/HSC Constructs. *Invest Ophthalmol Vis Sci,* 62, 17.
[http://dx.doi.org/10.1167/iovs.62.3.17] [PMID: 33704360]

Bellezza, AJ, Rintalan, CJ, Thompson, HW, Downs, JC, Hart, RT & Burgoyne, CF (2003) Deformation of the lamina cribrosa and anterior scleral canal wall in early experimental glaucoma. *Invest Ophthalmol Vis Sci,* 44, 623-37.
[http://dx.doi.org/10.1167/iovs.01-1282] [PMID: 12556392]

Fuwa, M, Toris, CB, Fan, S, Taniguchi, T, Ichikawa, M, Odani-Kawabata, N, Iwamura, R, Yoneda, K, Matsugi, T, Shams, NK & Zhang, JZ (2018) Effects of a Novel Selective EP2 Receptor Agonist, Omidenepag Isopropyl, on Aqueous Humor Dynamics in Laser-Induced Ocular Hypertensive Monkeys. *J Ocul Pharmacol Ther,* 34, 531-7.
[http://dx.doi.org/10.1089/jop.2017.0146] [PMID: 29989843]

Fuwa, M, Toris, CB, Fan, S, Taniguchi, T, Ichikawa, M, Odani-Kawabata, N, Iwamura, R, Yoneda, K, Matsugi, T, Shams, NK & Zhang, JZ (2018) Effects of a Novel Selective EP2 Receptor Agonist, Omidenepag Isopropyl, on Aqueous Humor Dynamics in Laser-Induced Ocular Hypertensive Monkeys. *J Oculharmacol Ther.*
[http://dx.doi.org/10.1089/jop.2017.0146]

Lee, PY, Podos, SM, Howard-Williams, JR, Severin, CH, Rose, AD & Siegel, MJ (1985) Pharmacological testing in the laser-induced monkey glaucoma model. *Curr Eye Res,* 4, 775-81.
[http://dx.doi.org/10.3109/02713688509020033] [PMID: 3861296]

Marx, MS, Podos, SM, Bodis-Wollner, I, Howard-Williams, JR, Siegel, MJ, Teitelbaum, CS, Maclin, EL & Severin, C (1986) Flash and pattern electroretinograms in normal and laser-induced glaucomatous primate eyes. *Invest Ophthalmol Vis Sci,* 27, 378-86.
[PMID: 3949466]

May, JA, McLaughlin, MA, Sharif, NA, Hellberg, MR & Dean, TR (2003) Evaluation of the ocular

hypotensive response of serotonin 5-HT1A and 5-HT2 receptor ligands in conscious ocular hypertensive cynomolgus monkeys. *J Pharmacol Exp Ther,* 306, 301-9.
[http://dx.doi.org/10.1124/jpet.103.049528] [PMID: 12676887]

Pederson, JE & Gaasterland, DE (1984) Laser-induced primate glaucoma. I. Progression of cupping. *Arch Ophthalmol,* 102, 1689-92.
[http://dx.doi.org/10.1001/archopht.1984.01040031373030] [PMID: 6541902]

Podos, SM, Camras, CB & Serle, JB (1989) Experimental compounds to lower intraocular pressure. *Aust N Z J Ophthalmol,* 17, 129-35.
[http://dx.doi.org/10.1111/j.1442-9071.1989.tb00502.x] [PMID: 2569320]

Quigley, HA & Hohman, RM (1983) Laser energy levels for trabecular meshwork damage in the primate eye. *Invest Ophthalmol Vis Sci,* 24, 1305-7.
[PMID: 6885314]

Sasaoka, M, Nakamura, K, Shimazawa, M, Ito, Y, Araie, M & Hara, H (2008) Changes in visual fields and lateral geniculate nucleus in monkey laser-induced high intraocular pressure model. *Exp Eye Res,* 86, 770-82.
[http://dx.doi.org/10.1016/j.exer.2008.02.004] [PMID: 18378230]

Toris, CB, McLaughlin, MA, Dworak, DP, Fan, S, Havens, S, Zhan, GL, Horan, N & Prasanna, G (2016) Effects of Rho Kinase Inhibitors on Intraocular Pressure and Aqueous Humor Dynamics in Nonhuman Primates and Rabbits. *J Ocul Pharmacol Ther,* 32, 355-64.
[http://dx.doi.org/10.1089/jop.2015.0116] [PMID: 27266531]

Toris, CB, Zhan, GL, Camras, CB & McLaughlin, MA (2005) Effects of travoprost on aqueous humor dynamics in monkeys. *J Glaucoma,* 14, 70-3.
[http://dx.doi.org/10.1097/01.ijg.0000146361.15163.ea] [PMID: 15650608]

Toris, CB, Zhan, GL, Feilmeier, MR, Camras, CB & McLaughlin, MA (2006) Effects of a prostaglandin DP receptor agonist, AL-6598, on aqueous humor dynamics in a nonhuman primate model of glaucoma. *J Ocul Pharmacol Ther,* 22, 86-92.
[http://dx.doi.org/10.1089/jop.2006.22.86] [PMID: 16722794]

Toris, CB, Zhan, GL, Wang, YL, Zhao, J, McLAUGHLIN, MA, Camras, CB & Yablonski, M (2000) Aqueous humor dynamics in monkeys with laser-induced glaucoma. *J Ocul Pharmacol Ther,* 16, 19-27.
[http://dx.doi.org/10.1089/jop.2000.16.19] [PMID: 10673127]

Yablonski, ME, Cook, DJ & Gray, J (1985) A fluorophotometric study of the effect of argon laser trabeculoplasty on aqueous humor dynamics. *Am J Ophthalmol,* 99, 579-82.
[http://dx.doi.org/10.1016/S0002-9394(14)77963-2] [PMID: 4003496]

Zhang, Y, Toris, CB, Liu, Y, Ye, W & Gong, H (2009) Morphological and hydrodynamic correlates in monkey eyes with laser induced glaucoma. *Exp Eye Res,* 89, 748-56.
[http://dx.doi.org/10.1016/j.exer.2009.06.015] [PMID: 19591828]

CHAPTER 34

Protocol for Assessment of Aqueous Humor Dynamics in the Living Mouse

J. Cameron Millar[1,*] and **Wei Zhang**[1]

[1] *North Texas Eye Research Institute (NTERI), Department of Pharmacology & Neuroscience, University of North Texas Health Science Center (UNTHSC), 3500 Camp Bowie Boulevard, Room IREB-511, Fort Worth, TX 76107, USA*

Abstract: A protocol is described in detail to make an assessment in a mouse model in an experimental session of all principle parameters of aqueous humor dynamics (AHD), specifically intraocular pressure (IOP), aqueous flow rate (F_{in}), uveoscleral outflow rate (F_u), total aqueous outflow facility (C_{tot}), and episcleral venous pressure (EVP). Using the technique described, direct measurements of IOP, C_{tot}, and EVP can be made. On the basis of these measurements, by utilizing the modified Goldmann equation, values for F_{in} and F_u can then be derived. These measurements have relevance in the mouse, as the anterior segment of the mouse eye has many anatomic, physiologic, and pharmacologic features in common with the human eye. The mouse has found much use over the last two decades as an animal model for the study of primary open-angle glaucoma (POAG), a progressive optic neuropathy and a leading cause of irreversible blindness globally. POAG is very often associated with elevated IOP and disturbances in other parameters of AHD. Thus, an ability to quantify these parameters in this species has much relevance to research into POAG, especially when considering (1) animal model validation, and (2) effects of experimental compounds designed to modify AHD.

Keywords: Anterior chamber, Aqueous flow, Aqueous humor dynamics, Aqueous outflow facility, Eye, Episcleral venous pressure, Glaucoma, Intraocular pressure, Mouse, Posterior chamber, Protocol, Uveoscleral outflow.

INTRODUCTION

Glaucomas are a group of optic neuropathies in which there is a progressive loss of retinal ganglion cell somas and their axons, as well as damage to the optic nerve and certain centers involved in the relay of visual impulses in the brain. Primary open-angle glaucoma (POAG) accounts for ~86% of all glaucomas in the

* **Corresponding author J. Cameron Millar:** North Texas Eye Research Institute (NTERI), Department of Pharmacology & Neuroscience, University of North Texas Health Science Center (UNTHSC), 3500 Camp Bowie Boulevard, Room IREB-511, Fort Worth, TX 76107, USA; Tel: (817) 735-2682; E-mail: Cameron.Millar@unthsc.edu

Najam A. Sharif and Sunny E. Ohia (Eds.)

world (Tham *et al.,* 2014). It is estimated that by 2040, there will be 111,800,000 cases of glaucoma globally, an increase of ~47% since 2020 (Tham *et al.,* 2014). In the USA alone, 150,000 people have been bilaterally blinded by the condition. In POAG, there is pathological damage to the trabecular meshwork (TM), which forms part of the principal outflow pathway for aqueous humor. This damage, which often develops slowly over a period of many years, involves endoplasmic reticulum (ER) stress in TM cells, as well as increased synthesis and deposition of the insoluble structural proteins, fibronectin, laminin, elastin, and collagen types I, III, IV, and VI, as well as increased expression of various glycosaminoglycans and the cross-linking enzymes transglutaminase and lysyl oxidase (Kasetti *et al.,* 2017; Raychaudhuri, Millar & Clark, 2017). This leads to a gradually increased resistance beyond normal values to aqueous humor outflow *via* this route. Since the eye is a closed system, the pressure required to drive the aqueous out of the anterior chamber often slowly increases. Thus, the intraocular pressure (IOP) is often increased from equilibrated values of 10 to 15 mmHg (healthy eye) to a higher equilibrated value in excess of 21 mmHg (after POAG has developed over several years). It does still hold true, however, that at equilibrated IOP, whatever its value, the total aqueous humor secretion rate must be equal to the total aqueous humor outflow rate. If the former exceeds the latter, IOP will continue to rise until the increased total outflow rate with increasing IOP finally equals the total inflow rate, and then IOP stabilizes at a new, higher value. If the former is less than the latter, then IOP will drop until the reduction in total outflow rate with dropping IOP finally equals the total inflow rate, and then IOP stabilizes at a new, lower value. Indeed, this positive correlation between changes in total aqueous humor outflow rate with corresponding changes in IOP is what constitutes total aqueous outflow conductance or facility (represented by $C_{(tot)}$, mathematically the reciprocal of total aqueous humor outflow resistance). Healthy eyes or eyes with POAG exhibit higher or lower values of $C_{(tot)}$, respectively.

This situation is qualitatively different from the situation seen in complete 360° angle closure, whereby all of the TM is completely covered by the peripheral iris, and aqueous humor cannot access the trabecular outflow pathway. In such cases, no amount of increase in IOP will increase the trabecular outflow rate of aqueous humor (which is zero), and thus, IOP will spike very rapidly (within a matter of a few hours) to values of around 50 to 100 mmHg, or sometimes even greater. In such cases, the alternative aqueous humor outflow pathway, the uveoscleral pathway, which exhibits a very minimal capacity for increase in outflow rate with increasing IOP (*i.e.*, very minimal facility), can make up the required total aqueous outflow (to equal total aqueous humor inflow), but only when IOP rises very rapidly to very high levels, not typically seen in POAG. In such cases, where IOP is extremely high, there is likely also a significant reduction in total aqueous humor inflow rate (Bill, 1971; Todd & Woodhouse, 1973). However, in POAG, where IOP rises only moderately, there is no significant reduction in the total aqueous humor inflow rate (Martin, Fernández-Vila & Pérez, 1995).

An ability to measure $C_{(tot)}$ is therefore of importance when establishing, validating, or utilizing animal models of POAG. The mouse has been utilized for the study of this disease for over two decades at this point. The reasons for this are several-fold. Mice are relatively inexpensive and easy to house. Their relatively brief life span means that desired conditions can be developed rapidly, and they can be aged out within a reasonable time frame. There are more than 20,000 transgenic strains of mice now commercially available, and thus, many genes can be knocked in, knocked out, knocked up, or knocked down, thus facilitating studies on the disease at the genetic level. Further, there are many similarities between the mouse and human genomes. The anterior segment of the mouse eye has many features in common with the human eye in terms of structural anatomy, physiological function, innervation, pharmacological receptor expression, and blood supply. Also, the mouse TM and aqueous outflow pathway distal to the TM is structurally and functionally very similar to that of the human (Millar *et al.,* 2015; Lopez *et al.,* 2017), which sets mice apart from most other placental mammals, with the exception of non-human primates and rats. Until the advent of the 21st century, POAG studies on mice were limited as accurate and repeatable measurements of IOP in these animals were difficult to perform, and reliable measurements of aqueous humor dynamics (AHD) were thought to lie outside of the limits of available instrumentation due to the small size of the eyes of this species and the relatively tiny volumes of fluid involved. However, improvements in instrumentation have now led to the ability to perform both of these tasks in these animals routinely.

Here, we describe a protocol for the measurement of $C_{(tot)}$ in living mouse eyes using a technique of constant flow rate infusion of perfusate into the aqueous chamber of the eye (Millar, Clark & Pang, 2011; Millar *et al.,* 2015). For illustrative purposes, some representative data obtained using this technique is also presented. During infusion, pressure developed within the system is monitored *via* a pressure transducer. The apparatus may also be utilized to obtain a value for episcleral venous pressure (EVP). Using this data, it is then also possible to derive estimates for aqueous humor formation rate (F_{in}) and uveoscleral outflow (F_u) by substitution into the modified Goldmann equation (Goldmann, 1955; Gabelt & Kaufman, 2011), which specifies a good approximation of a value for IOP in terms of F_{in}, F_u, C_{tot}, and EVP:

$$IOP = \left[\frac{Fin - Fu}{Ctot}\right] + EVP$$

If F_{in} and F_u are specified in units of μL/min, C_{tot} is specified in units of μL/min/mmHg and EVP is specified in mmHg, then the calculated value of IOP will also be cited in mmHg above ambient air pressure.

Thus all parameters of AHD can be obtained in a single experimental session.

EXPERIMENTAL PROTOCOLS

The following procedures were performed in compliance with the Statement for the Use of Animals in Ophthalmic and Visual Research published by the Association for Research in Vision and Ophthalmology (ARVO) and also the regulations of the Institutional Animal Care and Use Committee (IACUC) of the University of North Texas Health Science Center.

Preparation of Perfusate Solution

Phosphate Buffered Saline (PBS) solution, Balanced Salt Solution (BSS), or Balanced Salt Solution with added glutathione (BSS-Plus) are available for purchase as sterile preparations available from a number of different suppliers. We use Ultra-Pure PBS, USP sterile supplied at 10 × concentration (VWR Chemicals, LLC; 28600 Fountain Parkway, Solon, OH 44139, USA). Of these three solutions specified, only BSS-Plus has added D-glucose at a concentration of 5.1 mM (which closely matches the concentration found in normal aqueous humor). Nevertheless, we find that for short-term perfusions (lasting no more than 2 to 3 hours), any of these solutions are sufficiently similar in composition to aqueous humor that they may be used at 1× concentration as perfusate solutions. As an alternative, Bárány's mock aqueous humor solution (BAH, Bárány's) (Bárány, 1964) can be used. However, although BAH better mimics the essential composition of aqueous humor, it is not commercially available and so must be made up fresh prior to each experimental session from pre-purchased chemical components. However, 10× stock (without added $CaCl_2$) can be prepared and stored. Following dilution to 1× concentration immediately prior to each perfusion session, $CaCl_2$ may be added dropwise. Dulbecco's Modified Eagle's Cell Culture Medium (DMEM) may also be utilized, although, for such a short-term perfusion, we find that this offers no particular advantage. For detailed components of each solution, see Tables **1** - **4** (Appendix).

200 mL of perfusate should be prepared prior to each experiment. Before use, the perfusate should be filtered to remove any particulate material that could clog the TM. Currently, we use sterile 0.2 μm Cellulose Acetate Membrane Syringe Filters (VWR USA, North American Catalog Number: 28145-477). In the past, we used 0.2 μm Acrodisc® Syringe Filters (HT Tuffryn®Membrane Low Protein Binding Non-Pyrogenic, REF: 4454) supplied by PALL Gelman Laboratory, Port

Washington, NY, USA. However, any sterile syringe filter of the same pore size would be suitable for this purpose.

Perfusion Apparatus

A perfusion apparatus should be constructed from the list of components, as shown in Table **5** (Appendix). Many components produced by alternative manufacturers other than the ones we have suggested may be used. However, because of the very low flow rates involved during infusion, if an alternative infusion pump is used, it should be capable of a minimum pusher advance per ½-step of 88 nm or less (Lopez *et al.,* 2017). This is necessary to minimize the issue of inducing pulsatile flow, especially at the lower flow rates specified. The list given includes apparatus sufficient to perfuse 2 animals (thus 4 eyes) simultaneously. The apparatus should be assembled as shown in the diagram and the photograph shown in Fig. **1**. The apparatus can be duplicated if more than 2 animals are to be perfused together. We have two such set-ups in our laboratory and can routinely perfuse 4 animals (8 eyes) simultaneously.

Methods

Filling of Perfusion Lines and Manometers

Freshly prepared and filtered perfusate should be used to fill all perfusion lines and manometers. First, use a clean, sterile 3 mL syringe to fill the perfusion tubing (ensuring that no bubbles are present). After the tube is filled, pour perfusate from a beaker into the manometer reservoirs. Then disconnect the distal tubing of the manometers from the 3-way valves to allow perfusate to run from the manometer reservoirs to the distal end of the manometer tubing, taking care to ensure that the manometer reservoirs do not completely empty during this process. Once again, it is important to ensure that no bubbles are present. Finally, reconnect the distal manometer tubing to the 3-way valves and top up the manometer reservoirs once more.

To fill the glass microsyringes placed in the microdialysis infusion pumps, move the pump pusher block back to allow movement of the syringe plunger all the way out of the syringe. Open the manometer reservoir to the syringe and allow the syringe to fill. Remove the plunger and allow perfusate to flow from the proximal end of the syringe until satisfied that no bubbles are present. Then, replace the plunger and move the pump pusher block up just far enough to prevent the plunger from being ejected from the syringe by the pressure induced on the plunger by the manometer, ensuring the syringe remains filled. Relieve the pressure in the syringe barrel by closing the manometer to the syringe using the 3-

way valve. Then, repeat this process to fill the other syringes. When all syringes are filled, wipe up any spilled perfusate from the pump housing.

Finally, switch on the TBM4M Transducer Amplifier Manifold (thus energizing BLPR2 Pressure Transducers). Also, switch on the Microdialysis Infusion Pumps, but set them to idle (so that they are not pumping fluid). Leave the apparatus undisturbed for at least 30 minutes.

Animal Anesthesia

For animal anesthesia, we use a cocktail of ketamine (10 mg/mL) and xylazine (1 mg/mL). Camras *et al.* (2010) reported that these anesthetic agents, when co-administered, do not affect $C_{(tot)}$ in mice, even after 2 hours of duration. We do not incorporate acepromazine into the mixture because we have found that acepromazine carries a small but significant risk of causing premature animal death. For induction, animals are given 100 µL of cocktail intraperitoneally (I.P.) for every 10 g body weight, thus a dose of ketamine (100 mg/kg) and xylazine (10 mg/kg). For maintenance, animals receive ½ × to ¼ × the induction dose. For the preparation of animals for the procedure, each animal is weighed and then receives one induction dose I.P. After each animal becomes quiescent, it is then placed on the energized warming pad to maintain body temperature. Fifteen minutes thereafter, each animal receives ½ × the induction dose I.P. Fifteen minutes following that, each animal receives ¼ × the induction dose I.P. Five minutes following that, animals are assessed for a lack of a flexor withdrawal response to a painful toe-pinch, a lack of a response to a painful tail pinch, and the absence of a blink reflex in response to brief light stroking of the eyes with a surgical sponge. If the animal lacks these responses at this stage, it is judged to be in a suitable plane of surgical anesthesia. A value for anesthetized IOP is then obtained for each eye using a TonoLab™ impact tonometer. We take the IOP value as the mean of 6 individual valid readings. Following this, cannulation of the eyes can proceed.

Zeroing of Transducer Output and Cannulation of Eyes

Immediately prior to cannulation of ocular aqueous chambers, the apparatus should be zeroed. To achieve this, the software should be set to record. With the transducers positioned at the same level from the laboratory floor as the eyes to be cannulated and ensuring that the microdialysis infusion pumps are not running, bridge switches on the TBM4M Transducer Amplifier Manifold corresponding to all relevant channels should be moved to the Diff position. At that point, the Position Adjust Knob above the Gain Switch should be rotated one way or the other, as necessary, until both red LED indicators (low indicator and high indicator) are illuminated. At that point, the output is zeroed, *i.e.*, the chart recorder trace indicates zero when the signal from the transducer is zero volts. If only the low LED is illuminated, the output is negative, and the Position Adjust Knob should be rotated clockwise. If only the high LED is illuminated, the output is positive, and the Position Adjust Knob should be rotated counter-clockwise.

Once each channel output has been zeroed, eyes may be cannulated. Under × 30 magnification, the anterior chamber of each eye is cannulated with a 32G ½-inch steel needle (we use STERiJECT™, The Hague, The Netherlands, and also Tochigi-Shi, Tochigi-Ken, Japan) as shown in Fig. (**1b**) (Panel G). For cannulation, the globe is first stabilized with forceps and proptosed. The tip of the cannulating needle is then held approximately 0.5 mm from the limbus over the peripheral cornea. The needle is then inserted through the peripheral cornea and pushed through the anterior chamber until it approaches the aspect of the chamber angle opposite the point of cannulation, with the opening of the needle tip facing the anterior part of the iris. During this procedure, it is important not to allow the needle to damage the anterior surface of the iris, the corneal endothelium, the lens capsule, or the lens. Also, it is important to follow the described cannulation procedure such that the needle tip ends up positioned in the anterior chamber with the bevel facing towards (but without touching) the iris. This will minimize any tendency towards partial blockade of the needle tip (Fig. **2a**). The tubing to which the needle is attached is supported in a holder (we make ours from a small block of modeling clay (Fig. **1b**, Panel G) so that the needle will remain in place in the eye after cannulation. The contralateral eye is then cannulated in the same manner. 30G steel needles can be used when working with fully mature animals, but juvenile animals have less space available in their anterior chambers, and therefore, it may not be possible to cannulate them with 30G needles without deforming the chamber. Glass microneedles can also be used but we have found that these exhibit a greater tendency to become blocked during the course of the perfusion. In addition, one must be careful that the tips of such microneedles are not so narrow as to induce a significant resistance to flow at the flow rates to be utilized during the experiment.

It is also possible to cannulate the posterior chambers of the eyes, as shown in Fig. **2b**. If posterior chamber cannulation is desired, the eye should be proptosed and stabilized with forceps. The tip of the cannulating needle should be placed approximately 1mm behind the limbus over the sclera. It should then be pushed through the sclera and underlying pars plicata to enter the posterior chamber. The needle tip should be advanced slowly until it just becomes visible to the pupil as it emerges from behind the iris. The needle should then be withdrawn until the tip disappears behind the iris and is now fully within the posterior chamber.

Topical anesthesia may optionally be given immediately prior to cannulation. We use oxybuprocaine 0.5% (Alcaine®, Alcon Laboratories, Fort Worth, TX USA) and apply it as 1-2 drops to each eye, allowing 5 minutes for effect prior to cannulation. The use of mydriatics, however, should be avoided as these can influence $C_{(tot)}$ by (1) causing the iris to crowd the outflow angle and (2) if the mydriatic is a muscarinic receptor blocker (cyclopentolate, homatropine, atropine, or tropicamide), it will promote cycloplegia, which may reduce $C_{(tot)}$.

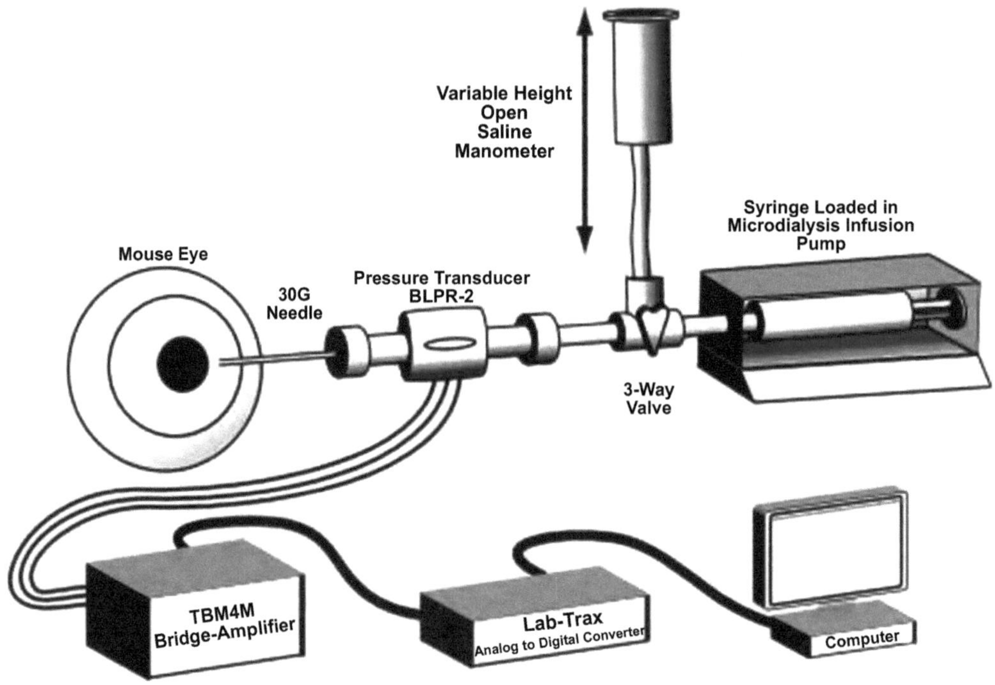

Fig. (1A). Constant Flow Infusion Apparatus (Schematic Representation). The anterior or posterior aqueous chamber of the living mouse eye is cannulated with a 32G steel needle or a glass microneedle. If working with fully mature mice, a slightly larger 30G steel needle may be used instead. Using this system, a supported enucleated eye can also be cannulated (see text). The needle is connected via tubing to a flow-through BLPR2 Pressure Transducer (WPI Instruments, Sarasota, FL, USA) for continuous determination of pressure within the system. The opposing end of the transducer is connected to a 3-way valve, which in turn is connected to (1) a 50 uL or 100 uL glass microsyringe loaded into a SP101i Microdialysis Infusion Pump (WPI) and an open-ended, variable height, raised reservoir manometer. The pressure transducer is connected electrically to a TBM4M Transducer Amplifier Manifold (WPI). A Lab-Trax Analog-to-Digital Converter (WPI) is included in the circuit. Pressure data as a function of time is displayed and stored on a computer. Voltage output from the transducers can be related to IOP by using the manometers to calibrate the apparatus, on the principle that for every 13.6 cm, the manometer reservoir perfusate meniscus is elevated above the transducer chamber corresponds to a pressure of 10 mmHg. Calibration may also be confirmed using a sphygmomanometer attached to the transducer chamber (Adapted from Millar, Clark & Pang, 2011).

(Panel A)

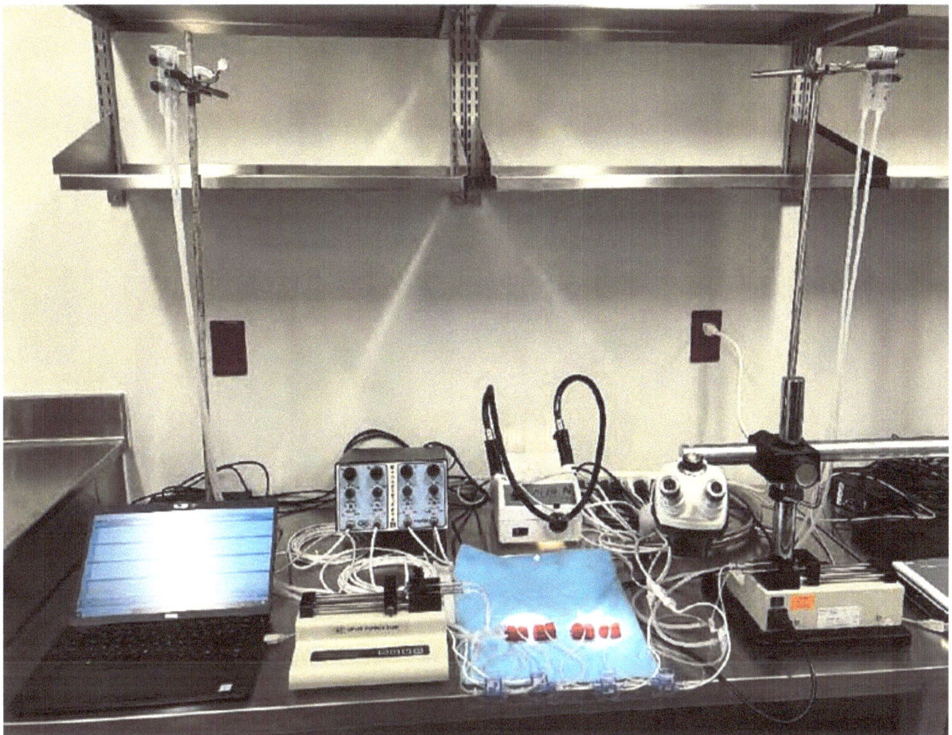

(Panel B)

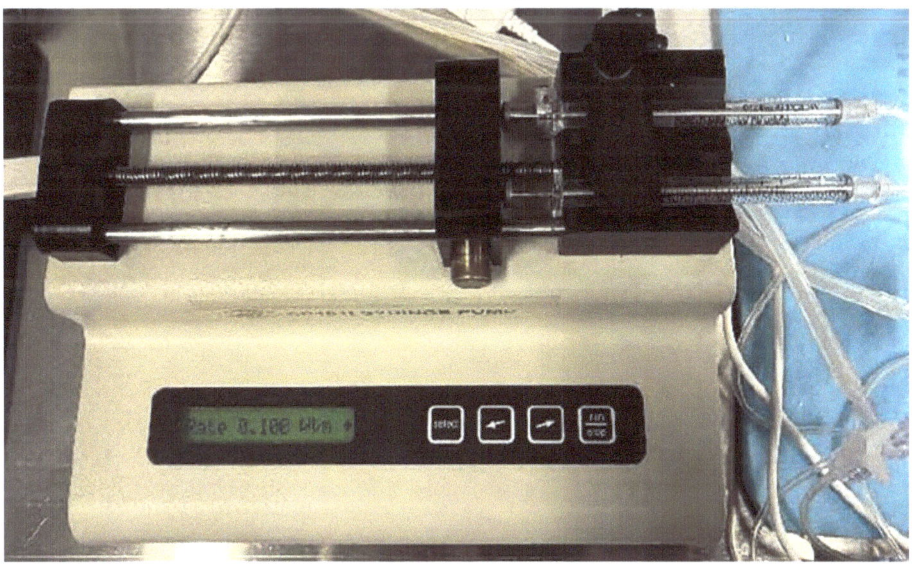

(Panel C)

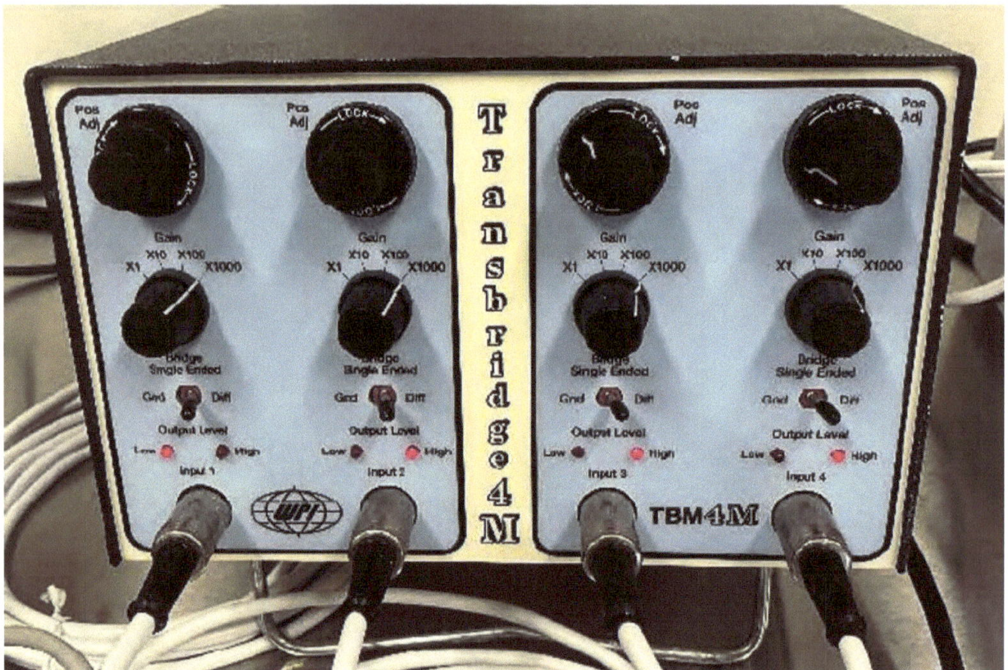

(Panel D)

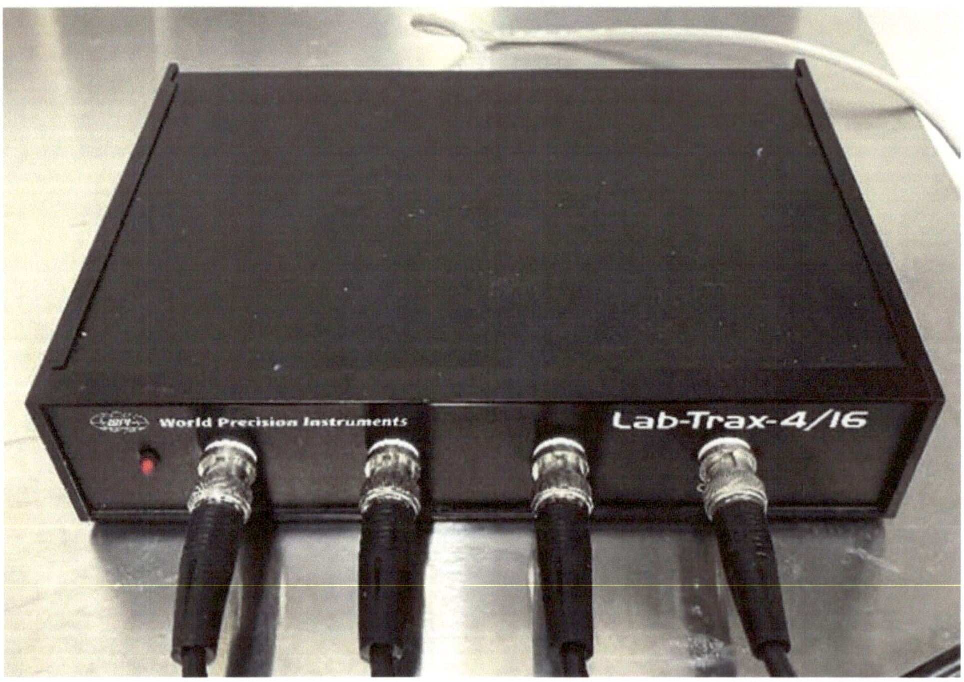

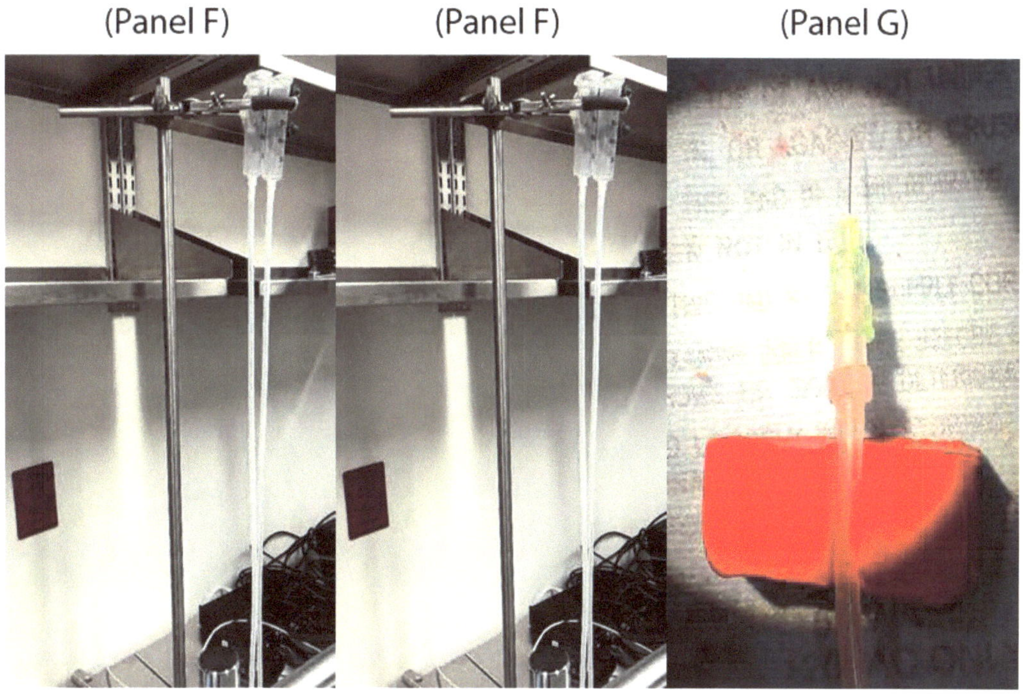

Fig. (1B). Photographs of Constant Flow Infusion Apparatus. Panel A: Overview of set-up. A dissection microscope and illuminator are included. Notice the BLPR2 pressure transducers are affixed to the edge of the bench such that their fluid chambers are levelled with the mouse eyes when they are cannulated. An electrical warming pad (with a blue cloth cover) is also included to prevent animals from becoming hypothermic when under anesthesia. The apparatus shown is sufficient to infuse 2 mice (thus 4 eyes) simultaneously. Panel B: SP101i Microdialysis Infusion Pump (WPI, Sarasota, FL, USA), loaded with 100 mL capacity glass microsyringes (Hamilton Co., Reno, NV, USA). Panel C: Transbridge TBM4M Transducer Amplifier Manifold (WPI). Panel D: Lab-Trax 4/16 Analog-to-Digital Converter (WPI). Panel E: BLPR2 flow-through Pressure Transducer (WPI). Panel F: Variable-height open-ended manometer, made up of a 20 mL plastic syringe barrel connected to the tubing. The distal end of the tubing is connected to a 3-way valve. Panel G: Close-up view of 32G ½" needle connected to luer attachment and supported in a block of modeling clay.

Following anterior chamber or posterior chamber cannulation, the eye should be examined for evidence of any post-cannulation bleeding into the chamber. If bleeding occurrs, then that eye should be considered lost for measurement of the facility, as red blood cells will clog the TM and reduce the aqueous outflow facility. Also, there is a very high likelihood that the cannulating needle tip will become blocked with fibrin. With practice and careful placement of the needle tip, however, bleeding should not be an issue. Also, as a rule, one has only one attempt to cannulate each eye. Multiple needle sticks into the globe (through both the cornea and especially the sclera) will lead to a high probability of leakage, which will artificially increase the outflow facility to supra-physiological values.

After cannulation is complete, a drop of perfusate should be applied topically to each eye to prevent corneal drying. Care should be taken to ensure that further drops are added if necessary as the experiment proceeds.

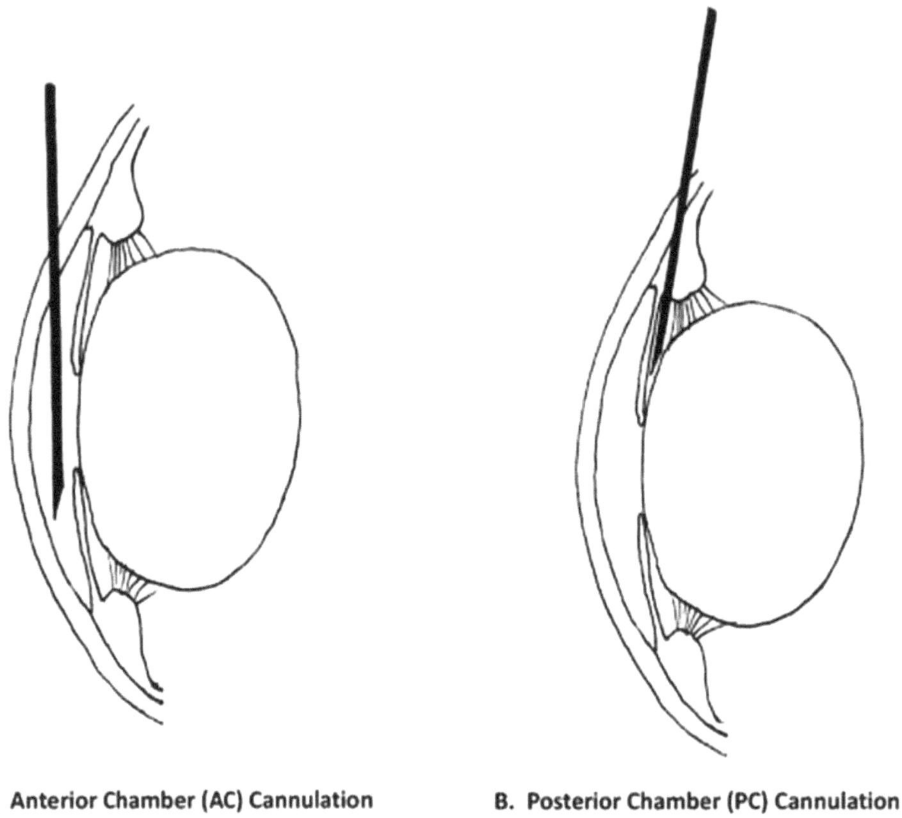

Fig. (2). Cannulation of Eyes. (A) Anterior Chamber (AC) Cannulation. In AC cannulation, under high illumination and × 30 magnification, a 32G steel needle is passed through the cornea ~1 mm from the limbus (bevel facing down) and pushed across to the opposing end of the anterior chamber, taking care not to strike the corneal endothelium, anterior lens capsule, or iris. (B) Posterior Chamber (PC) Cannulation. In PC cannulation, under high illumination and ×30 magnification, a 32G steel needle is passed through the region of the anterior sclera overlying the pars plicata and advanced into the posterior chamber under the iris until the tip of the needle is just visible under the iris at the pupillary margin (thus confirming that the PC is cannulated). The needle tip is then carefully and slowly withdrawn back under the iris just until it ceases to be visible and the pupil margin has settled back into a normal anatomic position. (Adapted from Lopez *et al.*, 2017).

Obtaining a Value for Episcleral Venous Pressure (EVP)

After cannulation, the manometers are opened to the circuit, and each eye of the animal is returned to its anesthetized but pre-cannulated tonometrically-indicated

IOP by adjusting the height of each reservoir accordingly. Pressure in the eye is read from the output from the BLPR2 pressure transducers. Each eye is then given 5 minutes to allow pressure to stabilize. Following that, the IOP is artificially lowered in 1 mmHg increments, at a rate not exceeding 1 mmHg/min, by lowering the manometer reservoir. Following the establishment of each new lowered IOP value, the anterior segment (in particular, Schlemm's canal and the episcleral veins) should be visualized using a direct ophthalmoscope or a dissection microscope. At least a full minute should be allowed at each new lowered pressure. At the point when IOP is lowered sufficiently, the episcleral veins, and then, as pressure is lowered marginally more, Schlemm's canal will be seen to swell and redden as a result of retrograde flow from the episcleral veins, which lack valves. When this is seen to occur, the value of IOP at this point represents a close approximation of EVP. At that point, the eye is returned manometrically to its pre-cannulation but post-anesthesia tonometrically-indicated IOP, and the manometer is then closed to the perfusion line. To practice this method of obtaining a value for EVP, we suggest practicing on albino mice first, as it is easier to see the reddening and swelling of the episcleral veins and Schlemm's canal in such non-pigmented animals. This method of estimating EVP was first described by Aihara, Lindsey, and Weinreb (2003).

Perfusion of Live Animals

The microdialysis infusion pump is then switched on at a flow rate of 100 nL/min (0.1 μL/min), and the cannulated eyes are allowed 30 minutes for pressure equilibration. Initially, upon switching on the perfusion pumps, pressure output from the BLPR2 transducers will start to rise but should have stabilized to a reasonably consistent plateau by 30 minutes. Pressure stabilization may be considered to have been achieved when the initial sharp rate of increase in pressure at each successively higher flow rate has tailed off to less than 15% of the original increase and then starts to move both upward and downward but by no more than 2 mmHg in each direction. A perfectly flat plateau, especially with a living eye, is almost impossible to obtain due to small but continuous changes in IOP, aqueous outflow resistance, and EVP, probably secondary to sympathetic and parasympathetic autonomic nervous inputs. At that point, stabilized pressure should be recorded for a period of 15 minutes. The flow rate should then be increased in 50 nL/min to 100 nL/min increments (0.05 μL/min to 0.1 μL/min increments) until reaching a flow rate of 400nL/min (0.4 μL/min). The flow is allowed to continue at each new flow rate for 15 minutes before moving on to the next higher flow rate to allow for pressure stabilization. Flow rates of greater than 400 nL/min (0.4 μL/min) can also be utilized. It should be understood, however, that at these higher flow rates (450 nL/min and 500 nL/min (0.45 μL/min and 0.5 μL/min) in a proportion of eyes, Schlemm's canal will constrict to the point that total aqueous outflow resistance will sharply increase, and thus $C_{(tot)}$ will sharply decrease (Li *et al.,* 2014). Thus, at this point, in some animals, the linear relationship between Pressure (P) and Pump Flow Rate (F) may be lost. And indeed, if F is increased beyond 500 nL/min (0.5 μL/min), then we have found that the linear relationship will certainly be lost (Millar *et al.,* ARVO Abstract, 2018).

Following completion of perfusion, the experiment can be ended (if only values for $C_{(tot)}$ and EVP are required). Infusion pumps should be switched off, and needles should be rapidly withdrawn from each eye. Care should be taken to ensure that output from the transducers returns to zero, thus confirming that needles are not blocked. For further confirmation, the manometers can be opened to the needles to ensure that perfusate drips from the tips of the needles. If, at this stage, needles are found to be blocked, then data from the involved eye(s) should be discarded. Insertion of a needle through the cornea of a live eye (a procedure called paracentesis) can lead to a degree of breakdown of the blood-aqueous barrier. Obviously, it would be desirable that this did not happen, but it is probably impossible to eliminate completely. A degree of secretion of protein-bearing plasmoid aqueous may then occur (Millar, Gabelt & Kaufman, 1998), which can lead to fibrin clots blocking the lumen of the needle. Bleeding into the chamber can also occur. The effect is minimized by rapid and skilled insertion of the needle into the target location within the aqueous chamber without damaging any collateral structures or blood vessels.

If it is desired to estimate F_{in} and F_u, then animals should be perfused dead as described below in section 3.6.

Perfusion of Dead Animals

Following completion of perfusion of live anesthetized animals, the animals can be euthanized *in situ* by administration of a ketamine/xylazine anesthesia cocktail at 5 × the induction dose. While performing euthanasia in this way, care should be taken to avoid disturbing the placement of the cannulating needles in the aqueous chambers of the eyes. Animals should be observed until all breathing has ceased, which typically takes between 5 and 15 minutes. To confirm cessation of heartbeat, ophthalmoscopic examination of the retina should also be performed to establish that blanching of the retinal vessels has taken place. At this point, the microdialysis infusion pumps should be switched off. The eyes should then be opened to the reservoirs of the manometers by adjustment of the respective 3-way valves. Pressures in each eye should then be adjusted by lowering the reservoirs until the readout from the BLPR2 pressure transducers indicates zero mmHg (*i.e.*, ambient air pressure). We do so because following the cessation of heartbeat and aqueous humor secretion, we assume that both F_{in} and EVP approximate zero, and thus, by Goldmann considerations, IOP also approximates zero. Eyes should be given 2 to 3 minutes to equilibrate. The manometer reservoirs should then be close to the eyes by adjustment of the 3-way valves once again. At this point, the microdialysis infusion pumps should be switched on at a flow rate of 100 nL/min (0.1 µL/min), and the eyes should be given 15 minutes at this flow rate to equilibrate. Following this, eyes should be perfused once again at each flow rate utilized while the animals were alive in a manner identical to that described in Section 3.5 (Perfusion of Live Animals).

During the perfusion of dead animals, care should be taken to ensure that all corneas are given an additional drop of perfusate topical ocular to ensure that eyes do not dry out.

Following this second perfusion, the experiment is over. The needle should be removed from each eye. As previously described in Section 3.5, it should be established that upon doing so, pressure indicated by the transducers returns to zero. Further confirmation can be obtained by opening the manometers to the needle to ensure that perfusate drips from the needles. If needles are found to be blocked, then data from the involved eye(s) should be discarded.

Animal carcasses should be disposed of in an approved manner. All perfusion lines, manometer lines, reservoirs, and microsyringes should be flushed with sterile water to remove all traces of salt solution, which will otherwise tend to cause blockages as it dries and salts precipitate out of the solution. As a precaution, at this stage, we turn off and disconnect all electrical apparatus.

Calculations

Total Outflow Facility ($C_{(tot)}$)

Mean Stabilized Perfusion Pressure (P) in mmHg as ordinate against each Infusion Flow Rate (F) as abscissa should be plotted (Fig. **3b**). The plot is fitted by simple linear regression. A statistical rationale for doing so is discussed by Lopez *et al.* (2017). Intersection through the origin should not be assumed. The slope of the curve is equal to Total Outflow Resistance ($R_{(tot)}$). The reciprocal of R(tot) is equal to the total outflow facility ($C_{(tot)}$). $C_{(tot)}$ should be calculated for each eye studied while live and (if appropriate) also following euthanasia. Thus, a population of values for $C_{(tot)}$ (live) and $C_{(tot)}$ (euth) will be generated. In our experience, there is no significant difference between the means of $C_{(tot)}$ (live) and $C_{(tot)}$ (dead), although, on occasion, individual eyes will show variation between these two parameters. In a small proportion of eyes, the curve may deviate significantly from linearity at values of F > 400 nL/min (> 0.4 µL/min). In these cases, high-pressure values at such relatively high flow rates should be discarded (bearing in mind that the natural aqueous secretion rate in a healthy mouse eye lies between 100 and 200 nL/min (0.1 and 0.2 µL/min)), as this most likely corresponds to a constriction of Schlemm's canal and a sharp increase in R(tot) (Li *et al.,* 2014) which is not reflective of R(tot) during day-to-day life of the animal.

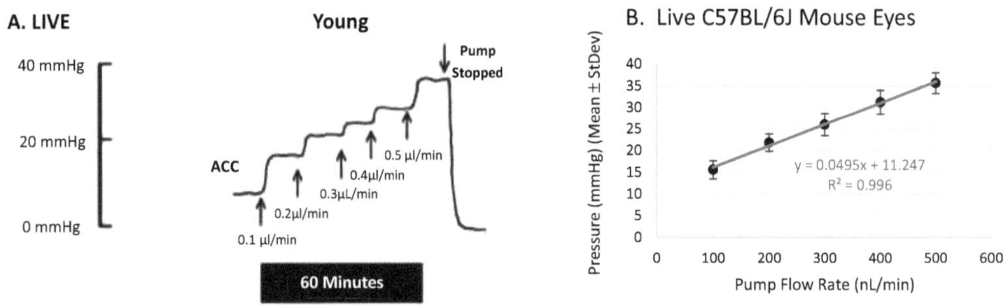

Fig. (3). Panel A: Example Pressure-Time Trace from a single experiment with a live C57BL/6J mouse (age 14 weeks). Panel B: Mean Pressure-Flow Rate curve derived from N=8 live C57BL/6J animals (aged 16-20 weeks). The curve has been fitted by simple linear regression (solid gray line). The Y-intercept of 11.2 mmHg indicates a good approximation for resting intraocular pressure under ketamine/xylazine anesthesia. Total outflow resistance (R(tot)) over this range of pump flow rates is given by slope (= 0.0495 mmHg/nL.min). $C_{(tot)}$ is given by the reciprocal of the slope (= 20.2 nL/min/mmHg). In living animals, we found no significant difference between Pressure-Flow Rate curves plotted for animals perfused with the tip of the cannulating needle placed in the AC or the PC (Lopez *et al.,* 2017). This, however, may not be the case when perfusing enucleated eyes perfused *ex vivo* (Millar *et al.,* ARVO Abstract, 2018). (Panel A adapted from Millar *et al.,* 2015).

Uveoscleral Outflow Rate (Fu)

In an euthanized animal, aqueous humor formation rate (F_{in}) and episcleral venous pressure (EVP) can both be assumed to be zero. Thus, by Goldmann considerations, a mathematical estimation of uveoscleral outflow rate (F_u) is given by:

$$Fu = F - (P\ (at\ that\ value\ of\ F) \times C(tot)\ (euth))$$

Values for F_u are calculated at each value of F. The resultant population of calculated values is averaged to obtain a final value for F_u.

Aqueous Humor Formation Rate (F_{in})

By Goldmann considerations, a mathematical estimation of aqueous humor formation rate (F_{in}) during life is given by:

$$Fin = [(C(tot)\ (live) \times (IOP - EVP)] + Fu$$

(IOP, in this case, is given by post-anesthesia but pre-cannulation IOP as determined by TonoLab impact tonometry). Note: IOP – EVP is a good approximation of the more accurate but currently unquantifiable (in a mouse eye) expression;

Pressure in Anterior Chamber Angle – Pressure in the lumen of Schlemm's canal

This is related to the facts that (1) actual pressure in the aqueous chamber is higher at the point of secretion into the posterior chamber, from where it flows down a pressure gradient into the anterior chamber and then to the anterior chamber angle, and (2) pressure in the lumen of Schlemm's canal is higher than pressure in the scleral collector channels, which in turn is higher than pressure in the aqueous veins, which in turn is higher than episcleral venous pressure. However, the degree of error introduced in this case by simply subtracting EVP from IOP is likely very minimal in percentage terms.

These calculations are outlined in greater detail by Millar, Clark & Pang (2011).

Perfusion of Enucleated Eyes

Murine eyes can also be perfused *ex vivo* using the apparatus and techniques described following the enucleation of whole globes from animals. When doing this, we set the eyes up immediately following enucleation in an eye holder made from a small block of modeling clay, with an indentation (forming a well) made upon its upper surface large enough to hold a murine globe. The eye is grasped by its optic nerve using forceps, and then the AC or PC (as desired) is cannulated. Following cannulation, the eye is placed in the well, which can be filled with perfusate (*i.e.*, the eye is completely immersed in perfusate to eliminate evaporation from the ocular surface, which will then tend to take place in the absence of adnexal tissue that normally surrounds the globe and the tear film (which normally incorporates a lipid layer and inhibits evaporation from the ocular surface). Alternatively, if desired, the well can be left empty, and thus, the eye can be perfused in air. In this scenario, evaporation from the globe may occur, creating additional fluid outflow, which could potentially lead to significantly reduced pressures at any given flow rate (Madekurozwa *et al.,* 2022). It should also be remembered that, since there is no aqueous humor secretion in an enucleated eye, and the episcleral veins are now directly opened to the exterior (thus EVP will approximate to zero), prior to switching on the microdialysis perfusion pumps, the pressure inside the eye will be equal to air pressure, and hence IOP will register as zero. Pressures at any given flow rate will also be correspondingly reduced.

Sources of Error

When conducting the procedure described, it is assumed that the infusion at various flow rates has no effect on F_{in}, F_u, C, or EVP. F_{in} is probably not much affected as the pressures in the eye invariably end up (even at their highest levels) between 30 and 40 mmHg, which is insufficiently high to cause a large reduction in aqueous secretion rate (Todd & Woodhouse, 1973). F_u is likely not much affected either, as uveoscleral outflow exhibits only 5 - 10% of the facility of the trabecular pathway (Kaufman, 2003). An error of 10% in the calculation of $C_{(tot)}$ can lead, in our experience, to an error in the calculated value of F_u of as much as 36%. It is important to proceed through all steps with care and due diligence and to eliminate spurious data that may arise as a result of poor cannulation technique, bleeding into the chamber, or subsequent blockage of the cannulating needles. When using the technique described to estimate EVP, it should be remembered that the value obtainable is likely to be marginally lower than actual EVP, as the technique requires a degree of retrograde flow of blood from the episcleral veins into Schlemm's canal, which can only occur down a pressure gradient (*i.e.*, when intracameral pressure is artificially lowered to a value that is actually slightly lower than true EVP). A small (~ 1 mmHg) error in the measurement of EVP can potentially lead to a ~10% error in computed F_{in}. Leakage from a cannulated eye is also a possibility, and indeed, in some eyes, there will be obvious leakage as pressures will not build or stabilize as expected. If desired, fluorescein isothiocyanate (FITC) dextran can be incorporated into the perfusate and, in combination with ophthalmoscopy, microscopy, or even use of a slit lamp suitable mounted on the apparatus, as well as with the darkening of the laboratory and ultra-violet illumination, detailed searching for leakage during perfusion can be undertaken.

CONCLUSION

We aimed to provide sufficient detail of the protocol described above such that the procedures can be adequately replicated. However, readers are strongly encouraged to review in detail the original publications (Aihara, Lindsey & Weinreb, 2003; Millar, Clark & Pang, 2011; Millar *et al.,* 2015; Millar, Lopez *et al.,* 2017; Millar, Phan & Pang, 2018) where such methods have been described. Additional literature searches may also prove to be of benefit, especially if the experimenter is interested in attempting to modify or refine the procedures described herein. Measurement of $C_{(tot)}$ in the mouse eye is difficult and requires considerable practice, care, patience, and attention to detail. Even in the hands of the experienced experimenter, a certain proportion of eyes will fail to yield meaningful data. Indeed, when beginning to learn the technique, it is reasonable to expect that most eyes will fail. One also must expect a certain degree of variation within resultant data sets, such that for statistical significance between treated and control groups, we recommend obtaining good data from a minimum of 5 to 7 eyes per group.

ACKNOWLEDGEMENTS

The authors would like to thank Dr. AF Clark for many discussions, as well as the North Texas Eye Research Institute (NTERI) for continued and invaluable support.

APPENDIX

Table 1. Phosphate-buffered saline solution (PBS).

Compound	Mol. Weight	g/L for 10× Stock	g/L	Concentration (mM)
NaCl	58.4	80.1	8.01	137
KCl	74.6	2.0	0.20	2.7
Na_2HPO_4	142.0	14.2	1.42	10
KH_2PO_4	136.1	2.4	0.24	1.8

Table 2. Balanced salt solution (BSS).

Compound	Mol. Weight	g/L for 10× Stock	g/L	Concentration (nM)
NaCl	58.4	71.4	7.14	122.0
KCl	74.6	3.8	0.38	5.1
$MgCl_2$	95.2	2.0	0.2	2.1
$CaCl_2$	111.0	1.54	0.154	1.4
NaH_2PO_4	120.0	4.2	0.42	3.5

Table 3. Balanced salt solution with oxidized glutathione (BSS-Plus).

Compound	Mol. Weight	g/L for 10× Stock	g/L	Concentration (mM)
NaCl	58.4	71.4	7.14	122.0
KCl	74.6	3.8	0.38	5.1
$MgCl_2$	95.2	2.0	0.2	2.1
$CaCl_2$	111.0	1.54	0.154	1.4

(Table 3) cont.....

Compound	Mol. Weight	g/L for 10× Stock	g/L	Concentration (mM)
NaH_2PO_4	120.0	4.2	0.42	3.5
$NaHCO_3$	84.0	21.0	2.1	25.0
D-Glucose (Dextrose)	180.2	9.2	0.92	5.1
Glutathione disulfide (oxidized glutathione)	612.6	1.84	0.184	0.3

Table 4. Bárány's mock aqueous humor solution (MAH, Bárány's). [a]Add 1.53 mL from 1M stock solution drop-wise after adding all other components for a final solution. Do NOT add $CaCl_2$ to 10× stock. [b]Ascorbic acid is optional. After adding $CaCl_2$ and ascorbic acid (if desired) to the final solution, pH should be adjusted to 7.4 with 1M HCl and/or 1M NaOH added dropwise, as required.

Compound	Mol. Weight	g/L for 10× Stock	g/L	Concentration (mM)
NaCl	58.4	80	8	137
KCl	74.5	3.5	0.35	4.7
$MgCl_2$	95.2	0.64	0.064 = 64 mg	0.67
$CaCl_2$	111.0	-	0.17[a]	1.53
Na_2HPO_4	142.0	0.69	0.069 = 69 mg	0.49
NaH_2PO_4	120.0	0.137	0.0137 = 13.7 mg	0.11
D-Glucose (Dextrose)	180.2	10	1	5.55
Ascorbic Acid	176.1	88.1 mg	0.00881 = 8.81 mg	50

Table 5. Apparatus required to perfuse 2 mice (thus 4 eyes) simultaneously.

Item	Number Required	Model/Catalog #	Supplier	Comment
Blood Pressure Transducer	4	BLPR2	World Precision Instruments (WPI), Sarasota, FL USA	Each transducer supplied with a Luer-fitted 3-way valve
Microdialysis Infusion Pump	2	SP101i	WPI	-
Transducer Amplifier Manifold	1	Transbridge TBM4M	WPI	-
Analog-to-Digital Converter	1	Lab-Trax 4	WPI	-
Data Collection Software	1	LabScribe2	WPI	Supplied as a free download with Lab-Trax 4 unit
Electric Warming Pad	1	CAT94B E12107 or similar	VWR North America	-

(Table 5) cont.....

Item	Number Required	Model/Catalog #	Supplier	Comment
High-Intensity Illuminator	1	83365; 31804443434	Nikon Instruments, Inc.	-
Dissecting Microscope	1 or 2	-	Nikon, or Bausch & Lomb, or similar	-
Cables	4	-	WPI	-
Cables	4	-	WPI	-
USB Cable	1	-	WPI	-
Tubing	10 m (~33 ft)	PE60	VWR	-
Computer	1	-	-	-
Luer Connectors (Male & Female)	1 pack of 100 of each size required	-	VWR	-

REFERENCES

Aihara, M, Lindsey, JD & Weinreb, RN (2003) Episcleral venous pressure of mouse eye and effect of body position. *Curr Eye Res,* 27, 355-62.
[http://dx.doi.org/10.1076/ceyr.27.6.355.18194] [PMID: 14704919]

Bill, A (1971) Effects of longstanding stepwise increments in eye pressure on the rate of aqueous humor formation in a primate (Cercopithecus ethiops). *Exp Eye Res,* 12, 184-93.
[http://dx.doi.org/10.1016/0014-4835(71)90089-3] [PMID: 5000887]

Camras, LJ, Sufficool, KE, Camras, CB, Fan, S, Liu, H & Toris, CB (2010) Duration of anesthesia affects intraocular pressure, but not outflow facility in mice. *Curr Eye Res,* 35, 819-27.
[http://dx.doi.org/10.3109/02713683.2010.494241] [PMID: 20795864]

Gabelt BT, Kaufman PL. (2011). Production and flow of aqueous humor. In: Adler's Physiology of the Eye (11th edition). Levin LA, Nilsson SFE, Ver Hoeve J, Wu SM (eds). Saunders Elsevier. Edinburgh, London, New York, Oxford, Philadelphia, St. Louis, Sydney, Toronto. Ch. 11, pp. 274-307
[http://dx.doi.org/10.1016/B978-0-323-05714-1.00011-X]

Goldmann, H (1955) Un nouveau tonomètre d'applanation. (A new applanation tonometer). *Bull Soc Ophtalmol Fr,* 67, 474-8. [Article in French].

Kasetti, RB, Maddineni, P, Millar, JC, Clark, AF & Zode, GS (2017) Increased synthesis and deposition of extracellular matrix proteins leads to endoplasmic reticulum stress in the trabecular meshwork. *Sci Rep,* 7, 14951.
[http://dx.doi.org/10.1038/s41598-017-14938-0] [PMID: 29097767]

Kaufman, PL (1996) Pressure-dependent outflow. In: Ritch, R., Shields, M.B., Krupin, T., (Eds.), *The Glaucomas* CV Mosby Yearbook, St. Louis, MO, USA 307.

Kaufman, PL (2003) Some thoughts on the pressure dependence of uveoscleral flow. *J Glaucoma,* 12, 89.
[http://dx.doi.org/10.1097/00061198-200302000-00018] [PMID: 12619645]

Li, G, Farsiu, S, Chiu, SJ, Gonzalez, P, Lütjen-Drecoll, E, Overby, DR & Stamer, WD (2014) Pilocarpine-induced dilation of Schlemm's canal and prevention of lumen collapse at elevated intraocular pressures in living mice visualized by OCT. *Invest Ophthalmol Vis Sci,* 55, 3737-46.
[http://dx.doi.org/10.1167/iovs.13-13700] [PMID: 24595384]

Lopez, NN, Patel, GC, Raychaudhuri, U, Aryal, S, Phan, TN, Clark, AF & Millar, JC (2017) Anterior

chamber perfusion versus posterior chamber perfusion does not influence measurement of aqueous outflow facility in living mice by constant flow infusion. *Exp Eye Res,* 164, 95-108.
[http://dx.doi.org/10.1016/j.exer.2017.08.011] [PMID: 28822760]

Madekurozwa, M, Reina-Torres, E, Overby, DR & van Batenburg-Sherwood, J (2022) Measurement of postmortem outflow facility using iPerfusion. *Exp Eye Res,* 220, 109103.
[http://dx.doi.org/10.1016/j.exer.2022.109103] [PMID: 35525299]

Millar, JC, Clark, AF & Pang, IH (2011) Assessment of aqueous humor dynamics in the mouse by a novel method of constant-flow infusion. *Invest Ophthalmol Vis Sci,* 52, 685-94.
[http://dx.doi.org/10.1167/iovs.10-6069] [PMID: 20861483]

Millar, JC, Gabelt, BT & Kaufman, PL (1998) Aqueous humor dynamics. In: Tasman, W., Jaeger, E.A., (Eds.), *Duane's Clinical Ophthalmology* Lippincott-Raven Publishers, Philadelphia 1-34.

Millar, JC, Lopez, NN, Raychaudhuri, U & Clark, AF (2018) Mouse eye perfusion *in-vivo* versus *ex-vivo:* influence on aqueous outflow facility (Abstract). *Annual Meeting of the Association for Research in Vision and Ophthalmology (ARVO).*

Millar, JC, Phan, TN, Pang, IH & Clark, AF (2015) Strain and age effects on aqueous humor dynamics in the mouse. *Invest Ophthalmol Vis Sci,* 56, 5764-76.
[http://dx.doi.org/10.1167/iovs.15-16720] [PMID: 26325415]

Millar JC, Phan TN, Pang I-H. (2018). Assessment of aqueous humor dynamics in the rodent by constant flow infusion. Methods in Glaucoma Research, in Methods in Molecular Biology 1695 (Laboratory Protocol Series). Springer, Humana Press, Chapter 11, pp109-120. ISBN: 978-1-4939-7406-1; ISBN (eBook): 978--4939-7407-8.
[http://dx.doi.org/10.1007/978-1-4939-7407-8_11]

Beneyto Martin, P, Fernández-Vila, PC & Pérez, TM (1995-1996) Determination of the pseudofacility by fluorophotometry in the human eye. *Int Ophthalmol,* 19, 219-23.
[http://dx.doi.org/10.1007/BF00132690] [PMID: 8737702]

Raychaudhuri, U, Millar, JC & Clark, AF (2017) Tissue transglutaminase elevates intraocular pressure in mice. *Invest Ophthalmol Vis Sci,* 58, 6197-211.
[http://dx.doi.org/10.1167/iovs.17-22236]

Todd, R & Woodhouse, D (1973) Pseudofacility: a method of measurement using suction-cup tonography. *Exp Eye Res,* 17, 173-82.
[http://dx.doi.org/10.1016/0014-4835(73)90207-8] [PMID: 4759534]

CHAPTER 35

Aqueous Humor Dynamic Measurements in Nonhuman Primates

Carol B. Toris[1,*] and **Shan Fan**[2]

[1] *Havener Eye Institute, Department of Ophthalmology and Visual Sciences, The Ohio State University Wexner Medical Center, Columbus, OH 43212, USA*

[2] *Department of Ophthalmology and Visual Sciences, The University of Nebraska Medical Center, Omaha, Nebraska, USA*

Abstract: This chapter describes the protocols to noninvasively measure the parameters of aqueous humor dynamics (AHD) in nonhuman primates (NHPs). These parameters define intraocular pressure (IOP) as described in the modified Goldmann equation, and changes to these parameters can alter IOP. Methods to access these parameters are used to study glaucoma and to examine new treatment ideas to lower IOP. The methods to access AHD include measurements of IOP by pneumatonometry, aqueous flow by fluorophotometry, and outflow facility by two methods, tonography and fluorophotometry. Uveoscleral outflow and episcleral venous pressure cannot be measured noninvasively in NHPs. Instead, episcleral venous pressure values in NHPs are obtained from the literature, and uveoscleral outflow is mathematically calculated using the modified Goldmann equation. These methods have been used in NHPs with ocular normotension, naturally occurring glaucoma, and experimental ocular hypertension. Preclinical studies of AHD are often conducted on NHPs before progressing to phase I clinical trials.

Keywords: Aqueous humor dynamics, Aqueous flow, Fluorophotometry, Intraocular pressure, Ocular hypertension, Outflow facility, Tonography, Tonometry, Uveoscleral outflow.

INTRODUCTION

The anatomy and physiology of nonhuman primates (NHPs) are similar to humans in many ways, making the NHP an important model in defining and understanding the pathogenesis of human disease. They respond to pharmacological drugs in a manner similar to humans and are often used to study

* **Corresponding author Carol B. Toris:** Havener Eye Institute, Department of Ophthalmology and Visual Sciences, The Ohio State University Wexner Medical Center, Columbus, OH 43212, USA; Tel: +614-688-9573; E-mail: carol.toris@osumc.edu

Najam A. Sharif and Sunny E. Ohia (Eds.)

novel treatments for human conditions. One important disease in humans that NHPs have helped to understand is glaucoma, a potentially blinding ocular disease of humans around the world. Elevated intraocular pressure (IOP) is the primary modifiable risk factor for glaucoma; lowering IOP by surgical or pharmacological means is its primary treatment.

Intraocular pressure is maintained by the fluid dynamics in the anterior segment of the eye. The key equation describing the factors involved in aqueous humor dynamics (AHD) and their relationships to each other is the Goldmann equation. It was developed over 70 years ago (Brubaker, 2004), and the modified Goldmann equation remains an important research tool today. It defines IOP as (Fa - Fu)/C + EVP. Fa (µl/min) is the rate of flow of aqueous humor from the posterior chamber, where it is secreted into the anterior chamber, where it circulates and drains. Fa is an estimate of the rate of aqueous humor production. C (µl/min/mmHg; the inverse of resistance) is the facility of outflow of aqueous humor from the eye. C is primarily, but not solely, located within the trabecular outflow pathway. Fu (µl/min) is uveoscleral outflow, the flow rate of aqueous humor around and through uveal tissues and sclera. EVP (mmHg) is the episcleral venous pressure, the pressure in the vessels that drain aqueous humor from the trabecular outflow pathway. Numerous methods, both invasive and noninvasive, have been developed to assess these parameters (Toris *et al.*, 2021). Although the noninvasive methods tend to be less accurate than invasive methods, they cause no lasting effects and can be repeated, which is essential for studies with a longitudinal design.

The purpose of this report is to describe the noninvasive methods to measure parameters of AHD in nonhuman primates, primarily cynomolgus and rhesus macaques. These methods have been performed with the approval of the Institutional Animal Care and Use Committees at the institute where the primate research was done and in compliance with the Statement for the Use of Animals in Ophthalmic and Visual Research from the Association for Research in Vision and Ophthalmology (ARVO).

EXPERIMENTAL PROTOCOLS

Three of the parameters in the Goldmann Equation can be measured noninvasively in monkeys, preferably on the same day. IOP is measured by tonometry, Fa by fluorophotometry, and C by tonography and/or a fluorophotometric method. EVP cannot be measured noninvasively in the cynomolgus macaque because the vessels are not visible under the heavily pigmented conjunctiva of this species. Fu is not measurable noninvasively but is assessed mathematically by the rearranged Goldmann equation: Fu = Fa - C(IOP-

EVP). IOP, Fa, and C are the measured values, and EVP is taken from a paper by Maepea and Bill (Maepea and Bill, 1989). They measured EVP directly using microneedles and reported EVP at several different IOPs set experimentally. Fu is a highly variable term because it is calculated from parameters with their own inherent variability. Changes in Fu from an experimental manipulation may not be detectable unless the changes and/or sample size are large (Fig. **1**).

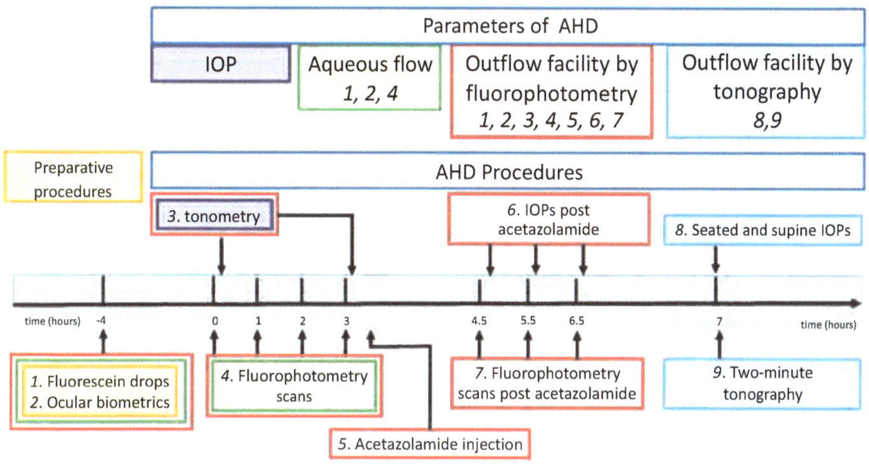

Fig. (1). Timeline (grey box) of study procedures to measure IOP (purple), aqueous flow (green), outflow facility by fluorophotometry (red), and outflow facility by tonography (blue). Numbers in the parameters boxes indicate the numbers of the procedures that are needed to make the parameter assessment. Color-coded outlines around procedure boxes indicate measurements needed for a particular procedure. Preparative procedures are in gold, and they can be performed 4 or more hours before the first fluorophotometry scan. AHD, aqueous humor dynamics; IOP, intraocular pressure.

Tonometry

The pneumatonometer, Tonolab, and Tonopen tonometers can be used in NHPs. These instruments are used in humans in accordance with the manufacturer's instructions.

a. Equipment: Our preference is the pneumatonometer for several reasons. The pressure readings can be saved in a digital format. Pressures are collected for multiple seconds to minutes and graphed. A section of the IOP graph can be deleted if there is excessive movement during data collection. This happens frequently with awake, curious animals. An IOP measurement of a supine sedated animal is shown in Fig. (**2**). Under anesthesia, there is not much of a pulse wave.
b. Supplies: Artificial tears, such as EyeStream (Alcon), proparacaine hydrochloride, 0.5% (Alcaine; Alcon, Ft. Worth, TX), report forms (one for each animal), pen, soft tissue wipes, and pen light.

c. Preparation:
   i. Preferably, animals are trained to sit in specially designed chairs and remain still during the reading. Training requires 3 to 5 months and is not described further herein. Untrained animals can be measured with strong physical or chemical restraints, but these methods can affect the IOP reading.
   ii. The corneas are anesthetized with a drop of proparacaine.
      1. If an experiment requires multiple IOP readings in a day, it is preferable to dilute proparacaine 1:10 with artificial tears or equivalent to reduce the anesthetic exposure, which can irritate the cornea and increase the risk of cornea abrasion.

d. Procedure:
   i. Apply the tonometer probe to the eye for several seconds until characteristic waveforms are collected. IOP data are digitally captured at 40 Hz. An average of 3 or more waveforms are used to obtain one IOP reading.
   ii. Take a second reading.
   iii. If the two readings are not within 3 mmHg of each other, collect a third reading. The closest two readings are averaged.

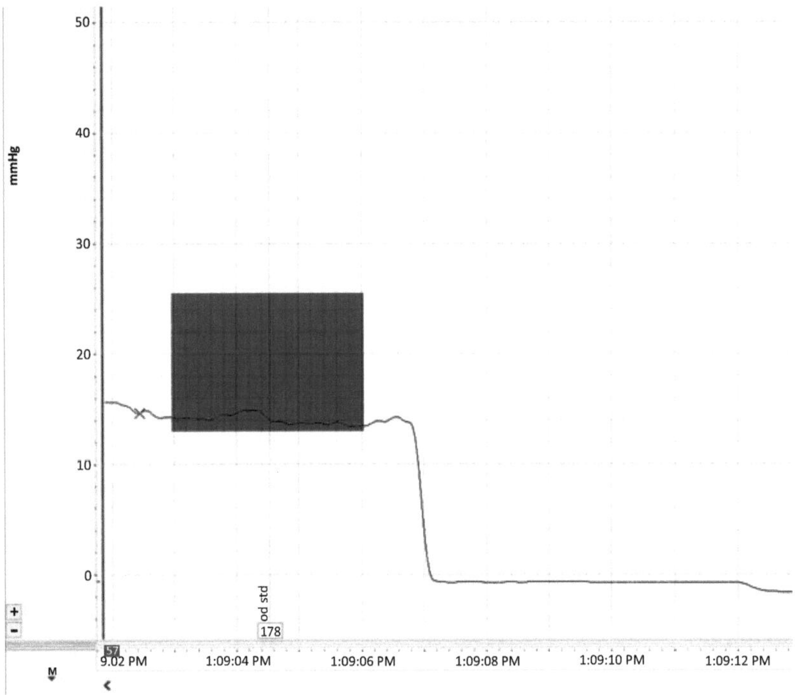

Fig. (2). Screenshot of the IOP of the right eye taken with pneumatonometer in a supine, sedated monkey. Data were plotted in PowerLab (LabChart V8) and saved digitally. The data selected for averaging is shown in the grey box. IOP was 11.9 mmHg.

Fluorophotometry

a. Equipment:
   i. Fluorotron Master Fluorophotometer, Laboratory Animal Edition with anterior chamber adaptor (Ocumetrics, Palo Alto, CA), computer with FM software to run the fluorophotometer, and red light lamp. The Fluorotron detects changes in fluorescence of the cornea and anterior chamber over a 2 to 3-hour period. A fluorescence decay slope is generated from 4-5 sets of scans.
   ii. Ultrasound pachymeter (Sonomed or equivalent). This unit measures the central cornea thickness (CCT) and anterior chamber depth (ACD). Two different probes are needed.
   iii. Calipers (Fine Science Tools). This tool measures the cornea diameter, also known as white-to-white (WTW).
   iv. An alternative instrument to measure white-to-white (WTW), CCT, and ACD is the IOL Master (Zeiss). This instrument or an equivalent is routinely used in eye clinics but cannot be shared with NHPs. It must be dedicated to animal use exclusively.

b. Supplies: 10% fluorescein, soft tissue wipes, artificial tears, saline solution

c. Preparative procedures (sedation is not needed in trained animals).
   i. Ocular biometrics
      1. Measurements of cornea thickness, anterior chamber depth, and cornea diameter are necessary for the calculation of cornea volume and anterior chamber volume for the individual animal. These numbers are used by the Fluorotron software to calculate aqueous turnover (aqueous flow). Do not use the default values.
      2. Collect these measurements just before administering the fluorescein (step ii below). Do not take these measurements during the time needed to collect the 4 to 5 sets of fluorophotometry scans or after tonography. Tonography can change the thickness of the cornea.
      3. Calculate cornea and anterior chamber volumes using the following formulas.

$$V_{as} = \pi/6(d + t)[(d + t)^2 + 3/4y^2]$$

$$V_{ac} = \pi/6d^2[3/4y^2/(d + t) + d - 3t]$$

$$V_c = V_{as1} - V_{ac}$$

Where:

y = cornea diameter, t = cornea thickness, d = anterior chamber depth,

V_{as} = volume of a segment of a sphere bordered by the anterior surface of the cornea and an imaginary plane at the anterior surface of the lens,

V_{ac} = anterior chamber volume,

V_c = cornea volume.

d. Fluorescein administration
   1. At least four hours before the first fluorophotometry scan, apply one drop of proparacaine HCl 0.5% and three to five 10 µl drops of 10% fluorescein to each eye. The proparacaine makes the cornea more permeable and increases the absorption of the fluorescein.
   2. Administer the fluorescein drops at 5-minute intervals. The goal is to achieve levels of fluorescein in the cornea and anterior chamber that are measurable for a minimum of 10 hours after administration. No sedation is needed in trained animals.
   3. Five minutes after the last drop, gently and thoroughly wash the face with warm water until no fluorescein can be seen on the lids, lashes, or washcloth.
   4. Wait a minimum of 4 hours for the fluorescein to traverse the cornea, enter the anterior chamber, and become well mixed.
   5. Just before the first fluorophotometry scan, thoroughly wash the face again. Dab dry. Washing removes fluorescein from the lids and lashes that potentially could be deposited on the cornea during the fluorophotometry scans, which would invalidate the results.
   6. Ideally, begin with a fluorescence signal in the range of 500-2000 ng/ml in the cornea and 50-200 ng/ml in the anterior chamber. Too little means background noise cannot be separated from the fluorescence signal. Too much causes quenching, and fluorescence levels do not change over time. In this case, collect scans for more hours until a linear decay curve is generated.
      i. Sedation
         1. Administer an intramuscular injection of ketamine (20 mg/kg).
         2. Remove the animal from the cage and place an intravenous catheter for administration of ketamine, saline, and acetazolamide throughout the day.
         3. Just before each fluorophotometry scan, inject enough ketamine (5-10 mg/kg) to keep the animal calm, followed by 5-10 ml of saline through the catheter. The saline is for hydration.
            a. Procedures
               i. Instructions for the use of the Fluorotron Master are found on the Ocumetrics website, http://ocumetrics.com/. Do not

be confused with the http://ocumetics.com/ website.

ii. Check that the anterior chamber adaptor is installed on the eyepiece of the Fluorotron.
iii. Move the eyepiece to the right to measure the right eye first.
iv. Open the Fluorotron Master program. In the main menu, enter the patient ID and select the aqueous turnover program, Yablonski Routine.
v. In the tabs on the top, select Scan.
vi. Place sedated animal in a prone position with the right eye aligned with the eyepiece. Observe proper alignment by looking through the portal window on the side of the Fluorotron.
vii. Turn off all room lights. Keep the room as dark as safely possible.
viii. Hit any key on the keyboard to run the scan.
ix. Take 2 to 3 scans and check cornea and anterior chamber fluorescein levels on the graph. If the fluorescence levels are too variable or there is too much eye movement, collect more scans until you have three good ones.
x. Move the eyepiece to the left using the top left knob on the left side of the Fluorotron. Collect scans of the left eye as was done on the right eye.
xi. Forty-five minutes to one hour later, repeat scans of both eyes.
xii. Collect sets of scans two more times at 45-60 minute intervals for a total of four sets.
xiii. Select the Analysis tab on the top right of the screen. Follow directions on the screen and in the Fluorotron manual. Run an Analysis. In Fig. (**3**), the scans before the vertical intervention blue line are used to calculate aqueous flow (aqueous turnover).
    1. Fill in cornea volume, anterior chamber volume, and cornea thickness (upper right cells on the screen) before completing the analysis. A graph should be generated with two parallel straight lines having negative slopes. The upper line is the cornea fluorescence over time, and the lower line is the anterior chamber fluorescence over time.
    2. Ideally, the Cornea Correlation Coefficient and Anterior Chamber Correlation Coefficient should be above 0.8. If not, there may be too much scatter in the data.
    3. Outliers should be removed. Outliers can occur from eye

movements during the scan or if the fluorescein is not evenly distributed in the cornea and anterior chamber.

xiv. If the correlation coefficients are below 0.8 after removing outliers, then collect a fifth set of scans 45-60 minutes after the fourth. Run another Analysis.

xv. Aqueous flow is the Aqueous Turnover value found at the bottom right on the Analysis screen.

xvi. The fluorophotometry procedure can be repeated on another day, and data from the two days can be compared as long as the time of day is the same for each assessment.

1. Aqueous flow has distinctive nyctothemeral rhythms, which should be taken into consideration when designing research experiments.

Tonography

Outflow facility is based on the principle that at a set intraocular pressure, fluid drains from the anterior chamber at a constant rate. When the IOP is changed, the fluid outflow changes accordingly. The ratio of the change in flow to the change in pressure yields an outflow facility. Tonography is a method to change the pressure in the eye by pushing on the cornea with a weighted probe for 2 or 4 minutes. The weighted probe increases the IOP and the aqueous humor outflow rate. The outflow of aqueous humor cannot be measured with this method but can be estimated by assessing the Friedenwald tables developed in the 1950s. Several important assumptions should be considered when doing tonography. These assumptions are described elsewhere (Chan, 2021).

Two instruments (pneumatonometer and Schiotz) have been used historically to measure outflow facility. Pneumatonography (Model 30, Reichert, Inc., Depew, NY) has higher intersubject and interobserver measurement variability than Schiotz tonography because it is more sensitive to movements from the subject and operator holding the probe. Pneumatonography outflow facility values are lower than Schiotz values, and the two methods cannot be compared directly (Kazemi *et al.*, 2017). The Schiotz tonographer is no longer manufactured and is difficult to obtain. The pneumatonographer is the only device commercially available for tonography. The use of this instrument is described below.

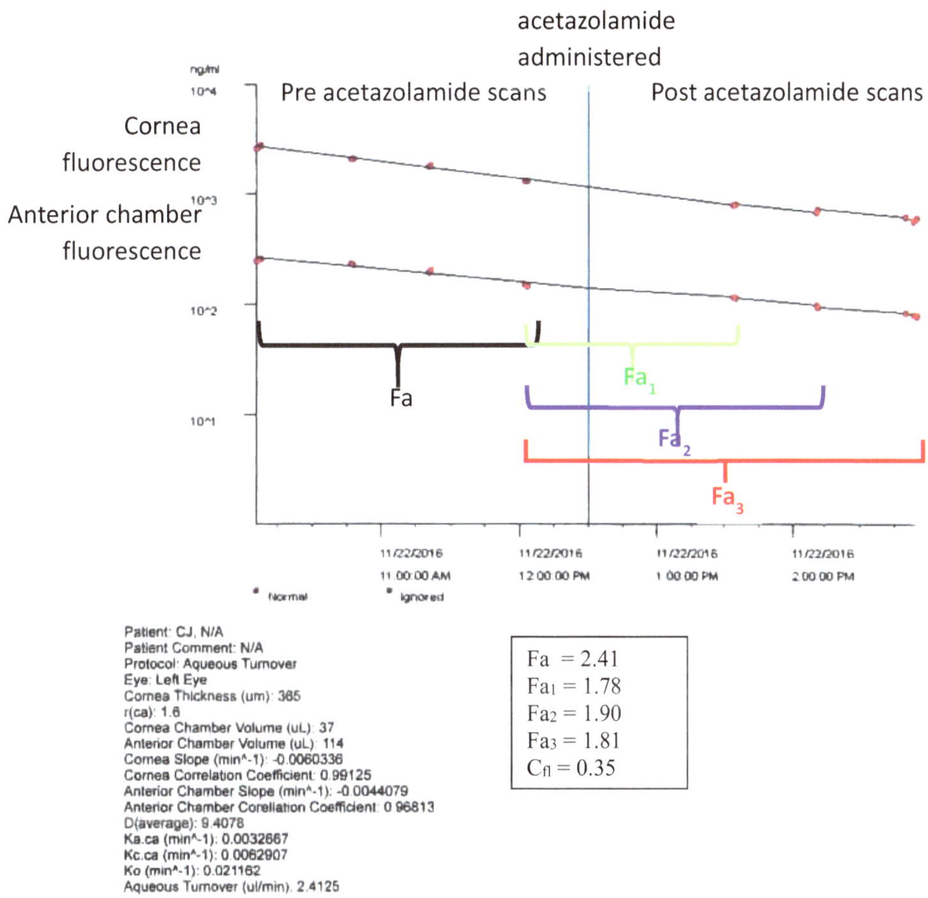

Fig. (3). Screenshot of the Analysis screen of the Fluorotron software with overlayed labels. These data are from the left eye of an NHP at baseline. Fa is the aqueous turnover (aqueous flow) calculated from four sets of fluorescence scans to generate two parallel lines with negative slopes. These slopes, along with the cornea thickness, cornea volume, and anterior chamber volume, are used to calculate Fa. The vertical blue line is the time of administration of acetazolamide, a carbonic anhydrase inhibitor that slows the Fa. Three sets of scans are collected after acetazolamide administration (intervention). A change in Fa is calculated three times (Fa-Fa_x) where x= time 1, 2, or 3 post-administration. This change is used to calculate outflow facility (C) three times. The three values are averaged to give one C_{fl}.

a. Equipment: Pneumatonometer with tonography option and ten-gram weight. The tonography option requires the Tonography Kit, P/N 16033. Details of the pneumatonometer with tonography mode can be found on the Reichert website. https://www.reichert.com/en/products/model-30
b. Supplies: Artificial tears, proparacaine, soft facial tissue.
c. Preparation

   i. Lightly sedate the animal with ketamine.
   ii. Apply a drop of proparacaine topically to the cornea.

d. Procedure
   i. Place the animal in a seated position.
   ii. Take seated IOP reading.
   iii. Place the animal in a supine position for 5 minutes. Support the head on a cushioned platform to minimize movements.
   iv. Take supine IOP reading. Seated and supine IOPs are needed for the tonography calculation.
   v. Select the tonography setting on the pneumatonometer.
   vi. Select the two-minute test.
   vii. Snap the 10-gram weight (supplied with the instrument) to the shaft of the probe.
   viii. Place the probe on the center of the cornea and press down until the shaft is between the black and red lines on the shaft.
   ix. Begin the test by pressing the foot pedal or by touching the Tonography icon on the tonometer screen.
   x. End the test at two minutes. The tonographer generates a beep when the test is done. An example of a tonography test is shown in Fig. (**4**).
   xi. Repeat the procedure on the left eye.
   xii. The outflow facility value is the C value on the tonometer screen. If this value is displayed as two question marks (??), it means the starting IOP is lower than the ending IOP, and the value cannot be calculated. The value can be recalculated by following the instructions and using the Calculator Mode on the instrument.
   xiii. The measurement can be repeated an hour later if needed by the study design or if the first attempt failed.

Outflow Facility by a Fluorophotometric Method

To circumvent the need for the antiquated Friedenwald tables and determine aqueous flow directly on an individual basis, a fluorophotometric method to access the outflow facility was developed by Michael Yablonski (Hayashi *et al.*, 1989). This method has its benefits but also its problems. A discussion of the pros and cons of the technique has been published recently (Toris *et al.*, 2021).

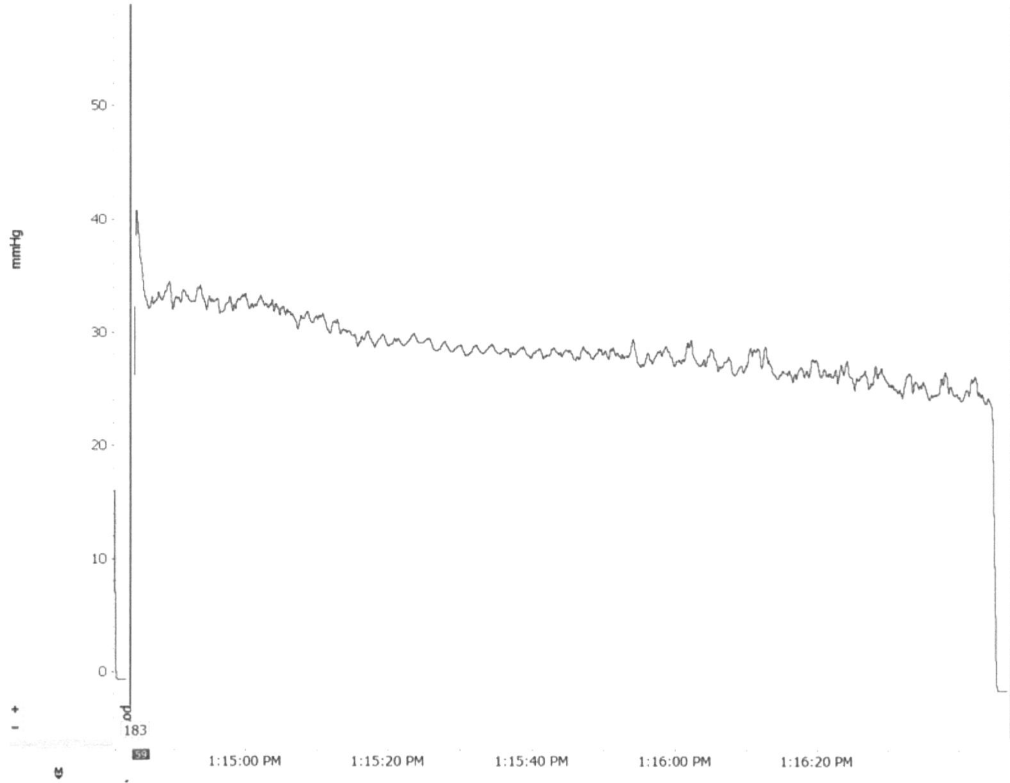

Fig. (4). Two-minute tonography trace of the normotensive right eye in a supine sedated NHP treated with a test drug that increases C. Initial IOP=32.5mmHg, Final IOP=25.5mmHg, C=0.52 microliters/min/mmHg.

a. Equipment: Pneumatonometer (described above), fluorophotometer (described above)
b. Supplies: Artificial tears, proparacaine, fluorescein, soft facial tissues
c. Procedure
    i. Measure aqueous flow by fluorophotometry (Aqueous turnover) as described above. This is done between 8 AM and noon.
    ii. Immediately after the final scan, measure IOP with the pneumatonometer (described above). Record the time.
    iii. Administer an intravenous dose of acetazolamide (12.5 mg/kg) through the previously placed catheter.
        1. Each animal responds differently to acetazolamide, therefore, for future experiments, the drug dosage may need to be adjusted for each animal to assure a minimum 2 mmHg IOP decrease.
    iv. Wait one hour.
    v. Take one set of fluorophotometric scans.
    vi. Take IOP.

vii. Repeat scans and IOPs two more times at 45 to 60-minute intervals.
viii. Record the aqueous turnover value from the fluorophotometer.
ix. Calculate C at each of the three sets of scans.
x. Record the aqueous turnover value from the intervention section on the Analysis tab of the fluorophotometer. You now have one aqueous turnover value and one IOP value before acetazolamide and three turnovers and IOPs after.
xi. Calculate C as follows.
1. C_{fl1} =(Fa-Fa_1)/(IOP-IOP_1)
2. C_{fl2} =(Fa-Fa_2)/(IOP-IOP_2)
3. C_{fl3} =(Fa-Fa_3)/(IOP-IOP_3)
4. Cfl = (Cfl_1 + Cfl_2 + Cfl_1)/3. This is the value for the outflow facility by fluorophotometry.
5. Keep in mind that C=ΔFa/ΔIOP, fl signifies fluorophotometry, Fa = aqueous flow (or aqueous turnover in the Fluorotron), IOP = intraocular pressure, and x = time interval 1, 2, or 3, after acetazolamide administration.

6. Omit values in which Fa-Fa_x is negative, IOP-IOP_x is negative, or C_{flx} values are outliers. An example of data from an NHP is found in Fig. (**3**).

Animal Recovery

a. Remove catheter.
b. Apply lubricating ointment to the eyes.
c. Return the animal to its cage just prior to consciousness.
d. Monitor the animal until fully awake.

CONCLUSION

The protocols described above are noninvasive methods to assess aqueous humor dynamics in nonhuman primates. These are well-established methods used by numerous primate labs around the world. With modifications, the methods can be used in humans or animals with eyes of similar size (mainly cats, dogs, and rabbits). Invasive methods are also available, but they require surgery and sacrifice, which is not preferred for numerous reasons. The invasive methods are not described herein. Refinements to these methods are ongoing and completely new approaches to evaluate the parameters of aqueous humor dynamics are under investigation. A literature review must be conducted before designing and commencing a new study on aqueous humor dynamics in nonhuman primates.

REFERENCES

Brubaker, RF (2004) Goldmann's equation and clinical measures of aqueous dynamics. *Exp Eye Res,* 78, 633-7.
[http://dx.doi.org/10.1016/j.exer.2003.07.002] [PMID: 15106943]

CHAN, E. T., C.B. (2021). Tonography and ocular rigidity. In: PALLIKARIS, I. T., M.; DASTIRIDOU, A. (ed.) Ocular Rigidity, Biomechanics and Hydrodynamics of the Eye. Switzerland: Springer International Publishing.

Hayashi, M, Yablonski, ME & Novack, GD (1989) Trabecular outflow facility determined by fluorophotometry in human subjects. *Exp Eye Res,* 48, 621-5.
[http://dx.doi.org/10.1016/0014-4835(89)90004-3] [PMID: 2737260]

Kazemi, A, McLaren, JW, Lin, SC, Toris, CB, Gulati, V, Moroi, SE & Sit, AJ (2017) Comparison of Aqueous Outflow Facility Measurement by Pneumatonography and Digital Schiøtz Tonography. *Invest Ophthalmol Vis Sci,* 58, 204-10.
[http://dx.doi.org/10.1167/iovs.16-20754] [PMID: 28114581]

Mäepea, O & Bill, A (1989) The pressures in the episcleral veins, Schlemm's canal and the trabecular meshwork in monkeys: Effects of changes in intraocular pressure. *Exp Eye Res,* 49, 645-63.
[http://dx.doi.org/10.1016/S0014-4835(89)80060-0] [PMID: 2806429]

Toris, CB, Gagrani, M & Ghate, D (2021) Current methods and new approaches to assess aqueous humor dynamics. *Expert Rev Ophthalmol,* 16, 139-60.
[http://dx.doi.org/10.1080/17469899.2021.1902308]

CHAPTER 36

Protocols for Pre-Clinical Testing Microshunts to Drain AQH for Glaucoma

Yasushi Kato[1,*] and **Len Pinchuk**[1]

[1] *Research & Development, InnFocus Inc. (A Santen Co.), 12415 S.W. 136 Ave., Unit 3, Miami, FL 33186, USA*

Abstract: This chapter summarizes and describes most of the test methods used for pre-clinical testing of a permanently implantable glaucoma drainage device called the PRESERFLO® MicroShunt (InnFocus Inc./A Santen Co.) The tests are required by most medical device regulatory authorities as technical files or experimental data to demonstrate safety and subsequently to advance testing in humans to demonstrate efficacy and final approval for commercialization. There are many international standards and guidelines, such as the International Organization for Standardization (ISO), American Society for Testing and Materials (ASTM), United States Pharmacopeia (USP), and American National Standard Institute (ANSI), to name a few, which help in the harmonization of testing required to show the device is designed and functions as expected. Glaucoma drainage devices are typically shunts that divert aqueous humor from the anterior chamber to the exterior spaces of the eye by bypassing some of the common pathways, such as the trabecular meshwork or choroidal space. Some devices attempt to enhance the obstructed pathways and are made of metal, plastic, or degradable materials. The test methods described herein are compiled to educate the reader of pre-clinical tests required, with the understanding that each device model is unique, requiring customization of methods and/or tooling to accommodate the test requirements using the design at hand.

Keywords: Anterior chamber, Biocompatibility, Bond test, Compression test, Carcinogenicity test, Ethylene oxide residual test, Eye, Flow test, Exhaustive extraction test, Genotoxicity test, Glaucoma drainage device, Genotoxicity test, Intraocular pressure, Leachable test, Microshunt, Pre-clinical test, Protocol, Pyrogen test, Shelf-life test, Transportation test, Test method, Visual inspection.

INTRODUCTION

Pre-clinical testing of glaucoma drainage devices has been ongoing since 1976, when the first devices began to be regulated by the governing agencies, such as

* **Corresponding author Yasushi Kato:** Research & Development, InnFocus Inc. (A Santen Co.), 12415 S.W. 136 Ave., Unit 3, Miami, FL 33186, USA; Tel: +(786) 679-6650; E-mail: yasushi.kato@santen.com

Najam A. Sharif and Sunny E. Ohia (Eds.)

the Food and Drug Administration (FDA). Since then, there have been efforts to come up with guidance and recommendations that are recognized by regulatory bodies to harmonize and help companies to design safe implantable devices. One such organization in the medical ophthalmic field is the Z80 committee, accredited by the American National Standard Institute Inc. (ANSI), founded in 1956, and further vision council subcommittees formed in 2009. The original and first American Glaucoma device standard came about in 2001, and a revised version was released in 2014 as ANSI Standard Z80.27-2014, American National Standards for Ophthalmics-Implantable Glaucoma Devices.

This section will describe some general test methods or protocols that were developed to demonstrate the safety of the PRESERFLO MicroShunt. By no means do these protocols represent standard test methods; however, they were designed to demonstrate and satisfy the guidelines and recommendations at that time of development. It should be understood that new implantable glaucoma devices, whether designed as permanent devices or degradable devices, may have unique properties or characteristics where new test methods must be developed to satisfy the guidance or supplemented to show the device is safe to proceed first in human and clinical studies, thereof.

EXPERIMENTAL PROTOCOLS

Although these protocols will help guide, for example, the type of testing required for pre-clinical testing of glaucoma drainage devices, it must be understood that depending on the design of the device, test methods need to be developed by the developer, which may be necessary and unique to its design. For example, a device that may have electronic components or has been designed to be active rather than passive devices will likely need additional testing and test methods not described here. It is the responsibility of the developer to assess the pre-clinical tests necessary to show safety and efficacy before moving onto human clinical trials.

Physical and Mechanical Assessments

Visual Inspection

- Prepare a stereo microscope or microscope that has a magnification of 10X and obtain forceps and a clean Petri dish filled with a 1-2 mm depth of isopropyl alcohol. Also, prepare a separate dish for reject devices.
- Obtain the device to be inspected and immerse it in the isopropyl alcohol, allowing the lumen to be filled with fluid as opposed to air bubbles.

- Inspect the device from one end to the other at 10X. Refer to standard photos for acceptable and non-acceptable defects and sort accordingly. These defects can range from surface roughness to lumen defects and inclusions.
- Record the type of un-accepted defects for each of the rejected units.

Compression Test

- Set up the material tester machine (*e.g.*, Instron Machine) with a 50N load cell with a custom top and bottom compression tool held by the pneumatic or mechanical flat grips. Set an automatic stop to 10N to prevent accidental over-compression, which can damage the load cell. Set compression test speed at 700 μm/min.
- Manually, by jogging the machine, bring the top grip down until the top and bottom compression tools touch. Reset or zero that position on the machine, as this will be the reference position.
- Move the top grip up to leave space to place the device onto the bottom compression tool and place the device into position.
- Manually jog down the top grip until the top compression tool is just touching the device (usually the tube). This should be a position reading close to the outer diameter of the tube.
- Start the compression test until 50% of the tube is compressed or until ½ of the outer diameter is compressed. Record the load at 50% compression.

Gravimetric Flow Test

- Set up the gravimetric flow test apparatus, which consists of a weight balance, a water reservoir connected to a tube to a 3-way connector, and an adjustable platform for the water reservoir.
- The 3-way connector is mounted with a clamp holder at a fixed height, and the water reservoir is filled with clean water and checked to ensure there are no air bubbles throughout the tube and connector.
- The water reservoir height is adjusted on the platform to achieve a head pressure of 20 ± 1 mmHg using a calibrated manometer connected to the 3-way connector.
- The front end of the MicroShunt is mounted into a 21G 10 mm long needle and glued with silicone rubber adhesive to prevent a leak. This needle with a device is then primed with filtered water to be mounted onto the 3-way connector facing down.
- The needle with the device is carefully connected to the 3-way connector, avoiding any air bubbles. A small glass vial with water is placed on the balance. The 3-way connector mounted on the stand is placed inside the balance chamber such that the water drips into the vial. Add water in the vial such that the tip of

the device is almost touching the meniscus. Minimize the surface area of the vial to minimize evaporation.

- Tear the balance to zero, start a timer, and measure the weight after 30 minutes. Assuming 1g = 1mL, calculate the mL/min or uL/min.
- Repeat the test after adjusting the head pressure to 5 ± 1 mmHg with the same device and calculate the flow rate.

Bond Test

- Set up the material tester machine (*e.g.*, Instron Machine) with a 50N load cell and pneumatic or mechanical flat grips and set the tensile speed of testing at 1 in/min.
- Obtain a Microshunt sample and feed it through the small hole in the custom rig such that the fin is touching the rig.
- Mount the custom rig with the device onto the bottom grip material tester machine such that the exposed tube is vertical, and manually bring the top grip to clamp the exposed tube.
- Close the top grip to clamp the tube and start the test, where the fin is pulled through the small hole, which causes the fin to tear from the tube. Record the ultimate tensile strength as the fin bond strength.

Biological Assessment

Note: The biological assessment or biocompatibility tests follow ISO 10993-1 (2018) for biological evaluation of medical devices and premarket studies on implantable Minimally Invasive Glaucoma Surgical (MIGS) Devices (FDA 2015). Depending on the material and size of the device, the testing requires using extracted material or facsimile to be made under the same conditions as the final product.

Cytotoxicity

- For this testing, ISO 10993-5 is referenced, and the medium elution method is used instead of the solid direct contact or percent cell growth inhibition.
- 0.38g (60 cm^2) of the test article is prepared, and ethylene oxide is sterilized under production conditions. For the positive control article, latex is used, and for the negative control, high-density polyethylene is used. For the control vehicle, a single-strength minimum essential medium supplemented with 5% fetal bovine serum, 2% antibiotics, and 1% L-glutamine (1X MEM) is used. A mammalian cell culture monolayer consisting of L-929 mouse fibroblast cells free from mycoplasma is used for the in vitro assessment.

- Each of the test articles, the negative control article and the positive control article are all extracted at 37 ^{0}C for 24 hours using 10 mL of the control vehicle (1X MEM).
- Immediately after extraction, in triplicates, 2 mL of growth medium solution in the cell culture wells is replaced with 2 mL of extract solution and incubated at 37 ^{0}C for 48 hours.
- Following incubation, the cells are examined microscopically at 100X to evaluate cellular characteristics and lysis scoring as none (discrete intracytoplasmic granules, no cell lysis), slight (<20% round cells), mild (<50% round cells), moderate (<70% round cells), and severe (nearly complete destruction of cell layers).

Genotoxicity and Carcinogenicity

Note: The genotoxicity and carcinogenicity tests can be very extensive and time-consuming, ranging from 6 months using transgenic mice to 2 years using rodents. They include in vitro and *in vivo* tests dependent on the material characteristics (degradable and non-degradable), physical characteristics, such as the shape and roughness of a medical device, and mode of action (passive or active device). A general guide on methodology is discussed here with references that have more information on tests and protocols to be considered.

- Genotoxicity tests are for detecting gene mutations and chromosomal damage and no single test can detect genotoxic agents. A battery of in vitro tests is conducted, and in some cases, *in vivo* tests usually use extracts from the test article. There are several steps to consider, such as identification of confounding factors, identification of metabolic effect, identification of impurities, and weight of evidence assessment with mechanism and mode of action to be considered ISO 10993-3 (2014). Hence, not all tests are necessary, and therefore, the information obtained from Leachable tests and Exhaustive extraction tests becomes a basis for performing a risk analysis and justifying if tests are required and scientifically justified.
- When genotoxicity testing is performed, one of the following three tests for gene mutations in bacterial modified for medical devices OECD 471 (1997) is needed: an in-vitro test with the cytogenetic evaluation of chromosomal damage with mammalian cells OECD 473 (2016), a mouse lymphoma tk assay modified for medical devices OECD 476 (2016), or a mammalian cell micronucleus test from chromosomal damage and aneugenicity OECD 487 (2016) modified for medical devices. An *in vivo* test for chromosomal damage in rodent hemopoietic cells may be necessary if the developer can not demonstrate that the quantity of extractable from the test article is less than the amount of material that would

induce a positive response with a potent, well-characterized *in vivo* micronucleus genotoxin, such as cisplatin.

- Carcinogenicity tests are needed if carcinogenic hazards can be presumed from genotoxicity. A flowchart to decide whether further tests are needed based on confounding factors and mode of action in genotoxicity results is presented in Annex B of ISO 10993-3 (2014) for follow-up evaluation. A typical test in mice can take 2 years to evaluate carcinogenicity. Pre-screening in vitro cell transformation systems are now available, such as the Syrian hamster embryo cell transformation assay and Balb3T3 cell transformation assay (Schectaman, 2012).
- Since the animal model (rodents) for carcinogenicity is usually small compared to the medical device to be tested, device material extracts or an implant in a form representative of the finished device state is used, and then tissues are evaluated according to OECD 451 (2018) or OECD 453 (2018). If the risk analysis suggests that chronic toxicity and carcinogenicity are considered relevant, then testing must be performed in accordance with OECD 453 (2018). If only carcinogenicity is considered relevant, then testing must be performed in accordance with OECD 451 (2018).

Sensitization

- 1. 0.57g (90 cm^2) of the test article is prepared, and ethylene oxide is sterilized under production conditions. 0.9% USP sodium chloride (SC) is used to extract the test article at a ratio of 6 cm^2: 1 mL at 50 ^{0}C for 72 hours. Similarly, sesame oil (SO) is used to extract the test article at a ratio of 6 cm^2: 1 mL at 37 ^{0}C for 72 hours. If the material swells substantially in oil, to minimize damage to the test article, the extraction in sesame oil is at 37 ^{0}C. Freund's Complete Adjuvant (FCA) is needed in Induction I, and 10% (w/w) sodium lauryl sulfate (SLS) suspension in petrolatum is needed in Induction II. Hartley guinea pig weighing 300-500g in weight is used as the test animal (ISO 10993-10).
- The care of animals follows Institutional Animal Care and Use Committee (IACUC) guidelines, and animals will undergo acclimations, husbandry, and all veterinary care, including analgesics and euthanasia procedures.
- Induction I: Three pairs of intradermal injections are administered within a 2 x 4 cm area over the dorsal scapular region as follows:

For control animals: (A) 0.1 mL of 50:50 (v/v) mixture of FCA and the chosen vehicle. (B) 0.1 mL of vehicle. (C) 0.1 mL of a 1:1 mixture of the 50:50 (v/v) vehicle/FCA mixture and the vehicle.

For test animals: (A) 0.1 mL of 50:50 (v/v) mixture of FCA and the chosen vehicle. (B) 0.1 mL of test extract. (C) 0.1 mL of a 1:1 mixture of the 50:50 (v/v) vehicle/FCA mixture and the test extract.

- Induction II: After 6 days of Induction I, the fur is carefully removed using clippers and SSL suspension to coat the skin and left uncovered. At 24 hours, any SLS residue is wiped, and a 2 x4 cm section of filter paper saturated with 0.3 mL of the test extract preparation (test animals) or vehicle (control animals) is applied over the same injection area. Each patch is secured with tape and elastic bandage. At 48 hours, bandages and patches are removed.
- Challenge: At 14 days after unwrapping Induction II, the fur is removed carefully with clippers. A nonwoven cotton disk backed by a flexible Hill Top Chamber® and semi-occlusive hypoallergenic tape is saturated with 0.3 mL of freshly prepared test material extract and applied to the right flank or dorsum of each animal. In addition, the vehicle control is patched to the left flank or dorsum of each animal. An approximate 2 x 2 cm section of test material is applied to the right flank.
- The trunk of each animal is wrapped to maintain occluded sites. At 24 hours, the wraps and Hill Toop Chambers® are removed. Additionally, the test article patches are removed.
- Observations for dermal reactions are conducted at 24 and 48 hours after patch removal in accordance with the grading scale: (0) no visible change; (1) discrete or patchy erythema; (2) moderate and confluent erythema; (3) intense erythema and swelling. Grades (1) or greater observed in the test group generally indicate sensitization, provided grades less than (1) are observed on the control animals. The overall pattern, intensity, duration, and character reactions of the test as compared to the control conditions are considered. The control conditions are (1) the control vehicle on the test animals, (2) the test on the control animals, and (3) the control vehicle on the control animals.

Immunotoxicity Test

- For this testing, *ANSI Z80.27-2014* recommends the use of Guidance for Industry and FDA Reviewers - Immunotoxicity Testing Guidance, May 6, 1999, as a reference and is applicable only for devices made from or containing animal or plant-derived sources. The MicroShunt does not contain nor is it made of animal or plant sources.

Ocular Implantation Test

- For intraocular irritation assessment, 0.38g (60 cm^2) of the test article is prepared, and ethylene oxide is sterilized under production conditions. Balanced saline solution (BSS) is used to extract the test article at a ratio of 6 cm^2: 1 mL at 50 ^{0}C for 72 hours. New Zealand white rabbits not less than 2.5 kg in weight are used as test animals.

- The care of animals follows Institutional Animal Care and Use Committee (IACUC) guidelines, and animals will undergo acclimations, husbandry, and all veterinary care, including anesthesia and euthanasia procedures.
- Following appropriate surgical procedures under anesthesia, 0.15 mL of extract is injected into the rabbit eye after 0.15 mL of aqueous humor is removed using a 27G needle on a 1 mL sterile syringe. On the contralateral control eye, a similar injection is performed but with an extract that does not include the test article.
- Eyes are examined at the end of the treatment day (day 0), and on days 1, 2, and 3 for evidence of irritation, and ocular changes will be scored according to the McDonald-Shadduck Score System modified to exclude fluorescein and lens examination. After the test is complete, the animals are euthanized by intravenous injection of sodium pentobarbital-based solution according to IACUC guidelines.
- In addition to the ocular irritation test in rabbits, a 6-month chronic implant study is conducted on rabbits following IACUC guidelines with follow-ups at post-operative days 0, 1, 7, 14, 21, 30, 60, 90, and 180 days. The implant procedure should follow the recommended surgical procedure for the device.
- Immediately after induction of anesthesia at each follow-up period, pachymetry and tonometry readings are performed, and the animal is placed under the surgical microscope with a slit lamp.
- The examination consists of an ophthalmic exam, describing the appearance of the ocular adnexa, anterior segment, and lens with the help of a gonio lens to visualize the drainage angle and/or the retina. Observations are documented, including photographs.
- After ophthalmic exams and at terminal points of 1, 3, and 6 months, the animals are euthanized, and eyes are enucleated to be preserved in 10% buffered formalin for histopathological analysis around the test device.

Pyrogen Test

- This test follows USP-31-NF26<151> guidelines, and the test solution is prepared by extracting solution using injection grade 0.9% balanced sodium chloride from the device at 35±2 ^{0}C for 72±2 hours (See Leachable Test). Treat all solutions and assemblies, such as glass vials, to ensure that they are sterile and pyrogen-free.
- Use healthy mature rabbits that have been acclimated for 5 days and use a rectal thermometer with an accuracy of ± 0.1 ^{0}C to take a controlled temperature not more than 30 minutes before the injection and do not use any rabbit having a temperature exceeding 39.8 ^{0}C.
- Inject 10 mL of test solution per Kg of body weight (solution should be warmed to 37 ± 2 ^{0}C) into the ear vein of each of the 3 rabbits within 10 minutes and

record the rabbits' temperature at 30 minutes intervals between 1 to 3 hours. If no rabbits show a rise in temperature of 0.5 ^{0}C from the control temperature, the product meets the requirements for the absence of pyrogens. If any rabbits show a temperature rise of 0.5 ^{0}C, then another 5 rabbits are tested. If the sum of the 8 maximum temperature rises does not exceed 3.3 ^{0}C, the test article meets the non-pyrogenic requirements.

Physicochemical Assessment

Note: There are no specific guidelines as to the extractable and leachable limits. Hence, biocompatibility tests are performed to assess the safety of the finished device, and a biological risk assessment (ISO 10993-1, 2018) is conducted considering the type of device contact and potential hazards of the materials that make up the device.

Extractables and Exhaustive Extraction

- Two groups of test articles, approximately 400 mg per group, are prepared after rinsing in deionized water for 15 minutes, and each sample is introduced to a Teflon thimble to dry in a room temperature vacuum for 15 minutes and then placed in a desiccant chamber and allowed to dry overnight to obtain an initial mass. This is repeated until 2 consecutive masses are equivalent to within ±0.0001 g.
- A mini Soxhlet extraction apparatus is assembled with a Teflon mesh thimble charged with LCMS-grade isopropanol alcohol (IPA). A 2-hour cleaning run is performed, and solvents are discarded.
- The Soxhlet is re-assembled with the thimble and no sample is loaded and run for 4 hours at 4-6 flushes per hour to produce a solvent blank.
- A group of test samples is placed into the Teflon mesh extraction thimble, dried in a vacuum oven, and weighed to ± 0.00001 g, after which the apparatus is filled with LCM-grade IPA so the test samples can be extracted for 4 hours. All solvent extracted is transferred and stored refrigerated until further analysis.
- The Teflon mesh thimble with test samples is removed and dried to constant mass in the vacuum oven at 60 ^{0}C and recorded to ± 0.00001 g as mass after extraction. The percent extractable is calculated based on initial mass and mass after extraction.
- Acquire the UV/VIS absorbance spectra of the test extract and solvent blanks in the 200-800 nm wavelength using a 1 cm path quartz cuvette and identify absorbances in the test extract spectra not found in the solvent blank spectra.
- Acquire UPLC/PDA-UV chromatograms of the test extracts and solvent blanks for wavelengths 220, 250, 280, and 330 nm and 'stack' them for comparison with the objective of identifying valid residual peaks. Similarly, mas spectral

base peak intensity (BPI) chromatograms of the IPA extracts and solvent blanks are analyzed in 'stack' format.

- Run a split GC/MS analysis at 250 ^{0}C on IPA extracts and solvent blanks to acquire total ion chromatograms and run a performance standard lipophilic 3 mix to demonstrate sensitivity and selectivity for a range of volatile/semi-volatile analytes.
- Prepare dry spot residues of IPA extracts by drop-wise application of extract to a KBr IR card, leaving non-volatile residue on the card, and acquire an FTIR-ATR spectrum of the spot residue.

Hydrolytic Degradation

- The evaluation of hydrolytic degradation of the device is based on ISO 11979 (2006), immersed at 55±2 ^{0}C for 15 months in HPLC-grade water, equivalent to 5 years in the eye.
- After incubation, examine samples at 10X and 40X for surface changes, discoloration, lumen changes, and other signs of degradation. Compare with non-incubated control samples and document photographically.
- After incubation, examine samples by scanning electron microscopy (SEM) at 75-500X magnification for surface changes and other signs of degradation. Compare with non-incubated control samples and document photographically.

Leachables Test

- The evaluation of leachables is based on ISO 11979-5 (2006) incubated at 35±2 ^{0}C for 72±2 hours in aqueous and lipophilic solvents and analytical tests using GC/FID, GC/MS, HPLS-PDS, and UV-VIS.
- Prepare in 4 borosilicate clean glass vials: 2 groups for duplicate aqueous (HPLC grade water) extractions and 2 groups for duplicate lipophilic (HPLC isopropanol) extractions. Determine the mass of each group using tared samples to set the amount of solvent required for each group. Submerge in a 10:1 solvent-to-sample ratio.
- Similarly, prepare control solvent blank vials with duplicate aqueous and duplicate lipophilic solvents.
- Incubate all vials in a constant shaker at 35 ± 2 ^{0}C for 72 ± 2 hours.
- Standards are to be used for each of the analytical methods to verify performance and sensitivity and selected from the group of monomers used in the formulation of the device and solvent and process aids used during the production of the device.
- Measure the absorbances that are amenable to the UV/VIS analysis spectra spanning the 200-800 nm range, compare with test leachates and solvent blanks, and report detection limits.

- Perform reverse-phase HPLC with photodiode array (PDA) UV detection on the test leachates and solvent blanks and report any peaks found in the test chromatograms not present in the solvent blank chromatograms.
- Acquire GC/FID chromatograms on the test leachates and solvent blanks and identify peaks present in the test leachates not present in the blanks. Acquire GC/FID chromatograms for volatile and semi-volatile monomer standards and quantify reporting detection limits.
- Acquire GC/MS chromatograms of the water and IPA test leachates and solvent blanks and discuss any peaks found that are not detected in the solvent blanks. Examine significant peaks and attempt to identify them using the NIST standard mass spectral library. Acquire GC/MS chromatograms for any volatile or semi-volatile species that might be necessary to verify NIST assignments or to aid in quantification.

Sterility and Packaging Assessment

Note: There are many ways to sterilize medical devices, such as Gamma or E-beam sterilization, heat or steam sterilization, nitrogen dioxide sterilization, *etc*. Ethylene oxide sterilization is a common sterilization for medical devices and is the focus of this section.

Ethylene Oxide Residuals

- Ethylene oxide (EO) and ethylene chlorohydrin (ECH) residuals after EO sterilization are tested using the liquid exhaustive extraction methods (ISO 11135, 2014).
- After EO sterilization, the samples are stored in a freezer until testing and tested within 24 hours. The device is considered as permanent contact >30 days to be tested at $37 \pm 2\ ^0$C using single extraction and exhaustive extraction.
- For single extraction, water is used with headspace above the immersed sample to be less than 10% of the total volume of fluid used for extraction.
- For exhaustive extraction, methanol is used, and after initial extraction, the sample is collected and transferred to a GC vial and stored frozen if testing is not completed right away. New extraction fluid is drained from the sample after the prior remaining extraction fluid is drained from the sample. The extraction is repeated until the amount of EO or ECH in subsequent extractions is less than 10% of that detected in the first extraction or until there is no analytically significant increase in the cumulative residual levels detected.
- The amount of sample in contact with the volume of extraction fluid (multiplication ratio = g of sample: mL of solvent) is 1:1, 1:5, or 1:10 depending on the nature of the sample, detection limit of the analytical instrumentation, and the sensitivity required by the analyte.

- Extraction solution is prepared by diluting to an internal standard concentration of approximately 50 µg/g (50 ppm). Extraction time is 24 hours at 37 ± 2 ^{0}C and continues until criteria are achieved as described above.
- EO and ECH spiked samples for recovery analysis are prepared by spiking untreated samples with each of the standard solutions in order to determine procedural recovery for each compound. The 'sample to extract' ratio is maintained at 1 part sample to 5 parts extraction fluid (*e.g.*, 10 µg/g spike, 25 µg/g spike, 100 µg/g spike). The weight of the spiked standard is recorded in order to determine the extract concentration for the spiking solution calculated as µg/g of sample = weight of standard used x concentration of standard divided by sample weight. Spiked samples are extracted and analyzed the same way testing samples are analyzed.
- The extracted fluid is analyzed using GC in units of ppm (w/v) for ethylene oxide and ethylene chlorohydrin.
- Ethylene oxide residues must not exceed 0.5 µg per device per day and not exceed 1.25 µg in total per device. Ethylene chlorohydrin residues must not exceed 2.0 µg per device per day and not exceed 5.0 µg in total per device.

Bacterial Endotoxin (Pyrogen test)

Note: The method below is based on the Kinetic-Chromogenic Limulus Amebocyte Lysate (LAL) test kit (Endosafe®) using Escherichia coli 055:B5 as the endotoxin standard and microplate LAL Reader. A 0.50 EU/mL Product Positive Control (PPC) is the Food and Drug Administration (FDA) recommended concentration for devices with a pass/fail criteria of 0.5 EU/mL.

- Prepare the test article solution by incubating the test article in 120 mL of sterile nonpyrogenic water for 40-60 minutes at 37-40 °C on a shaker.
- Prepare a standard stock solution of endotoxin according to the instructions by adding 3.0 mL of LAL reagent water to one vial of endotoxin and vortexing for 5 minutes (50 EU/mL).
- Using a de-pyrogenated test tube containing 2.70 mL of LAL reagent water, prepare 4 standard solutions by adding 0.30 mL of 5.0, 0.5, 0.05, and 0.005 EU/mL concentrations in each tube and vigorously vortexing for 1 minute.
- Duplicate 100 µL aliquots of water blank (negative control), and dispense each of the four standards into the microplate. Similar aliquots of each test extract are dosed to quadruplicate wells (2 wells for endotoxin quantification and 2 wells for positive product control (PPC) testing). PPC testing evaluates the potential for the test article to interfere with the reaction (inhibiting or enhancing the reaction). To each well designated for PPC testing, spike with a 10 µL aliquot of 5.0 EU/mL standard.

- Place the filled plate into the LAL Reader and pre-incubate for 10 minutes. Near the end of the pre-incubation period, reconstitute the LAL reagent with LAL reagent water, and after the incubation period, add 100 μL of the LAL reagent into the wells of the microplate to initiate the assay in the reader.
- The standard curve shall consist of at least 4 reference standard endotoxin or control standard endotoxin concentrations in water that extend over the desired range. The absolute value of the linearity of the standard curve must be $0.980 < r \leq 1.000$. The slope of the standard curve must be $-0.1 < m < -1.0$. The detected amount of endotoxin in the spiked extract must be within plus or minus 50% of the known PPC concentration for the extract to be considered to neither enhance nor inhibit the assay. If the undiluted extract shows inhibition or enhancement, the extract can be diluted, not exceeding the maximum value of dilution, and the test must be repeated.

Shelf Life and Transport Assessment

Note: Transportation and shelf life tests are usually considered in tandem as the product is typically shipped to a contract service sterilizer and later to a warehouse or customer for storage. There are several standard guides and methods, such as the ASTM F1980-21, Standard Guide for Accelerated Aging of Sterile Barrier Systems for Medical Devices, ASTM D4169-22, Standard Practice for Performance Testing of Shipping Containers and Systems, ASTM D4332-22, Standard Practice for Conditioning Containers Packages, or Packaging Components for Testing in Accordance with Special Atmospheres, ASTM F1886/F1886M-22; Standard Test Method for Determining Integrity of Seals for Flexible Packaging by Visual Inspection, and ASTM F2096-19; Standard Test Method for Detecting Gross Leak in Packaging by Internal Pressurization (Bubble Test). The ISO 11979-6 (2014) shelf-life and transport stability testing guidance should be referenced even though it is for intra-ocular lenses.

Transportation Test

- Shipper boxes and fillers come in different sizes and configurations depending on the size of the product and must be chosen to protect the contents from transportation handling and transportation conditions. Corrugated card boxes are most commonly used due to their availability and cost. Each manufacturer must choose and tailor the tests based on the assurance level desired. Typically, a level II assurance level is chosen for medical devices. Special equipment, such as a vibration table/platform, is usually required to perform these tests.
- Manual handling drop sequence 13" with different impact orientations assurance level II.
- Vehicle stacking is based on computed load or displacement of 10% reached.

- Loose load vibration frequency is increased until 1/16" metal shim can be moved intermittently underneath the shipping unit with a dwell time of 10-20 minutes on 3 faces assurance level II.
- Vehicle Vibration acceleration level intensities at High for 5", medium for 15", and low for 40"; maximum frequency of 200Hz.
- Concentration impact drop of cylindrical mass at a height of 32" on 6 faces.

Accelerated Shelf-Life Test

Note: Accelerated shelf-life tests are typically performed to simulate 6 months, 1 or 3 years, and up to 5 years of storage, depending on the need by the manufacturer to demonstrate packaging and device stability. They should be followed by real-time shelf-life tests to substantiate the accelerated test.

- Final packaged devices in shippers are subjected to simulated distribution hazards as per ASTM D4169-22 Standard Practice for Performance Testing of Shipping Containers and Systems at assurance level II.
- Shippers are subject to temperature conditioning as per ASTM D4332-22 Standard Practice for Conditioning Containers, Packages, or Packaging Components for Testing in accordance with special atmospheres for frozen storage at -18 ± 2 ^{0}C for 72 hours and special atmospheres tropical conditions at 40 ± 2 ^{0}C and 90% ± 5% RH for 72 hours.
- After packages are subjected to the distribution and temperature conditioning, accelerated shelf-life is performed according to ASTM F1980-21 based on the Arrhenius equation with Q_{10} equal to 2 as a common conservative means of calculating and accelerating aging factor (AAF), where Taa = accelerated aging temperature (55^{0}C) and Trt = representative ambient temperature (25^{0}C). AAF = Q_{10}^[(Taa-Trt)/10] = 5.657. As an example, using the AAF and a desired shelf-life of 5 years (5 x 365.25 = 1826.25 days), the accelerating aging time would be 323 days.
- Determining the accelerating aging temperature and relative humidity (RH) conditions is dependent on the product material (degradable versus non-degradable) and packaging materials used since higher temperatures will shorten the accelerating aging time but may affect the materials. Typically, accelerated aging temperatures of 45-55 ^{0}C and RH is 20-40% are used for medical devices.
- During post accelerated period, the test product undergoes testing as described in section 1, 'Physical and Mechanical Assessment', and in section 4, 'Sterility and Packaging Assessment', to verify all specifications are met.

Real-Time Shelf-Life Test

- Real-time shelf-life tests are essentially the same as the accelerated shelf-life test, with the exception that the product is stored under recommended storage conditions for the equivalent time as tested during the accelerated test in real time. This can typically range from 2, 3, and 5 years for medical devices.

- After conditioning, the main points to consider for a real-time shelf-life test are to test for sterility integrity, pyrogens, and device integrity, especially if the device is made or contains degradable materials.

CONCLUSION

The protocols described above were pre-clinical testing examples taken from a unique glaucoma drainage device developed by InnFocus Inc. called the PRESERFLO MicroShunt prior to a first–in-human use. Every new device has its unique characteristics, which need to be assessed by the designing team, and guidelines must be referred to demonstrate to regulatory agencies the safety of such devices prior to being implanted in humans. To demonstrate efficacy, usually, some type of clinical testing or usability testing is ultimately required as in vitro and animal models have their limitations. Readers are encouraged to check out literature on similar devices to understand how a protocol may not fit one for all. Additional literature searches and referring to references within guidelines may also be beneficial to find suitable modifications or refinements to the procedures described herein.

CONFLICT OF INTEREST STATEMENT

The authors declare that they were involved in the development of the PRESERFLO MicroShunt. However, the authors have no conflict of interest in the contents of this chapter as these protocols were solely used for the development of the glaucoma device and do not bring any financial benefit to the authors or company.

ACKNOWLEDGEMENTS

The authors would like to thank all the engineers, operators, quality technicians, and other supporting staff who took part in the preparation of test samples and execution of many of the protocols and test methods described herein.

REFERENCES

American Standards of Testing Materials. (2016) Standard Test Method for Determining Integrity of Seals for Flexible Packaging by Visual Inspection. ASTM F1886/F1886M-16

American Standards of Testing Materials. (2019) Standard Test Method for Detecting Gross Leak in Packaging by Internal Pressurization (Bubble Test). ASTM F2096-19

American Standards of Testing Materials. (2021) Standard Guide for Accelerated Aging of Sterile Barrier Systems for Medical Devices. ASTM F1980-21

American Standards of Testing Materials. (2022) Standard Practice for Performance Testing of Shipping Containers and Systems. ASTM D4169-22

American Standards of Testing Materials. (2022) Standard Practice for Conditioning Containers. Packages, or Packaging Components for Testing in Accordance with Special Atmospheres. ASTM D4332-22

Food and Drug Administration. (1999) Guidance for Industry and FDA Reviewers - Immunotoxicity Testing Guidance

Food and Drug Administration. (2012) Guidance for Industry-Pyrogen and Endotoxin Testing: Question and Answers

Food and Drug Administration. (2015) Premarket Studies of Implantable Minimally Invasive Glaucoma Surgical (MIGS) Devices. Document 1400049

International Organization for Standardization. (2008) Biological evaluation of medical devices Part 7: Ethylene oxide sterilization residuals. ISO 10993-7 2008

International Organization for Standardization. (2014) Biological evaluation of medical devices – Part 3: Tests for genotoxicity, carcinogenicity, and reproductive toxicity. ISO 10993-3:2014

International Organization for Standardization. (2014) Biological evaluation of medical devices – Part 33: On Tests to evaluate genotoxicity - Supplement to ISO 10993-3. ISO 10993-33:2015

International Organization for Standardization. (2018) Biological evaluation of medical devices - Part 1: Evaluation and testing within a risk management process. ISO 10993-1:2018

International Organization for Standardization. (2021) Biological evaluation of medical devices – Part 10: Tests for skin sensitization. ISO 10993-10:2021

International Organization for Standardization. (2014) Sterilization of health-care products - Ethylene oxide - Requirements for the development, validation, and routine control of a sterilization process for medical devices. ISO 11135:2014

International Organization for Standardization. (2014) Ophthalmic implants - Intraocular lenses, Part 6: Shelf-life and transport stability testing. ISO 11979-6:2014(E)

International Organization for Standardization. (2020) Ophthalmic implants – Intraocular lenses, Part 5: Biocompatibility. ISO 11979-5:2020(E)

Organization for Economic Co-operation and Development (OECD). (2016) Test No. 473 In Vitro Mammalian Chromosomal Aberration Test, Guidelines for the Testing of Chemicals, Section 4 [http://dx.doi.org/10.1787/9789264264649-en]

Organization for Economic Co-operation and Development (OECD). (2016) Test No. 476 In Vitro Mammalian Cell Gene Mutation Test using the Hprt and xprt genes, Guidelines for the Testing of Chemicals, Section 4
[http://dx.doi.org/10.1787/97892642664809-en]

Organization for Economic Co-operation and Development (OECD). (2016) Test No. 487 In Vitro Mammalian Cell Micronucleus Test, Guidelines for the Testing of Chemicals, Section 4 [http://dx.doi.org/10.1787/9789264264861-en]

Organization for Economic Co-operation and Development (OECD). (2018) Test No. 451 Carcinogenicity Studies, OECD Guidelines for the Testing of Chemicals, Section 4
[http://dx.doi.org/10.1787/9789264071186-en]

Organization for Economic Co-operation and Development (OECD). (2018) Test No. 453, Combined Chronic Toxicity/Carcinogenicity Studies, OECD Guidelines for the Testing of Chemicals, Section 4
[http://dx.doi.org/10.1787/9789264071223-en]

Organization for Economic Co-operation and Development (OECD). (1997) Test No. 471 Bacterial Reverse Mutation Test, OECD Guidelines for the Testing of Chemicals. Available from: https://oecd.org/chemicalsafety/risk-assessment/1948418.pdf

Schechtman, LM (2012) Rodent cell transformation assays—A brief historical perspective. *Mutat Res Genet Toxicol Environ Mutagen,* 744, 3-7.

[http://dx.doi.org/10.1016/j.mrgentox.2011.12.018] [PMID: 22230428]

United States Pharmacopeia. (2023) General Chapter 151 Pyrogen Test. USP-31-NF26

The Vision Council Secretariat. (2014) American National Standards for Ophthalmics-Implantable Glaucoma Devices. ANSI Z80.27-2014: 1-41

SPONTANEOUSLY/NATURALLY OCCURRING AND GENETICALLY ENGINEERED ANIMAL MODELS OF OCULAR HYPERTENSION (OHT)/GLAUCOMA

CHAPTER 37

Protocols for the Use of DBA/2J Mice for Pigmentary Glaucoma Research

Abdelrahman Anter[1], **Betsy Benitez**[2] and **Sanjoy K. Bhattacharya**[3,*]

[1] *Bascom Palmer Eye Institute, University of Miami Miller School of Medicine, Miami, FL 33136, USA*

[2] *Miami Integrative Metabolomics Research Center, Miami, FL 33136, USA*

[3] *University of Miami Miller School of Medicine, 1638 NW 10th Avenue, Suite 707Am Miami, FL 33136, USA*

Abstract: Pigmentary glaucoma (PG) is a subtype of secondary open-angle glaucoma defined by iris melanin granules or pigment deposits in the trabecular meshwork. Morphological and functional changes in the aqueous humor outflow pathways lead to increased intraocular pressure and progressive damage to the optic nerve, which could lead to vision loss. The DBA/2J mouse has become an indispensable resource in scientific research, providing insights into the underlying pathophysiology of PG. In this chapter, we describe three methods pertinent to the study of PG utilizing the DBA/2J mouse model: intraocular pressure (IOP) measurement, pattern electroretinography (PERG) as a measurement of inner retinal functional assessment of vision, and a modified Fontana-Masson staining (FMS) technique for quantitative measurement of melanin pigments.

Keywords: Fontana-Masson stain, Pigmentary glaucoma, Pattern electroretinogram, Trabecular meshwork, Intraocular pressure.

INTRODUCTION

Pigmentary glaucoma (PG) is a type of secondary open-angle glaucoma characterized by the accumulation of pigment granules in the trabecular meshwork (TM), leading to increased intraocular pressure (IOP) and optic nerve damage. It typically affects males in their third to fifth decades of life (the male-female ratio is around 3:1) and is more prevalent in myopic patients (Niyadurupola and Broadway, 2008; Potash *et al.*, 1994; Di Pippo *et al.*, 2020).

* **Corresponding author Sanjoy K. Bhattacharya:** University of Miami Miller School of Medicine, 1638 NW 10th Avenue, Suite 707Am Miami, FL 33136, USA; Tel: +3054824103; E-mail: SBhattacharya@med.miami.edu

Najam A. Sharif and Sunny E. Ohia (Eds.)

Pigment dispersion syndrome (PDS) and PG reflect different stages on a spectrum of the same condition. PDS occurs when anomalous iridozonular contact leads to rubbing between the posterior iris epithelium and lens structures (Liebmann *et al.*, 1995; Okafor *et al.*, 2017; Campbell, 1979). This rubbing leads to the liberation and dispersion of pigment particles that accumulate in the TM, causing TM endothelial cell necrosis (Niyadurupola and Broadway, 2008). The clinical presentation of PDS is defined by the triad of dense pigmentation of the TM, pigment localized on the corneal endothelium called Krukenberg's spindle and radial mid-periphery iris transillumination defect (Liebmann *et al.*, 1995; Okafor *et al.*, 2017). PG is defined when these characteristics cause an increase in IOP and glaucomatous optic neuropathy (Fig. **1**) (Scuderi *et al.*, 2019; Okafor *et al.*, 2017). Not all cases of PDS progress to develop PG. The risk of developing PG as a result of PDS has been estimated to be between 35-50% (Okafor *et al.*, 2017).

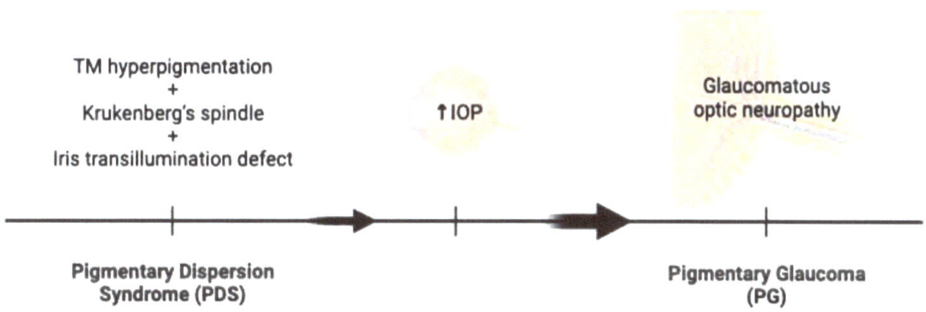

Fig. (1). Pigment dispersion syndrome and pigmentary glaucoma constitute stages of a spectrum of the same disease. PDS is characterized by the triad of TM hyperpigmentation, Krukenberg's spindle, and iris transillumination defect. PG is defined when PDS characteristics progress to cause glaucomatous optic neuropathy.

When diagnosing PG, the standard workup procedures for glaucoma are performed, including fundoscopy, optical coherence tomography (OCT), slit-lamp examination, and gonioscopy. In cases of PG, fundoscopy reveals glaucomatous optic nerve neuropathy, OCT shows retinal nerve fiber layer (RNFL) thinning, slit-lamp examination exhibits the presence of Krukenberg's spindle and iris transillumination defects, and gonioscopy displays homogenous pigmentation on the TM (Scuderi *et al.*, 2019). In addition to these standard procedures, ultrasound biomicroscopy (UBM) and anterior segment OCT (AS-OCT) are performed to confirm the presence of iridozonular contact (Scuderi *et al.*, 2019; Okafor *et al.*, 2017; Potash *et al.*, 1994).

The DBA/2J mouse strain (John *et al.*, 1997; John *et al.*, 1998) is a widely used animal model for studying PDS and PG. Mutations in the *Tyrp1* and *Gpnmb* genes, which code for melanosomal proteins, contribute to iris atrophy and pigment dispersion in DBA/2J mice (Wang and Dong, 2016; Anderson *et al.*, 2002). As a result, DBA/2J mice develop an age-related form of glaucoma that displays the clinical features of PDS and PG, with most of these mice beginning to develop iris pigmentation abnormalities or dispersion by six months and optic nerve damage by eight months (Lu *et al.*, 2011; Pu *et al.*, 2022).

There are a variety of experimental techniques that can be used to study the pathogenesis of PG in DBA/2J mice. These include pharmacological interventions, such as topical or systemic administration of drugs to lower intraocular pressure, and genetic manipulations, such as using CRISPR-Cas9 to knock out or knock in specific genes. Additionally, histological techniques, such as immunohistochemistry and electron microscopy, can be used to study the accumulation of pigments in the trabecular meshwork and the subsequent changes in the structure and function of the meshwork. In this chapter, we describe three protocols relevant to studying PG in DBA/2J mice: IOP measurement, pattern electroretinography (PERG), and a modified Fontana-Masson staining (FMS) technique.

INTRAOCULAR PRESSURE MEASUREMENT

Measuring IOP in DBA/2J mice is an essential step in assessing the development and progression of PG. Several methods can be used to measure IOP in mice, including invasive and non-invasive methods.

Invasive methods for measuring IOP in mice include cannulation of the anterior chamber and micro-tip manometry. Cannulation of the anterior chamber involves inserting a small tube through the cornea and into the anterior chamber and measuring the pressure directly. Micro-tip manometry involves inserting a small probe into the eye through a small incision and measuring the pressure directly. These methods are more accurate than non-invasive methods but require anesthesia and have a higher risk of complications such as opacity and perforation (Morris *et al.*, 2006; Danias *et al.*, 2003).

One of the most commonly used non-invasive methods for measuring IOP in mice is the Tono-Pen, which uses a small probe to measure the resistance to indentation of the cornea. Another non-invasive method is the rebound tonometer, which measures the rebound of the cornea after a small impact. Both of these methods are quick, easy to perform, and have a lower risk than invasive methods (Morris *et al.*, 2006). Anesthesia can be used, but it is important to consider the potential effects of anesthesia on IOP measurements, as certain anesthetics can lower IOP (Danias *et al.*, 2003). In the following section, we describe the steps to measure IOP using a TonoLab tonometer, which has been found to accurately measure IOP in normal and DBA/2J mice (Pease *et al.*, 2011).

IOP MEASUREMENT PROTOCOL

1. Fixate the TonoLab tonometer (Colonial Medical Supplies) to a ring stand using a three-prong swivel clamp.
2. Make sure the central groove is in a horizontal position.
3. Set a platform of adjustable height next to the tonometer.
4. Press the measuring button of the tonometer to turn it on.
5. Once the display shows *"Load"* on "*mice setting*" showing *"letter N"* insert a probe into the probe base.
6. Anesthetize or restrain the mouse.
   a. Anesthetized:
      i. Anesthetize the mouse with an intraperitoneal injection (0.5– 0.7 mL/kg) of Ketamine/Xylazine solution (1mL Ketamine/ 1mL Xylazine/ 4.6mL H_2O).
      ii. Verify mouse is anesthetized by checking foot reflexes with tweezers.
   b. Restrained:
      i. Place the mouse in a clear plastic decapicone so that the mouse's head is outside of the cone.
      ii. Cut the small end of the decapicone to accommodate the mouse's head size if necessary.
      iii. Place the mouse held in a decapicone onto a custom-made restrainer and tighten each Velcro.
      iv. Make sure the mouse's eyes are easily accessible by pushing the mouse forward; adjust Velcro as necessary.
7. Once anesthetized or restrained, place the mouse on the platform.
8. Adjust the height of the platform so that the probe is at the mouse's eye level (Fig. **2A** and **2B**).
9. Align the probe to the optical axis of the mouse's eye, 1-4 mm away from the center of the cornea (Fig. **2C**).
10. Press the measuring button of the tonometer one time.
11. Once the display shows "00," the tonometer is ready for measurement.
12. Press the measuring button six times.
    a. If an error occurs, clear the "error" message by pressing the measuring button and continue measuring.
13. Once the six measurements are done, the IOP will be shown on the display.

Notes

a. Ensure the mouse is calm; otherwise, the IOP measurement could be elevated.
b. Take measurements at the same time of the day, as IOP is affected by day/night cycles.

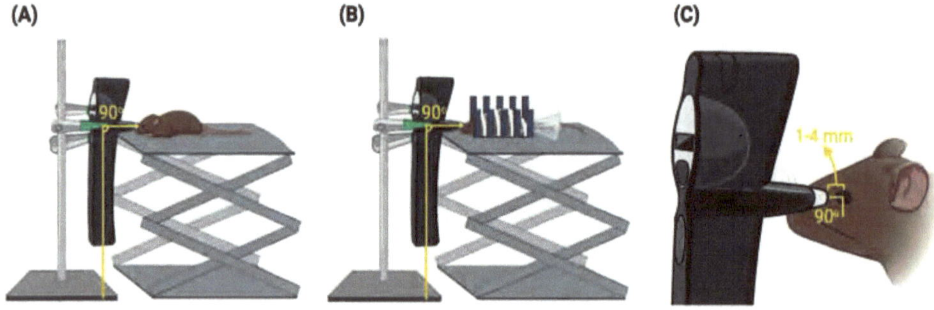

Fig. (2). Experimental setup for IOP measurement using a TonoLab tonometer. Anesthetized (A) or restrained (B) mouse is placed on an adjustable platform. (C) The tonometer should be at a 90° angle and 1-4 mm away from the center of the mouse's cornea.

Pattern Electroretinography

The retina is a complex neural network that converts light into electrical signals transmitted to the brain. The retinal ganglion cells drive this process and are particularly vulnerable in glaucoma. The increased IOP associated with this disease can damage these cells and is thought to be commensurate with visual field loss (Germano *et al.*, 2022).

Pattern electroretinography (PERG) is a non-invasive technique used to evaluate the function of retinal ganglion cells. It is considered to be a valuable tool in the diagnosis and management of PG. PERG can detect the dysfunctional visual function or the inner retinal function. It is thought to capture electrophysiological signals when retinal ganglion cells are alive but dysfunctional, allowing the initiation of treatment in some situations before irreversible damage occurs (Senger *et al.*, 2020; Turkey *et al.*, 2019; Ventura and Porciatti, 2006).

PERG is based on the principle that the electrical activity of the retinal ganglion cells can be measured by recording the response of the retina to a patterned stimulus. The technique involves the application of a patterned stimulus, such as a checkerboard, to the retina and recording the electrical activity of the retina using electrodes placed on the cornea or the skin. The results of a PERG study are typically reported as the amplitude and implicit time of the pattern-evoked response. A reduction in the response amplitude or an increase in the implicit time indicates retinal ganglion cell dysfunction, which is often associated with glaucoma (Bach and Hoffmann, 2008; Salgarello *et al.*, 2018).

PERG has been shown to be a sensitive and specific technique for detecting early glaucomatous damage. It has also been used to monitor disease progression and evaluate treatment response. However, a limitation of the technique is that it only assesses the function of the retinal ganglion cells/inner retinal function and does not provide information about the health of the other cells in the retina or the optic nerve (Jung *et al.*, 2020; van Lith *et al.*, 1984). In addition, the technique can be affected by factors such as cataracts, macular degeneration, and diabetic retinopathy, leading to false-positive results (van Lith *et al.*, 1984).

As in human subjects, PERG amplitude and latency are affected in DBA/2J mice with increased damage to the optic nerve (Ventura and Porciatti, 2006; Porciatti, 2007; Porciatti, 2015; Porciatti *et al.*, 2007). In the following section, we include a protocol for PERG in mouse models.

PERG Protocol

1. Set the heater to 37°C.
2. Place the mouse cage on the heater.
3. Anesthetize the mouse with an intraperitoneal injection (0.5– 0.7 mL/kg) of Ketamine/Xylazine solution (1mL Ketamine/ 1mL Xylazine/ 4.6mL H_2O).
4. Turn on the power source, anal probe heater, and computer.
5. Open "PERG Animal Research Software" on the computer.
6. Set up mouse information by clicking "Patient" and "New Patient." Include mouse identifiers such as cage number, tag number, age, gender, and gender.
7. Check the mouse's foot reflexes with tweezers to verify it is anesthetized.
8. Once the mouse is fully anesthetized, place the mouse on stage in a prone position with the mouth on the bite bar.
9. Place the rectal heater probe under the mouse's abdomen to keep a constant body temperature of 37 °C.
10. Place one drop of BSS onto each eye to prevent corneal dryness.
11. Insert subcutaneous probes (Fig. **3A**).
    a. Insert the Reference probe subcutaneously near the root of the tail.
        i. Use tweezers to grip the skin upwards.
        ii. Position the needle to point cranially.
    b. Insert the Cranial probe subcutaneously in the center between the two ears.
        i. Position the needle end in the center between the two eyes.
    c. Insert the Rostral probe subcutaneously in the center between the two eyes.
        i. Position the needle end at the edge of the snout without piercing through.
        ii. Ensure each probe is inserted completely without piercing through the skin a second time.
12. Align the mouse's body on the stage, ensuring each eye is directed to its corresponding monitor.
13. Verify connections using a resistance meter.
14. Check probe signals by clicking "EEG & Amplifier" on the PERG software program.

   a. Verify blue signal does not extend onto the red areas for Channel A. Repeat for Channel B.
   b. If the signal extends onto the red area, the probes are not placed correctly.
   c. Close the "EEG & Amplifier" window.
15. Dry the BSS on the mouse's eyes using Kimwipe.
16. Turn off all lights in the room.
17. Click "Acquire" in the bottom left corner.
18. Wait for the PERG to finish running (372 sweeps).
19. Once the first acquisition is complete, repeat the acquisition two more times to obtain a total of three replicates.
20. Once three replicates are obtained, create an average graph for each eye, record the Latency and Amplitude values, and export files (Fig. **3B**).
21. Once files are exported, remove the probes from the mouse and return the mouse to the heated cage until it wakes up.
22. Sanitize probes and stage using alcohol.
23. Turn off all equipment when finished.

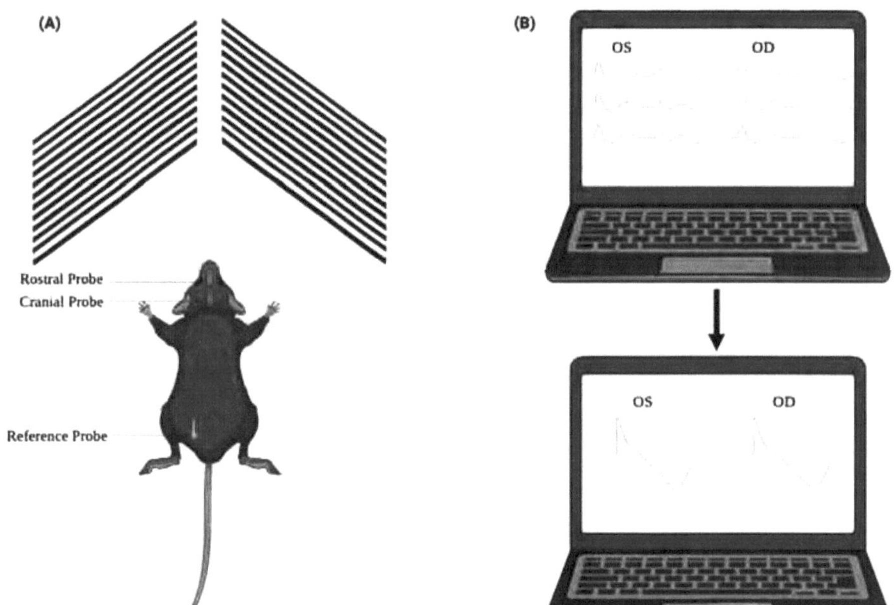

Fig. (3). Experimental setup for mice PERG. (A) Dorsal view with marked positions of subcutaneous probe placements. (B) Example of PERG replicates and final averaged graphs. Graphs are obtained separately for each eye but are shown together for simplicity. Latency and amplitude values are obtained by scrolling below the averaged graph.

Fontana-Masson Staining

Fontana-Masson staining (FMS) is a histological technique that can be used to study the accumulation of melanin granules in the iridocorneal angle of DBA/2J mice. The staining is based on the principle that melanin reacts with silver nitrate to form a brownish-black precipitate, which can be visualized under a microscope, allowing for the identification and quantification of pigmented cells (Barbosa *et al.*, 1984).

The FMS method can detect the presence of melanin in tissue samples that have been fixed and embedded in paraffin, which is a common procedure in histology. The use of other techniques that can specifically target melanin, such as immunohistochemistry, can be used in conjunction with Fontana-Masson staining to confirm the presence of melanin or dispersed pigment in the iridocorneal angle (Sundaram *et al.*, 2014).

An analysis of the existing literature revealed the need for more quantification methods of pigments. In response, we modified the standard FMS protocol utilizing spectrophotometry to impart a more quantitative approach (Fig. **4**) (Edwards *et al.*, 2020). In the following sections, we present the classic Fontana-Masson staining method followed by our modified approach.

Classic FMS Protocol (Semi-Quantitative)

1. Obtain fresh or fixed tissue samples of experimental and control mouse eyes.
    a. For the experimental (PG) group, use DBA/2J mice over six months of age.
    b. For control (non-PG) groups, use CD-1 mice of the same age as the experimental group or DBA/2J mice below five months of age.
    c. For fixed tissue, use 4% formaldehyde (10% formalin) for 24 hours.
2. Embed in tissue in paraffin and cryosection at 30 µm.
    a. Tissues *must* be sectioned at the same size and within the same approximate location to accurately compare between samples.
3. Stain sections using FMS.
    a. Prepare a silver nitrate solution by dissolving 0.1g of silver nitrate in 100 mL of distilled water.
    b. Immerse the tissue samples in the silver nitrate solution for 30 minutes.
    c. Rinse the tissue samples with distilled water and then with ethanol.
    d. Immerse the tissue samples in a 5% hydrochloric acid solution for 5 minutes.
    e. Rinse the tissue samples with distilled water and then with ethanol.
    f. Dehydrate the tissue samples by immersing them in a series of ethanol solutions (70%, 80%, 90%, and 100%).
    g. Clear the tissue samples by immersing them in xylene.

h. Mount with a coverslip using a mounting medium.

4. Examine the tissue samples under a microscope and count the number of pigmented cells in at least five different fields of view.
5. Measure by densitometry using Image J (Fig. **4A**).

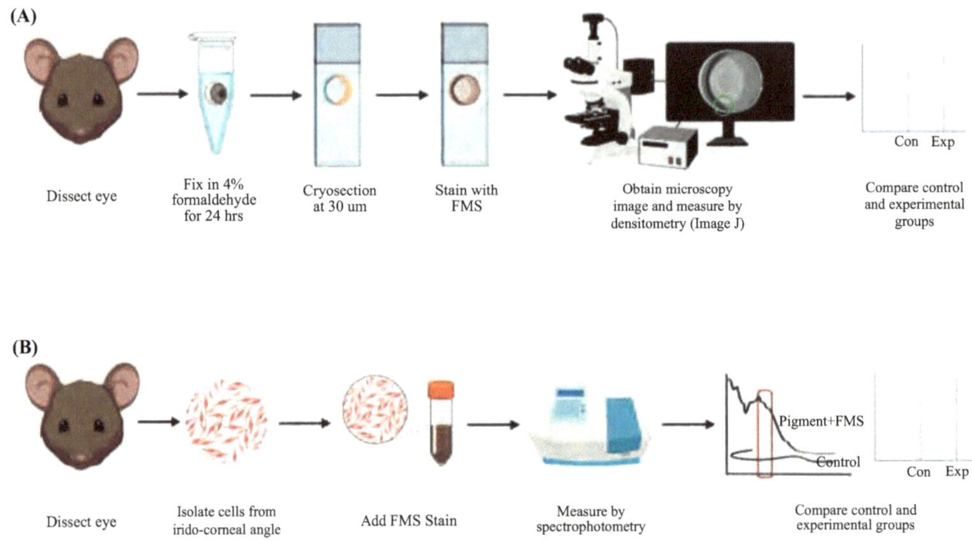

Fig. (4). Fontana Masson Staining Techniques. (A) Semi-quantitative FMS approach. After dissecting the eye, quickly wash it in saline and either keep the tissue fresh or fix it in 4% formaldehyde for 24 hours. Embed eye in paraffin, cryosection at 30 µm, and stain with FMS. Obtain a microscopy image of the iridocorneal angle and use Image J to measure by densitometry. Compare control (non-PG) and experimental (PG) groups. A limitation of this approach is the variability in area between tissue sections. (B) Modified quantitative FMS approach. After dissecting the eye, isolate cells from the iridocorneal angle and stain with FMS. Measure by spectrophotometry, recording the absorbance at 480 nm. Compare control (non-PG) and experimental (PG) groups.

Modified FMS protocol (Quantitative)

1. Obtain fresh tissue samples of experimental and control mouse eyes.
   a. For the experimental (PG) group, use DBA/2J mice over six months of age.
   b. For control (non-PG) groups, use CD-1 mice of the same age as the experimental group or DBA/2J mice below five months of age.
2. Isolate cells from an iridocorneal angle.
3. Prepare fresh tissue extract in 25 mmol L^{-1} Tris-HCl pH 7.8, 50 mmol L^{-1} NaCl, and 0.1% Genapol C100.
4. Measure the extract so the concentration does not exceed 10 µg/µL.
5. Incubate extract in preheated 60°C ammoniacal silver solution until it becomes yellowish-brown.
6. Rinse in deionized water for 1 minute.
7. Add 100 µL of 0.1% gold chloride solution and incubate for 1 minute.

8. Treat with 10 μL of 5% sodium thiosulfate solution.
9. Measure by spectrophotometry and record the absorbance at 480 nm (Fig. **4B**).

Representative measurements of the parameters described above for DBA/2J mice (equal gender distribution) are given in the Table **1** below:

Table 1. Representative data of IOP, PERG, and FMS staining from the right eye of DBA/2J mice. Data was gathered from 3 male and 3 female DBA/2J mice at 5 months, 6 months, and 9 months.

Age	IOP (mmHg) Mean (n=6)	PERG (μV) Mean (n=6)	Amount of Pigment (μg) Range (n=6)
5 months	12 ± 4	15 ± 3	0.5 – 0.8
6 months	15 ± 2	12 ± 3	0.8 – 1.6
9 months	26 ± 4	10 ± 4	3.2 – 3.5

CONCLUSION

Protocols have been presented here to allow the detection and quantification of retinal damage caused by PDS as in the prototypic mouse model of PG, the DBA/2J mouse. Using this mouse model, researchers have tested compounds which may lower and control IOP (Arcuri *et al.*, 2023), and in other studies where compounds may provide neuroprotection to help preserve RGCs (Boodram and Lim, 2024). Hence, the DBA/2J mouse model is a useful animal model of glaucoma/glaucomatous optic neuropathy

ACKNOWLEDGEMENTS

The authors would like to acknowledge support from an unrestricted grant from Research to Prevent Blindness to the University of Miami.

REFERENCES

Anderson, MG, Smith, RS, Hawes, NL, Zabaleta, A, Chang, B, Wiggs, JL & John, SWM (2002) Mutations in genes encoding melanosomal proteins cause pigmentary glaucoma in DBA/2J mice. *Nat Genet,* 30, 81-5. [http://dx.doi.org/10.1038/ng794] [PMID: 11743578]

Arcuri J, Elbaz A, Sharif NA, Bhattacharya SK. Ocular Treatments Targeting Separate Prostaglandin Receptors in Mice Exhibit Alterations in Intraocular Pressure and Optic Nerve Lipidome. J Ocul Pharmacol Ther. 2023 Oct;39(8):541-550.

Bach, M & Hoffmann, MB (2008) Update on the pattern electroretinogram in glaucoma. *Optom Vis Sci,* 85, 386-95.
[http://dx.doi.org/10.1097/OPX.0b013e318177ebf3] [PMID: 18521020]

Barbosa, AJA, Castro, LPF, Margarida, A & Nogueira, MF (1984) A simple and economical modification of the Masson-Fontana method for staining melanin granules and enterochromaffin cells. *Stain Technol,* 59, 193-6.
[http://dx.doi.org/10.3109/10520298409113855] [PMID: 6208641]

Boodram V, Lim H. Differential protection by nicotinamide in a mouse model of glaucoma DBA/2J revealed by second-harmonic generation microscopy. PLoS One. 2024 Sep 10;19(9):e0309400.

Campbell, DG (1979) Pigmentary dispersion and glaucoma. A new theory. *Arch Ophthalmol,* 97, 1667-72. [http://dx.doi.org/10.1001/archopht.1979.01020020235011] [PMID: 475638]

Danias, J, Kontiola, AI, Filippopoulos, T & Mittag, T (2003) Method for the noninvasive measurement of intraocular pressure in mice. *Invest Ophthalmol Vis Sci,* 44, 1138-41.
[http://dx.doi.org/10.1167/iovs.02-0553] [PMID: 12601041]

Di Pippo, M, Ciancimino, C, Scuderi, L & Perdicchi, A (2020) An Iconic Case of Pigmentary Glaucoma: Brief Review of the Literature. *Case Rep Ophthalmol,* 11, 377-84.
[http://dx.doi.org/10.1159/000508605] [PMID: 32884553]

Edwards, G, Arcuri, J, Wang, H, Ziebarth, N, Zode, G, Lee, RK & Bhattacharya, SK (2020) Endogenous ocular lipids as potential modulators of intraocular pressure. *J Cell Mol Med,* 24, 3856-900.
[http://dx.doi.org/10.1111/jcmm.14975] [PMID: 32090468]

Germano, RAS, Germano, CS, Susanna, FN & Susanna, R (2022) Patterns of Visual Field Loss in Early, Moderate, and Severe Stages of Open Angle Glaucoma. *J Glaucoma,* 31, 609-13.
[http://dx.doi.org/10.1097/IJG.0000000000001986] [PMID: 35019874]

John, SW, Hagaman, JR, MacTaggart, TE, Peng, L & Smithes, O (1997) Intraocular pressure in inbred mouse strains. *Invest Ophthalmol Vis Sci,* 38, 249-53.
[PMID: 9008647]

John, SW, Smith, RS, Savinova, OV, Hawes, NL, Chang, B, Turnbull, D, Davisson, M, Roderick, TH & Heckenlively, JR (1998) Essential iris atrophy, pigment dispersion, and glaucoma in DBA/2J mice. *Invest Ophthalmol Vis Sci,* 39, 951-62.
[PMID: 9579474]

Jung, KI, Jeon, S, Shin, DY, Lee, J & Park, CK (2020) Pattern Electroretinograms in Preperimetric and Perimetric Glaucoma. *Am J Ophthalmol,* 215, 118-26.
[http://dx.doi.org/10.1016/j.ajo.2020.02.008] [PMID: 32087144]

Liebmann, JM, Tello, C, Chew, SJ, Cohen, H & Ritch, R (1995) Prevention of blinking alters iris configuration in pigment dispersion syndrome and in normal eyes. *Ophthalmology,* 102, 446-55. [http://dx.doi.org/10.1016/S0161-6420(95)31001-9] [PMID: 7891984]

Lu, H, Wang, X, Pullen, M, Guan, H, Chen, H, Sahu, S, Zhang, B, Chen, H, Williams, RW, Geisert, EE, Lu, L & Jablonski, MM (2011) Genetic dissection of the Gpnmb network in the eye. *Invest Ophthalmol Vis Sci,* 52, 4132-42.
[http://dx.doi.org/10.1167/iovs.10-6493] [PMID: 21398278]

Morris, CA, Crowston, JG, Lindsey, JD, Danias, J & Weinreb, RN (2006) Comparison of invasive and non-invasive tonometry in the mouse. *Exp Eye Res,* 82, 1094-9.
[http://dx.doi.org/10.1016/j.exer.2005.12.001] [PMID: 16466714]

Niyadurupola, N & Broadway, DC (2008) Pigment dispersion syndrome and pigmentary glaucoma – a major review. *Clin Exp Ophthalmol,* 36, 868-82.
[http://dx.doi.org/10.1111/j.1442-9071.2009.01920.x] [PMID: 19278484]

Okafor, K, Vinod, K & Gedde, SJ (2017) Update on pigment dispersion syndrome and pigmentary glaucoma. *Curr Opin Ophthalmol,* 28, 154-60.
[http://dx.doi.org/10.1097/ICU.0000000000000352] [PMID: 27898469]

Pease, ME, Cone, FE, Gelman, S, Son, JL & Quigley, HA (2011) Calibration of the TonoLab tonometer in mice with spontaneous or experimental glaucoma. *Invest Ophthalmol Vis Sci,* 52, 858-64.
[http://dx.doi.org/10.1167/iovs.10-5556] [PMID: 20720229]

Porciatti, V (2007) The mouse pattern electroretinogram. *Doc Ophthalmol,* 115, 145-53.
[http://dx.doi.org/10.1007/s10633-007-9059-8] [PMID: 17522779]

Porciatti, V (2015) Electrophysiological assessment of retinal ganglion cell function. *Exp Eye Res,* 141, 164-70.
[http://dx.doi.org/10.1016/j.exer.2015.05.008] [PMID: 25998495]

Porciatti, V, Saleh, M & Nagaraju, M (2007) The pattern electroretinogram as a tool to monitor progressive retinal ganglion cell dysfunction in the DBA/2J mouse model of glaucoma. *Invest Ophthalmol Vis Sci,* 48, 745-51.
[http://dx.doi.org/10.1167/iovs.06-0733] [PMID: 17251473]

Potash, SD, Tello, C, Liebmann, J & Ritch, R (1994) Ultrasound biomicroscopy in pigment dispersion syndrome. *Ophthalmology,* 101, 332-9.
[http://dx.doi.org/10.1016/S0161-6420(94)31331-5] [PMID: 8115154]

Pu, L, Zhou, R, Li, Q & Qing, G (2022) Distribution of Pigment Particles in Aqueous Drainage Structures in a DBA/2J Mouse Model of Pigmentary Glaucoma. *Invest Ophthalmol Vis Sci,* 63, 2.
[http://dx.doi.org/10.1167/iovs.63.6.2] [PMID: 35648639]

Salgarello, T, Giudiceandrea, A, Calandriello, L, Marangoni, D, Colotto, A, Caporossi, A & Falsini, B (2018) Pattern Electroretinogram Detects Localized Glaucoma Defects. *Transl Vis Sci Technol,* 7, 6.
[http://dx.doi.org/10.1167/tvst.7.5.6] [PMID: 30221072]

Scuderi, G, Contestabile, MT, Scuderi, L, Librando, A, Fenicia, V & Rahimi, S (2019) Pigment dispersion syndrome and pigmentary glaucoma: a review and update. *Int Ophthalmol,* 39, 1651-62.
[http://dx.doi.org/10.1007/s10792-018-0938-7] [PMID: 29721842]

Senger, C, Moreto, R, Watanabe, SES, Matos, AG & Paula, JS (2020) Electrophysiology in Glaucoma. *J Glaucoma,* 29, 147-53.
[http://dx.doi.org/10.1097/IJG.0000000000001422] [PMID: 31809397]

Sundaram, C, Shantveer, GU, Umabala, P & Lakshmi, V (2014) Diagnostic utility of melanin production by fungi: Study on tissue sections and culture smears with Masson-Fontana stain. *Indian J Pathol Microbiol,* 57, 217-22.
[http://dx.doi.org/10.4103/0377-4929.134666] [PMID: 24943753]

Turkey, E, Elsanabary, ZSE, Elshazly, LHM & Osman, MH (2019) Role of Pattern Electroretinogram in Ocular Hypertension and Early Glaucoma. *J Glaucoma,* 28, 871-7.
[http://dx.doi.org/10.1097/IJG.0000000000001325] [PMID: 31306362]

van Lith, G, Ringens, P & de Heer, LJ (1984) Pattern electroretinogram and glaucoma. *Dev Ophthalmol,* 9, 133-9.
[http://dx.doi.org/10.1159/000409816] [PMID: 6526100]

Ventura, LM & Porciatti, V (2006) Pattern electroretinogram in glaucoma. *Curr Opin Ophthalmol,* 17, 196-202.
[http://dx.doi.org/10.1097/01.icu.0000193082.44938.3c] [PMID: 16552256]

Wang, J & Dong, Y (2016) Characterization of intraocular pressure pattern and changes of retinal ganglion cells in DBA2J glaucoma mice. *Int J Ophthalmol,* 9, 211-7.
[PMID: 26949637]

CHAPTER 38

Protocols for Creating Genetically-Transduced Animal Models of Ocular Hypertension and Glaucoma

Najam A. Sharif[1,*] and **Saima Chaudhry**[2]

[1] *Research & Development Nanoscope Therapeutics Inc., 2777 N. Stemmons Fwy, Suite 1102, Dallas, TX-75207, USA*

[2] *Univ N. Texas at Arlington, 701 S Nedderman Dr. Arlington, TX-76019, USA*

Abstract: Several animal models of ocular hypertension (OHT) have been developed over the last two decades. Some researchers simply use naturally available naïve mammals such as rodents, rabbits, dogs, and monkeys to evaluate the effects of test agents. Other OHT researchers have created rodent models by ablating episcleral veins on the corneal surface using lasers or clips or filling them with hypertonic saline. In monkeys, the trabecular meshwork, the major aqueous humor (AQH) drainage system from the anterior chamber of the eye, can be partially coagulated using a laser to increase intraocular pressure (IOP). With the advent of genetical techniques, scientists have created gene knockout models of OHT. In the current chapter, the authors describe methods to genetically deliver genes into the anterior chamber and/or specific tissues that transduce the production of fibrotic cytokines such a transforming growth factor-beta (TGF-β_2). This cytokine is abnormally elevated in AQH of OHT/glaucoma patients and is increasingly linked to the development of OHT/glaucoma.

Keywords: Genes, Glaucoma, Ocular diseases, Ocular hypertension, Viral vectors.

INTRODUCTION

Ocular hypertension (OHT) or elevated intraocular pressure (IOP) is one of the major culprits implicated in the pathogenesis of many forms of glaucoma, an insidious, asymptomatic silent thief of eyesight (Weinreb *et al*., 2014; Sharif, 2017, 2021). It is well known that the inflammatory and fibrosis-causing cytokine, transforming growth factor-beta (TGF-β2), is naturally elevated in the aqueous humor (AQH) of patients with OHT/glaucoma (Trapathi *et al*., 1994; Yamamoto

* **Corresponding author Najam A. Sharif:** Vice President and Head of Research & Development Nanoscope Therapeutics Inc., 2777 N. Stemmons Fwy, Suite 1102, Dallas, TX-75207, USA; Tel: +1(817)-565-7686; E-mail: nsharif@nanostherapeutics.com

et al., 2005) and is responsible for inducing the production and accumulation of collagen and fibronectin in and around the trabecular meshwork (TM) (Fuchshofer *et al.*, 2005; Shephard *et al.*, 2010). The clogging of the TM causes the subsequent excess accumulation of AQH in the anterior chamber of the eye, and this results in an increase in IOP (Weinreb *et al.*, 2014; Sharif, 2017, 2021). The resultant OHT over several decades damages the optic nerve and kills the retinal ganglion cells, which transmit electrochemical signals to the brain for decoding and visual perception. Chronic OHT leads to loss of vision and can lead to blindness if not diagnosed and treated in a timely manner (Weinreb *et al.*, 2014; Sharif, 2017, 2021).

In an effort to better understand the molecular and cellular mediators of OHT and how this affects the visual apparatus and the loss of vision, researchers have created many types of animal models of elevated IOP/OHT and many are described in this book. The topic of the current chapter is the way genetic techniques have been deployed to recapitulate a human version of OHT in a rodent model by applying the known involvement of TGF-beta in the process of IOP elevation. Such genetic manipulation has been successfully rendered in mice and rats and will be described below using adenoviral delivery (Shephard *et al.*, 2010) and lentiviral delivery methods (Patil *et al.*, 2022).

ANIMAL HANDLING

All animals should be treated in accordance with the Association for Research in Vision and Ophthalmology (ARVO), and the animal handling and testing protocols must be approved by the institutional Animal Care and Use Committee. It is recommended that Wistar rats (2– 4 months old) and BALB/cJ mice (2–5 months old) were acquired from Charles River Labs (Wilmington, MA) and Jackson Labs (Bar Harbor, ME). The rodents should be adequately housed, maintained on a 12/12 hours light/dark cycle, and offered food and water ad libitum.

VIRAL VECTOR PRODUCTION AND DELIVERY OF TGF-B2 TO ELEVATE IOP

1. Obtain wild-type (WT) human transforming growth factor β2 (hTGFβ2) cDNA (NM_003238) in the pCMV6-XL5 vector from a reputable source.
2. Next, generate the cDNA coding for the active form of hTGFβ2 by converting the cysteines at positions 226 and 228 to serines.
3. Synthesize the region extending from the HindIII site (nt 1976) to the PpuMI site (nt 2395) so that nucleotides 1985 and 1991 are changed from guanine to cytosine, converting the cysteines to serines at amino acids 226 and 228 of the hTGFβ2 protein as mentioned above.

4. Next, clone this fragment into pCMV6- XL5.hTGFβ2 and then subclone the wild-type and mutant coding region cDNAs into the pacAd5.CMV.KN.pA shuttle vector using EcoRI/Xba1 restriction.
5. Use CsCl gradient centrifugation to purify the viruses, and then dialyze against Tris-EDTA buffer containing 10% sucrose and store at -80°C. Test each virus for wild-type revertants and titer by polymerase chain reaction and A549 plaque assay. In all cases, use empty adeno-associated virus (AAV) (Ad.Empty) as a negative control.
6. Confirm that the animals to be used are free of any apparent ocular disorders by direct ophthalmoscopic examination.
7. Anesthetize rats *via* an intramuscular injection using a solution of acepromazine (3 mg/kg), ketamine (33 mg/kg), and xylazine (7 mg/kg). For mice, perform a single intraperitoneal injection of a solution containing acepromazine (1.8 mg/kg), ketamine (73 mg/kg), and xylazine (1.8 mg/kg;).
8. When performing intracameral injections, instill 1-2 drops of 1% cyclopentolate (Mydriacyl) to dilate the pupil. Topical ocularly instill 1-2 drops of 0.5% tropicamide (Alcaine) to locally anesthetize the ocular surface of the eye.
9. Then perform intravitreal or intracameral injection of a suspension of adenovirus of a specified titer in a volume of 5 μL for the rat eye and 2 μL for the mouse eye using a Hamilton glass microsyringe fitted with a custom-made 1-inch 33-gauge needle with a 10° bevel. The uninjected contralateral eye should be used as a control. The injections should be performed slowly over 30 seconds. Leave the needle in place after the injection is completed for a minute to prevent fluid reflux and then withdraw slowly from the eye. Allow the rats to recover from all the aforementioned procedures.
10. For taking the IOP measurements, ensure the investigator is masked to the treatment paradigm. Use a rebound tonometer (TonoLab; Tiolat Oy; Helsinki, Finland) to take several measurements for each eye at each time point (before and after the injections).
11. A pictogram of the procedure for the lentivirus-delivered TGFβ2 gene and its expression *in vivo* in mice is shown in Fig. (**1**). Furthermore, the elevation of IOP by this genetic means is shown in Fig. (**2**).

RNA Isolation from Rodent Tissues

1. Euthanize the animals at various times following AAV vector-genetic construct injection using the CO_2 asphyxiation method, enucleate the eyes, and dissect them into the anterior and posterior segments.
2. Place each segment in an individual microfuge tube that contains 1 mL Trizol reagent, 1 μL GlycoBlue (glycogen covalently coupled to blue dye), and one 5-

mm stainless steel ball. Homogenize each sample using a TissueLyser system (Qiagen) for 5 minutes at 25 Hz.

3. Isolate the RNA according to the manufacturer's guidelines (Invitrogen). Next, dissolve the isolated RNA in 10 μL nuclease-free water, followed by determining the concentration by absorbance (at A260).

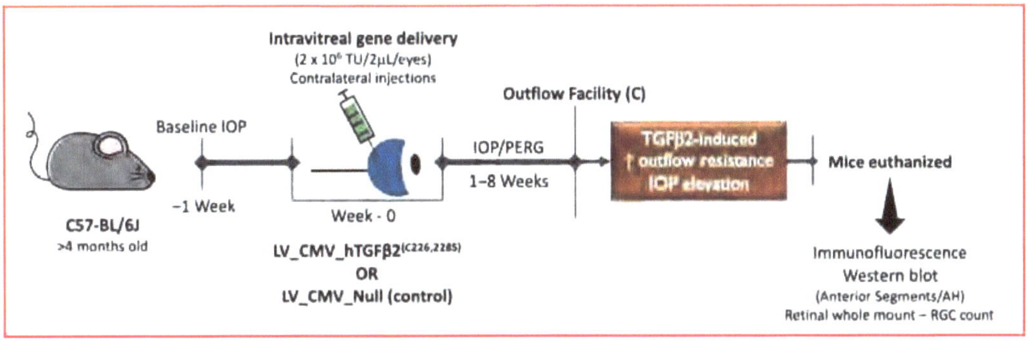

Fig. (1). A schematic diagram that depicts the lentiviral delivery of the TGF-β2 gene and its expression *in vivo* in mice to raise the IOP (Patil *et al.*, 2022).

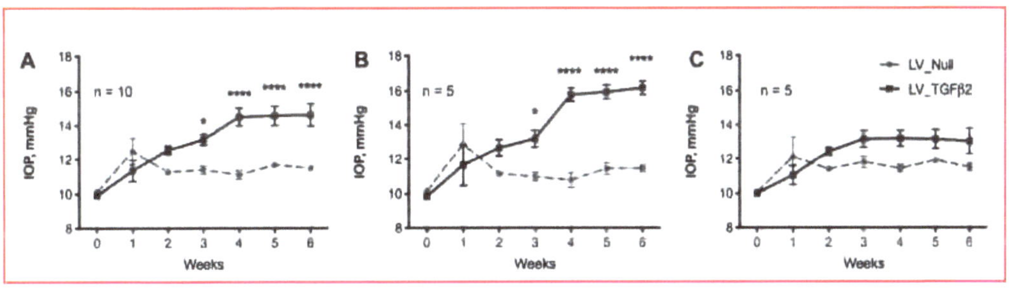

Fig. (2). Elevation of IOP in mice injected with lentivirus-delivered TGF-β2 genetic construct. IOP was significantly raised in LV_TGFβ2-injected eyes relative to controls (LV_Null), beginning 21 days following the injection (A). In (B), animals exhibiting IOPs >2.5 mmHg were isolated from those that possessed non-elevated IOPs (C). Statistical significance between the two groups of mice was found at * $p < 0.05$, **** $p < 0.0001$ at various time points after the injections (Adapted from Patil *et al.*, 2022). LV_Null denotes an empty vector.

Determination of AQH TGFβ2 Protein

1. Use a sensitive hTGFβ2 ELISA kit (R&D Systems, Minneapolis, MN) to determine the TGFβ2 protein concentrations in the AQH of the transduced animals and controls. Acid-activation of samples can then yield the total TGFβ2 levels.
2. The optical density of the samples should be determined on a spectrophotometer.
3. Fix enucleated eyes in 4% paraformaldehyde over 1 day at room temperature and embed in paraffin wax for tissue sectioning.

4. Cut 5 μm thick sections from the fixed eyes and collect them on microscope slides. Stain the sections with hematoxylin and eosin reagents and examine them under the microscope.

CONCLUSION

Our improved knowledge and understanding of the disease mechanisms and factors involved in the initiation and progression of ocular hypertension and glaucoma is due to the use of various animal models that mimic the diseases in humans. Although many genes have been implicated in OHT and glaucoma pathology (Sharif, 2023), the current chapter illustrated how delivering an excess of the fibrotic cytokine, TGFβ2, into the posterior segment of the eye of mice *via* a viral vector-gene construct can successfully reproduce the human OHT morphology and pathology. Such genetically created animal models can thus be used to test and find suitable drugs to lower and control the elevated IOP.

REFERENCES

Fuchshofer, R, Birke, M, Welge-Lussen, U, Kook, D & Lu¨tjen-Drecoll, E (2005) Transforming growth factor-beta 2 modulated extracellular matrix component expression in cultured human optic nerve head astrocytes. *Invest Ophthalmol Vis Sci,* 46, 568-78.
[http://dx.doi.org/10.1167/iovs.04-0649] [PMID: 15671284]

Patil, SV, Kasetti, RB, Millar, JC & Zode, GS (2022) A novel mouse model of TGFβ2-induced ocular hypertension using lentiviral gene delivery. *Int J Mol Sci,* 23, 6883.
[http://dx.doi.org/10.3390/ijms23136883] [PMID: 35805889]

Sharif, NA (2017) Ocular hypertension and glaucoma: a review and current perspectives. *Int. J Ophthalmol Vis Sci,* 2, 22-36.

Sharif, NA (2021) Therapeutic drugs and devices for tackling ocular hypertension and glaucoma, and need for neuroprotection and cytoprotective therapies. *Front Pharmacol,* 12, 729249.
[http://dx.doi.org/10.3389/fphar.2021.729249] [PMID: 34603044]

Sharif, NA (2023) Gene therapies and gene product-based drug candidates for normalizing and preserving tissue functions in animal models of ocular hypertension and glaucoma. *Mol Aspects Med,* 94, 101218.
[http://dx.doi.org/10.1016/j.mam.2023.101218] [PMID: 37976898]

Shepard, AR, Millar, JC, Pang, IH, Jacobson, N, Wang, WH & Clark, AF (2010) Adenoviral gene transfer of active human transforming growth factor-beta2 elevates intraocular pressure and reduces outflow facility in rodent eyes. *Invest Ophthalmol Vis Sci,* 51, 2067-76.
[http://dx.doi.org/10.1167/iovs.09-4567] [PMID: 19959644]

Tripathi, RC, Li, J, Chan, WA & Tripathi, BJ (1994) Aqueous humor in glaucomatous eyes contains an increased level of TGF-beta 2. *Exp Eye Res,* 59, 723-8.
[http://dx.doi.org/10.1006/exer.1994.1158] [PMID: 7698265]

Weinreb, RN, Aung, T & Medeiros, FA (2014) The pathophysiology and treatment of glaucoma: a review. *JAMA,* 311, 1901-11.
[http://dx.doi.org/10.1001/jama.2014.3192] [PMID: 24825645]

Yamamoto, N, Itonaga, K, Marunouchi, T & Majima, K (2005) Concentration of transforming growth factor beta2 in aqueous humor. *Ophthalmic Res,* 37, 29-33.
[http://dx.doi.org/10.1159/000083019] [PMID: 15637419]

CHAPTER 39

Protocol for Conditional Knockout Mouse Model of OHT and Glaucoma

Judith West-Mays[1,*] and **Fatima Shirazee**[1]

[1] *Department of Pathology and Molecular Medicine, McMaster University, Hamilton, Canada*

Abstract: This chapter describes the protocols used to create a conditional knockout mouse model to study partially closed-angle glaucoma where the intraocular pressure (IOP) is raised beyond normal levels. The Cre/loxP approach was employed as a strategy to conditionally inactivate the AP-2β gene from the developing periocular mesenchyme (POM) that is responsible for creating the trabecular meshwork (TM) (Taiyab *et al.*, 2022). The Mgp-Cre knock-in (Mgp-Cre.KI) mice, in combination with the AP-2β floxed mice, were utilized to create a targeted deletion of AP-2β to the TM area. The AP-2β TMR KO mutants exhibit an absent TM and underdeveloped Schlemm's canal (SC) and partial adherence of the iris to the cornea. The mutants have significantly higher IOP than their wild-type littermates by one month of age, and this is correlated with a progressive, significant loss of retinal ganglion cells, reduced retinal thickness, and reduced retinal function, as measured by electroretinography. Thus, these mutant mice can serve as a model for understanding and treating progressive human primary angle-closure glaucoma with associated ocular hypertension.

Keywords: Anterior segment dysgenesis, Conditional KO, Eye, Glaucoma, Intraocular pressure, Ocular hypertension, Optic nerve, Protocol, Retina.

INTRODUCTION

Appropriate development of structures in the anterior segment of the eye is critical for normal ocular functioning. Proper development of the aqueous humor outflow structures, including the trabecular meshwork (TM) and Schlemm's canal (SC), is necessary to ensure that there is a balance between aqueous humor (AQH) production and drainage, thus maintaining optimal intraocular pressure (IOP). Glaucoma due to ocular hypertension (OHT) can occur due to an imbalance of aqueous humor (AQH) generation and its egress, which can result in the building

* **Corresponding author Judith West-Mays :** Department of Pathology and Molecular Medicine, McMaster University, Hamilton, Canada; Tel: +905-525-9140; Ext: 26237; E-mail: westmayj@mcmaster.ca

Najam A. Sharif and Sunny E. Ohia (Eds.)

of IOP. This ultimately causes pressure and damages the optic nerve head (Dietze *et al.*, 2022). While there are many types of glaucoma, primary open-angle glaucoma and angle closure glaucoma are two major forms (Taiyab *et al.*, 2022). In primary open-angle glaucoma (POAG), there is a build-up of aqueous humor fluid in the anterior chamber due to an increased resistance to AQH flow through the trabecular meshwork (TM) and Schlemm's canal (SC) drainage structures responsible for conventional outflow. However, in primary angle closure glaucoma (PACG), these structures are completely blocked, causing the conventional pathway to become inaccessible. One of the underlying conditions that can cause angle closure glaucoma is referred to as peripheral anterior synechia (PAS), a condition in which the iris adheres to the cornea (Lee *et al.*, 2006). Additionally, aberrations in the development of the anterior structures (cornea, iris, lens, the cornea, ciliary body, trabecular meshwork, and Schlemm's canal) can lead to anterior segment dysgenesis (ASD) and disorders, and individuals with ASD are more susceptible to glaucoma (Taiyab *et al.*, 2022). Importantly, glaucoma is one of the leading causes of blindness in the world, with an estimated 76 million people affected by it, and this number is projected to increase by almost 30% over the next decade (Quigley & Broman, 2006).

Current treatments for primary angle closure glaucoma include topical treatments such as prostaglandin analogs that lower IOP by increasing outflow or aqueous suppressants that help reduce the production of aqueous humor. Although several medications assist in managing PACG during its early stages, severe conditions require laser or surgery to expand the drainage angle or create an opening in the iris to allow for outflow (Wright *et al.*, 2016).

Investigating the genetic pathways and mechanisms that govern the proper development of the tissues within the anterior segment of the eye will lead to a better understanding of the underlying cause of ASD and angle closure glaucoma. Anterior segment tissue development in mice is regulated by a collection of genes (*e.g.*, *Pitx2, Foxc1, Foxc2, Lmx1b, and Pax6)* (Chen & Gage, 2016; Cross *et al.*, 2014; Liu & Johnson, 2010; Romero *et al.*, 2011; Smith *et al.*, 2000; Tümer & Bach-Holm, 2009) and the activating protein 2 (AP-2) family of transcription factors (*e.g.*, AP-2α and AP-2β) (Barzago *et al.*, 2017; Bassett *et al.*, 2007, 2010, 2012; Chen & Gage, 2016; Kerr *et al.*, 2014; Pontoriero *et al.*, 2008; West-Mays *et al.*, 1999). AP-2α and AP-2β encoded by Tfap2a and Tfap2b genes, respectively, are both highly expressed in periocular mesenchyme (POM)-derived structures at earlier stages of embryogenesis, but only *Tfap2b* is specifically expressed within POM cells during the secondary migration phase (Bassett *et al.*, 2012)(West-Mays *et al.*, 1999). Importantly, we have demonstrated that the AP-2β family member, encoded by the *Tfap2b* gene, is present within POM cells that move to the area between the cornea and the anterior rim of the optic cup and subsequently develop into the TM and SC (Bassett *et al*., 2012; Martino *et al*., 2016). To ascertain the role of AP-2β in the creation of the latter, we recently used the Cre/loxP approach to conditionally delete AP-2β from the evolving POM. This conditional deletion enabled targeting of the TM area and avoided the perinatal death observed in the AP-2β germline KO mutants.

The Cre/loxP approach is a refined strategy for conditional gene inactivation that relies on the DNA recombinase Cre and its recognition (loxP) sites. For conditional mutagenesis, a target gene is modified by the insertion of two loxP sites that enable to excise the flanked (floxed) gene segment through Cre-mediated recombination. Conditional mutant mice are obtained by crossing the floxed strain with a Cre transgenic line such that the target gene becomes inactivated *in vivo* within the expression domain of Cre. Our laboratory employed this approach using the MgpCre transgenic mouse system (Borrás *et al*., 2015) combined AP-2β floxed mice (Martino *et al*., 2016; Van Otterloo *et al*., 2022) to target AP-2β from the POM cell population that creates the TM. These mice have been termed the AP-2β-TM-region knockout mice (AP-2β TMR-KO). Previous work has shown that the expression of MgpCre is confined to the iridocorneal angle and the peripapillary scleral region (Borras *et al*., 2015). Our lab was the first to demonstrate that the expression of MgpCre occurs earlier in the eye during embryonic development at E15 and, importantly, in the POM (Taiyab *et al*., 2022). This new knowledge inspired us to create a conditional KO model of AP-2β in the developing TM region using the MgpCre (Fig. **1**).

Deletion of AP-2β using the Mgp-Cre knock-in (Mgp-Cre.KI) from the developing TM area resulted in offspring with an absent TM and underdeveloped SC as ascertained by the reduction in key markers (*e.g*., αSMA, myocilin, Prox1, and endomucin) (Taiyab *et al*., 2022). There was a partial adherence of the iris to the cornea with the iridocorneal angle partially closed, and this resulted in significantly elevated IOP by 1-month of age. Moreover, elevated IOP correlated with decreased retinal thickness, progressive loss of RGCs, and thus decreased ERG responses. The elevated IOP was temporarily reduced following latanoprost treatment, thus indicating the functionality of the uveoscleral pathway in this model (Taiyab *et al*., 2022).

Although there are a variety of mouse models that have been developed to understand the progression of glaucoma (*e.g*., optic nerve crush model, microbead injection model, and DBA/2J model) (Johnson & Tomarev, 2010)), there are fewer models where genetic mutation/deletion has been applied. Some of these models include mice with mutations in *Sh3pxd2b* (Mao *et al*., 2011)), *Pitx2* (Chen & Gage, 2016), *Foxc1*, *Foxc2* (Smith *et al*., 2000), and *Lmx1b* (Liu & Johnson, 2010), as well as AP-2β NCC KO mice (Martino *et al*., 2016). All these models exhibit various forms of ASD and some glaucomatous pathophysiology. However, the AP-2β TMR KO model described herein exhibits defects that are more confined to the outflow structures associated with the conventional pathway and is an acute model of OHT/glaucoma that exhibits elevated IOP and glaucomatous features in a fully penetrant manner. We have also shown that the increased IOP in P30 AP- 2β mutant mice can be significantly lowered following topical ocular instillation of 0.005% latanoprost, an FP-receptor-selective prostaglandin analog that enhances uveoscleral outflow of AQH. This suggests our model is ideal for understanding and discovering treatment strategies for primary open-angle glaucoma with associated ocular hypertension.

The purpose of this chapter is to describe the key approaches and protocols to create the AP-2β TMR KO mouse model (Taiyab *et al*., 2022). As outlined above, the AP-2β TMR KO mutants exhibit significantly increased IOP than their wild-type littermates by one month of age, which correlates with a progressive significant loss of RGCs, decreased retinal thickness, and decreased functional responses of the retina. Key features of this model are shown in Figs. (**2** - **5**); however, a detailed description can be found in our recent publication (Taiyab *et al*., 2022).

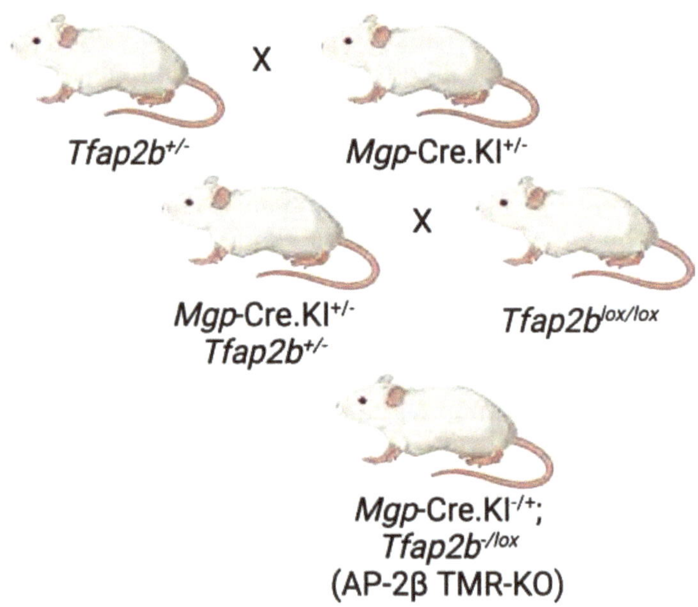

Fig. (1). Crossings of mouse lines.

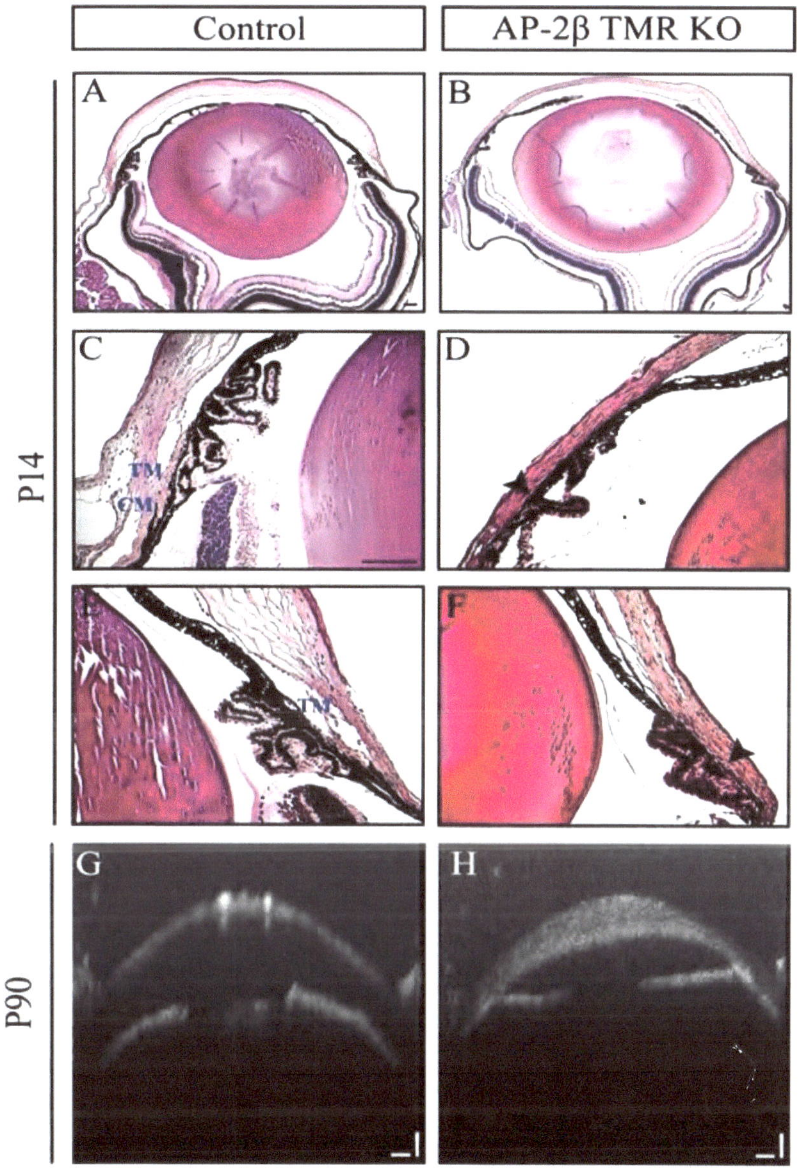

Fig. (2). Observation of abnormal anterior chamber morphology of AP-2β-TMR-KO mice. A) B) The TM area appeared to be present in the control mouse but not in the mutant mouse. Fig. (1G and H) OCT images demonstrate an open iridocorneal angle in the P45 control mouse (G); however, the angle was partially closed in the mutant mouse (H), similar to a PAS condition (Taiyab *et al.*, 2022).

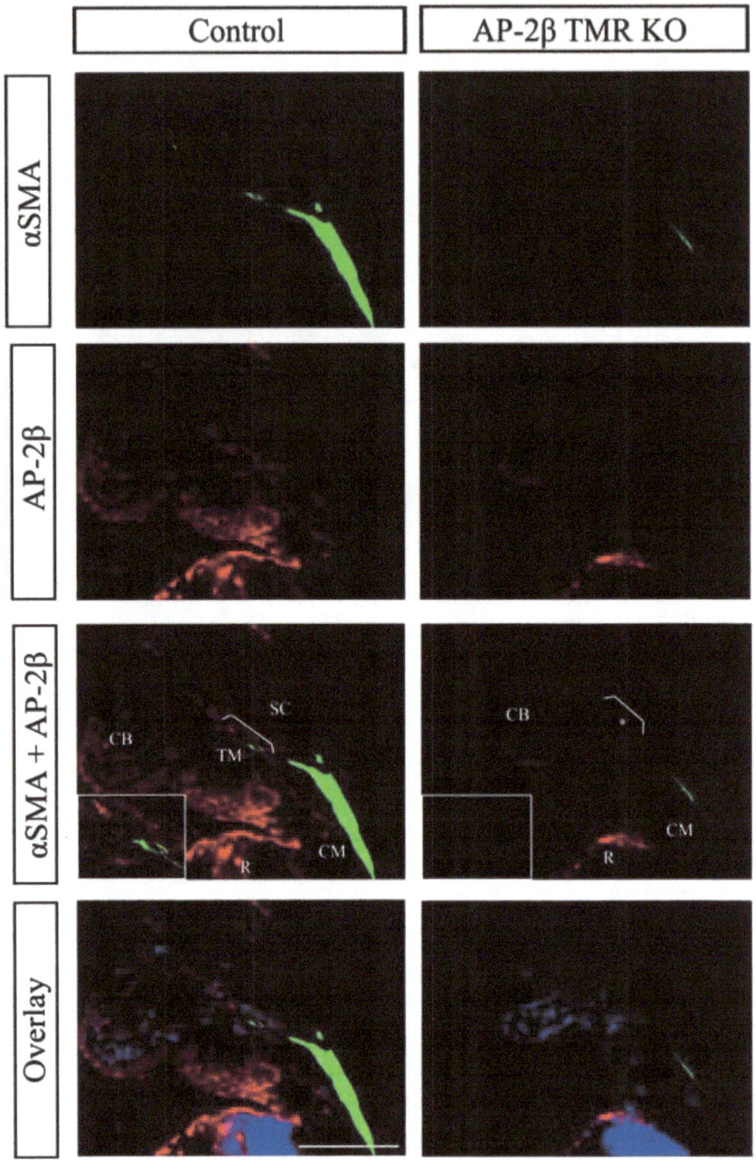

Fig. (3). Immunohistochemistry of key markers. AP-2β in TMR KO deletion resulted in a decreased expression of key markers of TM and SC. A) In P14 control mice, AP-2β was visible in the iridocorneal angle, ciliary body, and retina. However, in mutant mice, AP-2β was not observed in the iridocorneal angle, although it was present in the retina and the ciliary body. There also was a reduced expression of αSMA within the TM area of the mutant mouse compared to the control (Taiyab *et al.*, 2022).

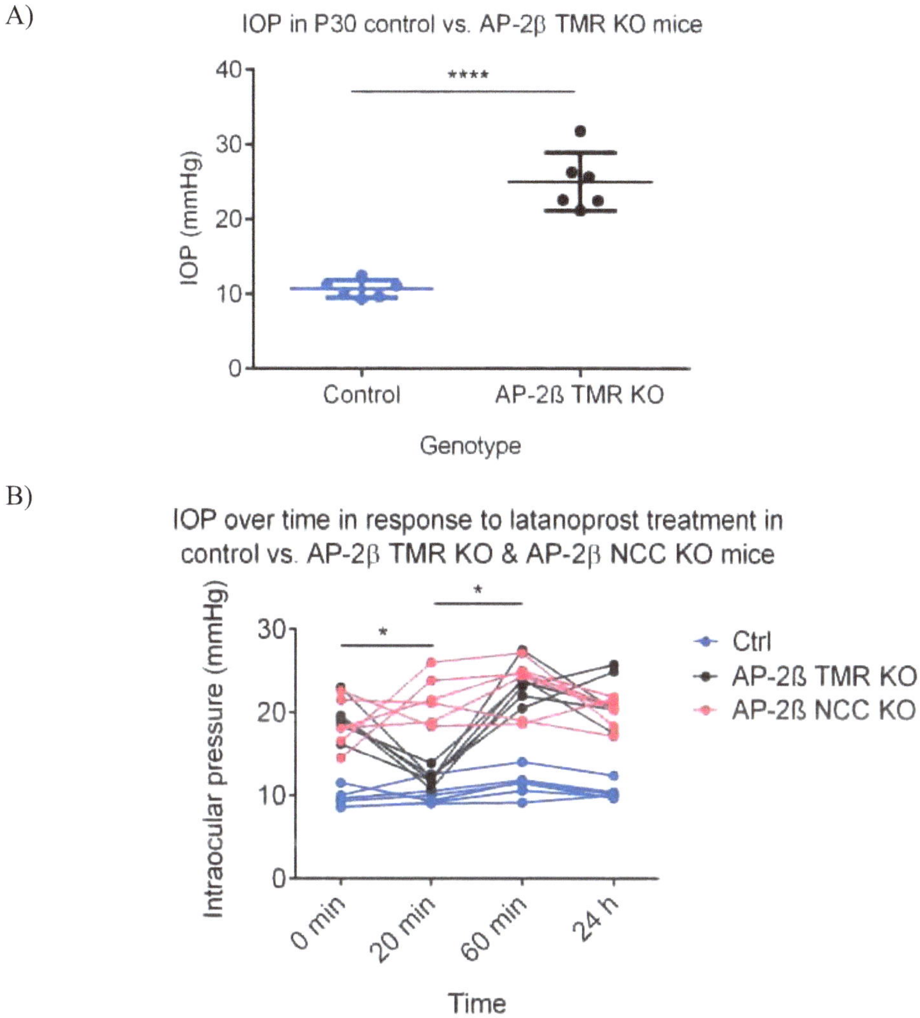

Fig. (4). Measuring the IOP of mutant mice as well as control littermates. Mutant mice have a significantly elevated IOP as compared to the control mice (A). Their IOP appears to have temporarily reduced at 20 minutes following latanoprost treatment and then goes back up to baseline at 1hr following treatment (Fig. **4B**). Whereas the AP-2β NCC KO mice (previously developed in our lab) demonstrate an elevated IOP prior to and after treatment across all time points (Taiyab *et al*., 2022). * $p < 0.05$; **** $p < 0.0001$.

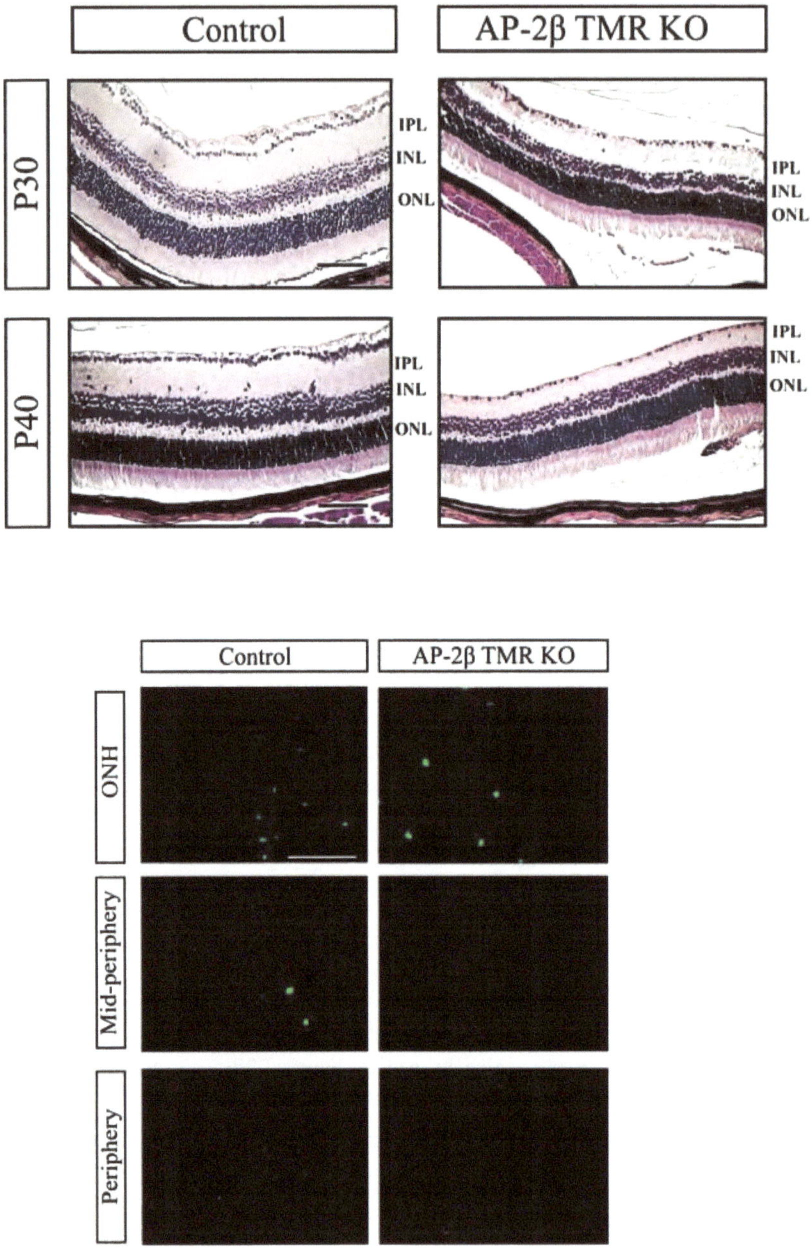

Fig. (5). H&E of retinal thickness, IHC of RGC cell counts. A) The total retinal thickness ($P<0.01$), the IPL ($P<0.05$), and the INL ($P<0.01$) thickness appear to be significantly reduced in our mutant model compared to the control at P30 and P40. Fig. 4B) There is a significant reduction ($P < 0.0001$) in Brn3a cell counts of the mutant mice compared to control mice (Taiyab *et al.*, 2022).

EXPERIMENTAL PROTOCOLS

The following animal procedures were performed in accordance with the Association for Research in Vision and Ophthalmology (ARVO) statement for the use of animals in ophthalmic and vision research. All experiments were performed at McMaster University, with animals housed in the Central Animal Facility in compliance with the guidelines of the Canadian Council on Animal Care for the Use of Experimental.

Lines of Mice and Genetic Crosses to Generate AP-2β TMR-KO Mice

The *Mgp*-Cre.KI mouse line was used to experimentally eliminate the iridocorneal area of the anterior segment using the protocol described below. The resulting mutant mice, termed AP-2β-TMR knock-out mice, exhibited a partial angle closure, significantly elevated IOP, and progressive loss of RGCs.

Cre Mice

- A line of mice was obtained from our collaborator, Dr. Terete Borras (University of N Carolina), in which Cre recombinase was expressed under the control of the promoter for the Matrix Gla Protein (Mgp) gene (Mgp-Cre.KI+/-) (Borras *et al.*, 2015).
- A line of mice heterozygous for a Tfap2b-null allele (Tfap2b+/-) (Moser *et al.*, 1997; Danielian *et al.*, 1998) was obtained from Dr. Trevor Williams (University of Colorado).
- Female Tfap2b+/- mice bred with male Mgp-Cre.KI+/- mice resulted in **Tfap2b+/-;Mgp- Cre.KI+/- mice***. Genotyping was used to identify the required mice from this crossing, as outlined in the genotyping section below.
    - It is important to note that the Cre transgene was passed on by male breeders in all crosses to minimize differences in Cre recombinase activity due to parent-of-origin, as has been reported previously (Heffner *et al.*, 2012).

Floxed Mice

- AP-2β floxed mice were generated by flanking exon 4 of the Tfap2b gene by loxP sites **(Tfap2b lox/lox)**(Martino *et al.*, 2016; Van Otterloo *et al.*, 2022). The mice were provided by Dr. Trevor Williams (University of Colorado).

Final Cross

- Male **Tfap2b+/-;Mgp- Cre.KI+/-** mice were crossed with female **Tfap2b lox/lox** mice to produce the final mutants, **Tfap2b-/lox; Mgp-Cre.KI+/- (AP-2β TMR KO**). Their genome contained one active copy of Tfap2b in all cells, except for Mgp-expressing cells, in which exon 4 of the second copy was excised by Cre recombinase to render a conditional deletion of AP-2β. Genotyping was used to identify the required mice from this cross, as outlined in the genotyping section below.

Control Littermate Mice

- Control littermates were identified that still contained at least one functional copy of Tfap2b on the Mgp-Cre background -**Tfap2b+/lox; Mgp-Cre.KI+/-.**

Additional Considerations

A number of mouse lines need to be maintained for the final cross to obtain the mutants. These include: BetaFlox (Tfap2blox/lox), Mgp.Cre.Ki (MgpCre.KI+/−; Tfap2b+/−), Mgp.Cre.KiβKO

(MgpCre.KI+/−; Tfap2b−/lox) x BFlpTomato (Tfap2blox/lox; tdTomatolox/lox), Tomato (tdTomatolox/lox), UbeCreβKO (UbCreERT2+/-; Tfap2b-/lox; tdTomatolox/+), Wnt1 (Wnt1Cre+/-; Tfap2b+/-), Wnt1 x βKO (Wnt1Cre+/-; Tfap2b-/lox), BFlp homoxTomatohomo (Tfap2b-/-; tdTomato), BFlpxTomato homo (Tfap2b+/-; tdTomato), and βKO (Tfap2b-/lox).

- For the final genetic crossings, inbreeding was avoided, and the background strain used for all genetic crosses was wild-type C57BL/6J (Charles River, Wilmington, MA).
- For the experiments, equal numbers of male and female mice generated from the final crossing were used.
- The mice were kept in environmentally enriched cages (up to 5/cage) under a 12/12hrs light/dark cycle at 25°C.

The breeding scheme deployed to create the AP-2β-TMR-KO mutant mice is depicted in Fig. (**1**).

Genotyping Mice

Genotyping for Tfap2b null, Tfap2b flox, and Mgp-Cre alleles was performed by PCR using DNA extracted from ear clippings using the EZNA Tissue DNA Kit (Omega Bio-Tek) with relevant primer sequences shown in Table **1**. Standard PCR protocols were followed (Martino *et al.*, 2016)

Table 1. PCR Primers for genotyping of AP-2β TMR-KO mice.

Alleles	Primers	PCR Conditions	Products
MgpCre	**Cre1** 5'-GCT GGT TAG CAG CGC AGG TGT AGA G-3' **Cre3** 5'-CGC CAT CTT CCA GCA GGC GCA CC-3'	33 cycles of: 45 seconds at 95 °C 1 minute at 67 °C 1 minute 10 sec at 72 °C	Cre transgene present at 420 bp
Tfap2b	**4 Exon DW** 5'-CCT CCC AAA TCT GTG ACT TCT-3' **PGK-PolyA** 5'-CTG CTC TTT ACT GAA GGC TCT TT-3' **4 Exon Rev** 5'-TTC TGA GGA CGC CCA GG-3'	37 cycles of: 45 sec at 95 °C 45 sec at 58 °C 1 min at 72 °C	Tfap2b– at 380 bp Tfap2b+ at 221 bp

Briefly, genes were amplified (Applied Biosystem 2720 Thermal Cycler) by:

- Heating the reaction mix to 95° C for 2 min for initial denaturation.
- Followed by 39 cycles of:
  - 95° C for 45sec for denaturation
  - 62° C for 45sec for annealing
  - 72° C for 60sec for extension
- Followed by 72° C for 10min for the final extension.
- Gel electrophoresis on a 2% agarose gel in Tris-base, acetic acid, and ethylenediaminetetraacetic acid (TAE) buffer containing fluorodye (fluorescent loading dye, green, from SMOBIO; run with 120V for 30min) was utilized to determine the PCR products. Imaging of the resultant gels was performed on a G:box Chemi-XRQ system (from VWR) using the GeneSys software (from VWR).

Histological Observation of AP-2β TMR-KO Mice

To observe the morphology of our mutant mice eyes, hematoxylin and eosin (H&E) staining was performed, which revealed a partially open angle phenotype. This information was further confirmed through optical coherence tomography (OCT). The procedure is as follows:

- Mice were anesthetized using 2.5% avertin, and eyedrops were applied to prevent corneal desiccation (Alcon, Mississauga, CA)

- To perform live imaging, the mouse cornea was placed 1-2 cm from an anterior chamber/segment imaging system using an OCT attachment (Phoenix Research Labs, Pleasanton, CA).

Histological Validation of AP-2β TMR-KO Mice

Immunohistochemistry was used to evaluate the successful deletion of AP-2β in the TM of the AP-2β-TMR-KO mice using specific antibodies for AP-2β and αSMA, the latter being a TM marker. The procedure used was as follows:

- Mice were euthanized with CO_2; their eyeballs were removed and fixed in 4% PFA for 2 h. These were then washed in PBS buffer and incubated in 70% ethanol overnight.
- After embedding in paraffin wax, 4 μm sections were cut and collected on microscope slides.
- The sections were then deparaffinized in xylene and rehydrated in decreasing ethanol concentrations (100%, 95%, and 70% ethanol) before a final wash in water.
- To block non-specific staining, the sections were incubated for 60-min with normal serum (5% in 1xPBS) from the host-animal of the secondary antibody.
- Sections were subsequently incubated overnight at 4^0C with the primary antibodies (AP-2β; at 1:50 dilution; Cell Signaling, Danvers, MA); αSMA, at 1:100 dilution; Sigma Aldrich, Oakville, ON).
- Alexa Fluor secondary antibodies (at1:200 dilution; Invitrogen, Molecular Probes, Burlington, ON) were utilized to detect the primary antibodies, and the slides were mounted with ProLong Gold containing DAPI (4′,6-diamidino-2-phenylindole) (from ThermoFisher, Waltham, MA).
- The stained section images were then acquired on a microscope equipped with bright-field or fluorescence capability, and photos of the sections were captured with a high-resolution camera and LasX imaging software.

Latanoprost Treatment on Control and Mutant Mice

Latanoprost is a prostaglandin analog that works to reduce IOP by increasing outflow through the uveoscleral pathway (Johnson *et al.*, 2010). We have previously established that the conventional pathway is inaccessible in our model due to the absence of key drainage structures (Taiyab *et al.*, 2022). To assess the functionality of the unconventional/uveoscleral pathway in our mutant model, latanoprost treatment was performed. The procedure is as follows:

- The eyes of mutant and control mice were anesthetized and topically treated with 10μL of 0.005% LTP ((Pfizer, New York, NY). The IOPs at baseline and at various intervals post-instillation of LTP (20 min, 60 min, and 24hrs) were recorded as previously described (Taiyab *et al.*, 2022).

IOP Measurements of c-KO Mice

Tonometry was the method used to determine IOP in the mice. Most tonometers (like the Tonolab) are calibrated to measure pressure in millimeters of mercury (mmHg).

- Adult AP-2β TMR-KO and control littermates were anesthetized with an intraperitoneal injection of 0.06mL of (75mg) Ketamine and (5 mg) Xylazine mixture per 10 grams of body weight.
- Eye drops (Alcon, Mississauga, ON, Canada) were applied to prevent corneal desiccation.
- Whiskers were trimmed to prevent interference with the probe, and a rebound tonometer (TonoLab, Vantaa, Finland) was used to obtain a minimum of 6 baseline IOP values. IOP values were then averaged (Martino *et al.*, 2016).
- Place the anesthetized animal on an adjustable platform provided by the Tonolab kit and clamp the tonometer to a retort stand to keep it steady; lubricate the animal's cornea.
- Ensure that the area around the tonometer is not wet, turn on the tonometer, and insert a fresh probe (also provided in the kit).
- Place the tonometer with the retort stand about 2-3 mm from the animal's cornea at a slight angle (Chatterjee *et al.*, 2013). Please take caution not to open the tonometer's case, but the battery compartment can be opened for replacing batteries.
- Acquire consecutive measurements by pressing the "measure" button and record the average value that will be provided by the tonometer. Get as many readings as necessary.
- Potential statistically significant differences in IOPs in control and AP-2β-T-R-KO mice following LTP instillation can then be determined using appropriate software programs. Differences in corrected total fluorescence between AP-2β TMR-KO and control mice of all treatment conditions should be analyzed using a 2-way ANOVA analysis.

Assessment of other Glaucomatous Features in the Mutant Mouse Model: Retinal Thickness

Previous studies found that elevated IOP was correlated with reduced thickness of the retina (Tu *et al.*, 2019). To assess IOP correlation with retinal thickness, we looked at the retinal thickness of the three different layers of the retina. The procedure was as follows:

- Retinal thickness was assessed via H&E stain of eye sections of our mutant and control mice.
- Analysis of retinal thickness was performed via a two-sided independent t-test.

Assessment of other Glaucomatous Features in Mutant Mouse Model: RGC Cell Count

There is a well-established idea that increased IOP causes changes at the optic nerve head, and this ultimately leads to retinal ganglion cell death (Guo *et al.*, 2005). To assess for IOP correlation with retinal ganglion cell death in our mouse model, we performed IHC on paraffin sections and flat-mounted retinas of mutant and control mice. The procedure was as follows:

- IHC staining of Brn3a on P60 paraffin tissue sections was similar to the IHC protocol listed above.
- For IHC of retinal wholemounts, the eyes were first fixed using 4% PFA overnight and then washed with 1xPBS 3 times over 10 minutes.
- The retinae were then dissected out and permeabilized in 0.3% Triton X mixed in PBS (PBST) overnight, then blocked with a mixture of serum (5%)-containing PBST for 3hr at 24 ºC. They were gently agitated side-to-side in a mixture of Brn3a antibody (Santa Cruz, CA) (1:100 dilution) along with normal serum (5%) and 1% DMSO in PBST at 4 ºC for 72hrs.
- The retinae were then rinsed in PBST and agitated in a mixture of secondary antibody (1:200 dilution), 1% DMSO, and serum (2.5%) in PBST 24ºC for 4hr. Lastly, the retinae were washed with 1xPBS, flat-mounted with DAPI, and coverslipped for microscopic examination.
- Cell counts were performed using the Image J software and analyzed. Statistical analyses were performed using an independent two-sided t-test.

Assessment of other Glaucomatous Features in a Mutant Mouse Model: ERG

To confirm that the changes in retinal thickness, along with an increase in retinal cell death in our mutant model, affected their overall retinal function, we performed an electroretinogram (ERG). The procedure was as follows:

- Retinal function was assessed via full-field ERG.
- The pupils of anesthetized mice were dilated using topically instilled 0.5% tropicamide.
- Eye drops were applied to prevent corneal drying.
- Electrodes were placed in the tail, scalp, and eye, and the retinal response to flashes of light at specific intensities was recorded.
- Analysis of results was performed via Tukey's post hoc test.

CONCLUSION

Based on the information presented above, it can be concluded that the AP-2--TMR KO mouse model is an attractive transgenic OHT/glaucoma model that exhibits a partially open angle phenotype and increases IOP in a relatively acute manner compared to other animal models. Additionally, the glaucomatous features are consistent, and there is a 100% penetrance across all cohorts. We have also confirmed that the unconventional outflow pathway is accessible and active in this model through our experiments with latanoprost treatment, which promotes AQH egress between ciliary muscle bundles. This model resembles the human condition of PACG in the sense that these mice develop a similar PAS phenotype, increased IOP, and retinal damage that corresponds to a reduction in RGCs, which is also observed in humans (Wright *et al.*, 2016). Thus, these characteristics suggest that our model is useful for understanding and treating progressive human PACG. This model can also be exploited in developing treatment strategies that are more convenient and less invasive than current treatment regiments for PACG.

The experimental methodology described herein was outlined in detail and deemed sufficient to successfully create and characterize the AP-2β TMR KO mice. It is, however, recommended that the readers refer to original publications where necessary and explore recent publications for additional refinements to the procedure, as mouse genetic experimentation is continuously evolving.

ACKNOWLEDGEMENTS

The authors would like to acknowledge the funding support for this research from the National Institutes of Health, Grant/Award Number: R01 EY025789.

REFERENCES

Barzago, MM, Kurosaki, M, Fratelli, M, Bolis, M, Giudice, C, Nordio, L, Cerri, E, Domenici, L, Terao, M & Garattini, E (2017) Generation of a new mouse model of glaucoma characterized by reduced expression of the AP-2β and AP-2δ proteins. *Sci Rep,* 7, 11140.
[http://dx.doi.org/10.1038/s41598-017-11752-6] [PMID: 28894266]

Bassett, EA, Korol, A, Deschamps, PA, Buettner, R, Wallace, VA, Williams, T & West-Mays, JA (2012) Overlapping expression patterns and redundant roles for AP-2 transcription factors in the developing mammalian retina. *Dev Dyn,* 241, 814-29.
[http://dx.doi.org/10.1002/dvdy.23762] [PMID: 22411557]

Bassett, EA, Pontoriero, GF, Feng, W, Marquardt, T, Fini, ME, Williams, T & West-Mays, JA (2007) Conditional deletion of activating protein 2alpha (AP-2alpha) in the developing retina demonstrates non-cel--autonomous roles for AP-2alpha in optic cup development. *Mol Cell Biol,* 27, 7497-510.
[http://dx.doi.org/10.1128/MCB.00687-07] [PMID: 17724084]

Bassett, EA, Williams, T, Zacharias, AL, Gage, PJ, Fuhrmann, S & West-Mays, JA (2010) AP-2α knockout mice exhibit optic cup patterning defects and failure of optic stalk morphogenesis. *Hum Mol Genet,* 19, 1791-804.

[http://dx.doi.org/10.1093/hmg/ddq060] [PMID: 20150232]

Borrás, T, Smith, MH & Buie, LK (2015) A Novel *Mgp* -Cre Knock-In Mouse Reveals an Anticalcification/Antistiffness Candidate Gene in the Trabecular Meshwork and Peripapillary Scleral Region. *Invest Ophthalmol Vis Sci,* 56, 2203-14.
[http://dx.doi.org/10.1167/iovs.15-16460] [PMID: 25711639]

Chen, L & Gage, PJ (2016) Heterozygous *Pitx2* Null Mice Accurately Recapitulate the Ocular Features of Axenfeld-Rieger Syndrome and Congenital Glaucoma. *Invest Ophthalmol Vis Sci,* 57, 5023-30.
[http://dx.doi.org/10.1167/iovs.16-19700] [PMID: 27654429]

Cross, S H, Macalinao, D G, McKie, L, Rose, L, Kearney, A L, Rainger, J, Thaung, C, Keighren, M, Jadeja, S, West, K, Kneeland, S C, Smith, R S, Howell, G R, Young, F & Robertson, M (2014) A dominant-negative mutation of mouse Lmx1b causes glaucoma and is semi-lethal via LDB1-mediated dimerization. *PLoS Genet,* 10, e1004359.
[http://dx.doi.org/10.1371/journal.pgen.1004359] [PMID: 24809698]

Danielian, PS, Muccino, D, Rowitch, DH, Michael, SK & McMahon, AP (1998) Modification of gene activity in mouse embryos in utero by a tamoxifen-inducible form of Cre recombinase. *Curr Biol,* 8, 1323-S2.
[http://dx.doi.org/10.1016/S0960-9822(07)00562-3] [PMID: 9843687]

Dietze, J, Blair, K & Havens, SJ Glaucoma. *StatPearls.*StatPearls Publishing.Available from: http://www.ncbi.nlm.nih.gov/books/NBK538217/ (2022)

Guo, L, Moss, SE, Alexander, RA, Ali, RR, Fitzke, FW & Cordeiro, MF (2005) Retinal ganglion cell apoptosis in glaucoma is related to intraocular pressure and IOP-induced effects on extracellular matrix. *Invest Ophthalmol Vis Sci,* 46, 175-82.
[http://dx.doi.org/10.1167/iovs.04-0832] [PMID: 15623771]

Johnson, TV & Tomarev, SI (2010) Rodent models of glaucoma. *Brain Res Bull,* 81, 349-58.
[http://dx.doi.org/10.1016/j.brainresbull.2009.04.004] [PMID: 19379796]

Johnson TV, Fan S, Zhan G, Camras CB, Toris CB. Efficacy and mechanisms of intraocular pressure reduction with latanoprost and timolol in participants with ocular hypertension: a comparison of 1 and 6 weeks of treatment. J Glaucoma. 2010 Aug;19(6):356-64.

Kerr, CL, Zaveri, MA, Robinson, ML, Williams, T & West-Mays, JA (2014) AP-2α is required after lens vesicle formation to maintain lens integrity. *Dev Dyn,* 243, 1298-309.
[http://dx.doi.org/10.1002/dvdy.24141] [PMID: 24753151]

Lee, JY, Kim, YY & Jung, HR (2006) Distribution and characteristics of peripheral anterior synechiae in primary angle-closure glaucoma. *Korean J Ophthalmol,* 20, 104-8.
[http://dx.doi.org/10.3341/kjo.2006.20.2.104] [PMID: 16892646]

Liu, P & Johnson, RL (2010) Lmx1b is required for murine trabecular meshwork formation and for maintenance of corneal transparency. *Dev Dyn,* 239, 2161-71.
[http://dx.doi.org/10.1002/dvdy.22347] [PMID: 20568247]

Mao, M, Hedberg-Buenz, A, Koehn, D, John, SWM & Anderson, MG (2011) Anterior segment dysgenesis and early-onset glaucoma in nee mice with mutation of Sh3pxd2b. *Invest Ophthalmol Vis Sci,* 52, 2679-88.
[http://dx.doi.org/10.1167/iovs.10-5993] [PMID: 21282566]

Martino, VB, Sabljic, T, Deschamps, P, Green, RM, Akula, M, Peacock, E, Ball, A, Williams, T & West-Mays, JA (2016) Conditional deletion of AP-2β in the cranial neural crest results in anterior segment dysgenesis and early-onset glaucoma. *Dis Model Mech,* 9, dmm.025262.
[http://dx.doi.org/10.1242/dmm.025262] [PMID: 27483349]

Moser, M, Pscherer, A, Roth, C, Becker, J, Mücher, G, Zerres, K, Dixkens, C, Weis, J, Guay-Woodford, L, Buettner, R & Fässler, R (1997) Enhanced apoptotic cell death of renal epithelial cells in mice lacking transcription factor AP-2β. *Genes Dev,* 11, 1938-48.
[http://dx.doi.org/10.1101/gad.11.15.1938] [PMID: 9271117]

Pontoriero, GF, Deschamps, P, Ashery-Padan, R, Wong, R, Yang, Y, Zavadil, J, Cvekl, A, Sullivan, S,

Williams, T & West-Mays, JA (2008) Cell autonomous roles for AP-2α in lens vesicle separation and maintenance of the lens epithelial cell phenotype. *Dev Dyn,* 237, 602-17.
[http://dx.doi.org/10.1002/dvdy.21445] [PMID: 18224708]

Quigley, HA & Broman, AT (2006) The number of people with glaucoma worldwide in 2010 and 2020. *Br J Ophthalmol,* 90, 262-7.
[http://dx.doi.org/10.1136/bjo.2005.081224] [PMID: 16488940]

Romero, P, Sanhueza, F, Lopez, P, Reyes, L & Herrera, L (2011) c.194 A>C (Q65P) mutation in the LMX1B gene in patients with nail-patella syndrome associated with glaucoma. *Mol Vis,* 17, 1929-39.
[PMID: 21850167]

Smith, RS, Zabaleta, A, Kume, T, Savinova, OV, Kidson, SH, Martin, JE, Nishimura, DY, Alward, WL, Hogan, BL & John, SW (2000) Haploinsufficiency of the transcription factors FOXC1 and FOXC2 results in aberrant ocular development. *Hum Mol Genet,* 9, 1021-32.
[http://dx.doi.org/10.1093/hmg/9.7.1021] [PMID: 10767326]

Taiyab, A, Akula, M, Dham, J, Deschamps, P, Sheardown, H, Williams, T, Borrás, T & West-Mays, JA (2021) Deletion of transcription factor AP-2β from the developing murine trabecular meshwork region leads to progressive glaucomatous changes. *J Neurosci Res*
[http://dx.doi.org/10.1002/jnr.24982] [PMID: 34822722]

Taiyab, A, Akula, M, Dham, J, Deschamps, P, Sheardown, H, Williams, T, Borrás, T & West-Mays, JA (2022) Deletion of transcription factor AP-2β from the developing murine trabecular meshwork region leads to progressive glaucomatous changes. *J Neurosci Res,* 100, 638-52.
[http://dx.doi.org/10.1002/jnr.24982] [PMID: 34822722]

Tu, S, Li, K, Ding, X, Hu, D, Li, K & Ge, J (2019) Relationship between intraocular pressure and retinal nerve fibre thickness loss in a monkey model of chronic ocular hypertension. *Eye (Lond),* 33, 1833-41.
[http://dx.doi.org/10.1038/s41433-019-0484-1] [PMID: 31227788]

Tümer, Z & Bach-Holm, D (2009) Axenfeld–Rieger syndrome and spectrum of PITX2 and FOXC1 mutations. *Eur J Hum Genet,* 17, 1527-39.
[http://dx.doi.org/10.1038/ejhg.2009.93] [PMID: 19513095]

Uveoscleral Pathway—An overview | ScienceDirect Topics. (n.d.). Retrieved February 12, 2023, Available from: https://www.sciencedirect.com/topics/neuroscience/uveoscleral-pathway

Van Otterloo, E, Milanda, I, Pike, H, Thompson, JA, Li, H, Jones, KL & Williams, T (2022) AP-2α and AP-2β cooperatively function in the craniofacial surface ectoderm to regulate chromatin and gene expression dynamics during facial development. *eLife,* 11, e70511.
[http://dx.doi.org/10.7554/eLife.70511] [PMID: 35333176]

West-Mays, JA, Zhang, J, Nottoli, T, Hagopian-Donaldson, S, Libby, D, Strissel, KJ & Williams, T (1999) AP-2alpha transcription factor is required for early morphogenesis of the lens vesicle. *Dev Biol,* 206, 46-62.
[http://dx.doi.org/10.1006/dbio.1998.9132] [PMID: 9918694]

Wright, C, Tawfik, MA, Waisbourd, M & Katz, LJ (2016) Primary angle-closure glaucoma: an update. *Acta Ophthalmol,* 94, 217-25.
[http://dx.doi.org/10.1111/aos.12784] [PMID: 26119516]

DRUG FORMULATION, PHARMACOKINETICS, AND TOXICOLOGY STUDIES FOR COMPOUNDS

CHAPTER 40

Protocols to Study the Drug Formulation and Stability Aspects of Anti-Ocular Hypertension and Anti-Glaucoma Drugs

Onkar N. Singh[1,*]

[1] *CMC/Manufacturing/Technical Operations, Alentia Therapeutics Inc., Fort Worth, 2648 Gosling Way, Fort Worth, TX-76118, USA*

Abstract: In order to dissolve and make dilutions of test compounds for topical ocular delivery, a suitable formulation needs to be created that will deliver the molecule without causing ocular discomfort. Additionally, it is important to ensure that the formulation will not cause inflammation or induce serious ocular or systemic side effects. The physiochemical properties of the compound dictate the choice of the formulation that, in turn, will endeavor to control the pH, stability (solution, thermal, photo), and the overall characteristics of the drug in solution or suspension. Furthermore, the route of delivery of the test agent will also influence the choice of the formulation. Excipients may be added to enhance the ocular retention time and thus enhance the penetration of the drug across the cornea/conjunctiva in order to allow the active moiety to reach the aqueous humor in the anterior chamber of the eye.

Keywords: Drug delivery systems, Eye drops, Eye anatomy and physiology, Formulations, Glaucoma research, Inserts, ICH, Nanosuspension, Ocular barrier, Solution, Suspension, Stability, Topical delivery.

INTRODUCTION

This section describes a protocol to study the drug formulation and stability aspects of glaucoma research on the human eye. First of all, in order to develop an effective formulation for glaucoma research, it is important to understand the anatomy and physiology of the eye. The anterior segment of the eye includes the aqueous humor (AQH), cornea, iris, pupil, ciliary body, conjunctiva, and lens. However, the posterior segment contains the sclera, choroid, and retina, with the vitreous cavity containing the vitreous humor.

* **Corresponding author Onkar N. Sing:** CMC/Manufacturing/Technical Operations, Alentia Therapeutics Inc., Fort Worth, 2648 Gosling Way, Fort Worth, TX-76118, USA; Tel: +(817) 899-6031; E-mail: Onsingh2@yahoo.com

Najam A. Sharif and Sunny E. Ohia (Eds.)

Most anti-glaucoma drug formulations are developed as solution or suspension eye drops to instill on the anterior segment of the eye, the cornea. Anatomical (*e.g.*, conjunctiva, cornea) and physiological (*e.g.*, choroidal blood flow, efflux transporters) barriers limit the bioavailability and, thus, the efficacy of these conventional drug forms (Agrahari *et al.*, 2017; Barar *et al.*, 2016; Gaudana *et al.*, 2010; Janagam *et al.*, 2017). The most potent glaucoma drugs are BCS class 2 drugs (possess low aqueous solubility and high permeability) or BCS class IV drugs (possess low aqueous solubility and low permeability). The latter features of the drugs limit the efficacy of the topical ocularly delivered compounds. Also, an ideal ocular formulation should be easily self-administered to the eye, not cause ocular irritation, and garner patient acceptance/compliance. For this reason, eye drop solutions or suspensions are provided in easy-to-squeeze low-density polyethylene (LDPE) bottles with LDPE round or oval tips and polypropylene (PP) plastic caps, which are easy to remove for self-administration.

The bioavailability of topical formulations of drugs is adversely affected by many factors, such as solution drainage, blinking, tear turnover, and corneal/conjunctival tissue barriers. Consequently, perhaps only 1-7% of topical ocularly instilled drugs enter the AQH (Janagam *et al.*, 2017; Ghate and Edelhauser, 2006). Moreover, tear drainage facilitates the removal of the drug from the eye. Consequently, ~ 5% of the instilled eye drop drug actually comes in contact with tissues within the anterior chamber of the eye to evoke the desired intraocular pressure lowering (Gaudana *et al.*, 2010; Ali *et al.*, 2016). Hence, new drug dissolution and delivery methods (*e.g.*, liposomes, nanoparticles, nanomicelles, nanosuspensions, dendrimers, implants, microneedles, and *in situ* thermo-sensitive gels) need to be developed beyond the existing suspensions, emulsions, ointments, and aqueous gels to treat ocular diseases impacting the front and the back of the eye (Barar *et al.*, 2016).

To deliver drugs to the posterior eye segment, a variety of routes of administration have been developed, such as suprachoroidal and intravitreal, periocular (subconjunctival, sub-Tenon, and retrobulbar), and topical and systemic (Agrahari *et al.*, 2017, Peptu *et al.*, 2015). Topical ocular delivery is the least invasive and thus is the most used method, but the drawback is minimal delivery to the back of the eye (Barar *et al.*, 2016). Not surprisingly, the most efficient and effective way for drugs to reach the retinal and optic nerve head tissues is when they are intravitreally delivered (Peptu *et al.*, 2015).

Drug Formulations for Anti-Glaucoma Drug Research

There are many factors to consider when generating a good target product profile (TPP) for a drug to be formulated for ophthalmic application. The TPP attributes under such consideration should include as many of the following as possible: patient population, intended target tissue, single or multi-dose medication, duration of therapy, ease of manufacturing and scalability, formulation, route of delivery, sterility, shelf-life, storage, pH, endotoxin levels, addition or omission of preservatives, dosing frequency, safety and efficacy, and package type (*e.g.*, bottle size, fill volume, and types of plug).

Generally, early formulations are either solutions or suspensions of eye drops. For solution formulation, drug concentration, solubility, pH, osmolality, solubility, sterility, preservative efficacy (PET), and stability (physical and chemical) are very important. For suspension formulation, appearance, pH, osmolality, viscosity, resuspension time, and settling are important parameters in addition to sterility, PET, and stability. As mentioned above, eyedrops are the easiest to formulate for topical ocular administration. However, limited efficacy is often the result of low bioavailability for drugs that need to penetrate the cornea/conjunctiva to reach their intended target tissue(s) (Jumelle *et al.*, 2020; Souto *et al.*, 2019). This is where the use of suitable excipients such as polyalcohol, hydroxymethyl cellulose, sodium carboxymethyl cellulose, or a combination of the latter can be used to enhance the ocular surface retention times and thus aid in an overall greater penetration to the anterior chamber (Patel *et al.*, 2013; Achouri *et al.*, 2013). Drug permeation can also be enhanced using certain preservatives (benzalkonium chloride), chelating compounds (*e.g.*, EDTA), and mild detergents/surfactants (*e.g.*, polyethylene glycol; bile salts). However, many studies have shown these agents to cause ocular surface irritation (Achouri *et al.*, 2013).

Drug Substances (Active Pharmaceutical Ingredient)

Appropriate dose strength is critical due to poor bioavailability in ocular tissues, limitations and dosing volume, and ocular residence time. The physicochemical properties that are most common for the drug substance include molecular weight, logP, pKa, pH-solubility profile, solubility in co-solvent systems, solubility at various pH, chemical stability, degradation kinetics, and permeability. Key considerations for suspension formulations include crystallinity, particle size, melting point, hygroscopicity, surface area, polymorphism, density, non-homogeneity, aggregation and settling, and cake formation. Since the un-ionized form of the drug determines bioavailability, the ionization constant of the compound is an important determinant to consider. Hence, to obtain maximal un-ionization of the target compound at a pH close to 7.4, functional group selection present on the compounds is an important factor. Ultimately, such parameters should not impact the desired drug solubility, stability, and *in vitro* and *in vivo* potency. Additionally, knowledge and experience in improving the interfacial characteristics of drug suspension are also important. While water can help with the low interfacial tension particles, those with high interfacial tension require surfactants to enhance the wettability of the particles. Last but not least, the planned medication storage conditions, like ambient humidity and temperature, and the packaging materials also need serious consideration to avoid the loss of active drugs caused by reduced stability and other issues.

It is well known that the particle size of the active product ingredient (API) affects the final product appearance, drug dissolution, overall solubility, stability, potential settling of the compound, and absorption by ocular tissues. Evidence suggests that API particle size <10 μm is ideal for generating comfortable topical ocularly instilled drug suspensions that the patients can easily tolerate (Kaur and Kanwar, 2002; Missel, 2012). As drug particles can exist in polymorphic crystal types, inappropriate storage or manufacturing processes can thus change drug solubility, leading to aggregation and reduced bioavailability when the medication is delivered to the corneal surface. Thus, the development of crystallization and aggregation of the API in the formulation for topical ocular drugs should be explored and prevented. In the case of injectable drug formulations for retinal disease treatments, the preferred particle shape is rod-like, and the preferred size is around 30-100 μm to help retain the medication over a longer period of time (Thackaberry *et al.*, 2017). However, each drug's characteristics need to be considered and optimized for such formulation and for the specific route of administration desired.

Inactive Excipients

The choice of inactive excipients in the drug formulation affects the product's stability, comfort, and *in vivo* efficacy. However, ophthalmic solutions/ suspensions may contain several inactive excipients that are beneficial (Ibrahim, 2019). These include preservatives (*e.g.*, anti-microbials), suspending agents, dispersing agents, wetting agents, buffering agents, and tonicity agents. Thus, based on the physicochemical properties of the inactive excipients, such as surface-active agents, the excipients can add value by acting as stabilizers, preservatives (*e.g.*, antimicrobial agents), solubilizers, wetting agents, and potential drug penetration enhancers (Ibrahim, 2019).

Preservative and Preservative Aid

Commonly used preservatives are benzalkonium chloride (BAC), benzethonium bromide (BAB), and polyquaternium-1 (PQ-1; Polyquad). Commonly used preservative aids are edetate disodium (EDTA) and pentasodium edetate (PDTA). These agents are critical and essential for the inhibition of the growth of microbial contaminants in multi-dose bottles of topical ocularly instilled medications. An ideal preservative should be effective at low concentrations against a wide spectrum of microorganisms, soluble in the formulation at the desired concentration, nontoxic, compatible with formulation and packaging components, and stable over a wide pH range and temperatures. The aforementioned preservatives are cationic in nature, surface active, and ionizable. Hence, their effectiveness is influenced by formulation ionic strength, pH, ionized components, and the potential adsorption of the preservative on the suspended solid particles' surface. Consequently, preservative compatibility with excipients and the drug molecules needs careful evaluation using a wide range of pH conditions, ionic strength variations, surfactants, and possible polymers in order to accelerate the finalization and production of a stable formulation. Also, the use of preservatives needs to be carefully optimized to achieve appropriate effectiveness with minimal ocular surface toxicity. Moreover, since preservatives can bind to the eyedrop plastic due to adsorption, additional precautions to control the formulation pH and temperature in process development and the sequence of component addition and mixing need to be considered to ensure preservative effectiveness. These many facets have been recently reviewed and discussed in different studies, and readers are encouraged to consult these publications (Missel, 2012; Kulshreshtha *et al.*, 2010; Ibrahim, 2019; Jones, 2016).

Formulation Sterility

Whilst sterility of topical ocular drug formulations is of utmost importance, due consideration is also needed regarding the buffering capacity, viscosity, osmolality, and final packaging. Since the sterilization processes can drastically affect the chemical composition, stability, and overall efficacy of the API, the choice of the sterilization procedure is important. Many methods exist for sterilizing ophthalmic drug formulations (*e.g.*, gamma irradiation, ethylene oxide treatment, autoclaving, or dry heat or aseptic filtration), but the type of drug and the composition of the formulation should dictate the final choice since each method offers advantages as well as many disadvantages. Thus, for instance, only thermostable products should be autoclaved or dry heat sterilized. The aseptic filtration method (generally through a 0.22 μm filter) can only be effectively used for completely soluble APIs, which are in clear solution forms and not viscous. Likewise, the ethylene oxide (EO) sterilization process is ideal for thermo-labile APIs, but the process of removing the residual EO from the product is laborious and can be time-consuming and somewhat challenging. Lastly, the gamma irradiation process for sterilization is not used much since it can create harmful degradation byproducts.

Packaging for Ophthalmic Eye Drops formulations

The plastic bottles for packaging ophthalmic products are generally made of low-density polyethylene (LDPE) with LDPE dispensing tips either with or without any colorants or with opacifying agents. Also, middle-density polyethylene (MDPE), high-density polyethylene (HDPE), or polypropylene (PP) are also used to meet specific product requirements.

Key Steps to Formulate Anti-Glaucoma Drug Research Formulations

The following are key steps to follow for developing a solution or suspension formulation for glaucoma research.

- Find pKa, Log P, and Log D of the drug substance.
- Determine the equilibrium aqueous solubility of the drug substance through literature or experiments.
- Determine solubility and stability of the drug substance with respect to various pH, ionic strength, and temperature in the absence or presence of polymeric material if necessary. These parameters may be available in literature if the drug substance is established.
- The first preference is to select excipients that are listed in compendia, such as USP/NF, Pharm. Eur, and JP. If compendia material is not available, then attempts should be made to use GRAS material. GRAS stands for "Generally Recognized As Safe".
- Table **1** below summarizes typical key formulation composition for solution and suspension formulation based on optimal pH, solubility, and physical /chemical stability.

Table 1. Formulation composition of drug solutions and suspensions.

Components	Solution	Suspension	Commonly Used Ingredients
Drug Substance	√	√	API
Tonicity agent	√	√	NaCl, glycerine, PG
Solubilizer /stabilizer	√	√	PEG, PG, Glycerine, polymeric agents (CMC, HPMC), Cyclodextrins
Surface active agent	X	√	Surfactant (Tweens, Tylaxapol)
Viscosity Agent	X	√	Polymeric agents (CMC, HC, NACMC, HPMC)
Preservative	√	√	BAC, Polyquaternium
Preservative AID	√	√	EDTA
Buffering agent	√	√	Phosphate, Citrate, Acetate buffer

(Table 1) cont.....

Components	Solution	Suspension	Commonly Used Ingredients
pH adjusting agent	√	√	HCl, NaOH
Aqueous Solvent to QS to 100% W/W	√	√	Purified Water

(√) = Present; (X)= Absent

- Generally, ophthalmic solution formulations are filtered through a 0.2μ filter inside the sterile laminar hood to ensure sterility if API is temperature sensitive (thermally unstable).
- Sterile suspension formulation is compounded in two parts. Thermally stable portions are mixed in water until solubilized and autoclaved in a glass bottle. Thermally labile portions are solubilized in a sterile container aseptically inside the laminar hood. Both portions are mixed inside the laminar hood.
- Determine microbiological antimicrobial preservative efficacy through PET. The formulation must pass USP for USA jurisdiction (FDA), EPB and EPA for European jurisdiction, and JP for Japanese jurisdiction. In terms of robustness, meeting EPA is the most robust, followed by EPB, USP, and JP. A formulation meeting EPA will meet all EPB, USP, and JP. A formulation meeting EPB will meet USP and JP and fail EPA. A formulation meeting USP will fail EPB and EPA. Therefore, one must try to meet EPA, and if EPA is not achievable, then EPB should be met to develop formulation meeting the global requirement of preservation.
- Ensure that the sterility result is passed in order to confirm sterility.
- Assess the physical and chemical stability of the filled formulation in semipermeable (LDPE or MDPE) DropTainers.
- Submit sample for preclinical animal efficacy testing in rabbits
- Assess preclinical GLP tox in rabbits of the stable formulation.

Stability Storage Conditions and Duration [As per ICH Q1A(R2) Guidance]

Aqueous-based products packaged in semipermeable containers need to be assessed for potential water loss and checked for chemical, biological, physical, and microbiological stability. This assessment should be performed in a low relative humidity (RH) environment. Other methods can also be established for solvent-based products and nonaqueous products (Table **2**).

If significant loss of water from the bottle is detected when protracted studies are conducted at 25°C ± 2°C with 40% RH (± 5% RH) during 6-months' testing at the accelerated storage condition, additional testing at the intermediate storage conditions needs to be performed at 30°C. Even though water loss alone at the accelerated storage conditions does not necessarily require testing at the intermediate storage condition, data needs to be gathered to show that the drug product will not suffer significant water loss during the proposed shelf-life if stored at 25°C with 40% relative humidity. A 5% water loss from baseline is considered a significant change for a drug product packaged in a semi-permeable container after an equivalent of 3 months' storage at 40°C/NMT + 25% relative humidity. However, for small droptainers (1 mL or less) or unit-dose products, a water loss of ≥5% after an equivalent of 3 months' storage at 40°C/NMT 25% RH may be appropriate if justified. Key quality considerations are shown in Table **3**.

Table 2. Storage conditions and stability testing period accepted by health agencies.

Study	Storage Condition	Minimum Time Period Covered By Data At Submission
Long-term *	25°C ± 2°C/40% RH ± 5% RH or 30°C ± 2°C/35% RH ± 5% RH	12 months
Intermediate**	30°C ± 2°C/65% RH ± 5% RH	6 months
Accelerated	40°C ± 2°C/not more than (NMT) 25% RH	6 months

* It is up to the applicant to decide whether long-term stability studies are performed at 25°C ± 2°C/40% relative humidity (RH) ± 5% RH or 30°C ± 2°C/35% RH ± 5% RH.

** If 30°C ± 2°C/35% RH (± 5% RH) is the long-term condition, there is no intermediate condition required.

Table 3. Quality requirement for formulations.

Requirement	Attributes
Identification	Test to identify the presence of the drug in the formulation (HPLC, TLC, or IR)
Assay	Stability indicating specific test (HPLC) for drug content verification
Impurities	Degradation products Assay (HPLC)
pH	Normally, a neutral pH is ideal (7.0 ±4). PH can be changed based on the stability and solubility of the drug substance between 3.5 to 7.8
Osmolality	Normally acceptable range is 260 -340 mOsm/kg. The formulation should be preferred at a target osmolality of 275 to 290 mOsm/Kg (near the iso-osmolar range).
Viscosity	For suspension
Re-suspendability	For suspension
Particulate and foreign matter	Essentially free from particulate matter
Antimicrobial preservative Test (AET) or Preservative Effectiveness test (PET)	Required for multidose and not required for unit dose. Meet Global requirements EPA >EPB>USP>JP
Sterility	Pass (meet USP requirement)

Other Dosage forms Including Novel Drug Delivery Systems

Ointments

Ointments, due to their homogeneous semisolid condition, are sterile topical ocular drug preparations for placement on the cornea/conjunctiva or eyelid to enhance residence time for faster penetration to the AQH (Bao and Burgess, 2018). The other unique benefits of ointments are that their melting points are close to body temperature, they cause minimal ocular irritation upon topical ocular administration, they offer tunable viscosity, and, importantly, they are relatively cheap to manufacture.

Emulsion

Emulsions of drugs are mixtures of two immiscible phases (*e.g.*, oil in water or the reverse), which are well tolerated by patients due to reduced irritancy potential (Souto *et al.*, 2019; Peng *et al.*, 2011). These formulation types for drugs offer the advantage of improving drug absorption by the ocular surface tissues and sustaining the release of the API over an extended period of time.

Nanoparticles

Nanoparticle and microparticle formulations allow the API to be encapsulated, entrapped, adsorbed/absorbed, or attached to permit the API to pass through to the AQH after topical ocular delivery in a more efficient manner (Bucolo *et al.*, 2012).

Nanomicelles

Amphiphilic monomers make up nanomicelles that self-assemble to produce micelles ranging in size from 20-200 nm (Lynch *et al.*, 2019). Here, the amphiphilic polymers form with a hydrophobic core and a hydrophilic outer layer, which encapsulate and transport compounds with low aqueous solubility (Vaishya *et al.*, 2014).

Hydrogels

Crosslinkers in hydrogels permit tunable regulation of swelling, porosity, and mechanical strength. They also change their form in response to the local environment, be it pH, certain chemicals in close proximity, and/or temperature. They offer solution-to-gel transition capability and thus the ability to provide a means for sustained drug delivery onto the ocular surface when dosing topical ocularly (Fathi *et al.*, 2015; Lynch *et al.*, 2020).

Intravitreal implants

Biodegradable or non-biodegradable drug delivery platforms, such as intravitreal implants or antibody formulation complexes, can be used to provide long-term and sustained release of the active drugs to the retina and optic nerve-head tissues (Bourges *et al*., 2006; Cao *et al*., 2019). Such entities are surgically implanted in the vitreous humor, away from the direct line of vision, to continuously deliver the desired amount of API to the surrounding tissues. Recently, specific implants containing FP-receptor agonist drugs, such as bimatoprost and travoprost, have been developed and shown to lower intraocular pressure over several months (Weinreb *et al*., 2023).

CONCLUSION

The formulation of a drug for ocular delivery requires certain key properties to ensure compliance with the morphology and physiology of the ocular tissues. The target is to achieve a comfortable formulation that is close to neutral pH and that causes the least amount of transient stinging or burning upon instillation. The optimization of the formulation requires attention regarding the maintenance of overall stability, and when needing a long duration of action, the use of particular excipients may be necessary. Examples of these and other formulation characteristics have been provided in this chapter.

REFERENCES

Achouri, D, Alhanout, K, Piccerelle, P & Andrieu, V (2013) Recent advances in ocular drug delivery. *Drug Dev Ind Pharm,* 39, 1599-617.
[http://dx.doi.org/10.3109/03639045.2012.736515] [PMID: 23153114]

Agrahari, V & Singh Onkar, N (2022) Ocular formulation and novel drug delivery systems. *Handbook of Basic and Clinical Ocular Pharmacology and Therapeutics* Ohia SE, Sharif NA (Eds), Elsevier , Academic Press, Sub-Chapter 4.1; 155-78.

Agrahari, V, Agrahari, V, Mandal, A, Pal, D & Mitra, AK (2017) How are we improving the delivery to back of the eye? Advances and challenges of novel therapeutic approaches. *Expert Opin Drug Deliv,* 14, 1145-62.
[http://dx.doi.org/10.1080/17425247.2017.1272569] [PMID: 27967247]

Ali, J, Fazil, M, Qumbar, M, Khan, N & Ali, A (2016) Colloidal drug delivery system: amplify the ocular delivery. *Drug Deliv,* 23, 710-26.
[PMID: 24892625]

Bao, Q & Burgess, DJ (2018) Perspectives on physicochemical and *in vitro* profiling of ophthalmic ointments. *Pharm Res,* 35, 234.
[http://dx.doi.org/10.1007/s11095-018-2513-3] [PMID: 30324424]

Barar, J, Aghanejad, A, Fathi, M & Omidi, Y (2016) Advanced drug delivery and targeting technologies for the ocular diseases. *Bioimpacts,* 6, 49-67.
[http://dx.doi.org/10.15171/bi.2016.07] [PMID: 27340624]

Bucolo, C, Drago, F & Salomone, S (2012) Ocular drug delivery: a clue from nanotechnology. *Front Pharmacol,* 3, 188.
[http://dx.doi.org/10.3389/fphar.2012.00188] [PMID: 23125835]

Bourges, JL, Bloquel, C, Thomas, A, Froussart, F, Bochot, A, Azan, F, Gurny, R, BenEzra, D & Behar-Cohen, F (2006) Intraocular implants for extended drug delivery: Therapeutic applications. *Adv Drug Deliv Rev,* 58, 1182-202.
[http://dx.doi.org/10.1016/j.addr.2006.07.026] [PMID: 17107737]

Cao, Y, Samy, KE, Bernards, DA & Desai, TA (2019) Recent advances in intraocular sustained-release drug delivery devices. *Drug Discov Today,* 24, 1694-700.
[http://dx.doi.org/10.1016/j.drudis.2019.05.031] [PMID: 31173915]

Fathi, M, Barar, J, Aghanejad, A & Omidi, Y (2015) Hydrogels for ocular drug delivery and tissue engineering. *Bioimpacts,* 5, 159-64.
[http://dx.doi.org/10.15171/bi.2015.31] [PMID: 26929918]

Gaudana, R, Ananthula, HK, Parenky, A & Mitra, AK (2010) Ocular drug delivery. *AAPS J,* 12, 348-60.
[http://dx.doi.org/10.1208/s12248-010-9183-3] [PMID: 20437123]

Ghate, D & Edelhauser, HF (2006) Ocular drug delivery. *Expert Opin Drug Deliv,* 3, 275-87.
[http://dx.doi.org/10.1517/17425247.3.2.275] [PMID: 16506953]

Ibrahim, SS (2019) The role of surface active agents in ophthalmic drug delivery: a comprehensive review. *J Pharm Sci,* 108, 1923-33.
[http://dx.doi.org/10.1016/j.xphs.2019.01.016] [PMID: 30684539]

Janagam, DR, Wu, L & Lowe, TL (2017) Nanoparticles for drug delivery to the anterior segment of the eye. *Adv Drug Deliv Rev,* 122, 31-64.
[http://dx.doi.org/10.1016/j.addr.2017.04.001] [PMID: 28392306]

Jumelle, C, Gholizadeh, S, Annabi, N & Dana, R (2020) Advances and limitations of drug delivery systems formulated as eye drops. *J Control Release,* 321, 1-22.
[http://dx.doi.org/10.1016/j.jconrel.2020.01.057] [PMID: 32027938]

Pal Kaur, I & Kanwar, M (2002) Ocular preparations: the formulation approach. *Drug Dev Ind Pharm,* 28, 473-93.
[http://dx.doi.org/10.1081/DDC-120003445] [PMID: 12098838]

Kulshreshtha, A.K., Singh, O.N., Wall, G.M., (2010). Pharmaceutical Suspensions, From Formulation Development to Manufacturing. Springer publication

Lynch, C, Kondiah, PPD, Choonara, YE, du Toit, LC, Ally, N & Pillay, V (2019) Advances in biodegradable nano-sized polymer-based ocular drug delivery. *Polymers (Basel),* 11, 1371.
[http://dx.doi.org/10.3390/polym11081371] [PMID: 31434273]

Lynch, CR, Kondiah, PPD, Choonara, YE, du Toit, LC, Ally, N & Pillay, V (2020) Hydrogel biomaterials for application in ocular drug delivery. *Front Bioeng Biotechnol,* 8, 228.
[http://dx.doi.org/10.3389/fbioe.2020.00228] [PMID: 32266248]

Missel, MCJCLAP (2012) *Remington: Essentials of Pharmaceutics.*Pharmaceutical Press.

Moiseev, RV, Morrison, PWJ, Steele, F & Khutoryanskiy, VV (2019) Penetration enhancers in ocular drug delivery. *Pharmaceutics,* 11, 321.
[http://dx.doi.org/10.3390/pharmaceutics11070321] [PMID: 31324063]

Patel, A, Cholkar, K, Agrahari, V & Mitra, AK (2013) Ocular drug delivery systems: An overview. *World J Pharmacol,* 2, 47-64.
[http://dx.doi.org/10.5497/wjp.v2.i2.47] [PMID: 25590022]

Peng, CC, Bengani, LC, Jung, HJ, Leclerc, J, Gupta, C & Chauhan, A (2011) Emulsions and microemulsions for ocular drug delivery. *J Drug Deliv Sci Technol,* 21, 111-21.
[http://dx.doi.org/10.1016/S1773-2247(11)50010-3]

Peptu, C, Popa, M, Savin, C, Popa, R & Ochiuz, L (2015) Modern drug delivery systems for targeting the posterior segment of the eye. *Curr Pharm Des,* 21, 6055-69.

[http://dx.doi.org/10.2174/1381612821666151027151847] [PMID: 26503152]

Souto, EB, Dias-Ferreira, J, López-Machado, A, Ettcheto, M, Cano, A, Camins Espuny, A, Espina, M, Garcia, ML & Sánchez-López, E (2019) Advanced formulation approaches for ocular drug delivery: state-o--the-art and recent patents. *Pharmaceutics,* 11, 460.
[http://dx.doi.org/10.3390/pharmaceutics11090460] [PMID: 31500106]

Thackaberry, EA, Farman, C, Zhong, F, Lorget, F, Staflin, K, Cercillieux, A, Miller, PE, Schuetz, C, Chang, D, Famili, A, Daugherty, AL, Rajagopal, K & Bantseev, V (2017) Evaluation of the toxicity of intravitreally injected PLGA microspheres and rods in monkeys and rabbits: effects of depot size on inflammatory response. *Invest Ophthalmol Vis Sci,* 58, 4274-85.
[http://dx.doi.org/10.1167/iovs.16-21334] [PMID: 28850638]

Weinreb, RN, Bacharach, J, Brubaker, JW, Medeiros, FA, Bejanian, M, Bernstein, P & Robinson, MR (2023) Bimatoprost Implant Biodegradation in the Phase 3, Randomized, 20-Month ARTEMIS Studies. *J Ocul Pharmacol Ther,* 39, 55-62.
[http://dx.doi.org/10.1089/jop.2022.0137] [PMID: 36378864]

CHAPTER 41

Protocol for an Ocular Pharmacokinetic Study in Rabbits for an Ocular Anti-hypertensive Drug

James E. Chastain[1,*]

[1] *Novartis Institutes for BioMedical Research (Retired), The Woodlands, 26 Dawning Flower Dr., The Woodlands, TX 77375, USA*

Abstract: Ocular pharmacokinetics (PK) is an essential component of drug research and development, leading to the understanding of drug or drug candidate absorption, distribution, and elimination firstly in tissues targeted for efficacy and secondly in tissues/fluids that may be relevant to off-target effects (*e.g.*, toxicity). Rabbits are one species of choice for ocular PK due to greater eye size relative to rodents and lower expense relative to dogs or monkeys, as well as the wealth of published ocular PK data (and use in regulatory submissions). This chapter describes a generic protocol for assessing ocular PK for glaucoma and anterior eye segment research. The collection procedure is detailed but will vary depending on the objective of the PK study or the lab performing the study. As such, this is one, albeit relatively common, approach one can consider for studying ocular PK in rabbits.

Keywords: Drug distribution, Eye, Glaucoma, Ocular tissue, Ocular, Pharmacodynamics, PK/PD, Pharmacokinetics, Rabbit.

INTRODUCTION

Pharmacokinetic (PK) and pharmacokinetic/pharmacodynamic (PK/PD) studies have become essential for confirming drug exposure in target tissues and the relationship between drug exposure and efficacy. These assist the translational process of defining an efficacious dose in humans based on animal data. In the case of glaucoma research, ocular PK can be a stand-alone study or as part of a PK/PD study in an appropriate animal model. For compounds targeting the anterior eye segment (*e.g.*, control of intraocular pressure), one target tissue likely includes an iris-ciliary body (ICB or specifically the ciliary body). ICB is therefore collected and analyzed, along with the cornea, which is assessed for drug exposure at this ocular barrier, and aqueous humor from the anterior chamber, essentially representing a central compartment within the eye. Drug

* **Corresponding author James E. Chastain:** Novartis Institutes for BioMedical Research (Retired), The Woodlands, 26 Dawning Flower Dr., The Woodlands, TX 77375, USA; Tel: +1 817-680-2066;
E-mail: james.chastain3@gmail.com

Najam A. Sharif and Sunny E. Ohia (Eds.)

levels in the lens may be useful to assess accumulation within the lens for potential toxicity effects. Assessment of drug distribution to the posterior segment (behind the lens) can be useful to understand potential exposure to the retina (which can, at times, be collected as well). For reference, rabbit ocular anatomy is illustrated in Fig. (**1**). Various reviews of ocular PK and drug delivery, including application to glaucoma research and beyond, are available (Agrahari *et al.*, 2016; Gaudana R *et al.*, 2010; Urtti, 2006).

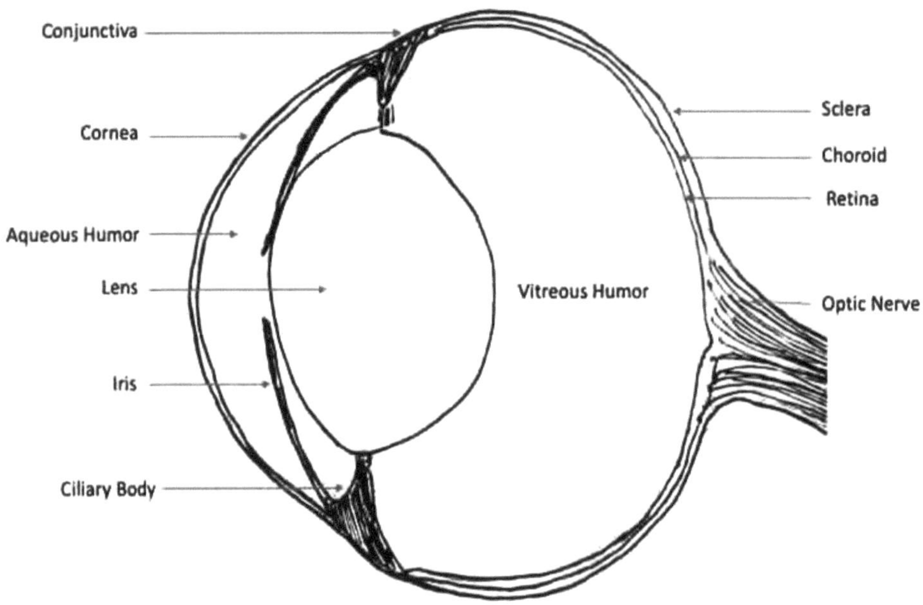

Fig. (1). Rabbit ocular anatomy.

The following describes a generic protocol for assessing ocular PK for glaucoma and anterior segment research. The collection procedure is detailed but can vary depending on the ultimate goal of the PK study or the particular requirement of the lab performing the study. Examples of ocular PK studies are those by Fayyaz *et al.* (2021), assessing the ocular PK of a beta-blocker cocktail, Shen *et al.* (2017), studying the ocular PK of topical bimatoprost, and Savinainen *et al.* (2019), studying the PK and intraocular pressure lowering activity of a drug candidate (PK/PD based on aqueous humor levels).

EXPERIMENTAL PROTOCOLS

The following procedures are performed for PK at predetermined time points following drug administration within a stand-alone ocular PK study or as part of a PK/PD study.

Materials

Isotonic saline (0.9%), gauze, 1cc tuberculin syringes with and without affixed needle (*e.g.*, 27G), weigh boat/paper, dissecting microscope (as needed), and pre-weighed (or tared) cryogenic polypropylene sample tubes with screw-caps (*e.g.*, 1.5mL and 15mL) are used. In addition, a weighing balance with at least 5-place precision with the goal of providing at least three significant figures for tissue weights is used. If blood is collected, a centrifuge for the separation of plasma fraction is needed.

Instruments

Tissue forceps with teeth, slightly curved microdissection forceps with teeth, slightly curved serrated microdissection forceps, curved corneal scissors (blunt tips), curved iris scissors (sharp tips), curved blunt scissors (enucleation scissors), eye scissors (straight or slightly curved with pointed tips), disposable scalpel with blade and Gill knife. These may be substituted as needed with similar instruments as required.

Animals and Treatment

Rabbits are commonly used due to the larger size of their eyes compared to rats and substantial published literature on ocular PK available for rabbits. This is despite differences between rabbit and human eyes, *e.g.*, the rabbit eye is slightly half the size of the human eye, substantially slower blink rate in rabbits, presence of a nictitating membrane, and only one punctum in the rabbit. Rabbits for PK can be non-pigmented (*e.g.*, New Zealand White) or pigmented (*e.g.*, Dutch-belted), depending on the degree to which the compound/drug is known or suspected to bind to melanin (pigment).

Investigative compounds are formulated as solutions or suspensions, preferably already tested for ocular compatibility and tolerance, and are administered by eye drop using a dropper (*e.g.*, droptainer) or a positive displacement pipet. The latter better ensures accurate volume, which is typically administered in the range of 35-40 microliters. Dosing is bilateral, *i.e.*, OS (left) and OD (right) eyes, except in the case where an undosed fellow eye is required for comparison, *e.g.*, in the case of safety assessment or to determine the contribution from systemic drug levels to ocular tissue levels *via* redistribution. Although drugs can be distributed from systemic circulation to the eye, this is less relevant for anterior segment tissues, for which the majority of drugs derive from local distribution from the ocular surface tissues, *e.g.*, cornea and conjunctiva. For the indication of glaucoma and IOP reduction, generally the anterior segment tissues are considered the drug target and are of primary interest for PK. As such, dosing is typically bilateral, and each eye (OD or OS) is considered an independent measure. Thus, for example, N = 2 rabbits yields N = 4 eyes, and it is the N=4 that is used for the calculation of summary statistics, *e.g.*, mean and standard deviation. Because sampling is terminal, each rabbit is associated with only one time point (an exception is if OD and OS eyes are dosed at different times, leading to collection representing two different time points – one for OD and another for OS).

Assessed Tissues and Sampling Time Points

Commonly evaluated ocular tissues for drugs targeting the anterior segment include the cornea, conjunctiva, anterior sclera, aqueous humor, iris-ciliary body (ICB), lens, and vitreous humor. As needed, the cornea can be further separated into its three layers, epithelium, stroma, and endothelium, and ICB can be separated into the iris and ciliary body. If the focus of the study is on pharmacological target tissues, tissues may only include cornea, aqueous humor, and ICB, or only aqueous humor. Where there is an interest in distribution to the back of the eye, retina, RPE/choroid, and, in some cases, the optic nerve may be collected. Time points post-dose can vary depending on the study objective. Ideally, there should be enough time points to characterize the absorption and elimination phases. However, this may require a substantial number of animals, especially around the absorptive phase. In practice, around 5 time points are selected to capture maximal concentration (Cmax) and preferably the elimination phase for calculation of terminal half-life. Intensive sampling time points may include 0.5, 1, 2, 4, 8, 12, 24, and, if needed, 48 hours (depending on the half-life, with the goal of capturing 3-5 half-lives and at least three data points in the terminal phase). Earlier time points, *e.g.*, 0.25 hour, are included if better characterization of the absorption phase is required (*e.g.*, comparing ocular bioavailabilities between formulations). More typically, sparse sampling is employed, with screening studies tending to use only up to three time points, which are selected within the region of Cmax (Tmax) and a portion of distribution and elimination phases, allowing a perhaps rough estimation of area under the concentration-time curve (AUC).

Ocular Tissue Collection

Details of tissue collection are given below. Variations of these techniques can be found in the published literature (Fayyaz *et al.*, 2021; Shen *et al.*, 2017; Savinainen *et al.*, 2019). Dissection can be either frozen or unfrozen (fresh), with the former particularly employed to collect the vitreous as a whole versus a portion of liquid vitreous collected. The latter, i.e., the fresh collection method, is described below.

Preparation of Workstation

The workstation should be clean and organized. Disposable pads are placed on the workstation surface. These should be changed between animals. Instruments should be cleaned and rinsed with saline first then with alcohol (ethanol) between animals and between tissue collections to prevent drug cross-sample contamination. Instruments should be wiped dry after rinsing. It is recommended to clean instruments with soap and water, followed by sonification between collection time points and for some drugs between animals at a given collection time, depending on the potential for cross-contamination. Instruments used for enucleation should be cleaned or rinsed thoroughly after each use.

In the case that one eye is dosed with a drug while the fellow eye is left undosed, two complete sets of instruments should be used – one for each eye. These sets should be kept separate and must have separate rinsing solutions. This process is to avoid drug cross-contamination of the undosed eye tissues.

Preparation of the Animal (Rabbit) for Ocular Tissue Collection

If required, a venous or arterial blood sample can be collected prior to euthanasia if needed using appropriate methods of restraint or sedation. Prior to tissue collection, the rabbit must be euthanized by an authorized and humane method. This is followed by placing the rabbit on its side opposite to the eye from which tissues will be collected. The eye is rinsed with isotonic saline (0.9%) and blotted with clean gauze to remove excess saline.

Collection of Aqueous Humor

The rabbit is oriented as indicated above, followed by positioning the eye by proptosing (pushing the eye globe out of the eye socket) using a needle cap or forceps handle. A 25-28G needle affixed to a 1cc tuberculin syringe is introduced (bevel up) at the limbus, and, observing through the cornea into the eye, it is carefully advanced into the anterior chamber until the tip is approximately in the center of the cornea. Care should be taken to avoid scraping the cornea, iris, or lens during insertion. Scraping these tissues could lead to drug cross-contamination of the aqueous humor sample, particularly from pigmented tissues (*e.g.*, iris), if the test drug binds to melanin.

Aqueous humor (typically 0.1 to 0.3 mL) is aspirated into the syringe. The needle is then slowly withdrawn, and the aqueous humor sample is expelled into a collection cryotube or vial (typically 1.5 mL). Pre-weighed or tared sample tubes are weighed again and placed on dry ice until transferred to cryostorage (typically approximately -70°C). If needed, *e.g.*, in case of drug instability, the sample can be flash-frozen by immersing the sample tube in a dry ice/ethanol bath or liquid nitrogen.

Collection of Conjunctiva

The conjunctiva consists of the palpebral and bulbar portions. The palpebral conjunctiva covers the inner surface of the eyelid and extends posteriorly to the fornix, then somewhat anteriorly along the globe/sclera, whereas the bulbar conjunctiva covers the eye globe extending to the limbus. Not all protocols require both sites – bulbar conjunctiva is the most common site collected.

To collect the bulbar conjunctiva, the conjunctiva over the sclera is grasped with forceps about 2-4 mm from the limbus. Starting at the temporal side and working around the inferior to nasal, the conjunctiva is cut away from the underlying Tenon's capsule and sclera as a ribbon approximately 2-4 mm in width. It is important not to cut too widely, which could result in connective tissue and muscle being included.

For the collection of palpebral conjunctiva, the conjunctiva lining the inferior eyelid is grasped with forceps at the temporal side, then cut away from the eyelid in a ribbon of approximately 2-4 mm in width. The depth of the cut should be limited to avoid the collection of connective tissue along with the conjunctiva.

Conjunctiva ribbons are rinsed thoroughly under a stream of isotonic saline, blotted dry with gauze, and transferred to an appropriate sample tube.

In Situ Collection of Cornea, Iris-Ciliary Body (ICB), Lens, and Vitreous Humor

As previously stated, for ocular PK studies related to glaucoma and anterior segment research, anterior segment tissues are most commonly collected and assessed for drug exposure/PK. These tissues usually include the cornea, ICB, and lens, along with aqueous humor from the anterior chamber (collection described above) and, in many cases, vitreous humor from the posterior segment. Collection of these tissues/fluids can be performed *in situ*, *i.e.*, without enucleating the eye.

For the *in situ* procedure, the eye is rinsed with normal saline and dabbed dry with clean gauze or microsponge. The cornea is collected using a disposable scalpel/blade or similar instrument to make a small 5 mm cut at the limbus. The cut is extended continuously with the limbus until the cornea is free from the eye, avoiding the collection of sclera attached to the perimeter. The cornea is then rinsed under a stream of normal saline and blotted dry with clear gauze. At this point, the ICB is removed as one tissue by grasping and pulling the iris and attached ciliary body with forceps and gently pulling these away from the sclera. The ICB is blotted with clean gauze to remove any adhering vitreous humor, rinsed with saline, and blotted dry.

Following removal of the ICB, if the lens is not protruding already, then gentle pressure is applied to the eye globe to protrude the lens from the eye. The lens is removed using forceps to scoop the lens, which is then rinsed with saline and gently blotted dry.

Vitreous humor is collected into a 1 cc tuberculin syringe without a needle attached. The syringe tip is gently inserted into the vitreous chamber (where the lens was removed), and about 0.2 to 0.6 mL is aspirated into the syringe. This is primarily liquid vitreous. Care is taken not to pull on the syringe plunger with too much force, as this can tug on the gelatinous portion of the vitreous and possibly detach the retina, resulting in tissue contamination.

Collection for Studies Requiring Anterior and Posterior Ocular Tissues PK

Enucleation of the Rabbit Eye

It is necessary to remove the entire eye globe by enucleation to obtain posterior segment ocular tissues in addition to those anterior. Aqueous humor and conjunctiva are obtained prior to enucleation, as described previously.

Initially, two cuts are made; one cut is made from the inner to outer the canthus, and the second cut in the same manner but below the eye. Holding eyelids closed with tissue forceps and using curved blunt scissors (enucleation scissors), the connective tissues and muscle attaching the eye globe in the socket are slowly cut away, being careful not to damage the posterior half of the eye. The globe is rinsed with saline, and if the optic nerve is to be collected, the globe is pulled out of the eye (proptosed) as much as possible before cutting the nerve.

Depending on the need to collect tissues surrounding the eye (adnexa), the eye is cleaned and prepared by cutting the conjunctiva, eyelids, muscle, and connective tissue from around the eye with eye or utility scissors (straight or slightly curved). To help maintain stability of analytes, the eye is placed in a chilled beaker or weigh boat with wet ice to maintain temperature at approximately 0°C.

Collection of Posterior Segment Tissues

If included in PK assessments, the optic nerve is collected by cutting approximately 1-2 mm above the sclera, avoiding cutting too close to the sclera as this will create a hole in the sclera. The optic nerve is cleaned of all muscle and connective tissue, rinsed thoroughly, blotted, and placed in an appropriate sample tube.

For the collection of vitreous humor, the eye is placed on its side, and a small cut (about 13 mm in length) is made with a disposable scalpel approximately 4-6 mm posterior to the limbus. Vitreous humor (typically 0.2 to 0.6 mL) is now aspirated into a 1 cc tuberculin syringe without an affixed needle. Pulling back too hard on the syringe plunger should be avoided, as this can detach the retina and break apart the lens. The vitreous humor sample is transferred to an appropriate collection vial/tube. This technique primarily collects the liquid phase of the vitreous, as opposed to the gelatinous portion, and as such, does not collect the whole vitreous. A frozen eye dissection method is employed for the collection of the entire vitreous, for example, as used by Struble *et al.* (2014).

Following the vitreous collection, the cut made for this collection is continued around the globe circumference using eye scissors. The posterior portion of the eye is gently pulled away from the anterior, and the eye is thus separated into two approximate halves.

For collection of the neuroretina (excludes retinal pigment epithelium (RPE)), remnants of vitreous humor attached to the retina must first be removed. This is done by gently turning the sclera over onto microsponges (sclera side up), patting the sclera, and dabbing the vitreous onto the microsponges. Alternatively, gauze may be used instead of microsponges, although this is less preferred. This is followed by holding the edge of the sclera with forceps while the neuroretina is gently pushed from the RPE/choroid to the center (optic nerve) using a Gill knife or equivalent. Forceps are used to grasp the neuroretina, and small iris scissors are used to cut the retina free from the optic nerve at the optic disc.

The tissues remaining on the sclera are the RPE and choroid, but these are typically collected together as RPE/choroid, which is initially rinsed under a stream of saline, followed by dabbing dry with clean gauze. The RPE/choroid is removed by scraping away from the sclera using a Gill knife. Forceps or the Gill knife can be used to transfer the tissue to an appropriate sample vial.

Following the collection of RPE/choroid, the sclera is rinsed thoroughly with saline. If not collected already, the optic nerve is sampled by holding the optic nerve head with toothed forceps and using eye scissors to cut the tissue free from the sclera. Care should be taken to avoid collecting scleral tissue along with the optic nerve.

Collection of Anterior Tissues: Cornea, Iris-Ciliary Body, and Lens

The lens is collected by scooping it from the anterior portion of the eye using a Gill knife while holding the edge of the sclera with forceps. The extraneous vitreous humor is then blotted from the lens with gauze prior to rinsing, drying, and transfer to an appropriate vial.

ICB is removed and collected as one whole tissue by grasping and pulling the iris, with attached ciliary process/body, from the sclera using forceps. The cornea is then cut from the sclera with scissors. Both ICB and cornea are rinsed with saline and blotted dry before placing them in their respective sample vials/tubes.

Preparation and Analysis of Ocular Tissues/Fluids

After dissection, each tissue/fluid is placed in an appropriate sample tube, weighed, and placed on dry ice until transfer to cryostorage (typically at approximately -70°C). If needed, *e.g.*, analyte or metabolite stability, the tissue can be flash-frozen by immersion of the sample tube in dry ice/ethanol or liquid nitrogen bath.

Tissues are individually homogenized in an appropriate buffer or buffer mixed with organic solvent (*e.g.*, acetonitrile) and homogenized using a sonifier probe or with a bead homogenizer unit. Following extraction and appropriate clean-up, an aliquot is analyzed using liquid chromatography-tandem mass spectrometry (LC-MS/MS) or another appropriate method for low molecular weight analytes. Protein therapeutics will typically be analyzed using enzyme-linked immunoassay (ELISA).

Pharmacokinetic Data Analysis

Levels of analytics in an ocular tissue/fluid matrix are normalized by tissue weight-yielding concentration, generally in ng/g (tissue) or ng/mL (fluid) units. Mean and standard deviation concentrations are typically determined at each time point based on eye replicates (N), as opposed to animal replicates. Time-concentration analysis yields pharmacokinetic parameters, *e.g.*, maximal concentration (Cmax), time to Cmax (Tmax), area under the concentration-time curve (AUC in units of ng·hr/g or ng·hr/mL), and, if possible, terminal half-life ($T_{1/2}$ in hours).

CONCLUSION

This generic protocol describes a relatively common method of studying ocular PK in rabbits, with details provided for the collection of tissues/fluids. Modifications of this protocol or alternative methods, *e.g.*, frozen eye technique or cyrosectioning with image analysis, have been employed with varying degrees of detail reported in the published literature.

REFERENCES

Agrahari, V, Mandal, A, Agrahari, V, Trinh, HM, Joseph, M, Ray, A, Hadji, H, Mitra, R, Pal, D & Mitra, AK (2016) A comprehensive insight on ocular pharmacokinetics. *Drug Deliv Transl Res,* 6, 735-54. [http://dx.doi.org/10.1007/s13346-016-0339-2] [PMID: 27798766]

Fayyaz, A, Vellonen, KS, Ranta, VP, Toropainen, E, Reinisalo, M, Valtari, A, Puranen, J, Ricci, GDA, Heikkinen, EM, Gardner, I, Ruponen, M, Urtti, A, Jamei, M & del Amo, EM (2021) Ocular pharmacokinetics of atenolol, timolol and betaxolol cocktail: Tissue exposures in the rabbit eye. *Eur J Pharm Biopharm,* 166, 155-62.
[http://dx.doi.org/10.1016/j.ejpb.2021.06.003] [PMID: 34139290]

Gaudana, R, Ananthula, HK, Parenky, A & Mitra, AK (2010) Ocular drug delivery. *AAPS J,* 12, 348-60. [http://dx.doi.org/10.1208/s12248-010-9183-3] [PMID: 20437123]

Savinainen, A, Prusakiewicz, JJ, Oswald, J, Spencer, E, Lou, Z, Cohen, ML, Rashidzadeh, H & Josiah, S (2019) Pharmacokinetics and intraocular pressure–lowering activity of TAK-639, a novel C-type natriuretic peptide analog, in rabbit, dog, and monkey. *Exp Eye Res,* 189, 107836.
[http://dx.doi.org/10.1016/j.exer.2019.107836] [PMID: 31626797]

Shen, J, Goodkin, ML, Tong, W & Attar, M (2017) Ocular pharmacokinetics and tolerability of bimatoprost ophthalmic solutions administered once or twice daily in rabbits, and clinical dosing implications. *Clin Ophthalmol,* 11, 1761-7.
[http://dx.doi.org/10.2147/OPTH.S143428] [PMID: 29026287]

Struble, C, Howard, S & Relph, J (2014) Comparison of ocular tissue weights (volumes) and tissue collection techniques in commonly used preclinical animal species. *Acta Ophthalmol,* 92, 0.
[http://dx.doi.org/10.1111/j.1755-3768.2014.S005.x]

Urtti, A (2006) Challenges and obstacles of ocular pharmacokinetics and drug delivery. *Adv Drug Deliv Rev,* 58, 1131-5.
[http://dx.doi.org/10.1016/j.addr.2006.07.027] [PMID: 17097758]

CHAPTER 42

Considerations for Ocular Toxicologic Pathology in Nonclinical Studies for the Development of Intraocular Biologics to Treat Glaucoma and Secondary Neurodegeneration

Vladimir Bantseev[1,*] and **Rachel N. Andrews**[1]

[1] *Therapeutic Area Lead for Ophthalmology, Safety Assessment – Toxicology, Genentech Research and Development, A Member of the Roche Group, 1 DNA Way, MS# 441A, South San Francisco, CA 94080, USA*

Abstract: Ocular hypertension (OHT) associated with many forms of glaucoma can be treated by traditional pharmaceutical drugs, surgery, and aqueous humor microshunt implants. More recently, however, attempts have been made to introduce gene and cell therapies and even biologics to treat OHT and IOP-independent glaucomatous optic neuropathies with various degrees of success. In order to ensure the safety of any test agent or product, it is imperative that a set of toxicological studies be conducted on the compound or test agent. Accordingly, in this section/chapter, we provide considerations for toxicologic pathology evaluation of intraocular biologic therapeutic candidates to treat glaucoma. These types of investigations can be applied not only to biologics but, with appropriate modifications, to any entity that is to be introduced into animals and perhaps in humans in due course as part of proof-of-concept studies.

Keywords: Anterior and posterior segments, Drug development, Glaucoma, Neuroprotection, Retina, Toxicology studies.

INTRODUCTION

Considerations for identifying and selecting the clinical therapeutic candidate [utilizing various *in vitro* approaches and establishing *in vivo* proof of concept (diseased animals, KO, or normal animals)] are described in this book/volume elsewhere. The purpose of this section/chapter is to provide points for consideration to characterize the local (ocular) and systemic effects of intraocular administered biologic therapeutic candidates and to enable first-in-human clinical

* **Corresponding author Vladimir Bantseev:** Therapeutic Area Lead for Ophthalmology, Safety Assessment – Toxicology, Genentech Research and Development, A Member of the Roche Group, 1 DNA Way, MS# 441A, South San Francisco, CA 94080, USA; Tel: +1.650.467.4971; E-mail: bantseev.vladimir@gene.com

Najam A. Sharif and Sunny E. Ohia (Eds.)

trials by executing a comprehensive toxicological program. Rather than being prescriptive and providing protocol-like settings, the goal of this chapter is to provide sufficient building blocks and considerations that can be adapted on a case-by-case basis for intraocularly (intracameral, IC or intravitreal, IVT) administered therapeutic biologic candidates/treatment modalities in an effort to treat glaucoma and provide neuroprotection.

The toxicology program is commonly performed in healthy animals (i.e., not a disease model) where only the potential ocular and systemic effects of the candidate therapeutic are characterized in the absence of other potentially confounding variables. The overall goal of the toxicological program is to characterize potential safety ocular and systemic safety risks for patients using nonclinical studies to build the weight of evidence, enable the clinical development plan (CDP), and initially enable first-in-human clinical trials. Thus, the CDP provides the foundation for toxicological program considerations in terms of dosing frequency and duration. This chapter will cover species selection, dose selection, study duration, dosing frequency, clinical ophthalmic and general toxicology endpoints, histopathology assessment, and integrated assessment of the totality of the toxicology data to interpret the data. In the absence of ocular-specific regulatory guidelines for intraocular biologic administration, guiding principles of ICH S6(R1) (preclinical safety testing requirements for biotechnological products) and ICH M3 (nonclinical safety studies recommended to support human clinical trials of a given scope and duration as well as marketing authorization for pharmaceuticals) will be applied as needed.

Species Selection

The nonclinical toxicology species selection is guided by pharmacological/pharmacodynamic assessment of the therapeutic candidate and includes (1) the evaluation of sequence homology, (2) binding, and (3) pharmacodynamic activity data for human vs. multiple laboratory species (*e.g.*, non-human primates (NHPs); minipig, dog, rabbit, rodent vs. human). Anatomical considerations include factors such as the size of the eye and the feasibility of intraocular dosing (intracameral, IC or intravitreal, IVT). These combined pharmacological and anatomic data support toxicology species selection to derive a relevant and accurate risk assessment for patients and establish a path forward. For intraocular administered biologics, NHPs are often the only pharmacologically relevant species. If the therapeutic candidate cross-react in multiple species, including NHPs, minipigs, or rabbits, lower species should be considered first rather than defaulting to NHP as the most relevant species. Rodents (when pharmacologically relevant) are not feasible for repeated intraocular (IC, IVT, *etc.*) toxicology studies due to ocular anatomical limitations (Rowe-Rendleman *et al.* 2014).

Dose Selection, Dosing Frequency, and Study Duration

From a toxicological standpoint, local intraocular administration offers the promise of the best combination of high local exposure and low systemic exposure. The eye of common laboratory species (*i.e.*, NHP, minipig, dog, or rabbit) is large enough to administer the clinically relevant dose volume via a clinically relevant route of administration and allow maximum feasible dose (MFD) administration. Administering the MFD allows the establishment of robust local safety margins to the human dose. Oftentimes, the MFD is achieved by administering two injections of a clinical dose volume. In the case of IVT, MFD is administered as 2x50ul injections administered approximately 10 min apart to allow the intraocular pressure (IOP) to return to baseline values (Dere *et al.* 2021; Bantseev *et al.* 2018). Stand-alone ocular pilot toxicology studies are done on a case-by-case basis and for cause only. When the target and modality are well characterized, information on ocular tolerability can be obtained via limited endpoints such as clinical ophthalmic exams and, in some cases, ocular imaging (i.e., optical coherence tomography (OCT) and fundus photos) as part of pharmacokinetics/pharmacodynamics (PKPD) studies. If a pilot toxicology ocular study is warranted, at least two doses should be administered to mimic periodic dosing in the clinic, as there is limited utility in characterizing ocular tolerability following a single intraocular administration. Dose-ranging (more than a single dose level) may be considered in the pilot toxicology to inform the dose selection and dosing frequency in the Good Laboratory Practices (GLP) toxicology ocular studies. If clinical formulation is available at the time of the pilot toxicology study, it should be used. In the absence of clinical formulation, a research-grade formulation may be considered for use in a pilot toxicology study. As already mentioned, the MFD should be considered a high dose in the pilot toxicology and GLP toxicology studies to establish robust local ocular safety margins to the human dose. The GLP toxicology study should be done with the clinical formulation. Short-duration bridging toxicology studies may be considered if the clinical formulation undergoes significant changes during the clinical development.

Dosing frequency in the pilot toxicology and GLP toxicology ocular studies is guided by the CDP. Differences in the ocular clearance in animals vs. humans are a guiding principle of PK modeling for dosing frequency selection. Dosing both eyes of each animal to the MFD typically allows for the achievement of at least 10-fold systemic margins (Cmax and AUC), as required by ICH S6(R1) for biologics *via* the clinical route of administration (*i.e.*, IVT) in an effort to identify and characterize potential systemic risk. When both eyes are dosed to the MFD, a subgroup of animals or a stand-alone study with a systemic route of administration (*i.e.*, IV or SubQ) to achieve at least 10-fold systemic margins is not warranted. The duration of the GLP toxicology ocular study is also guided by the CDP. The duration of repeat-administration intraocular GLP toxicology study ranges from 1-month to longer to enable FIH. A chronic GLP toxicology study of 6 months in duration typically enables registration.

Clinical Ophthalmic Endpoints and General Toxicology Endpoints on Ocular Toxicology Studies

Comprehensive clinical ophthalmic examinations (slit-lamp biomicroscopy, indirect ophthalmoscopy, ocular exams (OEs) should be performed pre-dose and at frequent time intervals during the study by qualified personnel. OEs and scoring of findings are generally performed as a mixture of semiquantitative grading systemic of ocular inflammation according to established and acceptable scoring systems (Eaton *et al.* 2017). During the OEs, the potential location and appearance of the injected therapeutic within the eye should be captured by detailed drawings. Intraocular pressure (IOP) measurements can be performed at the same frequency and in conjunction with OEs. In the pilot toxicology studies, OEs may be the only sufficient clinical ophthalmic endpoint. Other clinical ophthalmic assessments, such as scleral depression and gonioscopy, can be included on an as-needed basis. In addition to frequent OEs, imaging (fundus ocular photography, fluorescein angiography), optical coherence tomography (OCT), and electroretinography (ERG) should be performed pre-dose and periodically as part of the GLP toxicology studies.

General toxicology endpoints should include mortality, clinical signs, body weight, food consumption, TK, ADA, and clinical and full organ panel anatomical pathology evaluations. Safety pharmacology endpoints (neurological examinations and electrocardiography [ECG]) should be included as part of the ocular toxicology study rather than a stand-alone safety pharmacology study. Male fertility endpoints (i.e., stage-aware microscopic evaluation of spermatogenesis in the testes) should also be incorporated as part of the chronic ocular toxicology study.

Histopathology Assessment

There have been several guidance documents and position papers published to advise on the recommended best practices for the sampling and processing of ocular tissues in toxicologic studies. The optimal methods for tissue collection, fixation, trimming, histopathologic assessment, and secondary endpoints/ancillary testing should be carefully selected to best meet the needs of each individual study and should be determined in collaboration with the study pathologist. The preferred methods should be delineated in the study-design phase prior to initiation of the study, as suboptimal collection and sampling techniques may result in non-representative sampling, introduce undesirable tissue artifacts that may preclude thorough histopathologic assessment, hamper adequate evaluation of test-article biology, or impair downstream ancillary testing.

At all phases of tissue collection and processing, the eyes should be handled gently and with care to avoid damage to the tissue and artifactual changes (such as retinal detachment, lens displacement, and distortion of the globe) that may negatively affect histopathologic assessment.

Fixatives

An appropriate fixative should be selected that adequately preserves ocular morphology and is compatible with planned downstream analyses (*e.g.*, electron microscopy, immunohistochemistry, *in situ* hybridization, and additional molecular analysis). In general, immersion fixation in Davidson's or modified Davidson's solution is adequate for routine morphologic assessment (Chidlow *et al.*, 2011). As assessment of retinal cellularity and morphology is a key endpoint in glaucoma, fixation in 10% neutral buffered formalin (NBF) is generally discouraged due to suboptimal preservation of retinal cellular morphology and frequent artifactual retinal detachment. Further details are described in detail in different studies (Booler *et al.*, 2022; Ramos *et al.*, 2013; Bolon *et al.*, 2013), including specific considerations for compatibility with downstream analyses. Opinions are mixed regarding the necessity of the injection of fixatives into the eye to improve fixation under certain conditions and are dependent upon perimortem sampling procedures (*e.g.*, collection of vitreous humor) and individual study designs. It should be noted that the injection of fixatives into the globe may be a source of iatrogenic artifacts.

Trimming

Trimming of the globe should be custom-tailored to each study, taking into account the overall goals for that particular study, species-specific anatomic differences, route of test-article administration, and test-article behavior/biology. Furthermore, adequate sampling should also meet regulatory expectations for ocular therapeutics in nonclinical development. The Comparative Ocular Pathology Laboratory of Wisconsin recommends the immediate dissection of "all extraneous tissues from the globe unless directly involved in the pathologic process or considered important for orientation" (Dubielzig *et al.*, 2010). Identification of particular lesions of interest should be performed (*e.g.*, procedure sites, gross lesions), with the indication of the lesion location prior to fixation by the placement of a suture or a mark or provision of a simple drawing.

According to Per Booler *et al.* (2002), "the current regulatory expectations for ocular toxicity studies include (1) adequate microscopic assessment of a full range of ocular tissues; (2) microscopic evaluation of a sufficient number of eye sections, including assessment of the retinal cone-dense areas; (3) consideration of in-life observations, including ophthalmologic examination findings, with regard to sectioning the globe; and (4) the justification for the section/assessment approach by the study pathologist."

In general, for non-rodent species on ocular toxicologic studies, eyes from dogs, mini-pigs, and rabbits are trimmed and sectioned in the sagittal plane in order to capture the area centralis/visual streak, while non-human primate eyes are trimmed and sectioned in the horizontal plane due to the orientation of the macula and fovea. The Non-Rodent Ocular Trimming and Sectioning Working Group of the Society of Toxicologic Pathology (STP) suggests that for routine intracameral and intravitreal studies, sectioning and evaluation of 3 levels, including one that contains the retinal cone-dense areas (visual streak/macula, area centralis/fovea) should be sufficient to satisfy regulatory expectations.

Depending on the route of administration and test article biology, additional sections may be warranted to ensure this area is captured and evaluated on histopathology. Stepwise sections may be required to adequately sample regions of potential concern. Specific examples will be discussed below.

Intracameral injection is one of the primary routes of administration for glaucoma and is particularly relevant for IOP-lowering modalities. In the case of intracamerally delivered therapeutics, a minimum of three sections per eye should be evaluated: one section should include the cone-dense area for that species, as mentioned previously. Additional sections should capture the injection site, the site of test article deposition, and any relevant in-life findings (Booler *et al.*, 2022). In the case of IVT-administered therapeutics, a minimum of three sections should also be evaluated, including the cone-dense area and the site of injection, although, as noted by Booler *et al.* (2022), it is seldom necessary to utilize step-wise sectioning to visualize the injection site itself in the plane of section.

In the case of sustained-release/drug depot formulations, care should be taken to adequately sample the site of deposition to evaluate for local tolerability. Determination of the appropriate plane of the section may be identified by in-life observation of the site of the test article [ophthalmic examination and imaging (OCT, gonioscopy,], or in the case of IVT administration, trimming in the inferior calotte, as some compounds may settle ventrally over time. This is also true for intracamerally administered therapeutics, which may settle to the inferior iridocorneal angle.

Detailed trimming schematics for ocular toxicity studies and additional details are described by Booler *et al.* (2022).

Histopathologic Assessment

The study pathologist should be familiar with the comparative anatomical features of the animal model being used, including normal species-specific anatomic features, background findings, and anticipated changes that may be induced by procedural manipulation(s). Additionally, the study pathologist should be informed of key test-article characteristics *prior* to study initiation, including anticipated biological effects and known or suspected potential liabilities to aid in study planning, advise on potential ancillary evaluations/diagnostics, and assist in the interpretation of histopathologic findings.

Histopathologic Features of Glaucoma

In general, toxicology studies are performed on healthy animals to assess potential injurious effects of the test-article irrespective of disease status in order to de-risk the potential for harm to patients when transitioning into clinical trials. Thus, histopathologic assessment of tissues in this context emphasizes comparison to undosed control animals to evaluate whether the test article has induced deleterious effects independent of efficacy in a disease state. However, an understanding of the disease pathogenesis and test article biology may guide the pathologist to evaluate certain intraocular structures with more scrutiny.

Glaucomas are a complex of diseases of differing causal mechanisms (although most commonly caused by increased intraocular pressure) united by a common, clinically characteristic optic neuropathy ultimately resulting in progressive vision loss and blindness. Interference with axoplasmic flow in the optic nerve head, death of the retinal ganglion cells and their axons, and blindness are common features of glaucoma, regardless of etiology (Slatter *et al.*, 2008).

The key histopathologic changes of glaucoma, and thus, potential sites of interest associated with glaucoma therapeutics include (Dubliezig *et al.*, 2010; Maxie, 2016; Carioto 2014):

Retina

- Loss of retinal ganglion cells and nerve fiber layer, with later loss of neurons from the inner nuclear layer; increased prominence of the Müller cells
- Retinal atrophy with a predilection for ventral retina over dorsal

- Gliosis

Optic Nerve

- Necrosis/malacia
- Gliosis
- Optic nerve cupping*
- Loss of large-diameter axons

This is the pathognomonic lesion of glaucoma

Additional changes may be noticed within the:

Cornea and Sclera

- Corneal edema, fibrosis, and vascularization
- Descemet's streaks (Haab's striae)
- Limbal scleral atrophy
- Enlargement, thinning, and stretching and enlargement of the globe (buphthalmos) with desiccation or ulceration in end-stages of disease
- Equatorial and limbal staphyloma

Uvea

- Collapse of the ciliary cleft
- Atrophy of the corneoscleral trabecular meshwork
- Iris and ciliary body atrophy

Lens

- Cataract
- Lens subluxation/luxation

Bearing in mind that preclinical toxicological safety assessment is generally evaluated in healthy animals (*e.g.*, non-disease models), histopathological assessment should consider the potential effects of test-article biology and route of administration when evaluating the tissue for changes. Some considerations may include test-article biology-driven target tissue-specific responses (*e.g.*, retinal ganglion cell or optic nerve changes), the presence of procedure sites/injection tracts, procedurally-associated cellular infiltrate/inflammation, residual test-article depots and attending foreign body reaction or other cellular infiltrate/inflammation, retinal thickness, and changes to the optic nerve including degeneration, atrophy, or gliosis.

Evaluation of Late-Onset Ocular Inflammation

In preclinical toxicology studies, intravitreal administration of large molecule therapeutics has been associated with the development of late-onset, immune-mediated intraocular inflammation in animal species, detectable on both in-life ophthalmic examinations and, often, with histopathologic correlate. This entity is characterized by delayed-onset intraocular inflammation (generally after day 14; however may occur as early as day 8 in rabbits), which may be more severe after prolonged or repeat dosing. Histopathologically, this manifests as mononuclear (and less frequently mixed cell) infiltrate to inflammation, which occurs in the ciliary body, iris, pars plana, and optic nerve head and/or localizes to vascular/perivascular tissues. In some cases, there may also be evidence of immune complex disease (fibrinoid necrosis, plasma cells, and/or immune complexes).

This finding has been tentatively ascribed to the effects of anti-drug antibodies (ADA); however, not all animals with ADA develop late-onset ocular inflammation; ADA titers do not correlate with the severity of intraocular inflammation and the incidence of ADA in preclinical studies does not reliably predict translatable immunogenicity in the clinic. The appropriate evaluation of late-onset ocular inflammation and attribution of such findings to test-article immunogenicity requires a weight-of-evidence approach involving the integration of in-life data (ophthalmic examination, optical coherence tomography, and/or fluorescent angiography), ADA-data, and pathology findings.

Additionally, in rabbits, the IVT administration of ocular biologic therapeutics has been associated with marked intraocular inflammation and immunogenicity (de Zafra *et al.*, 2017), in some cases, resulting in early termination of the study due to animal welfare concerns. Additionally, these findings may preclude meaningful safety assessment. As such, assessment of IVT biologics in rabbits may be of limited interpretive value, and the decision to evaluate this species should be carefully considered, or this species should be avoided in favor of another preclinical animal model.

Ultimately, the determination of adversity and no-observed-adverse-effect level (NOAEL) should include the evaluation and integration of the totality of the data available for the toxicology program studies, including in-life observations (*e.g.*, clinical findings, ophthalmic examinations, ophthalmic imaging, ADA-titers, histopathology, and ancillary diagnostics). However, while these findings may be adverse in the context of the effects on animals within the specific study, translatability to humans may be limited due to differing ocular anatomy and relative ocular size, administration of a humanized protein to animal models, and other factors. Thus, it is recommended to add a statement to reports qualifying adversity and toxicologic findings within the context of translatability.

CONCLUDING REMARKS

In this chapter, we provided considerations for toxicologic pathology evaluation of intraocular biologic therapeutic candidates to treat glaucoma. A comprehensive toxicological program is designed to enable first-in-human clinical trials where, in relevant animal species models, the therapeutic candidate is administered via a clinically relevant route.

REFERENCES

Baldrick, P, Cosenza, ME, Alapatt, T, Bolon, B, Rhodes, M & Waterson, I (2020) Toxicology Paradise: Sorting Out Adverse and Non-adverse Findings in Animal Toxicity Studies. *Int J Toxicol,* 39, 365-78. [http://dx.doi.org/10.1177/1091581820935089] [PMID: 32618214]

Bantseev, V, Erickson, R, Leipold, D, Amaya, C, Miller, PE, Booler, H & Thackaberry, EA (2018) Nonclinical Safety Assessment of Anti-Factor D: Key Strategies and Challenges for the Nonclinical Development of Intravitreal Biologics. *J Ocul Pharmacol Ther,* 34, 204-13. [http://dx.doi.org/10.1089/jop.2017.0063] [PMID: 29148965]

Bolon, B, Garman, RH, Pardo, ID, Jensen, K, Sills, RC, Roulois, A, Radovsky, A, Bradley, A, Andrews-Jones, L, Butt, M & Gumprecht, L (2013) STP position paper: Recommended practices for sampling and processing the nervous system (brain, spinal cord, nerve, and eye) during nonclinical general toxicity studies. *Toxicol Pathol,* 41, 1028-48. [http://dx.doi.org/10.1177/0192623312474865] [PMID: 23475559]

Booler, HS, Lejeune, T, Sorden, S, Gruebbel, MM, Schafer, KA, Short, B, Farman, C, Ramos, MF, Bennet, B, Yekkala, K, Atzpodien, EA, Turner, OC, Brassard, J & Foley, G (2022) Scientific and Regulatory Policy Committee Points to Consider: Fixation, Trimming, and Sectioning of Nonrodent Eyes and Ocular Tissues for Examination in Ocular and General Toxicity Studies. *Toxicol Pathol,* 50, 235-51. [http://dx.doi.org/10.1177/01926233211047562] [PMID: 34693851]

Carioto, L (2014) *Can Vet J,* 55, 372.

Casson, RJ, Chidlow, G, Wood, JPM, Crowston, JG & Goldberg, I (2012) Definition of glaucoma: clinical and experimental concepts. *Clin Exp Ophthalmol,* 40, 341-9. [http://dx.doi.org/10.1111/j.1442-9071.2012.02773.x] [PMID: 22356435]

Chidlow, G, Daymon, M, Wood, JPM & Casson, RJ (2011) Localization of a wide-ranging panel of antigens in the rat retina by immunohistochemistry: comparison of Davidson's solution and formalin as fixatives. *J Histochem Cytochem,* 59, 884-98. [http://dx.doi.org/10.1369/0022155411418115] [PMID: 21832149]

Eaton, JS, Miller, PE, Bentley, E, Thomasy, SM & Murphy, CJ (2017) The SPOTS system: an ocular scoring system optimized for use in modern preclinical drug development and toxicology. *J Ocul Pharmacol Ther,* 33, 718-34. [http://dx.doi.org/10.1089/jop.2017.0108] [PMID: 29239680]

Dere, E, Crowell, S, Maia, M, Schuetz, C, Lai, P, Bantseev, V & Booler, H (2021) Nonclinical Safety Assessment of FHTR2163, An Antigen-Binding Fragment Against HTRA1 for the Treatment of Geographic Atrophy. *Toxicol Pathol,* 49, 610-20. [http://dx.doi.org/10.1177/0192623320976095] [PMID: 33297886]

de Zafra, CLZ, Sasseville, VG, Matsumoto, S, Freichel, C, Milton, M, MacLachlan, TK, Farman, C, Raymond, I, Gupta, S, Newton, R, Atzpodien, EA & Thackaberry, EA (2017) Inflammation and

immunogenicity limit the utility of the rabbit as a nonclinical species for ocular biologic therapeutics. *Regul Toxicol Pharmacol,* 86, 221-30.
[http://dx.doi.org/10.1016/j.yrtph.2017.03.013] [PMID: 28322894]

Dubielzig, RR, Ketring, K, McLellan, GJ & Albert, DM (2010) Veterinary ocular pathology: A comparative review. *Elsevier.*
[http://dx.doi.org/10.1016/C2009-0-32631-8]

Harmonised Tripartite Guideline, (2011). Accessed March, 2023. Available from: https://database.ich.org/sites/default/files/S6_R1_Guideline_0.pdf

ICH S6(R1). Preclinical safety evaluation of biotechnology-derived pharmaceuticals.

ICH M3(R2). (2009). Guidance on nonclinical safety studies for the conduct of human clinical trials and marketing authorization for pharmaceuticals. Harmonised Tripartite Guideline, Accessed March, 2023. Available from: https://database.ich.org/sites/default/files/M3_R2__Guideline.pdf

Jubb, Kennedy, and Palmer's pathology of domestic animals Maxie, M Grant. Sixth edition. St. Louis, Missouri : Elsevier, 2016. NLM ID: 101653265 [Book]

Maggs, D (2008) *Miller, P & Ofri, Ron.*Slatter's Fundamentals of Veterinary Ophthalmology.
[http://dx.doi.org/10.1016/B978-0-7216-0561-6.X5001-1]

Ramos, MF, Baker, J, Atzpodien, EA, Bach, U, Brassard, J, Cartwright, J, Farman, C, Fishman, C, Jacobsen, M, Junker-Walker, U, Kuper, F, Moreno, MCR, Rittinghausen, S, Schafer, K, Tanaka, K, Teixeira, L, Yoshizawa, K & Zhang, H (2018) Nonproliferative and Proliferative Lesions of the Ratand Mouse Special Sense Organs(Ocular [eye and glands], Olfactory and Otic). *J Toxicol Pathol,* 31 (Suppl.), 97S-214S.
[http://dx.doi.org/10.1293/tox.31.97S] [PMID: 30158741]

Rowe-Rendleman, CL, Durazo, SA, Kompella, UB, Rittenhouse, KD, Di Polo, A, Weiner, AL, Grossniklaus, HE, Naash, MI, Lewin, AS, Horsager, A & Edelhauser, HF (2014) Drug and gene delivery to the back of the eye: from bench to bedside. *Invest Ophthalmol Vis Sci,* 55, 2714-30.
[http://dx.doi.org/10.1167/iovs.13-13707] [PMID: 24777644]

NEW TECHNIQUES AND TECHNOLOGIES TO STUDY VARIOUS ASPECTS OF OCULAR HYPERTENSION/GLAUCOMA

CHAPTER 43

Gene Therapy Approaches and Protocols to Deliver Genes for IOP-Reduction in Animals

Adnan Dibas[1,*] and **Samarendra Mohanty**[1]

[1] *Nanoscope Technologies, 1312 Brown Trail, Bedford, TX 76022, USA*

Abstract: The glaucomas represent a heterogeneous group of optic neuropathies that result in progressive optic degeneration characterized by functional and structural impairment of ocular tissues. The two primary damaged ocular tissues in glaucoma are the trabecular meshwork in the front of the eye and the retinal ganglion cells in the back of the eye whose axons form the optic nerve. Elevated intraocular pressure (IOP) is the key risk factor for glaucoma, and drugs lowering IOP are the first line of defense in glaucoma therapy. Although self-administered topical ocular hypotensive eyedrops have been used for glaucoma management, patients encounter several problems, including non-compliance and incorrect drop instillation, especially patients suffering from motor function or coordination dysfunction. Unfortunately, as the majority of patients are asymptomatic, they become indifferent to the urgency of treatment. Even more problematic is that many patients require using multiple types of eye drops, and the likelihood of adherence decreases significantly, leading to worsening of the disease. Therefore, there is an urgent need for long-lasting IOP lowering therapy for glaucoma, and gene therapy offers such a possibility. Here, we describe several gene therapy approaches that are in development and protocols to deliver genes for IOP reduction in glaucomatous eyes.

Keywords: Adeno-associated virus, Gene, Intracameral, Intravitreal, Sonoporation, SiRNA, Therapy.

INTRODUCTION

Glaucoma is the second leading cause of irreversible blindness worldwide, affecting approximately 80 million people, and unfortunately, this number is expected to exceed 111 million by 2040 (Tham *et al.* 2014). It is estimated that there are more than 3 million people in America with glaucoma, with half of them undiagnosed, as glaucoma is frequently relatively asymptomatic until peripheral

* **Corresponding author Adnan Dibas:** Nanoscope Technologies, 1312 Brown Trail, Bedford, TX 76022, USA; E-mail: adibas@nanoscopetech.com

Najam A. Sharif and Sunny E. Ohia (Eds.)

vision deteriorates (Tham *et al.* 2014). It is estimated that the number of US glaucoma patients will reach 7.3 million by 2050 (Vajaranant *et al.* 2012). Sadly, the percentage of undiagnosed cases among Hispanics has reached > 80%, and it has been suggested that 50% of glaucoma patients in the US will be Hispanic by 2050 (Niraj and Joos 2016). Primary open-angle glaucoma (POAG) is the most prevalent form of glaucoma, affecting 90% of the USA's glaucoma patients. POAG is three to four times more common in African Americans than in non-Hispanic whites (Tielsh *et al.* 1991, Marshall 1989, Sommer *et al.* 1991, and Leske *et al.* 1994). Glaucoma is 6 times more common among African Americans than Whites and is 15 times more likely to cause irreversible blindness among them (Friedman *et al.* 2004 and Allison *et al.* 2019). Intriguingly, many of the population are not proactive about vision health, and even when diagnosed, medical intervention is not sought. Medication adherence is of great importance, especially in the early stages of glaucoma. A study has shown that an average of 27% of recently diagnosed POAG patients did not get any type of medical intervention (Stein *et al.* 2008). Further, the first line of treatment *via* self-administered topical ocular hypotensive eyedrops is associated with several issues, including incorrect drop instillation, adherence, and contamination. Davis *et al.* have shown that up to 80% of patients contaminate their eye drop bottle by accidently touching their eye or face, and up to 37% miss the eye completely. In another study, only 10% of glaucoma patients were found to be fully adherent to medications (Friedman 2007). Glaucoma causes an economic burden on patients with an estimated cost of 3 billion annually for the US economy (Rein *et al.* 2006). It appears that the cost of treatment depends on the severity of glaucoma, with early stages costing ~$623 compared to $2511 for severe cases (Lee *et al.* 2006). While it is common for drug therapy to be used as a 'first-option' treatment for glaucoma, surgical intervention is practiced when drug therapy fails. The cost of glaucoma surgery varies with the type of surgery and the area of the country where it is performed.

Potential Therapeutic Genes to Lower Intraocular Pressure

Microarray studies and genetic analysis have examined changes in gene expression in glaucomatous tissue versus nonglaucomatous tissues to identify genes that are either downregulated or upregulated, as well as mutated genes. Genome-wide association studies (GWAS) have identified important loci associated with primary open-angle glaucoma (POAG) risk (Gharahkhani *et al.* 2021). More importantly, the number of single nucleotide polymorphisms (SNPs) associated with glaucoma has continuously uncovered unknown genes that appear to affect aqueous humor (AH) (Abu-Amero *et al.* 2015). In addition, based on the physiology of AH outflow, scientists have examined genes that can alter AH flow rates. Lowering IOP by ~ 25% has been clinically effective in preserving the vision of glaucoma patients (Heijl *et al.* 2002), and such reduction in IOP may be considered as a standard for developing effective gene therapy for glaucoma.

Gene-knockout to Reduce IOP

The glaucoma association of an SNP identified caveolin-1 (CAV-1), not caveolin-2 (CAV-2), as a potential IOP-lowering therapeutic (Aga *et al.* 2014). Caveolin-1 knockout using short hairpin shRNAs resulted in increased outflow facility for CAV-1 but decreased facility for CAV-2 (Aga *et al.* 2014). On the contrary, Cav-1 knockout mice have shown reduced outflow facility and elevated IOP (Elliott *et al.*, 2016; Lei *et al.*, 2016; De Ieso *et al.*, 2020) due to permeant structural change and, therefore, may not be a good target to lower IOP. Another protein that appears to regulate the cytoskeletal actin network in TM is the GTPase-dependent rho kinase. Rho-kinase inhibitor is the latest IOP-lowering drug approved for glaucoma treatment, which functions to increase AH outflow (Batra *et al.* 2021). The inhibition of Rho-A gene expression using an adenoviral vector carrying a mutant dominant-negative RhoA protein that lacks the GTP binding site (AdhRhoA2) increased the outflow facility (Rao *et al.* 2005 and Vittitow *et al.* 2002). Borras *et al.* 2015 have shown that intracameral injection of scAAV2 expressing the dominant-negative RhoA also lowered IOP in rats at night (Borrás *et al.* 2015). The actin cytoskeleton in the TM can also be directly manipulated through the expression of caldesmon. Caldesmon, an actin-binding protein, can inhibit myosin binding to actin and calcium-dependent smooth muscle contraction. Gabelt *et al.* have shown that the overexpression of caldesmon using adenoviral viruses increased outflow in organ-cultured human and monkey anterior segments (Gabelt *et al.* 2006).

Gene Knockout Using CRISPR-Cas9 to Lower IOP

Clustered regularly interspaced short palindromic repeats (CRISPR) is one of the most exciting techniques that presents promising potential for glaucoma gene therapy targeting the anterior segment of the eye (Sander and Joung 2014). CRISPR-Cas9-mediated genome editing is driven by the binding of protein Cas9 to the targeted site and cleaving the target sequences of DNA. The protein 9 (Cas9) system can achieve efficient and precise gene editing ability, leading to permanent changes of only desired genes and, thus, effective IOP lowering treatment (Wu *et al.* 2020). While CRISPR-Cas9 gene-editing system has been successfully delivered to the retina by electroporation (Wang *et al.* 2014), a novel AAV serotype known as ShH10-AAV carrying the CRISPR cargo can transduce the ciliary epithelium following intravitreal injection. Disruption of aquaporin-1 (AQP1), a water channel involved in aqueous humor production in the ciliary epithelium, lowered IOP in two mouse models of glaucoma, the steroid and the microbead-induced ocular hypertension (OHT) (Wu *et al.* 2020). The study has shown that intravitreal injection of ShH10-AAV delivering a single vector CRISPR-Cas9 system disrupting AQP1 resulted in reduced IOP in treated eyes (~22% reduction). The group has not detected any off-target disruption of AQP1.

Gene Knockout Using RNA Interference (RNAi) to Lower IOP

RNA interference (RNAi) is a natural cellular mechanism utilized by eukaryotic cells to target foreign double-stranded RNA. Such a mechanism has been successfully used to degrade or downregulate the expression of genes as a therapeutic in numerous disorders. Topical siRNAs administered as eyedrops in phosphate-buffered saline solution (0.9% w/v) against the carbonic anhydrase A4 reduced IOP by ~14% (Jimenez *et al.* 2009). Since β2 adrenergic blockers such as timolol lower IOP, downregulation of β2-adrenergic receptors is expected to lower IOP. Jimenez *et al.* (2009) reported that siRNA against β2-adrenergic receptor lowered IOP by ~ 22% in rabbits. Similar IOP lowering was reported by downregulating β2 in rabbits by Loma *et al.* (2018). SYL040012, a chemically modified naked RNA, selectively inhibits the synthesis of β2-adrenergic receptor and reduces the production of AH-lowered intraocular pressure in rabbits (Moreno-Montanes *et al.,* 2014). Administration of SYL040012 (600 and 900 μg/eye/day) formulated as eye drops in phosphate-buffered saline (pH 7.2) has also been tested. Martınez *et al.* have shown that SYL040012 reduced IOP in a water load-induced glaucoma rabbit model (Martınez *et al.* 2014). Another targeted receptor is the purinergic 2Y ($P2Y_2$). siRNA downregulating the $P2Y_2$ receptor lowered IOP in rabbits (Martin-Gil *et al.* 2012). Liu *et al.* have shown that intracameral injection of the liposomal complex of siRNA against RhoA lowered IOP in mice (Liu *et al.* 2012). miR-21-5p is a known miRNA that is associated with cell adhesion and extracellular matrix formation in endothelial cells (Sabatel *et al.,* 2011). Since the trabecular meshwork (TM) and Schlemm's canal endothelium are involved in AH drainage, they were tested for their potential to affect IOP. Tan *et al.* (2020) have shown that the intracameral injection of PDA/PEI NPs/miR-21-5p (0.125 ng per eye, dissolved in sterilized PBS) significantly reduced IOP in mice by ~ 13% after 6 hrs post-injection, a reduction that lasted 48 hrs. As expected, the flow rate and conventional outflow facility were significantly increased in miR-21-5p overexpressing eyes. The mechanism of miR-21-5p appears to involve an increase in endothelial nitric oxide synthase enzyme (eNOS). The same group complexed miR-21-5p with nano-carrier Invivofectamine® 3.0 Reagent (IVF3001; Invitrogen) and performed intracameral injection in mice that also resulted in ~ 14% reduction in IOP, which lasted for 2 days. A similar enhancement of the conventional outflow facility was also observed (an increase of 60%) (Tan *et al.* 2021).

Gene-upregulation to Reduce IOP

Metallopeptidase 1 (MMP1), an interstitial collagenase that breaks down extracellular matrix (ECM) collagens, is downregulated by steroids in the TM. The injection of self-complementary AAV2 of MMP1 driven by a GRE promoter lowered IOP for up to one month (Borrás *et al.* 2016). Steroids also downregulate plasminogen tissue activator (PTA), a serine protease responsible for the conversion of plasminogen to plasmin, a known activator of MMPs. Kumar *et al.* (2013) have shown intracameral injection of an adenoviral vector expressing PTA reversed AH blockade in a mouse steroid-glaucoma model (Kumar *et al.* 2013). Overexpression of the prostaglandin biosynthesis enzyme cyclooxygenase-2 (the rate-limiting enzyme in PGF2α biosynthesis, COX-2) and the prostaglandin F 2α receptor (FPR) produces a sustained IOP lowering (Barraza *et al* 2010). A similar effect was observed in monkeys by overexpressing the prostaglandin F synthase (PGFS) gene following intracameral injection in monkeys (Lee *et al.* 2014). Recently, Chern *et al.* overexpressed both COX-2 and FPR using AAV2 with two 'off-type' tetracycline-responsive riboswitch elements (TC40 and TC45), driven by a ubiquitously expressing small chicken beta actin (CBA) promoter. Intracameral injections induced a dose-dependent reduction in intraocular pressure in normotensive Brown Norway rats that was sustained for more than 12 months.

The *Clostridium botulinum* C3 exoenzyme selectively ADP-ribosylates low molecular weight GTP-binding proteins RhoA, B, and C, leading to the inhibition of the Rho signaling pathway and changing actin network. Not surprisingly, an adenoviral vector expressing the clostridium botulinum-derived exoenzyme C3 transferase increased aqueous outflow in organ-cultured monkey eyes (Liu *et al.* 2005). Single-stranded DNA adeno-associated viruses (ssAAV) provide longer and sustained expression that can last for years (Borrás *et al.* 2006). A single intracameral injection of scAAV2-GFP in monkeys showed a positive fluorescent TM at 5 days that lasted for at least 2 years (Buie *et al.* 2010). scAAV transduction may be species-specific (Watakabe *et al.,* 2015; Asokan *et al.,* 2012). Among serotypes tested by intracameral injection, serotype 5 showed the maximum transduction of rat TM (Buie *et al.* 2008), and serotype 6 was highest in porcine (Ellliott *et al.* 2014). In contrast, scAAV2 showed the highest transduction in primary human TM cells (no to minimal transduction for 1, 8, and 9 serotypes). The triple mutation of the surface-exposed tyrosine in the capsid AAV protein further enhanced transduction *in vivo* (Bogner *et al.* 2015; Petrs-Silva *et al.* 2011, and Rodriguez-Estevez *et al.* 2020). Interestingly, intracameral injection of scAAV2-expressing Stanniocalcin-1, a naturally occurring hormone, lowered IOP for up to six months in a glaucoma model (Roddy *et al.,* 2022). A summary of genetic manipulation of genes to lower IOP by either downregulation or upregulation is shown in Table **1**.

Table 1. Gene targets for IOP lowering.

Gene Target for IOP Lowering	Mechanism of Action	Genetic Manipulation	Genetic Delivery Method	Gene Type	References
Aquaporin-1	Increases AH production	Knockout or downregulation	Intravitreal injection	ShH10-AAV delivering a single vector CRISPR-Cas9	Wu *et al.* 2020
carbonic anhydrase A4	Increases AH production	Knockout or downregulation	Topical eye drops	siRNA	Jimenez *et al.* 2009
β2-adrenergic receptor	Increases AH production	Knockout or downregulation	Topical eye drops	SYL040012, a chemically modified naked RNA	Loma *et al.* 2018, Moreno-Montanes *et al.* 2014, & Martınez *et al.* 2014
$P2Y_2$ receptor	Increases AH production	Knockout or downregulation	Topical eye drops	siRNA	Martin-Gil *et al.* 2012
RhoA kinase	Increases AH outflow, reduces AH production, and decreases episcleral venous pressure (EVP)	Knockout or downregulation	Intracameral injection	Liposomal complex of siRNA, scAAV2 expressing the dominant-negative RhoA	Liu *et al.* 2012, Borrás *et al.* 2015, respectively
Endothelial nitric oxide synthase enzyme (eNOS)	Increases aqueous humor outflow facility and inhibits aqueous humor production	Upregulation	Intracameral injection	Liposomal complex of siRNA (PDA/PEI NPs/miR-21-5p or Invivofectamine® 3.0)	Tan *et al.* 2020, Tan *et al.* 2021
Metallopeptidase 1 (MMP1)	Increases outflow	Upregulation	Intracameral injection	scAAV2-MMP1 driven by a GRE promoter	Borrás *et al.* 2016
Plasminogen tissue activator (PTA), a serine protease responsible for the conversion of plasminogen to plasmin, a known activator of MMPs	Increases outflow	Upregulation	Intracameral injection	Adenoviral vector	Kumar *et al.* 2013

(Table 1) cont.....

Gene Target for IOP Lowering	Mechanism of Action	Genetic Manipulation	Genetic Delivery Method	Gene Type	References
Cycloexogenase-2 (the rate-limiting enzyme in PGF2α biosynthesis, COX-2)	Stimulates the synthesis of MMPs to digest extracellular matrix and enhances uveoscleral outflow	Upregulation	Intracameral injection	Lentiviral vector	Barraza *et al* 2010
Prostaglandin F synthase (PGFS)	Stimulates the synthesis of MMPs to digest extracellular matrix and enhances uveoscleral outflow	Upregulation	Intracameral injection	Lentiviral vector	Lee *et al.* 2014
COX-2 and FPR	Stimulate the synthesis of MMPs to digest extracellular matrix and enhance uveoscleral outflow	Upregulation	Intracameral injection	AAV2	Chern *et al 2022*
Clostridium botulinum C3 exoenzyme	ADP-ribosylates GTP-binding proteins RhoA, B, and C, leading to the inhibition of the Rho signaling pathway and changing actin network	Upregulation	Intracameral injection	Adenoviral vector	Liu *et al.* 2005
Caldesmon	Increases outflow by disrupting the actin network and inhibiting muscle contraction	Upregulation	Intracameral injection	Adenoviral vector	Gabelt *et al.* 2006
Stanniocalcin-1	A stress-response protein	Upregulation	Intracameral injection	scAAV2	Roddy *et al.* 2022

Protocol for Intracameral Injection of Therapeutic Viruses in Mouse Eye to Lower IOP

Materials

Wild-type mice C57BL

scAAV2 Virus: scAAV can be produced in-house or *via* a commercial manufacturer.

Genes (to lower IOP following expression) to be packaged in scAAV2 include metallopeptidase 1 (MMP1), plasminogen tissue activator (PTA), prostaglandin biosynthesis enzyme cyclooxygenase-2 (the rate-limiting enzyme in PGF2α biosynthesis, COX-2), with or without the prostaglandin F 2α receptor (FPR), Stanniocalcin, and *Clostridium botulinum* C3 exoenzyme.

Betadine

70% ethanol

Insulin injection needles

Heating plate/mat

gloves

Glass needles (WPI, cat#: TIP01TW1F)

Dissecting microscope with appropriate light source

Cotton swabs

Injection pump (WPI, cat#:MCIRO21)

Animal Preparation

- Expose the adult mouse to 2.5-3.5% isoflurane in oxygen at a flow rate of 1 L/min in an induction chamber.
- After 5 min, transfer the animal to a head holder with a vaporizer/scavenger attachment. It is better to put animals on a heating pad.
- Dilate the pupils by applying one drop of tropicamide eye drops (1%) to each eye.
- Apply one drop of 0.5% proparacaine hydrochloride (local anesthetic, Alcon Laboratories Inc., Fort Worth, TX, USA) to each eye.

- Adjust the micromanipulator in a downward direction and install the Hamilton syringe containing the virus.
- Put the animal on its side to visualize the entire circumference of the eye under a surgical microscope.
- Remove any residual eye drops using tissue paper.
- Secure the eye by gripping both edges of the sclera using forceps and puncture the eye at a similar angle to the micromanipulator with a needle.
- Slowly remove the needle and release the forceps.
- Install the syringe loaded with the virus on the micromanipulator and align it to a similar angle to the puncture site on the corneal surface.
- Using the micromanipulator, advance the injection needle into the puncture site until the puncture site is sealed around the needle.
- Slowly press on the syringe pump to release the 1.5 μl vector solution (AAV~2 x 10^{9-11} viral genes (vg)/ml) into the eye (at a flow rate of 100 nl/sec). Wait for 1 min to minimize efflux.
- Slowly retract the micromanipulator to remove the needle from the eye and apply a drop of ciprofloxacin antibiotic (0.3%).
- Repeat the procedure for the animals using a control null vector as a negative control.
- After injection, clean the eyelid and inject the mouse subcutaneously with buprenorphine (0.1 mg/kg) to alleviate pain.
- Place the mouse back into its cage and place the cage onto a warm heating plate (37◦C) until the mouse is fully recovered.

Notes

Caldesmon is a large gene and cannot be packaged into the scAAV or even AAV due to packaging capacity limitations of 2.3 kb and 4.7 kb for scAAV and AAV, respectively.

The titer should be between 1×10^{12} to 1×10^{13} genome copies/ml.

Protocol for Intracameral Injection of Therapeutic SiRNAs in the Eye to Lower IOP

Animals are prepared as described above.

Materials

siRNA for purinoceptor $P2Y_2$ receptors, β2 adrenergic receptors, carbonic anhydrase, RhoA kinase, and aquaporin-1 can be purchased from Sant Cruz Inc, Origene Inc, or Dharmacon Inc.

Aquaporin 1 (AQP1) Human siRNA cat#: SR319368, Aqp1 Mouse siRNA cat#: SR407722, Aqp1 Rat siRNA cat#: SR503304, Carbonic Anhydrase IV (CA4) Human siRNA cat#: SR300532, β2 Adrenergic Receptor (ADRB2) Human siRNA cat#: SR319287, β2 Adrenergic Receptor Rat siRNA cat#: SR504103, are available from Origene Inc. Rat AQP1 siRNA (r): sc-156108, is available from Sana Cruz Inc. β2 adrenergic receptor-human siRNA (h): sc-39866, and control (scrambled) siRNA-A: sc-37007 can purchased from Santa Cruz Inc. The synthetic sequences of siRhoA are homologous between human and mouse (5'-3') 5' GAAGUCA AGCAUUUCUGUC dTdT 3' and (3'-5') 3' dTdT CUUCA GUUCGUAAAGACAG 5' and can be custom-made by companies. miR-21-5p is available from AcceGen Biotechnology.

Intracameral Injection

siRNAs are mixed with sterile PBS (to prepare:1 μg, 3 μg, 5 μg, 10 μg/2μl). Mice are injected with different doses of siRNA (1 μg, 3 μg, 5 μg, 10 μg/eye) as described above. Another set of mice is injected with Cy3-scrambled siRNA or PBS as a control.

Protocol for Intravitreal Injection of Therapeutic Viruses

Animal Preparation

Animals are prepared as described above.

Intravitreal Injection

- Intravitreal injection can be performed under an ophthalmic microscope with a 33-gauge beveled needle attached to a 10-μl syringe (Hamilton, Reno, NV). The injections are performed through the sclera, approximately 1 mm behind the limbus, and 1-2 μl of AAV (2 x 10^{9-11}) is slowly (~30 s) injected into the vitreous chamber of the eye.
- A 30 s interval is kept before removing the needle gently.
- One drop of 0.3% ciprofloxacin antibiotic is applied to the eye following injection.

Notes

Virus preparation: AAV serotype such as ShH10-AAV is recommended to package therapeutic genes such as MMP1, PLAT, COX-2, FPR, and *Clostridium botulinum* C3 exoenzyme that can be produced in-house or *via* a commercial manufacturer. Intravitreal ShH10 AAV injection successfully transduces the ciliary epithelium in the interior chamber.

Ocular Non-Viral Delivery Methods

Non-viral methods can be broadly classified into physical- and chemical-based methods. Chemical-based vectors are generally comprised of materials that are less immunogenic compared to viral vectors. The physical methods allow for spatial precision (*i.e.*, site-specific delivery of DNA, Al-Dosari and Gao 2009). Other methods, such as electroporation, sonoporation, and optoporation (Batabyal *et al.*, 2020), are also being increasingly used.

Transfection of Anterior Chamber By Sonoporation

Sonoporation, a procedure using ultrasound waves, may be an effective and safe method to move genes across the cornea and sclera. Similar to electroporation, sonoporation physically creates transient and localized pores within cell membranes *via* ultrasound waves, allowing the transfer of DNA to the nucleus (Wells 2004). Sonoporation uses ultrasonic waves to induce cell membrane permeabilization, allowing gene entry. In each ultrasonic cycle of radiation, part of the energy of the spreading acoustic waves is absorbed by the cells, rendering the cell membrane permeable. The use of contrast agents (*e.g.*, Optison and Sonovue), which are air-filled microbubbles, can greatly enhance gene transfer efficiency by making the membranes more fluidic (Endoh *et al.* 2002). Once activated by ultrasonic waves, cavitation microbubbles rapidly oscillate, then expand followed by shrinking and bursting, leading to local shock waves that efficiently and transiently perforate the membrane of nearby cells. Kowalczuk *et al.* (2011) successfully transfected rat ciliary epithelium *in vivo* using sonoporation, which was detected at 7 days post-transfection. However, the expression decreased significantly after one month.

Protocol for Transfection of Anterior Chamber by Sonoporation

Animal Preparation

Animals are prepared as described above.

Ultrasound Apparatus

Sonoporation can be performed using the sonoporator model SP100 (Sonidel Ltd., Dublin, Ireland). Another system has been described by Kowalczuk *et al.* (2011) from Artison (the Sonitron 2000). These systems have a 3-5 mm transducer (operating with 1 MHz or 3 MHz) that can be positioned directly above the mouse cornea following intracameral injection. The following settings can be tested as a start: 1 MHz, 2 W/cm^2, 50% DC, and a total insonation time of 5 min.

The advantage of a pulsed mode of ultrasound (US) application is that adverse thermal effects can be reduced. The treatment time is adjustable from 0 to 20 min.

Microbubbles (MB)

Commercially available, ready-to-use microbubbles are available from Artison Corp. (Inola, OK, USA) or from Targson (San Diego, CA, USA). MB can be purchased with neutral charge or cationic, with the latter providing better transfection when mixed with plasmid DNA. The MB solution is approximately composed of 1 $x10^8$ microspheres/ml. MB are prepared according to the manufacturer's instructions.

Preparation of Plasmid-MB Complex

MB are first re-dispersed by gently shaking the vial for 10 s until obtaining a homogenous milky white suspension, after which, the desired volume of the dispersion is withdrawn from the vial.

Then, the bubbles (5×10^4 and 5×10^6) are added to the plasmid solution (3-6 μg) and mixed gently for 10 s to allow their combination immediately prior to their injection.

In vivo Sonoporation of the Anterior Chamber

During treatment, the eye is held in position using a surgical sheet. 3 to 6 μg of plasmid DNA alone or mixed with MB is first injected intracamerally, as described in section 1.1, under a surgical microscope. Then, the ultrasound tip is applied directly over the ocular surface after the interposition of a transparent gel (Genteal, Alcon), and the region injected is exposed to the US. The US probe should not be moved during treatment. US plus MB-mediated gene transfer is conducted using the following setting: 1 MHz, 2 W/cm^2 for 2 min, a duty cycle of 50% with a pulse width of 5 ms (on-time), a pulse interval of 5 ms (off-time) and fixed pulse-repetition-frequency (PRF) of 100 Hz.

Protocol for Transfection of the Anterior Chamber with siRNA by Topical Application

Animal Preparation

Animals are prepared as described earlier.

siRNAs of targeted genes (see section 2) are prepared in sterile saline solution (0.9%).

The siRNAs are topically applied in one eye, and the contralateral eye receives the same volume of saline solution (0.9% NaCl).

The single eye treated with the siRNAs receives an amount of 1-10 μg (mice) of the siRNA dissolved in 5 μl of 0.9% NaCl daily in a single dose on four consecutive days.

For dose-response studies, concentrations of 10, 20, and 30 μg are dissolved in 5 μl of 0.9% NaCl.

Upregulation or downregulation of proteins following scAAV transduction or siRNA treatment is assessed by western blot and immunohistochemistry (Dibas *et al.* 2008).

IOP Measurement

IOP is measured in mice using a handheld rebound tonometer (Icare TonoLab).

Briefly, mice are anesthetized by nose cone delivery of isoflurane and oxygen. The probe of the Tonolab tonometer is positioned perpendicular and approximately 3 mm from the mouse cornea. Upon initiation, the probe extends out and rebounds off the cornea six times, each time taking a measurement. The internal software discards the highest and lowest values and shows the average of the remaining four values as a single measurement. For each IOP measurement, three sequential but independent readings are obtained, averaged, and recorded. Tonolab measurements obtain baseline IOP prior to treatment. These measurements are averaged and taken as a single baseline value. After treatment, IOPs are measured twice weekly for the duration of each experiment.

FUTURE DIRECTIONS

Ocular Electroporation

The process of applying electrical pulses or high-voltage electrical currents, known as electroporation, introduces transient nanopores in the cell membrane. This allows negatively charged DNA entry into the cell and has been successful in most cell types. Large-size DNA >100 kb can be delivered successfully by electroporation with sustained expression lasting more than one year (Magin-Lachmann *et al.* 2004; Molnar *et al.* 2004). Although the exact mechanism by which the genetic material enters the cells is not known, repeated pulses appear to run the genetic material by electrophoresis (Escoffre *et al.* 2009). The genetic material used is not limited to DNA, but also RNA, as well as oligonucleotides such as siRNA were introduced inside cells (Golzio *et al.* 2005). While electroporation may be difficult for most organs due to location-restricted access, the anterior segment of the eye is easily accessible and, therefore, represents an attractive method for treating eye diseases. Several studies have shown the successful introduction of genes in the cornea (Blair-Parks *et al.* 2002, Rosazza *et al.* 2016, and Yu *et al.* 2003). Blair-Parks *et al.* have shown that electroporation increased gene expression by 1000-fold without corneal damage or inflammation.

The combined treatment with EP and bleomycin was found to decrease IOP more prominently than electroporation or bleomycin treatment alone in filtering surgery (Sakamoto *et al.* 1997). Trabeculectomy following matrix metalloproteinase-3 (MMP-3) cDNA into rabbit conjunctiva by electroporation caused significantly longer survival of filtering bleb and decreased levels of IOP in comparison to both trabeculectomy alone or trabeculectomy with mitomycin C (Mamiya *et al.* 2004). Venkatesh *et al.* 2013 and Matsuda and Cepko 2004 developed an electroporation methodology to transfect the retina following subretinal injection in rodents. However, there are no current research studies using electroporation to transduce TM for sustained IOP reduction.

Optoporation

Photoporation or optical transfection is an exciting method for transfection of genetic materials. The method utilizes ultrafast and ultrashort femtosecond-pulsed/continuous lasers providing near-infrared (700-1100 nm) multiphoton pulses that generate small transient pores (optoporation) for gene entry with similar efficiency of electroporation (Batabyal *et al.* 2021, Stevenson *et al.* 2010, Yao *et al.* 2008, Li and Huang 2007). The laser is administered through a continuous wave (CW) or pulse laser irradiation (Mohan *et al.* 2005). Although one major disadvantage of optoporation is the penetration depth (~ 2 mm), it can be a problem for human use for trabecular meshwork (TM), ciliary epithelium (CE) and ciliary muscle (CM) transfection as the human cornea depth is ~ 0.5-0.66 mm (Stevenson *et al.* 2010). Optoporation has been used successfully *in vitro*, *in vivo*, and ex vivo for transfection of the cornea (Mohan *et al.* 2011, Bemelmans *et al.* 2009, and Jumelle *et al.* 2016). In fact, Satoh *et al.* (2005) have shown successful transfection of EGFP prepared with PEI in both adult and newborn mouse central nervous system using laser that achieved penetration depth of 1.5 mm and 3.5 mm into the cortex surface of adult and newborn mice, respectively. Zeira *et al.* (2007) have shown that a 2-minute irradiation of intradermal injected luciferase plasmid induced enhanced expression that lasted > 7 months without any observed expression in the nonirradiated mice. However, the optoporation of therapeutic genes to TM for sustained IOP reduction is still under development.

Is Suprachoroidal Injection of Viral Vectors to Target the Anterior Chamber for IOP Lowering Possible?

Another method to lower the IOP may involve the suprachoroidal space, which forms part of the uveovortex pathway in the circulation of aqueous humor. Suprachoroidal space (SCS) injection of hyaluronic acid (HA) hydrogel enabled IOP reduction for 4 months in rabbits (Chae *et al.* 2021). Lowering IOP may be in part due to the expansion of the suprachoroidal space in addition to the action of the drug. In fact, Pederson *et al.* have shown that SCS expansion with Ringer's solution lowered IOP by 3-7 mmHg in rhesus macaque (Pederson *et al.* 1979). Hao *et al.* performed SCS injection with polyzwitterionic polycarboxybetaine hydrogel to expand SCS to increase the drainage of aqueous humor from the eye *via* the uveovortex pathway in rabbits. Such a treatment lowered IOP for at least 8 weeks. The suprachoroidal injection has been adopted for lowering IOP in glaucoma patients (Bailey *et al.* 2014, Kaplowitz *et al.* 2014, and Laroche *et al.* 2020). However, suprachoroidal injection of viruses has successfully transduced photoreceptors and retinal pigment epithelium (RPE) without affecting the anterior chamber (You *et al.* 2020). Therefore, SC injection may not be used to target TM.

CONCLUSION

Several techniques have been described in this chapter that permit genetic manipulation and transduction of certain genes in targeted ocular tissues to lower and control IOP in animal models of ocular hypertension/glaucoma. Such gene therapeutics offer the advantages of long-term IOP control through minimal perturbation of the ocular environment and without causing long-term side effects. The gene therapies may be combined with more traditional pharmaceutical treatment paradigms to achieve an even greater duration of action and a higher overall efficacy.

REFERENCES

Aga, M, Bradley, JM, Wanchu, R, Yang, Y, Acott, TS & Keller, KE (2014) Differential effects of caveolin-1 and -2 knockdown on aqueous outflow and altered extracellular matrix turnover in caveolin-silenced trabecular meshwork cells. *Invest Ophthalmol Vis Sci,* 55, 5497-509.
[http://dx.doi.org/10.1167/iovs.14-14519] [PMID: 25103269]

Al-Dosari, MS & Gao, X (2009) Nonviral gene delivery: principle, limitations, and recent progress. *AAPS J,* 11, 671-81.
[http://dx.doi.org/10.1208/s12248-009-9143-y] [PMID: 19834816]

Allison, K Racial disparity in the prevalence of glaucoma in the United States. *Eye Rep,* 5, 1.Available from: https://www.eyereports.org/index.php/eyereports/article/view/73 (2019)

Asokan, A, Schaffer, DV & Jude Samulski, R (2012) The AAV vector toolkit: poised at the clinical crossroads. *Mol Ther,* 20, 699-708.
[http://dx.doi.org/10.1038/mt.2011.287] [PMID: 22273577]

Bailey, AK, Sarkisian, SR, Jr & Vold, SD (2014) Ab interno approach to the suprachoroidal space. *J Cataract Refract Surg,* 40, 1291-4.
[http://dx.doi.org/10.1016/j.jcrs.2014.06.013] [PMID: 25088626]

Barraza, RA, McLaren, JW & Poeschla, EM (2010) Prostaglandin pathway gene therapy for sustained reduction of intraocular pressure. *Mol Ther,* 18, 491-501.
[http://dx.doi.org/10.1038/mt.2009.278] [PMID: 19953083]

Batabyal, S, Gajjeraman, S, Tchedre, K, Dibas, A, Wright, W & Mohanty, S (2020) Near-Infrared laser-based spatially targeted nano-enhanced optical delivery of therapeutic genes to degenerated retina. *Mol Ther Methods Clin Dev,* 17, 758-70.
[http://dx.doi.org/10.1016/j.omtm.2020.03.030] [PMID: 32355865]

Batabyal, S, Kim, S, Wright, W & Mohanty, S (2021) Laser-assisted targeted gene delivery to degenerated retina improves retinal function. *J Biophotonics,* 14, e202000234.
[http://dx.doi.org/10.1002/jbio.202000234] [PMID: 33026157]

Batra, M, Gupta, S, Nair, AB, Dhanawat, M, Sandal, S & Morsy, MA (2021) Netarsudil: A new ophthalmic drug in the treatment of chronic primary open angle glaucoma and ocular hypertension. *Eur J Ophthalmol,* 31, 2237-44.
[http://dx.doi.org/10.1177/11206721211008783] [PMID: 33843288]

Bemelmans, A-P, Arsenijevic, Y & Majo, F (2009) Efficient lentiviral gene transfer into corneal stroma cells using a femtosecond laser. *Gene Ther,* 16, 933-8.
[http://dx.doi.org/10.1038/gt.2009.41] [PMID: 19387484]

Blair-Parks, K, Weston, BC & Dean, DA (2002) High-level gene transfer to the cornea using electroporation. *J Gene Med,* 4, 92-100.
[http://dx.doi.org/10.1002/jgm.231] [PMID: 11828392]

Bogner, B, Boye, SL, Min, SH, Peterson, JJ, Ruan, Q, Zhang, Z, Reitsamer, HA, Hauswirth, WW & Boye, SE (2015) Capsid Mutated Adeno-Associated Virus Delivered to the Anterior Chamber Results in Efficient Transduction of Trabecular Meshwork in Mouse and Rat. *PLoS One,* 10, e0128759.
[http://dx.doi.org/10.1371/journal.pone.0128759] [PMID: 26052939]

Borrás, T, Buie, LK & Spiga, MG (2016) Inducible scAAV2.GRE.MMP1 lowers IOP long-term in a large animal model for steroid-induced glaucoma gene therapy. *Gene Ther,* 23, 438-49.
[http://dx.doi.org/10.1038/gt.2016.14] [PMID: 26855269]

Borrás, T, Buie, LK, Spiga, MG & Carabana, J (2015) Prevention of nocturnal elevation of intraocular pressure by gene transfer of dominant-negative RhoA in rats. *JAMA Ophthalmol,* 133, 182-90.
[http://dx.doi.org/10.1001/jamaophthalmol.2014.4747] [PMID: 25412195]

Borrás, T, Gabelt, BT, Klintworth, GK, Peterson, JC & Kaufman, PL (2001) Non-invasive observation of repeated adenoviral GFP gene delivery to the anterior segment of the monkey eye *in vivo*. *J Gene Med,* 3, 437-49.
[http://dx.doi.org/10.1002/jgm.210] [PMID: 11601757]

Borrás, T, Rowlette, LL, Erzurum, SC & Epstein, DL (1999) Adenoviral reporter gene transfer to the human trabecular meshwork does not alter aqueous humor outflow. Relevance for potential gene therapy of glaucoma. *Gene Ther,* 6, 515-24.
[http://dx.doi.org/10.1038/sj.gt.3300860] [PMID: 10476211]

Bozoglu, T, Lee, S, Ziegler, T, Jurisch, V, Maas, S, Baehr, A, Hinkel, R, Hoenig, A, Hariharan, A, Kim, CI, Decker, S, Sami, H, Koppara, T, Oellinger, R, Müller, OJ, Frank, D, Megens, R, Nelson, P, Weber, C, Schnieke, A, Sperandio, M, Santamaria, G, Rad, R, Moretti, A, Laugwitz, KL, Soehnlein, O, Ogris, M & Kupatt, C (2022) Endothelial Retargeting of AAV9 *In Vivo*. *Adv Sci (Weinh),* 9, 2103867.
[http://dx.doi.org/10.1002/advs.202103867] [PMID: 35023328]

Buie, LK, Rasmussen, CA, Porterfield, EC, Ramgolam, VS, Choi, VW, Markovic-Plese, S, Samulski, RJ, Kaufman, PL & Borrás, T (2010) Self-complementary AAV virus (scAAV) safe and long-term gene transfer

in the trabecular meshwork of living rats and monkeys. *Invest Ophthalmol Vis Sci,* 51, 236-48.
[http://dx.doi.org/10.1167/iovs.09-3847] [PMID: 19684004]

Chae, JJ, Jung, JH, Zhu, W, Gerberich, BG, Bahrani Fard, MR, Grossniklaus, HE, Ethier, CR & Prausnitz, MR (2021) Drug-Free, Nonsurgical Reduction of Intraocular Pressure for Four Months after Suprachoroidal Injection of Hyaluronic Acid Hydrogel. *Adv Sci (Weinh),* 8, 2001908.
[http://dx.doi.org/10.1002/advs.202001908] [PMID: 33511001]

Chern, KJ, Nettesheim, ER, Reid, CA, Li, NW, Marcoe, GJ & Lipinski, DM (2022) Prostaglandin-based rAAV-mediated glaucoma gene therapy in Brown Norway rats. *Commun Biol,* 5, 1169.
[http://dx.doi.org/10.1038/s42003-022-04134-w] [PMID: 36329259]

Davis, SA, Sleath, B, Carpenter, DM, Blalock, SJ, Muir, KW & Budenz, DL (2018) Drop instillation and glaucoma. *Curr Opin Ophthalmol,* 29, 171-7.
[http://dx.doi.org/10.1097/ICU.0000000000000451] [PMID: 29140818]

De Ieso, ML, Gurley, JM, McClellan, ME, Gu, X, Navarro, I, Li, G, Gomez-Caraballo, M, Enyong, E, Stamer, WD & Elliott, MH (2020) Physiologic Consequences of Caveolin-1 Ablation in Conventional Outflow Endothelia. *Invest Ophthalmol Vis Sci,* 61, 32.
[http://dx.doi.org/10.1167/iovs.61.11.32] [PMID: 32940661]

Dibas, A, Yang, MH, He, S, Bobich, J & Yorio, T (2008) Changes in ocular aquaporin-4 (AQP4) expression following retinal injury. *Mol Vis,* 14, 1770-83.
[PMID: 18836575]

Elliott, MH, Ashpole, NE, Gu, X, Herrnberger, L, McClellan, ME, Griffith, GL, Reagan, AM, Boyce, TM, Tanito, M, Tamm, ER & Stamer, WD (2016) Caveolin-1 modulates intraocular pressure: implications for caveolae mechanoprotection in glaucoma. *Sci Rep,* 6, 37127.
[http://dx.doi.org/10.1038/srep37127] [PMID: 27841369]

Ellliott, R, Lane, B, Buie, LK & Borrás, T (2014) Increasing the efficiency of gene therapy in glaucoma by selecting an optimal scAAV serotype. *Invest Ophthalmol Vis Sci,* 55, E–5649.

Escoffre, JM, Portet, T, Wasungu, L, Teissié, J, Dean, D & Rols, MP (2009) What is (still not) known of the mechanism by which electroporation mediates gene transfer and expression in cells and tissues. *Mol Biotechnol,* 41, 286-95.
[http://dx.doi.org/10.1007/s12033-008-9121-0] [PMID: 19016008]

Friedman DS, Wolfs RC, O'Colmain BJ, Klein BE, Taylor HR, West S, Leske MC, Mitchell P, Congdon N, Kempen J, & Eye Diseases Prevalence Research Group (2004). Prevalence of open-angle glaucoma among adults in the United States. Archives of Ophthalmology (Chicago, Ill. : 1960), 122(4), 532–538
[http://dx.doi.org/10.1001/archopht.122.4.532]

Gabelt, BAT, Hu, Y, Vittitow, JL, Rasmussen, CR, Grosheva, I, Bershadsky, AD, Geiger, B, Borrás, T & Kaufman, PL (2006) Caldesmon transgene expression disrupts focal adhesions in HTM cells and increases outflow facility in organ-cultured human and monkey anterior segments. *Exp Eye Res,* 82, 935-44.
[http://dx.doi.org/10.1016/j.exer.2005.12.002] [PMID: 16442523]

Gharahkhani, P, Jorgenson, E, Hysi, P, Khawaja, AP, Pendergrass, S, Han, X, Ong, JS, Hewitt, AW, Segrè, AV, Rouhana, JM, Hamel, AR, Igo, RP, Jr, Choquet, H, Qassim, A, Josyula, NS, Cooke Bailey, JN, Bonnemaijer, PWM, Iglesias, A, Siggs, OM, Young, TL, Vitart, V, Thiadens, AAHJ, Karjalainen, J, Uebe, S, Melles, RB, Nair, KS, Luben, R, Simcoe, M, Amersinghe, N, Cree, AJ, Hohn, R, Poplawski, A, Chen, LJ, Rong, SS, Aung, T, Vithana, EN, Allingham, RR, Brilliant, M, Budenz, DL, Bailey, JNC, Fingert, JH, Gaasterland, D, Gaasterland, T, Haines, JL, Hauser, M, Lee, RK, Lichter, PR, Liu, Y, Moroi, S, Myers, J, Pericak-Vance, M, Realini, A, Rhee, D, Richards, JE, Ritch, R, Schuman, JS, Scott, WK, Singh, K, Sit, AJ, Vollrath, D, Weinreb, RN, Wollstein, G, Zack, DJ, Sharma, S, Martin, S, Zhou, T, Souzeau, E, Landers, J, Fitzgerald, JT, Mills, RA, Craig, J, Burdon, K, Graham, SL, Casson, RJ, Goldberg, I, White, AJ, Healey, PR, Mackey, DA, Hewitt, AW, Shiono, M, Misumi, K, Kaieda, R, Harada, H, Minami, S, Emi, M, Emoto, N, Daida, H, Miyauchi, K, Murakami, A, Asai, S, Moriyama, M, Takahashi, Y, Fujioka, T, Obara, W, Mori, S, Ito, H, Nagayama, S, Miki, Y, Masumoto, A, Yamada, A, Nishizawa, Y, Kodama, K, Kutsumi, H, Sugimoto, Y, Koretsune, Y, Kusuoka, H, Yanaiag, H, Nagai, A, Hirata, M, Kamatani, Y, Muto, K, Matsuda, K,

Kiyohara, Y, Ninomiya, T, Tamakoshi, A, Yamagata, Z, Mushiroda, T, Murakami, Y, Yuji, K, Furukawa, Y, Zembutsu, H, Tanaka, T, Ohnishi, Y, Nakamura, Y, Jalanko, A, Kaprio, J, Donner, K, Kaunisto, M, Mars, N, Dada, A, Shcherban, A, Ganna, A, Lehisto, A, Kilpeläinen, E, Brein, G, Awaisa, G, Harju, J, Pärn, K, Della Briotta Parolo, P, Kajanne, R, Lemmelä, S, Sipilä, TP, Sipilä, T, Lyhs, U, Llorens, V, Niiranen, T, Kristiansson, K, Männikkö, L, Jiménez, MG, Perola, M, Wong, R, Kilpi, T, Hiekkalinna, T, Järvensivu, E, Kaiharju, E, Mattsson, H, Laukkanen, M, Laiho, P, Lähteenmäki, S, Sistonen, T, Soini, S, Ziemann, A, Lehtonen, A, Lertratanakul, A, Georgantas, B, Riley-Gillis, B, Quarless, D, Rahimov, F, Heap, G, Jacob, H, Waring, J, Davis, JW, Smaoui, N, Popovic, R, Esmaeeli, S, Waring, J, Matakidou, A, Challis, B, Close, D, Petrovski, S, Karlsson, A, Schleutker, J, Pulkki, K, Virolainen, P, Kallio, L, Mannermaa, A, Heikkinen, S, Kosma, V-M, Chen, C-Y, Runz, H, Liu, J, Bronson, P, John, S, Lahdenperä, S, Eaton, S, Zhou, W, Hendolin, M, Tuovila, O, Pakkanen, R, Maranville, J, Usiskin, K, Hochfeld, M, Plenge, R, Yang, R, Biswas, S, Greenberg, S, Laakkonen, E, Kononen, J, Paloneva, J, Kujala, U, Kuopio, T, Laukkanen, J, Kangasniemi, E, Savinainen, K, Laaksonen, R, Arvas, M, Ritari, J, Partanen, J, Hyvärinen, K, Wahlfors, T, Peterson, A, Oh, D, Chang, D, Teng, E, Strauss, E, Kerchner, G, Chen, H, Chen, H, Schutzman, J, Michon, J, Hunkapiller, J, McCarthy, M, Bowers, N, Lu, T, Bhangale, T, Pulford, D, Waterworth, D, Kulkarni, D, Xu, F, Betts, J, Gordillo, JE, Hoffman, J, Auro, K, McCarthy, L, Ghosh, S, Ehm, M, Pitkänen, K, Mäkelä, T, Loukola, A, Joensuu, H, Sinisalo, J, Eklund, K, Aaltonen, L, Färkkilä, M, Carpen, O, Kauppi, P, Tienari, P, Ollila, T, Tuomi, T, Meretoja, T, Pitkäranta, A, Turunen, J, Hannula-Jouppi, K, Pikkarainen, S, Seitsonen, S, Koskinen, M, Palomäki, A, Rinne, J, Metsärinne, K, Elenius, K, Pirilä, L, Koulu, L, Voutilainen, M, Juonala, M, Peltonen, S, Aaltonen, V, Loboda, A, Podgornaia, A, Chhibber, A, Chu, A, Fox, C, Diogo, D, Holzinger, E, Eicher, J, Gormley, P, Mehta, V, Wang, X, Kettunen, J, Pylkäs, K, Kalaoja, M, Karjalainen, M, Hinttala, R, Kaarteenaho, R, Vainio, S, Mantere, T, Remes, A, Huhtakangas, J, Junttila, J, Tasanen, K, Huilaja, L, Luodonpää, M, Hautala, N, Karihtala, P, Kauppila, S, Harju, T, Blomster, T, Soininen, H, Harvima, I, Pihlajamäki, J, Kaarniranta, K, Pelkonen, M, Laakso, M, Hiltunen, M, Kiviniemi, M, Kaipiainen-Seppänen, O, Auvinen, P, Kälviäinen, R, Julkunen, V, Malarstig, A, Hedman, Å, Marshall, C, Whelan, C, Lehtonen, H, Parkkinen, J, Linden, K, Kalpala, K, Miller, M, Bing, N, McDonough, S, Chen, X, Hu, X, Wu, Y, Auranen, A, Jussila, A, Uusitalo-Järvinen, H, Kankaanranta, H, Uusitalo, H, Peltola, J, Kähönen, M, Isomäki, P, Laitinen, T, Salmi, T, Muslin, A, Wang, C, Chatelain, C, Xu, E, Auge, F, Call, K, Klinger, K, Crohns, M, Gossel, M, Palin, K, Rivas, M, Siirtola, H, Tabuenca, JG, Aslam, T, Barman, S, Barrett, J, Bishop, P, Bunce, C, Carare, R, Chakravarthy, U, Chan, M, Cipriani, V, Day, A, Desai, P, Dhillon, B, Dick, A, Egan, C, Ennis, S, Foster, P, Fruttiger, M, Gallacher, J, Garway-Heath, D, Gibson, J, Gore, D, Guggenheim, J, Hardcastle, A, Harding, S, Hogg, R, Keane, PA, Khaw, PT, Khawaja, A, Lascaratos, G, Lotery, AJ, Luthert, P, Macgillivray, T, Mackie, S, Mcguinness, B, Mckay, G, Mckibbin, M, Mitry, D, Moore, T, Morgan, J, Muthy, Z, O'Sullivan, E, Owen, C, Patel, P, Paterson, E, Peto, T, Petzold, A, Rahi, J, Rudnicka, A, Self, J, Sivaprasad, S, Steel, D, Stratton, I, Strouthidis, N, Sudlow, C, Thaung, C, Thomas, D, Trucco, E, Tufail, A, Vernon, S, Viswanathan, A, Williams, C, Williams, K, Woodside, J, Yates, M, Yip, J, Zheng, Y, Tapp, R, Atan, D, Doney, A, allen, N, Littlejohns, T, Sergouniotis, P, Black, G, Kanyaro, N, Ntomoka, C, Massaga, JJ, Ikungura, JK, Agee, M, Aslibekyan, S, Bell, RK, Bryc, K, Clark, SK, Elson, SL, Fletez-Brant, K, Fontanillas, P, Furlotte, NA, Gandhi, PM, Heilbron, K, Hicks, B, Hinds, DA, Huber, KE, Jewett, EM, Jiang, Y, Kleinman, A, Lin, K-H, Litterman, NK, McCreight, JC, McIntyre, MH, McManus, KF, Mountain, JL, Mozaffari, SV, Nandakumar, P, Noblin, ES, Northover, CAM, O'Connell, J, Pitts, SJ, Poznik, GD, Sathirapongsasuti, JF, Shastri, AJ, Shelton, JF, Shringarpure, S, Tian, C, Tung, JY, Tunney, RJ, Vacic, V, Zare, AS, Tamiya, G, Shiga, Y, Yamamoto, M, Nakazawa, T, Currant, H, Birney, E, Wang, X, Auton, A, Lupton, MK, Martin, NG, Ashaye, A, Olawoye, O, Williams, SE, Akafo, S, Ramsay, M, Hashimoto, K, Kamatani, Y, Akiyama, M, Momozawa, Y, Foster, PJ, Khaw, PT, Morgan, JE, Strouthidis, NG, Kraft, P, Kang, JH, Pang, CP, Pasutto, F, Mitchell, P, Lotery, AJ, Palotie, A, van Duijn, C, Haines, JL, Hammond, C, Pasquale, LR, Klaver, CCW, Hauser, M, Khor, CC, Mackey, DA, Kubo, M, Cheng, C-Y, Craig, JE, MacGregor, S & Wiggs, JL (2021) Genome-wide meta-analysis identifies 127 open-angle glaucoma loci with consistent effect across ancestries. *Nat Commun,* 12, 1258.
[http://dx.doi.org/10.1038/s41467-020-20851-4] [PMID: 33627673]

Golzio, M, Mazzolini, L, Moller, P, Rols, MP & Teissié, J (2005) Inhibition of gene expression in mice muscle by *in vivo* electrically mediated siRNA delivery. *Gene Ther,* 12, 246-51.
[http://dx.doi.org/10.1038/sj.gt.3302405] [PMID: 15592423]

Hao, H, He, B, Yu, B, Yang, J, Xing, X & Liu, W (2022) Suprachoroidal injection of polyzwitterion hydrogel

for treating glaucoma. *Biomaterials Advances,* 142, 213162.
[http://dx.doi.org/10.1016/j.bioadv.2022.213162] [PMID: 36279749]

Heijl A, Leske MC, Bengtsson B, Hyman L, Bengtsson B, Hussein M, & Early Manifest Glaucoma Trial Group (2002). Reduction of intraocular pressure and glaucoma progression: results from the Early Manifest Glaucoma Trial. Archives of ophthalmology (Chicago, Ill. : 1960), 120(10), 1268–1279
[http://dx.doi.org/10.1001/archopht.120.10.1268]

Ito, YA, Belforte, N, Cueva Vargas, JL & Di Polo, A (2016) A magnetic microbead occlusion model to induce ocular hypertension-dependent glaucoma in mice. *J Vis Exp,* e53731, e53731.
[http://dx.doi.org/10.3791/53731-v] [PMID: 27077732]

Jimenez, A, Mediero, A & Loma, P (2009) Efficacy of topically administered siRNAs in glaucoma treatment: *in vivo* results in hypertensive model. *IOVS,* 50, 4054.

Jumelle, C, Mauclair, C, Houzet, J, Bernard, A, He, Z, Forest, F, Perrache, C, Gain, P & Thuret, G (2016) Delivery of macromolecules into the endothelium of whole ex vivo human cornea by femtosecond laser-activated carbon nanoparticles. *Br J Ophthalmol,* 100, 1151-6.
[http://dx.doi.org/10.1136/bjophthalmol-2015-307610] [PMID: 27226345]

Kaplowitz, K, Schuman, JS & Loewen, NA (2014) Techniques and outcomes of minimally invasive trabecular ablation and bypass surgery. *Br J Ophthalmol,* 98, 579-85.
[http://dx.doi.org/10.1136/bjophthalmol-2013-304256] [PMID: 24338085]

Kee, C, Sohn, S & Hwang, JM (2001) Stromelysin gene transfer into cultured human trabecular cells and rat trabecular meshwork *in vivo*. *Invest Ophthalmol Vis Sci,* 42, 2856-60.
[PMID: 11687529]

Laroche, D, Nkrumah, G & Ng, C (2020) Combination microinvasive glaucoma surgery: 23-gauge cystotome goniotomy and intra-scleral ciliary sulcus suprachoroidal microtube surgery in refractory and severe glaucoma: A case series. *Indian J Ophthalmol,* 68, 2557-61.
[http://dx.doi.org/10.4103/ijo.IJO_892_20] [PMID: 33120691]

Lee, ES, Rasmussen, CA, Filla, MS, Slauson, SR, Kolb, AW, Peters, DM, Kaufman, PL, Gabelt, BAT & Brandt, CR (2014) Prospects for lentiviral vector mediated prostaglandin F synthase gene delivery in monkey eyes *in vivo*. *Curr Eye Res,* 39, 859-70.
[http://dx.doi.org/10.3109/02713683.2014.884593] [PMID: 24559478]

Lee PP, Walt JG, Doyle JJ, Kotak SV, Evans SJ, Budenz DL, Chen PP, Coleman AL, Feldman RM, Jampel HD, Katz LJ, Mills RP, Myers JS, Noecker RJ, Piltz-Seymour JR, Ritch RR, Schacknow PN, Serle JB, & Trick GL. (2006). A multicenter, retrospective pilot study of resource use and costs associated with severity of disease in glaucoma. Archives of Ophthalmology (Chicago, Ill. : 1960), 124(1), 12–19
[http://dx.doi.org/10.1001/archopht.124.1.12]

Lei, Y, Song, M, Wu, J, Xing, C & Sun, X (2016) eNOS Activity in CAV1 Knockout Mouse Eyes. *Invest Ophthalmol Vis Sci,* 57, 2805-13.
[http://dx.doi.org/10.1167/iovs.15-18841] [PMID: 27228562]

Johnson, LN (2002) Glaucoma: our role in reducing the burden of blindness. *J Natl Med Assoc,* 94, 908-11.
[PMID: 12408696]

Leske MC, Connell AM, Schachat AP, & Hyman L. (1994). The Barbados Eye Study. Prevalence of open angle glaucoma. Archives of ophthalmology (Chicago, Ill. : 1960), 112(6), 821–829
[http://dx.doi.org/10.1001/archopht.1994.01090180121046]

Li, SD & Huang, L (2007) Non-viral is superior to viral gene delivery. *J Control Release,* 123, 181-3.
[http://dx.doi.org/10.1016/j.jconrel.2007.09.004] [PMID: 17935817]

Liu, X, Hu, Y, Filla, MS, Gabelt, BT, Peters, DM, Brandt, CR & Kaufman, PL (2005) The effect of C3 transgene expression on actin and cellular adhesions in cultured human trabecular meshwork cells and on outflow facility in organ cultured monkey eyes. *Mol Vis,* 11, 1112-21.
[PMID: 16379023]

Loma, P, Guzman-Aranguez, A, de Lara, MJP & Pintor, J (2018) Beta2 adrenergic receptor silencing change intraocular pressure in New Zealand rabbits. *J Optom,* 11, 69-74.
[http://dx.doi.org/10.1016/j.optom.2017.08.002] [PMID: 29132913]

Magin-Lachmann, C, Kotzamanis, G, D'Aiuto, L, Cooke, H, Huxley, C & Wagner, E (2004) *In vitro* and *in vivo* delivery of intact BAC DNA – comparison of different methods. *J Gene Med,* 6, 195-209.
[http://dx.doi.org/10.1002/jgm.481] [PMID: 14978773]

Mamiya, K, Ohguro, H, Ohguro, I, Metoki, T, Ishikawa, F, Yamazaki, H, Takano, Y, Ito, T & Nakazawa, M (2004) Effects of matrix metalloproteinase-3 gene transfer by electroporation in glaucoma filter surgery. *Exp Eye Res,* 79, 405-10.
[http://dx.doi.org/10.1016/j.exer.2004.06.017] [PMID: 15336503]

Marshall, EC (1989) Racial differences in the presentation of chronic open-angle glaucoma. *J Am Optom Assoc,* 60, 760-7.
[PMID: 2685083]

Martínez, T, González, MV, Roehl, I, Wright, N, Pañeda, C & Jiménez, AI (2014) In vitro and *in vivo* efficacy of SYL040012, a novel siRNA compound for treatment of glaucoma. *Mol Ther,* 22, 81-91.
[http://dx.doi.org/10.1038/mt.2013.216] [PMID: 24025749]

Martin-Gil, A, de Lara, MJP, Crooke, A, Santano, C, Peral, A & Pintor, J (2012) Silencing of P2Y $_2$ receptors reduces intraocular pressure in New Zealand rabbits. *Br J Pharmacol,* 165, 1163-72.
[http://dx.doi.org/10.1111/j.1476-5381.2011.01586.x] [PMID: 21740413]

Matsuda, T & Cepko, CL (2004) Electroporation and RNA interference in the rodent retina *in vivo* and *in vitro*. *Proc Natl Acad Sci USA,* 101, 16-22.
[http://dx.doi.org/10.1073/pnas.2235688100] [PMID: 14603031]

Mohan, RR, Tovey, JCK, Sharma, A & Tandon, A (2012) Gene therapy in the Cornea: 2005–present. *Prog Retin Eye Res,* 31, 43-64.
[http://dx.doi.org/10.1016/j.preteyeres.2011.09.001] [PMID: 21967960]

Molnar, MJ, Gilbert, R, Lu, Y, Liu, AB, Guo, A, Larochelle, N, Orlopp, K, Lochmuller, H, Petrof, BJ, Nalbantoglu, J & Karpati, G (2004) Factors influencing the efficacy, longevity, and safety of electroporation-assisted plasmid-based gene transfer into mouse muscles. *Mol Ther,* 10, 447-55.
[http://dx.doi.org/10.1016/j.ymthe.2004.06.642] [PMID: 15336645]

Moreno-Montañés, J, Sádaba, B, Ruz, V, Gómez-Guiu, A, Zarranz, J, González, MV, Pañeda, C & Jimenez, AI (2014) Phase I clinical trial of SYL040012, a small interfering RNA targeting β-adrenergic receptor 2, for lowering intraocular pressure. *Mol Ther,* 22, 226-32.
[http://dx.doi.org/10.1038/mt.2013.217] [PMID: 24025752]

Morrison, JC, Cepurna Ying Guo, WO & Johnson, EC (2011) Pathophysiology of human glaucomatous optic nerve damage: Insights from rodent models of glaucoma. *Exp Eye Res,* 93, 156-64.
[http://dx.doi.org/10.1016/j.exer.2010.08.005] [PMID: 20708000]

Nathan, N & Joos, KM (2016) Glaucoma Disparities in the Hispanic Population. *Semin Ophthalmol,* 31, 394-9.
[http://dx.doi.org/10.3109/08820538.2016.1154165] [PMID: 27128326]

Pederson JE, Gaasterland DE, & MacLellan HM. (1979). Experimental ciliochoroidal detachment. Effect on intraocular pressure and aqueous humor flow. Archives of Ophthalmology (Chicago, Ill. : 1960), 97(3), 536–541
[http://dx.doi.org/10.1001/archopht.1979.01020010280020]

Petrs-Silva, H, Dinculescu, A, Li, Q, Deng, WT, Pang, J, Min, SH, Chiodo, V, Neeley, AW, Govindasamy, L, Bennett, A, Agbandje-McKenna, M, Zhong, L, Li, B, Jayandharan, GR, Srivastava, A, Lewin, AS & Hauswirth, WW (2011) Novel properties of tyrosine-mutant AAV2 vectors in the mouse retina. *Mol Ther,* 19, 293-301.
[http://dx.doi.org/10.1038/mt.2010.234] [PMID: 21045809]

Rao, PV, Deng, P, Maddala, R, Epstein, DL, Li, CY & Shimokawa, H (2005) Expression of dominant negative Rho-binding domain of Rho-kinase in organ cultured human eye anterior segments increases aqueous humor outflow. *Mol Vis,* 11, 288-97.
[PMID: 15889013]

Rein DB, Zhang P, Wirth KE, Lee PP, Hoerger TJ, McCall N, Klein R, Tielsch JM, Vijan S, & Saaddine J. (2006). The economic burden of major adult visual disorders in the United States. Archives of Ophthalmology (Chicago, Ill. : 1960), 124(12), 1754–1760
[http://dx.doi.org/10.1001/archopht.124.12.1754]

Roddy, GW, Chowdhury, UR, Monson, KJ & Fautsch, MP (2021) Stanniocalcin-1 Reduced Intraocular Pressure in Two Models of Ocular Hypertension. *Curr Eye Res,* 46, 1525-30.
[http://dx.doi.org/10.1080/02713683.2021.1899246] [PMID: 33757401]

Rodriguez-Estevez, L, Asokan, P & Borrás, T (2020) Transduction optimization of AAV vectors for human gene therapy of glaucoma and their reversed cell entry characteristics. *Gene Ther,* 27, 127-42.
[http://dx.doi.org/10.1038/s41434-019-0105-4] [PMID: 31611639]

Rosazza, C, Haberl Meglic, S, Zumbusch, A, Rols, MP & Miklavcic, D (2016) Gene Electrotransfer: A Mechanistic Perspective. *Curr Gene Ther,* 16, 98-129.
[http://dx.doi.org/10.2174/1566523216666160331130040] [PMID: 27029943]

Sabatel, C, Malvaux, L, Bovy, N, Deroanne, C, Lambert, V, Gonzalez, MLA, Colige, A, Rakic, JM, Noël, A, Martial, JA & Struman, I (2011) MicroRNA-21 exhibits antiangiogenic function by targeting RhoB expression in endothelial cells. *PLoS One,* 6, e16979.
[http://dx.doi.org/10.1371/journal.pone.0016979] [PMID: 21347332]

Sakamoto, T, Oshima, Y, Sakamoto, M, Kawano, YI, Ishibashi, T, Inomata, H & Ohnishi, Y (1997) Electroporation and bleomycin in glaucoma-filtering surgery. *Invest Ophthalmol Vis Sci,* 38, 2864-8.
[PMID: 9418741]

Sander, JD & Joung, JK (2014) CRISPR-Cas systems for editing, regulating and targeting genomes. *Nat Biotechnol,* 32, 347-55.
[http://dx.doi.org/10.1038/nbt.2842] [PMID: 24584096]

Satoh, Y, Kanda, Y, Terakawa, M, Obara, M, Mizuno, K, Watanabe, Y, Endo, S, Ooigawa, H, Nawashiro, H, Sato, S & Takishima, K (2005) Targeted DNA transfection into the mouse central nervous system using laser-induced stress waves. *J Biomed Opt,* 10, 060501.
[http://dx.doi.org/10.1117/1.2128432] [PMID: 16409064]

Sommer A, Tielsch JM, Katz J, Quigley HA, Gottsch JD, Javitt J, & Singh K. (1991). Relationship between intraocular pressure and primary open angle glaucoma among white and black Americans. The Baltimore Eye Survey. Archives of Ophthalmology (Chicago, Ill. : 1960), 109(8), 1090–1095
[http://dx.doi.org/10.1001/archopht.1991.01080080050026]

Stein, JD, Ayyagari, P, Sloan, FA & Lee, PP (2008) Rates of glaucoma medication utilization among persons with primary open-angle glaucoma, 1992 to 2002. *Ophthalmology,* 115, 1315-1319.e1, 1319.e1.
[http://dx.doi.org/10.1016/j.ophtha.2007.12.017] [PMID: 18321581]

Stevenson, DJ, Gunn-Moore, FJ, Campbell, P & Dholakia, K (2010) Single cell optical transfection. *J R Soc Interface,* 7, 863-71.
[http://dx.doi.org/10.1098/rsif.2009.0463] [PMID: 20064901]

Tan, C, Jia, F, Zhang, P, Sun, X, Qiao, Y, Chen, X, Wang, Y, Chen, J & Lei, Y (2021) A miRNA stabilizing polydopamine nano-platform for intraocular delivery of miR-21-5p in glaucoma therapy. *J Mater Chem B Mater Biol Med,* 9, 3335-45.
[http://dx.doi.org/10.1039/D0TB02881A] [PMID: 33881417]

Tan, C, Song, M, Stamer, WD, Qiao, Y, Chen, X, Sun, X, Lei, Y & Chen, J (2020) miR-21-5p: A viable therapeutic strategy for regulating intraocular pressure. *Exp Eye Res,* 200, 108197.
[http://dx.doi.org/10.1016/j.exer.2020.108197] [PMID: 32871166]

Tham, YC, Li, X, Wong, TY, Quigley, HA, Aung, T & Cheng, CY (2014) Global prevalence of glaucoma and projections of glaucoma burden through 2040: a systematic review and meta-analysis. *Ophthalmology,* 121, 2081-90.
[http://dx.doi.org/10.1016/j.ophtha.2014.05.013] [PMID: 24974815]

Tielsch, JM, Sommer, A, Katz, J, Royall, RM, Quigley, HA & Javitt, J (1991) Racial variations in the prevalence of primary open-angle glaucoma. The Baltimore Eye Survey. *JAMA,* 266, 369-74.
[http://dx.doi.org/10.1001/jama.1991.03470030069026] [PMID: 2056646]

Vajaranant, TS, Wu, S, Torres, M & Varma, R (2012) The changing face of primary open-angle glaucoma in the United States: demographic and geographic changes from 2011 to 2050. *Am J Ophthalmol,* 154, 303-314.e3.
[http://dx.doi.org/10.1016/j.ajo.2012.02.024] [PMID: 22541661]

Venkatesh, A, Ma, S, Langellotto, F, Gao, G & Punzo, C (2013) Retinal gene delivery by rAAV and DNA electroporation. Curr Protoc Microbiol. 2013; Chapter 14:Unit 14D.4.
[http://dx.doi.org/10.1002/9780471729259.mc14d04s28]

Vittitow, JL, Garg, R, Rowlette, LL, Epstein, DL, O'Brien, ET & Borrás, T (2002) Gene transfer of dominant-negative RhoA increases outflow facility in perfused human anterior segment cultures. *Mol Vis,* 8, 32-44.
[PMID: 11889464]

Wang, S, Sengel, C, Emerson, MM & Cepko, CL (2014) A gene regulatory network controls the binary fate decision of rod and bipolar cells in the vertebrate retina. *Dev Cell,* 30, 513-27.
[http://dx.doi.org/10.1016/j.devcel.2014.07.018] [PMID: 25155555]

Watakabe, A, Ohtsuka, M, Kinoshita, M, Takaji, M, Isa, K, Mizukami, H, Ozawa, K, Isa, T & Yamamori, T (2015) Comparative analyses of adeno-associated viral vector serotypes 1, 2, 5, 8 and 9 in marmoset, mouse and macaque cerebral cortex. *Neurosci Res,* 93, 144-57.
[http://dx.doi.org/10.1016/j.neures.2014.09.002] [PMID: 25240284]

Wu, J, Bell, OH, Copland, DA, Young, A, Pooley, JR, Maswood, R, Evans, RS, Khaw, PT, Ali, RR, Dick, AD & Chu, CJ (2020) Gene Therapy for Glaucoma by Ciliary Body Aquaporin 1 Disruption Using CRISPR-Cas9. *Mol Ther,* 28, 820-9.
[http://dx.doi.org/10.1016/j.ymthe.2019.12.012] [PMID: 31981492]

Yao, CP, Zhang, ZX, Rahmanzadeh, R & Huettmann, G (2008) Laser-based gene transfection and gene therapy. *IEEE Trans Nanobiosci,* 7, 111-9.
[http://dx.doi.org/10.1109/TNB.2008.2000742] [PMID: 18556259]

Yiu, G, Chung, SH, Mollhoff, IN, Nguyen, UT, Thomasy, SM, Yoo, J, Taraborelli, D & Noronha, G (2020) Suprachoroidal and Subretinal Injections of AAV Using Transscleral Microneedles for Retinal Gene Delivery in Nonhuman Primates. *Mol Ther Methods Clin Dev,* 16, 179-91.
[http://dx.doi.org/10.1016/j.omtm.2020.01.002] [PMID: 32055646]

Yu, WZ, Li, XX, She, HC, He, PY, Dong, JQ, Rui, M & Ma, DL (2003) Gene transfer of kringle 5 of plasminogen by electroporation inhibits corneal neovascularization. *Ophthalmic Res,* 35, 239-46.
[http://dx.doi.org/10.1159/000072143] [PMID: 12920335]

Zeira, E, Manevitch, A, Manevitch, Z, Kedar, E, Gropp, M, Daudi, N, Barsuk, R, Harati, M, Yotvat, H, Troilo, PJ, Griffiths, TG, II, Pacchione, SJ, Roden, DF, Niu, Z, Nussbaum, O, Zamir, G, Papo, O, Hemo, I, Lewis, A & Galun, E (2007) Femtosecond laser: a new intradermal DNA delivery method for efficient, long-term gene expression and genetic immunization. *FASEB J,* 21, 3522-33.
[http://dx.doi.org/10.1096/fj.06-7528com] [PMID: 17575264]

CHAPTER 44

Protocol for the Delivery of Stem Cells as Trabecular Meshwork

Anthonia Okolie[1], **Ya Fatou Njie Mbye**[1], **Fatima Muili**[1], **Catherine A. Opere**[2] and **Sunny E. Ohia**[1,*]

[1] *Department of Pharmaceutical Sciences, College of Pharmacy and Health Sciences, Texas Southern University, 3100 Cleburne Street, Houston, TX 77004, USA*

[2] *Department of Pharmacy Sciences, School of Pharmacy and Health Professions, Creighton University, Omaha, Nebraska, USA*

Abstract: In this chapter, the protocol for the delivery of stem cells as trabecular meshwork cell replacement therapy is described. There are several types of stem cells that have been investigated in ocular regenerative medicine, such as induced pluripotent stem cells, mesenchymal stem cells, tissue-specific stem cells (progenitor cells), and adipose tissue-derived stem cells. These stem cells have the capacity to differentiate into functional cells and have been used in various *ex vivo* and animal models of glaucoma to restore intraocular pressure (IOP) homeostasis and trabecular meshwork (TM) cellularity. The protocol provides a series of steps that can serve as a guide for researchers in the production and use of induced pluripotent stem cells (iPSCs) as cell replacement therapy for the TM, which is damaged and/or lost due to ocular hypertension-induced glaucomatous condition.

Keywords: Intraocular pressure, Induced pluripotent stem cells (iPSCs), Progenitor cells, Stem cells, Trabecular meshwork.

INTRODUCTION

The trabecular meshwork (TM) constitutes the main pathway for the drainage of aqueous humor (AQH) from the eye (Fan *et al.*, 2021). Anatomically, the TM is located within the iridocorneal angle (the recess between the cornea and the anterior surface of the attached margin of the iris). The role of the TM is to regulate the outflow of aqueous humor from the anterior chamber of the eye into the adjacent Schlemm's canal. A defect in this function leads to resistance to outflow, elevated intraocular pressure (IOP) (ocular hypertension [OHT]), and the

* **Corresponding author Sunny E. Ohia:** Department of Pharmaceutical Sciences, College of Pharmacy and Health Sciences, Texas Southern University, 3100 Cleburne Street, Houston, TX 77004, USA; E-mail: Sunny.Ohia@TSU.edu

Najam A. Sharif and Sunny E. Ohia (Eds.)

risk of glaucoma. Glaucoma is an optic neuropathy and one of the leading causes of vision loss worldwide. It is characterized by irreversible optic nerve damage and progressive vision loss (Fan *et al.*, 2021). Studies show that in glaucoma, there is decreased TM cellularity, TM cell loss, abnormal accumulation of extracellular matrix (ECM) components, and increased stiffness of TM (Weinreb and Khaw, 2004; Epstein, 2012). Treatment strategies to reduce IOP include drug therapies that target TM as therapeutics, such as Rho-kinase inhibitors, adenosine agonists, prostaglandin receptor agonists, and potentially inhibitors of SPARC (a fibrotic protein), as well as surgical interventions (Schehlein and Robin, 2019; Chan *et al.*, 2019). However, since OHT-induced glaucomatous damage primarily begins in the front of the eye, TM cells endeavor to correct the imbalance in ECM production/deposition by releasing proteases that digest the ECM and then phagocytosing the byproducts, thereby clearing the AQH outflow pathway and lowering IOP. Thus, the use of stem cells to regenerate lost or damaged TM tissue has been proposed as a novel means to treat OHT/glaucoma (Zhou *et al.*, 2020; Fan *et al.*, 2021; Coulon *et al.*, 2022). The purpose of this chapter is to provide a series of steps that can serve as a guide for researchers in the generation and use of induced pluripotent stem cells (iPSCs) to successfully deliver to the TM for TM regeneration and as cell replacement therapy.

EXPERIMENTAL PROTOCOLS

The following procedures were developed according to general considerations for the ethical use of stem cells in research. We focus mostly on methods adapted for human tissue-derived cells for brevity and relevance. Essentially, technology has advanced to a point where almost any somatic cell can be reprogramed into iPSCs by transfecting them with the specific Yamanaka factors (SOX2, KLF4, OCT4, and cMyc) (please see Kumar *et al.* (2020) and references therein for more information). Since the neural crest derivation of TM cells occurs during embryonic development, it was hypothesized that iPSCs could first be induced to differentiate into neural crest cells (NCCs) and then differentiate them into TM cells. Thus, human iPSCs were initially created by reprogramming human dermal fibroblasts, and their properties were determined as previously described (Lin *et al.*, 2012). In this study, human iPSCs were differentiated into TM cells via the NCC stage utilizing the conditioned media and ECM derived from cultured primary human TM cells.

Production and use of iPSCs for TM Repair

- Using the differentiated human iPSC-TM cells from the aforementioned procedures, culture them using mTeSR medium supplemented with fibroblast growth factor 2 (FGF2) (final concentration of FGF2 at 100ng/ml) on Matrigel

(Corning)-coated plates minus the feeder cells in an incubator at 37°C in an atmosphere of 5% CO_2 (Kumar *et al.*, 2020).

- The culture medium should be changed as soon as the cells reach 80-90% confluency.
- Use Accutase to dissociate the iPSC colonies, dilute the enzyme in the plate with fresh medium (5-10 ml) lacking any growth factors, centrifuge the mixture, and discard the medium containing the enzyme.
- Resuspend cells into a fresh mTeSR medium and dispense into A549 cell-derived ECM-coated plates for 3 days (Kumar *et al.*, 2020).
- Switch the medium after 3 days to N2B27 medium (DMEM/F12 (1:1) supplemented with 2% B27, 1% N2, 100X Glutamax, 100U/ml penicillin, and 100mg/ml streptomycin with 100 mM Rho kinase inhibitor Y27632 (to induce NCC differentiation) for 10 days.
- Upon establishing a pool of NCCs, differentiate them further into TM cells (see below).
- Following the above procedures, dissociate the NCCs with Accutase as mentioned above and seed onto new TM ECM-coated culture plates. The ECM should be created by lysing >90% confluent TM cells with 0.02 N ammonium hydroxide and 0.05% Triton X-100 for five minutes, decanting the fluid, and storing the plates at -20°C until needed.
- Use TM cell-conditioned culture medium (DMEM/F12 (1:1) with 10% FBS) to induce the cells over 10–14 days. Stain samples of cells to check for the appearance of some TM-cell membrane/cytosol markers such as tissue inhibitor of matrix metalloproteinase-3 (TIMP3), aquaporin-1 (AQP-1) and chitinase 3 like 1 (CHI3L1), thus indicating differentiation into TM cells. Additional checks on the cell identity may include responsiveness to a corticosteroid such as dexamethasone, which would induce ECM and myocilin production and induce cross-linking of actin networks detectable by immunofluorescence studies.
- The iPSC-TM cells can then be transplanted into the anterior eye chamber of animal model systems by intracameral injection to observe whether they integrate into the existing TM structure.

Induction of TM Cells from Mesenchymal Stem Cells

The protocol used for the induction of TM cells from mouse mesenchymal stem cells is described by Nadri *et al.* (2013).

- Isolate bone marrow mononuclear cells (BMMC) by aspiration from the femur and tibia of 2-month-old mice using density gradient centrifugation.
- Suspend the cells in Dulbecco's modified Eagle's medium (DMEM) containing 2 μM L-glutamine, 100 U/mL penicillin, 100 μg/mL streptomycin, and 20% heat-inactivated fetal bovine serum.

- Now plate the BMM cells in 75 cm^2 tissue culture flasks and incubate at 37°C in 5% CO_2 humidified air.
- After 48 hours, remove non-adherent cells and allow the adherent cells to grow to ~90% confluency.
- Passage the cells over the next 3–4 days using a fresh culture medium.
- Next, co-culture BMM cells with the TM cell line (MUTM-NEI/1) in 75 cm^2 adherent tissue culture flasks in TM cell medium containing Iscove's Modified Dulbecco's Medium supplemented with 20% FBSI and L-glutamine, penicillin, and streptomycin at 37°C.
- Identify the TM cell markers on the cultured cells using immunostaining procedures before transplantation into the anterior chamber of the recipient rodent as TM cell replacement therapy. Follow the progress of the transplantation and any IOP changes.

Induction of TM Cells from TM Progenitor Stem Cells

The methodology used for the induction of TM cells from TM progenitor stem cells was identical to that described by Fan *et al.* (2021) and Coulon *et al.* (2022).

- Dissect the TM tissue from human corneal rims.
- Treat tissue with collagenase for 1 hour to dissociate the tissue.
- Culture the isolated stroma tissue segments in low glucose DMEM medium supplemented with 20% serum and basic-fibroblast growth factor-2 for isolating the TM progenitor cells
- Passage the TM progenitor cells twice in the same medium.
- Perform cell sorting by neurosphere assay method for the generation of free-floating TM spheres by culturing TM cells in StemSpan™ Serum-Free Expansion Medium or the formation of cell populations using fluorescence-activated cell sorting.
- The cells produced by this method can now be checked for TM cell markers as previously described above and then can be used for transplantation.

Induction of TM Cells from Adipose Tissue-Derived Stem Cells

The methodology used for the induction of TM cells from adipose tissue-derived stem cells is essentially the same as described by Zhou *et al.* (2020).

- Isolate human adipose tissue-derived stem cells (ADSCs) from human lipoaspirate samples following digestion with collagenase, dilution with buffer to inactivate the enzyme, and then differential centrifugation.
- The washed and pelleted cells from above should be dispersed and then induced by co-culturing with primary human TM cells by seeding on TM-ECM-coated culture plates.

- Wash away the lysed cell debris with PBS and collect the TM-conditioned medium on the third day after TM cells are passaged at 5 x 10^3 cells/cm^2 (at passages 3-5).
- Seed the ADSCs at 2 x 10^3 cells/cm^2 and cultured on TM-secreted-ECM culture plates in culture medium containing 50% DMEM/F12%-10% and 50% conditioned medium for 10 days until clear morphological changes of TM differentiation are observed, as judged by the appearance of TM cell markers determined by immunofluorescence techniques.
- Change the culture medium every 3 days prior to harvesting of confluent cells. These can now be used for transplantation as necessary.

CONCLUSION

The protocols described here have been used in previous studies to successfully induce TM-like cells for TM restoration as stem cell-based therapy in animal models of OHT/glaucoma. The chapter does not contain an exhaustive report of all applicable methods, and readers are encouraged to consult some of the original publications on this subject.

REFERENCES

Chan, PP, Pang, JC & Tham, CC (2019) Acute primary angle closure–treatment strategies, evidences and economical considerations. *Eye (Lond),* 33, 110-9.
[http://dx.doi.org/10.1038/s41433-018-0278-x] [PMID: 30467424]

Coulon, SJ, Schuman, JS, Du, Y, Bahrani Fard, MR, Ethier, CR & Stamer, WD (2022) A novel glaucoma approach: Stem cell regeneration of the trabecular meshwork. *Prog Retin Eye Res,* 90, 101063.
[http://dx.doi.org/10.1016/j.preteyeres.2022.101063] [PMID: 35398015]

Epstein, DL (2012) Framing glaucoma questions: what are the opportunities for glaucoma treatment? A personal perspective. *Invest Ophthalmol Vis Sci,* 53, 2462-3.
[http://dx.doi.org/10.1167/iovs.12-9483c] [PMID: 22562840]

Fan, X, Bilir, EK, Kingston, OA, Oldershaw, RA, Kearns, VR, Willoughby, CE & Sheridan, CM (2021) Replacement of the trabecular meshwork cells—a way ahead in IOP control? *Biomolecules,* 11, 1371.
[http://dx.doi.org/10.3390/biom11091371] [PMID: 34572584]

Kumar, A, Cheng, T, Song, W, Cheuk, B, Yang, E, Yang, L, Xie, Y & Du, Y (2020) Two-step induction of trabecular meshwork cells from induced pluripotent stem cells for glaucoma. *Biochem Biophys Res Commun,* 529, 411-7.
[http://dx.doi.org/10.1016/j.bbrc.2020.05.225] [PMID: 32703444]

Nadri, S, Yazdani, S, Arefian, E, Gohari, Z, Eslaminejad, MB, Kazemi, B & Soleimani, M (2013) Mesenchymal stem cells from trabecular meshwork become photoreceptor-like cells on amniotic membrane. *Neurosci Lett,* 541, 43-8.
[http://dx.doi.org/10.1016/j.neulet.2012.12.055] [PMID: 23403103]

Schehlein, EM & Robin, AL (2019) Rho-associated kinase inhibitors: evolving strategies in glaucoma treatment. *Drugs,* 79, 1031-6.
[http://dx.doi.org/10.1007/s40265-019-01130-z] [PMID: 31134520]

Weinreb, RN & Khaw, PT (2004) Primary open-angle glaucoma. *Lancet,* 363, 1711-20.
[http://dx.doi.org/10.1016/S0140-6736(04)16257-0] [PMID: 15158634]

Zhou, Y, Xia, X, Yang, E, Wang, Y, Marra, KG, Ethier, CR, Schuman, JS & Du, Y (2020) Adipose-derived stem cells integrate into trabecular meshwork with glaucoma treatment potential. *FASEB J,* 34, 7160-77. [http://dx.doi.org/10.1096/fj.201902326R] [PMID: 32259357]

CHAPTER 45

Isolation and Characterization of Trabecular Meshwork Stem Cell Exosomes from the Conditioned Medium

Iswarya Radhakrishnan[1,2], Krishnadas Subbaiah[3], Muthukkaruppan Veerappan[1], Dharmalingam Kuppamuthu[2,4] and Gowri Priya Chidambaranathan[1,2,*]

[1] *Department of Immunology and Stem Cell Biology, Aravind Medical Research Foundation, Madurai, Tamil Nadu, India*

[2] *Department of Biotechnology, Aravind Medical Research Foundation - Affiliated to Alagappa University, Karaikudi, Tamil Nadu, India*

[3] *Glaucoma Services, Aravind Eye Hospital and Post Graduate Institute of Ophthalmology, Madurai, Tamil Nadu, India*

[4] *Department of Proteomics, Aravind Medical Research Foundation, Madurai, Tamil Nadu, India*

Abstract: Exosomes are nanovesicles (30-200nm) whose cargo includes proteins, RNA of different types, DNA, lipids, and small molecules. The exosome-based therapy is gaining significance in modern medicine due to the signal transduction capabilities and non-immunogenic properties of exosomes. In regenerative medicine, stem cell-derived exosomes are employed as an alternative in cell therapies. Currently, there are more than 35 ongoing clinical trials worldwide employing exosomes in various disease conditions, including two eye diseases. However, the efficacy of these nanovesicles in glaucoma therapy still remains unexplored. Trabecular meshwork (TM) is a tiny, porous tissue located in the iridocorneal angle of the eye that maintains intraocular pressure (IOP) homeostasis. The adult stem cells are located in the non-filtering region and are drastically reduced in glaucomatous conditions (Sundaresan *et al.*, 2021). Our previous TM stem cells (TMSC) transplantation studies on a human organ culture of anterior segment (HOCAS) model (Iswarya *et al.*, ISSCR 2021) and several other studies on animal models (Yun *et al.*, 2018; Xiong *et al.*, 2021,) promise the application of TMSCs in glaucoma therapy. To evaluate the efficacy of the TMSC exosomes as an alternative to cell-free therapy for glaucoma, we optimized a few *in vitro* assays, which give insights into the properties of isolated exosomes. This chapter describes protocols to isolate exosomes by ultracentrifugation, characterization by nan-

[*] **Corresponding author Gowri Priya Chidambaranathan:** Department of Immunology and Stem Cell Biology, Aravind Medical Research Foundation, Madurai, Tamil Nadu, India; Tel: +91452-4356550; Ext: 433/441; Fax: 91-452-2530984; E-mail: gowri@aravind.org

Najam A. Sharif and Sunny E. Ohia (Eds.)

oparticle tracking analysis (NTA), Western blot analysis, and transmission electron microscopy (TEM). Further, the functional efficacy of the exosomes was evaluated by *in vitro* wound healing assay and an anti-oxidant assay.

Keywords: Anti-oxidant, Conditioned medium, Exosomes, Glaucoma, *In vitro* wound healing, Nanoparticle tracking analysis (NTA), Trabecular meshwork stem cells, Transmission electron microscopy (TEM), Ultracentrifugation, Western blotting.

INTRODUCTION

Exosomes are nanovesicles (30-200nm) that contain a variety of biomolecules, such as proteins, lipids, and nucleic acids. The exosomes gained importance in therapeutic applications because of their size and ability to cross blood barriers as well as other barriers such as the blood-brain barrier (BBB), blood-cerebrospinal fluid barrier (BCSFB), blood–lymph barrier (BlyB), blood–air barrier (BAB), stromal barrier (SB), blood–labyrinth barrier (BLaB), blood-retinal barrier (BRB), and placental barrier (PB). Non-immunogenicity and the ability to transduce signals make them ideal nanocarriers. They can be engineered to carry specific cargo and deliver to specific targets. The exosomes mediate cell-to-cell communication and many other cellular processes through their cargo. The exosomes are excellent biomarkers as well. Mesenchymal stem cell (MSC) exosomes have gained significant attention in recent years as they can replace the need for MSC-based therapy. Currently, there are more than 35 ongoing clinical trials using MSC exosomes worldwide, including two eye diseases, which emphasize the efficacy of exosomes in cell-free therapy (https://www.clinicaltrials.gov/). However, there are no reports on the exosome-based therapy for glaucoma.

Trabecular meshwork (TM), a tiny, porous tissue located at the iridocorneal angle of the eye, is responsible for intraocular pressure (IOP) homeostasis. The stem cells for TM (TMSCs) are located in the non-filtering region (Sundaresan *et al.*, 2019), which is drastically reduced in glaucomatous conditions (Sundaresan *et al.*, 2021). Transplantation of TMSCs in cell loss human organ culture of anterior segment (HOCAS) model (Iswarya *et al.*, ISSCR 2021- unpublished data) and several other studies on animal models (Yun *et al.*, 2018; Xiong *et al.*,2021) enhanced TM cell proliferation and reducted in IOP, indicating the possibility of developing a stem cell therapy for glaucoma. Therefore, there is a huge potential for the use of TMSC exosomes for the treatment of glaucoma.

The purpose of this chapter is to describe our optimized, simple–to-use, and reliable methods to isolate and characterize exosomes from TMSC-derived conditioned medium since the use of proper isolation method is essential to maintain the integrity and functional competence of the exosomes.

TMSC Culture Establishment

Materials

Trabecular meshwork from donor eyes, 35mm dish, collagenase A (Roche, Germany), serum-free medium, pipettes, 15 ml falcon tubes, Stem Cell Growth Medium (SCGM- Opti-MEM, 5%FBS (Gibco- Thermofisher Scientific, USA), 200µg/ml calcium chloride, 0.08% chondroitin sulfate, 20µg/ml ascorbic acid, 100µg/ml bovine pituitary extract (Sigma-Aldrich, Darmstadt, Germany), 10ng/ml EGF (Invitrogen- Thermofisher Scientific, USA), pipettes, and tips.

Procedure

Sample: For TM tissues, whole globes (not suitable for transplantation) and corneoscleral rims (after removal of the cornea for transplantation) were obtained from the eye banks of Aravind Eye Hospitals.

- TM was carefully removed from the rims using fine forceps and digested with 4mg/ml collagenase A for 2 hours at 37°C in a CO_2 incubator (Stamer *et al.*, 1995).
- After incubation, the reaction was stopped by adding a complete medium and centrifuged at 1500g for 5 minutes.
- The cells were suspended in SCGM and cultured for 3-4 weeks (Du *et al.*, 2012) with the media change in alternative days.
- When the cells reached confluency, they were trypsinized and passaged in T75 flasks to obtain adequate cells for conditioned medium collection (Fig. **1**).

Conditioned Medium Collection

Materials

SCGM, Opti-MEM (31985-070- Thermofisher Scientific, USA), T75 flasks, serum-free medium, 10ml serological pipettes, culture grade PBS, exosome depleted FBS (System Biosciences, California, USA), and 50 ml falcon tubes.

Procedure

- Seed 2.1 $x10^6$ TMSCs in T75 flasks and maintain them for two days to reach confluency.
- Upon confluency, remove the medium with a sterile serological pipette and wash the adhered cells with PBS five times gently.

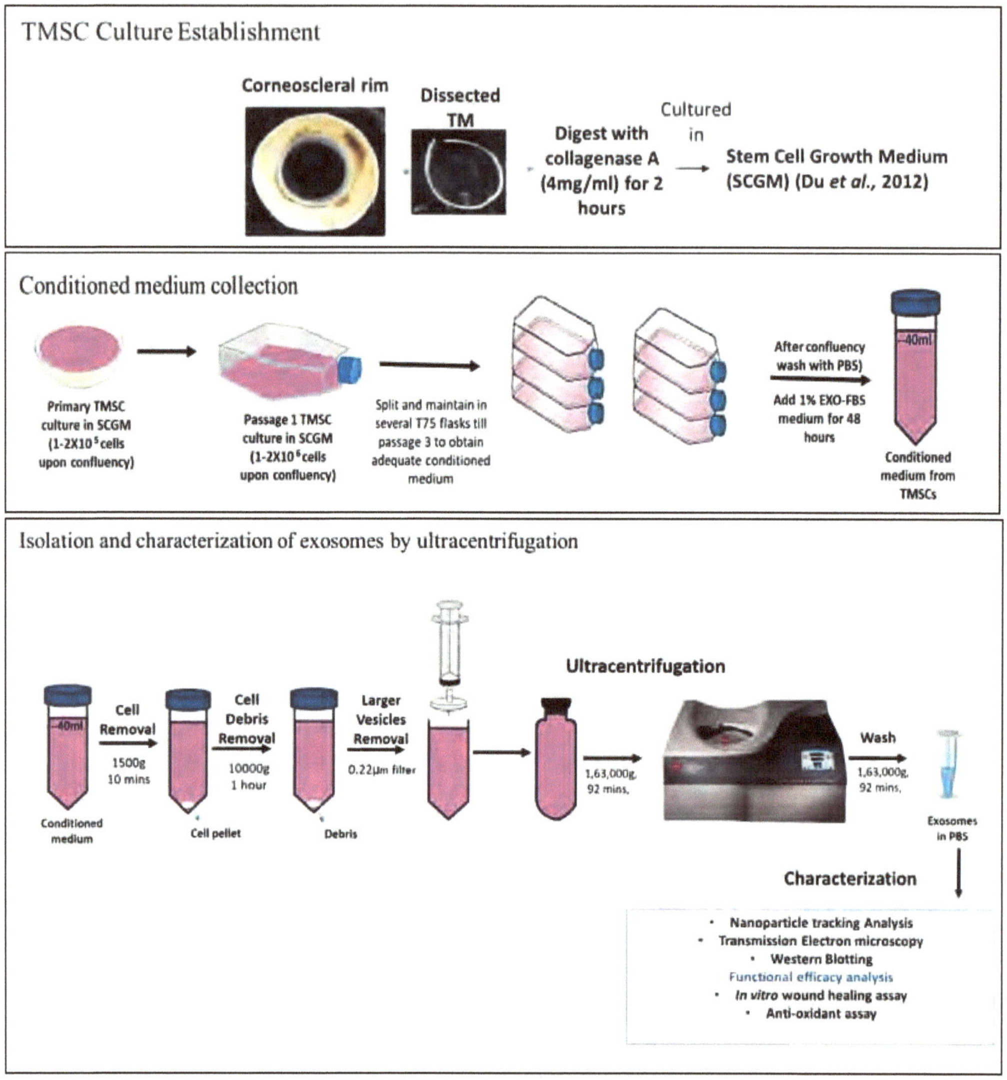

Fig, (1). Graphical representation of salient features explained under this protocol.

Note: Five PBS washes will be required to remove the interfering serum proteins, especially serum albumin.

Washing should be done gently as the confluent monolayer cells will detach easily upon mechanical damage compared to less confluent cultures.

- Add 10 ml of Opti-MEM with 1% exosome-depleted FBS.
- Incubate the cells for 48 hours with 5% CO_2 at 37° C.

- After incubation, collect the conditioned medium in 50ml falcon tubes, label them, and store the tubes at -80°C for further use.

Exosome Isolation by Ultracentrifugation

Note: To eliminate the other vesicles and debris, differential centrifugation followed by ultracentrifugation is recommended.

Materials

Ultracentrifuge (Optima MAX XP, Beckman Coulter, California, USA), Optiseal (29.9ml), 1 ml ultracentrifuge tubes (Beckman Coulter, California, USA-Cat#361625, 343778), MLA-50 and MLA-130 rotors, TMSC conditioned medium, filter sterilized PBS, and 0.22micron syringe filter.

Note: Keep the rotors at 4°C overnight before use for fast equilibration.

Procedure

- Thaw the conditioned medium and spin at 1500 g for 10 minutes at 4°C to remove cells.
- Transfer the supernatant to a fresh 50 ml tube and centrifuge at 10,000g for 60 minutes at 4° C to remove cell debris.
- Filter the supernatant using a 0.22 micron syringe filter to eliminate the larger vesicles.
- Transfer the filtrate to the ultracentrifuge tubes.
- Balance the tubes.

Note: A minimum of 40 ml of conditioned medium is needed for characterization experiments. This should be increased for analyzing low abundance protein markers in Western blotting.

Before ultracentrifugation, the opposite tubes should be balanced within a 5mg difference to avoid damage to the instrument. For this, label the tubes properly, weigh the tubes using a fine weighing balance, and remove or add medium according to the need. Avoid covering the writing with sellotape.

- Place the tubes in the MLA-50 rotor and follow instrument instructions for centrifugation. Centrifuge at 1,63,000 g for 92 minutes at 4°C.
- After completion of the run, remove the tubes from the rotor and place them in the proper holder; carefully remove the supernatant and suspend the pellet in one ml of sterile PBS.

Note: The pellet might not be visible in the majority of the samples. In such cases, mark the approximate pellet position in the ultracentrifuge tubes and gently aspirate the supernatant without disturbing the marked area.

If the pellets from multiple tubes are pooled after the first spin, make the total resuspension volume to one ml, which will minimize the loss by multiple pooling.

- Transfer the suspended exosomes to one ml ultracentrifuge tubes, place them in MLA-130 rotor, and repeat the centrifugation at 1,63,000 g for 92 minutes at 4°C. (Fig. **1**).

Note: The second spin is given to minimize protein contamination from the conditioned medium. If multiple tubes are pooled, a beige/white pellet might be visible at this point. Proceed to the next step, even if a pellet is not visible.

- Resuspend the pellet in 100µl of PBS and aliquot them for further experiments.

Note: *Multiple freeze-thaw cycles affect the nature of exosomes and hence aliquot the exosomes immediately after isolation, which are then stored at -80° C. It is reported that exosomes can be stored for long periods, but in our experience, we used exosomes stored for several weeks without any observable change.*

CHARACTERIZATION OF ISOLATED EXOSOMES

Nanoparticle Tracking Analysis (NTA)

Materials

NTA- instrument-NS300, 0.22-micron syringe filters, PBS, MilliQ water, one ml disposable syringe, 1.5 ml Eppendorf tubes, pipettes, and tips.

Procedure (Figs. **2** and **3**)

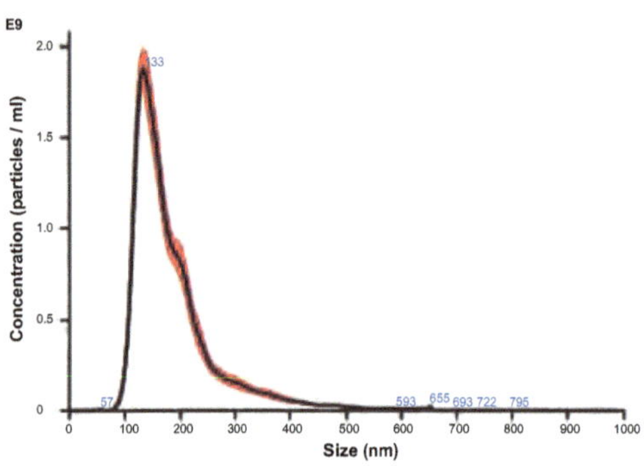

Results

Stats: Mean +/- Standard Error	
Mean:	188.7 +/- 1.6 nm
Mode:	136.5 +/- 2.7 nm
SD:	85.5 +/- 2.0 nm
D10:	120.2 +/- 0.7 nm
D50:	163.4 +/- 1.6 nm
D90:	296.3 +/- 6.5 nm
Concentration (Upgrade):	1.75e+11 +/- 5.62e+09 particles/ml
	42.6 +/- 1.4 particles/frame
	48.8 +/- 2.2 centres/frame

Fig, (2). Representative NTA graph and results of freshly isolated TMSC exosomes

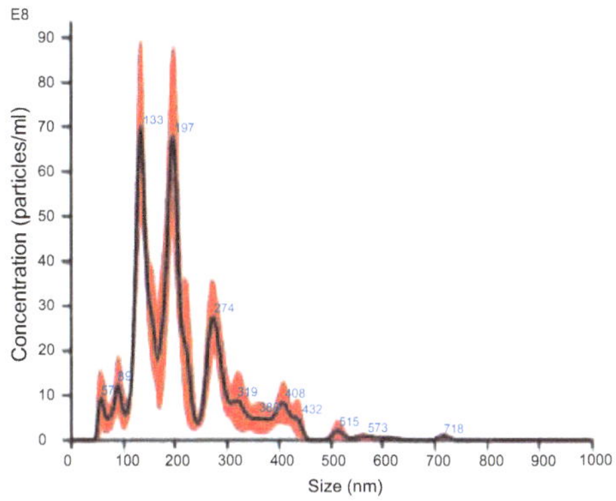

Results

Stats: Mean +/- Standard Error	
Mean:	213.6 +/- 6.0 nm
Mode:	184.8 +/- 14.8 nm
SD:	99.1 +/- 7.5 nm
D10:	117.0 +/- 7.3 nm
D50:	195.9 +/- 6.2 nm
D90:	330.1 +/- 15.4 nm
Concentration (Upgrade):	6.89e+10 +/- 4.69e+09 particles/ml
	17.6 +/- 1.5 particles/frame
	24.4 +/- 2.0 centres/frame

Fig, (3). Representative NTA graph and results of aggregated TMSC exosomes

- Thaw the exosome aliquot for NTA or use the fresh isolate.
- Filter sterilize the PBS and MilliQ water.
- Dilute the sample to 1:500 with filter-sterilized PBS and keep it at room temperature before use.

Note: Do the dilution just before injection into the NTA instrument to avoid aggregation, which will result in misinterpretation of the size.

- Wash the tubing thoroughly with MilliQ water, followed by filtered PBS several times.

Note: Inject one ml of filtered PBS using a syringe pump, switch on the camera, and measure it to ensure proper washing and a particle-free environment.

- Take one ml of diluted exosomes in the syringe and connect it with the syringe pump.
- Set the appropriate flow rate to avoid drift and take measurements in duplicates with a particular setting.

Example: Capture time: 60 seconds, number of capture: 2, Number of Frames: 1498, Temperature: 25.0°C, Viscosity: (Water) 0.888 - 0.889 cP, Dilution factor: 5 x 10e2, Syringe Pump Speed: 25.

Note: Setting a high syringe pump speed will create faster movement of particles and will result in drift error, leading to misinterpretation of the particle size,

The dilution factor will vary from sample to sample. If the concentration is low, then the dilution factor can be reduced and checked again.

If there are no errors and once settings are optimized, use the same settings for all replicates of a particular sample.

- After optimizing the settings, for poly-dispersive samples like exosomes from biological samples, 10-15 captures are essential, while mono-dispersive nanoparticles can be measured with 3-5 captures.

Note: Using fresh samples for NTA will give a single uniform peak in NTA as given above.

Freeze thaw cycles lead to aggregation, which will give multiple peaks with larger particle size and lower particle concentration (see below).

Protein Quantification by Qubit Protein Assay

Materials

Purified exosomes, buffer (PBS or diluent used to suspend exosomes), Qubit protein assay kit (Q33211), 0.5ml transparent thin wall PCR tubes, pipette, and tips.

Procedure

- Bring the reagents and exosome aliquots to room temperature before use.
- Dilute the sample five-fold in PBS.
  Note: Isolated exosomes can be used directly for protein estimation in the Qubit protocol.
- Prepare10 µl of buffer control (PBS)
- Prepare Qubit working solution by adding one µl of Qubit reagent with 199 µl of Qubit buffer.
  Note: 190 µl of this working solution is needed for each reaction; hence, prepare the volume according to the number of samples.
- Label the 0.5ml transparent thin wall PCR tubes for 3 standards, buffer control, and samples.
  Note: Always label the top of the tubes, as the light will pass through the sidewalls of the tubes during measurement.
- Add 10 µl of standard/samples to the corresponding tubes. Add 190 µl of Qubit working solution and mix well by vortexing for 2-3 seconds.
- Incubate the tubes in the dark at room temperature for 15 minutes.
- Measure the concentration using a Qubit Fluorometer (Fig. **4**).

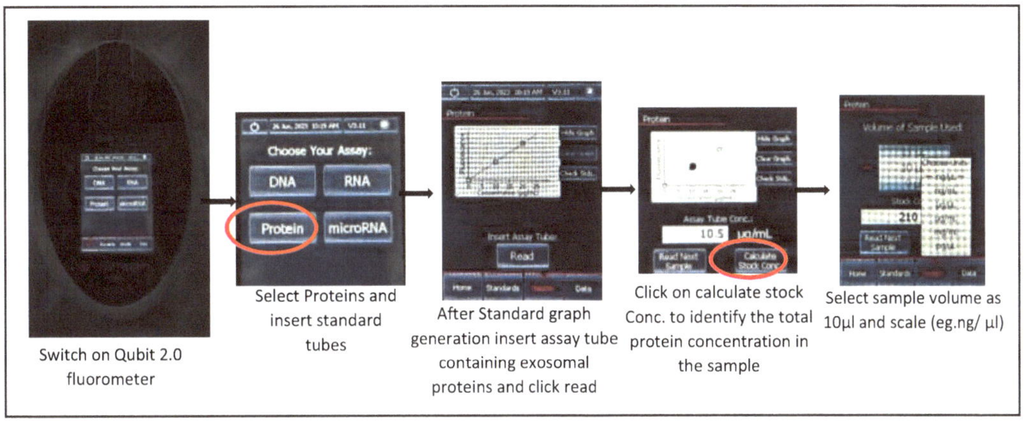

Fig, (4). Representative workflow of exosomal protein concentration measurement using Qubit 2.0 fluorometer.

CONCENTRATION MEASUREMENT USING QUBIT FLUOROMETER

Procedure

- Switch on the instrument and select protein as assay type on the home page.
- Click on read standards and place the standard tube 1 to proceed with taking readings. Follow the same procedure for all 3 standards. A standard graph will appear on the display.
- Click on run samples and measure the standards again as a sample to know the accuracy of the experiment.

Note: In the Qubit protein assay kit, the standard 1 = 0ng/ µl, *which will display as too low to measure, standard 2=200ng, and standard 3 = 400ng. Measure the same tube thrice and take the average for each sample.*

- Now measure the samples in triplicates and calculate the sample concentration by subtracting the buffer control value (Fig. **4**).

Western Blot Analysis

Materials

For SDS PAGE: Gel apparatus, exosomes, acrylamide: bisacrylamide 44:0.8(A: B), A:B 30:0.8, 10% SDS solution, 1.5M Tris-Cl buffer pH 8.8, 0.5MTris-Cl buffer PH 6.8, 10X Tris-glycine SDS-running-gel buffer, 10% ammonium persulfate, water-saturated butanol, 5X loading dye, TEMED,0.1% SDS, pipettes, and tips.

Note: For detailed chemical preparations, see the section – Chemical Preparation below

For Western blotting: Towbin buffer, Tris-buffered saline (TBS), TBS-T (add 0.1% tween 20 in TBS), blocking buffer, nitrocellulose membrane, filter papers, Trans-Blot® SD Semi-Dry Electrophoretic Transfer Cell, Pierce ECL western blotting substrate, X-ray films, fixer and developer for chemiluminescence detection.

Antibodies

In this protocol, the Western blot analysis for cytosolic protein Syntenin is given.

Syntenin (22399-1-AP rabbit anti-human antibody Proteintech, Illinois, USA), secondary mouse anti-rabbit HRP conjugate (Cell signaling Technology)

Note: As per the International Society of Extracellular Vesicles (ISEV) guidelines 2018, exosomes should be characterized for at least three positive markers, which include a minimum of one cytosolic and transmembrane protein. The isolated exosomes should also be characterized for the absence of a minimum of one negative marker. The negative marker will vary based on the source.

Preparation of chemicals:

Compositions are given below for the preparation of 100ml solution.

- *Acrylamide: Bisacrylamide(44:0.8) – for resolving gel*

Take 44g of acrylamide and 0.8g of bisacrylamide in 50 ml of MilliQ water. Dissolve the chemicals completely with the help of a magnetic stirrer and make up to 100ml.

Note: This can be stored in brown bottles at 4°C for months.

- *Acrylamide: Bisacrylamide (30:0.8)- for stacking gel*

Take 30g of acrylamide and 0.8g of bisacrylamide in 50 ml of MilliQ water. Dissolve the chemicals completely with the help of a magnetic stirrer and make up to 100ml.

Note: This can be stored in brown bottles at 4°C for months.

- *10% SDS*

Add 100g of SDS in 70ml MilliQ water. Stir gently to solubilize. Keep this at room temperature overnight to reduce the froth/foam formation. Make up to 100ml with MilliQ water.

Note: This can be stored at room temperature for months.

- *1.5M Tris-Cl(pH 8.8) (buffer for resolving gel)*

Note: Molecular weight of Tris base = 121.149

Dissolve 18.17 g in 75 ml of MilliQ water by stirring in a magnetic stirrer. Makeup to 90ml after complete solubilization. Adjust the pH to 8.8 using a concentrated HCl solution. Make up to 100ml with MilliQ water.

Note: This can be stored at 4°C for weeks.

- *0.5M Tris-Cl (pH 6.8) (buffer for stacking gel)*

Weigh 6.05g of Tris-base. Follow the same procedure mentioned above for 1.5M Tris-Cl buffer solution except adjust the pH to 7.0, and the final pH will be 6.8 after making up to 100 ml.

- *10X Tris-Glycine SDS buffer (running buffer)*

Weight 3g of Tris and 14.4g of glycine, and add 60 ml of MilliQ water. Dissolve completely and then add one gram of SDS. After complete solubilization, make up to 100ml.

Note: This can be stored at room temperature for weeks.

- *Towbin buffer (for semi-dry transfer)*

Add 0.3 g Tris and 1.44 g glycine in 60 ml of MilliQ water; after solubilization, add 30 mg SDS and make up to 80 ml. Keep methanol in a -20 °C freezer, and add 20 ml of ice-cold methanol in 80 ml of the above solution just before use.

Note: Prepare freshly. Do not store.

- *Tris-buffered saline –TBS*

Take 90 ml of MilliQ water in a bottle and add one ml of 1M Tris (pH 7.0) and 0.9 g sodium chloride. Mix well and make up to 100.

Note: Prepare freshly. Do not store.

- *Blocking Buffer-5% skim milk powder in TBST*

Add 100 µl of tween-20 with 100ml of TBS to obtain TBST. In 90ml of TBST, add 5g of skim milk powder, mix thoroughly, and make up to 100ml after complete solubilization.

Note: Prepare freshly. Do not store.

Other low-volume chemicals

- *10% ammonium persulfate- (one ml)*

Dissolve 100 mg ammonium persulfate in one ml of MilliQ water

Note: APS solution should be prepared fresh.

- *Water saturated butanol (1:1) 10ml*

Take 5 ml of butanol and 5 ml of MilliQ water in a centrifuge tube. Mix the tube by inverting it and allow phase separation. Layer the upper water-saturated butanol over the separating gel to obtain a uniform, smooth surface.

- *5X Loading Dye (10ml)*

Take a 15ml centrifuge tube and add 1.56ml of 0.5 M Tris-Cl solution (pH 6.8), 2.5ml of 10% SDS solution, 1.25ml glycerol, 3.1ml of 1% bromophenol blue, and 0.97ml MilliQ water. Mix thoroughly and aliquot this in 1.5ml Eppendorf tubes. Store the tubes at -80°C until use. Add 62.5µl/ml *ß*- mercaptoethanol immediately before use.

Note: This can be stored at -80°C for months. For better protein resolution, ß-mercaptoethanol should be added to each aliquot just before use as it is highly volatile.

Procedure

- Wipe the apparatus and glass plates with 70% ethanol and assemble the glass plates with an appropriate spacer on the casting setup.

  Note: The gel size and spacer size should be based on the final sample loading volume.

  Thaw all the chemicals to room temperature before use. Always keep APS on ice.
- Prepare 25ml of 10% SDS-PAGE separating gel mix in a side arm flask by adding the following: MilliQ water-12 .1ml, A:B 44:0.8- 5.57ml, 1.5M Tris-Cl pH8.8- 6.25ml, 10% SDS - 0.5ml.

- De-gas this solution for 5 minutes and keep it on ice for 20 minutes. Cooling will slow down the rate of polymerization.
- Prepare base seal by mixing 1ml of the above solution with 15 µl of 10%APS and 5 µl of TEMED in a 1.5ml Eppendorf tube and pour into the mold. This will form the base seal and avoid leaking.

  Note: This solution will polymerize within a few seconds. Add the solution in the base through the side walls and tilt the gel plates to form a uniform seal as quickly as possible.
- Further, add 63 µl of 10% APS and 50 µl of TEMED to the same side arm flask. Mix gently.
- Add it to the gel setup and overlay it with water-saturated butanol to form a uniform surface.
- Allow this to polymerize for two hours at room temperature, and then remove the butanol. After MilliQ water washes, overlay with 0.1% SDS and keep it in a refrigerator at 4°C overnight.
- Keep the gel at room temperature for an hour, remove the overlay solution and wash with MilliQ water.
- Prepare 10ml of 4% stacking gel by adding the following: MilliQ water-5.83ml, A:B (30:0.8) - 1.5ml, 0.5 M Tris-Cl pH 6.8 -2.5ml, 10% SDS -0.1ml, 10% APS-50µl, TEMED-20µl.
- Place the one mm comb and pour the gel carefully to avoid air bubbles.
- Allow it to polymerize and prepare the sample.

Sample Preparation

- Take 5µg of exosomal proteins and positive control cell lysates in labeled Eppendorf tubes. Make the volume equal in all tubes with MilliQ water.
- Add 5X cracking dye and heat the samples at 100 °C for 10 minutes in a heating block.
- Set the gel plates in the gel tank and add 1X running gel buffer.
- Load the protein standard (ladder) and the samples (cooled to room temperature) into the wells carefully.
- Allow it to run up to seven cm in the separating gel.

Transfer of Proteins from Gel to Nitrocellulose Membrane (Semi-Dry Method) (Fig. 5)

- Remove the gel from the apparatus and place it in the Towbin buffer.
- Soak the nitrocellulose membrane and filter papers in the Towbin buffer.
- Align the gel, nitrocellulose membrane, and filter paper in the order given below.

  Note: Remove the air bubbles by rolling a glass pipette to ensure proper transfer of proteins from gel to membrane.

- Turn on the power supply and set the voltage to 10-15V for minigels and 15-25V for larger gels. Run time is 30 -60 minutes.
  Note: The transfer time will be less for low molecular weight proteins, while maximum time is required for proteins with higher molecular weight. Syntenin 32kDa will take only 30 minutes to transfer completely.
- Transfer the membrane to a tray containing a blocking buffer and incubate for one hour at room temperature under rocking conditions.
- Add primary antibody (anti-syntenin ab 1:500) in blocking buffer and incubate overnight at 4ºC or at room temperature for 2 hours under rocking conditions.
  Note: The incubation time and antibody dilution will vary based on the antibody. All the incubations and washes should be carried out under rocking conditions.
- Remove the primary antibody solution and wash with TBS-T thrice, each for 15 minutes, followed by three TBS washes for 10 minutes each.
- Add a secondary antibody (prepared in TBS) and incubate for an hour at room temperature.
- After incubation, give three TBST washes and develop the bands by chromogenic or chemiluminescent method (Fig. **6**).
  Note: Since exosomal protein yield will be very low, the chemiluminescent method of detection will be more appropriate as it is more sensitive than chromogenic detection.
- For chemiluminescent detection, mix solution A –luminol and solution B developer given in the ECL kit and develop the bands on X-ray sheets by autoradiography.
- For chromogenic detection, substrates such as 3,3'Diaminobenzidine (DAB) or 3,3',5,5' tetramethylbenzidine (TMB) can be used to form brown or blue-coloured bands on the membrane.

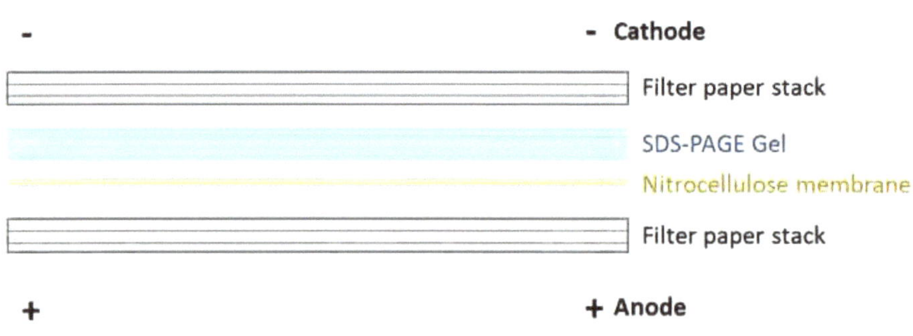

Fig. (5). *Schematic illustration of the gel and membrane set up for electrophoretic transfer.*

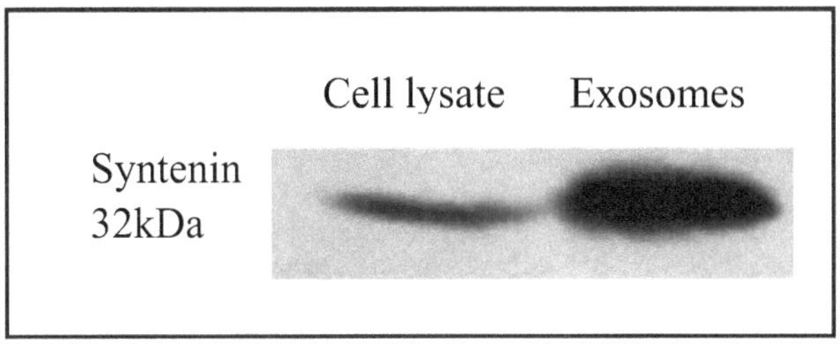

Fig. (6). *Characterization of exosomes by Western blotting. Expression of syntenin in trabecular meshwork stem cell lysate and exosomes. Detection: Chemiluminescence method*

Transmission Electron Microscopy

Materials

Exosome concentrated/dry pellet, PBS, 2% paraformaldehyde, 1% glutaraldehyde, uranyl-oxalate pH 7.0, uranyl acetate methyl cellulose solution, Formvar-carbon coated grid, Transmission Electron Microscope (TALOS 120C G2 –Thermo Fisher Scientific**)**, distilled water, parafilm, Whatmann. No.1 filter paper.

Procedure

- Add 50-100μl of 2% PFA to the concentrated exosome solution or pellet.
- Deposit 5 μl of this solution to the Formvar-carbon coated grid and allow it to dry for 20 minutes, which will allow better adsorption.
- Take 100 μl of PBS on a parafilm and wash the grids in this by holding them with thin forceps.

  Note: The membrane side should always be wet, while the opposite side should be dry. All the following fixation steps should be carried out in the same manner with parafilm.
- Take 50 μl of 1% glutaraldehyde in parafilm and place the grids in it for 5 minutes.
- Wash the grids several times with distilled water.
- Add 50 μl of uranyl-oxalate solution in a fresh parafilm and incubate the grids for 5 minutes.
- Place the grids in parafilm containing the uranyl acetate- methyl cellulose solution on ice for 10 minutes to contrast and then embed the samples.
- Remove the excess solution by blotting with Whatmann. No.1 filter paper.

  Note: The grids can be stored for a long time.
- After complete drying, observe and image using an electron microscope at 80kV-120kV (Fig. **7**).

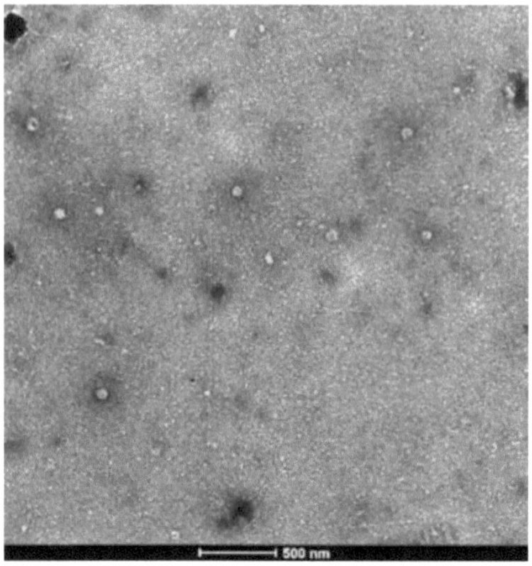

Fig. (7). Representative transmission electron microscopy image of TMSC exosomes. TEM analysis shows that the exosomes are spherical in shape and poly-dispersive in nature.

EVALUATING THE EFFICACY OF ISOLATED TMSC EXOSOMES

The main purpose of this experiment is to evaluate the efficacy of exosomes in therapeutic aspects. Before testing the efficacy of the isolated exosomes with animal models and clinical trials for a particular disease, it is crucial to confirm the efficacy with *in vitro* experiments.

In glaucomatous conditions, reduced TM cellularity and altered extracellular matrix lead to increased stiffness, oxidative stress, and increased IOP, thereby causing optic nerve damage and eventually blindness if untreated (Yun *et al.*, 2016, Wang *et al.*, 2019). Hence the therapeutic agent should have the regenerative potential as well as anti-oxidant capacity to combat IOP changes. Hence, the appropriate methods to evaluate the efficacy of the exosomes *in vitro* should incorporate these aspects.

In vitro Wound Healing Assay and Anti-oxidant Assay

In vitro Wound Healing Assay

Materials

TMSC exosomes, TM cells, DMEM low glucose medium, epidermal growth factor (EGF), 96 well flat bottom plates, 100µl and 20µl tips, Pipettes, Inverted phase contrast microscope with camera system, ImageJ software.

Procedure

- Seed 1 x 10^3 TM cells/well in 96 well plates
- Allow them to reach 90% confluency.
- At 90% confluency, wash thrice with PBS and create a wound in each well using a 20µl tip with constant pressure.
- After wound creation, wash with PBS to remove the wounded/detached cells.
- Add 100µl of complete medium or test component (TMSC exosomes or positive control EGF or sham) and incubate at 37°C. After wounding, record the images at regular intervals between 0- 72 hours (0, 24, 48, 72 hours)
- Measure the wound area using ImageJ (Fig. **8**):

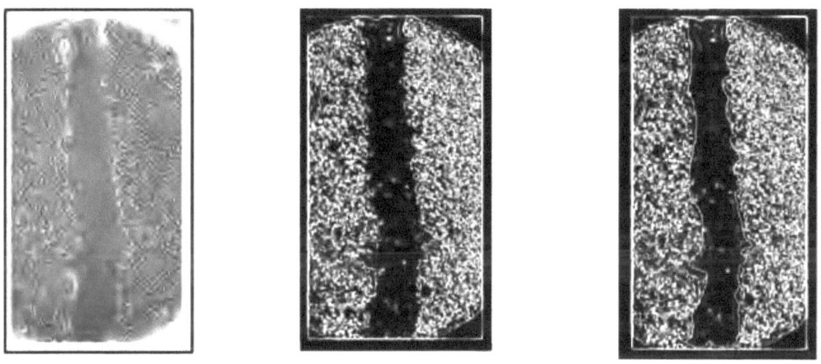
Step 1: Select image to be measured. Apply Grey scale, sharpen.
Step 2: In the process tab in software→ find edges
Step 3: Draw outline of wound using free hand tool- CTRL M to measure area

Fig. (8). Measurement of wound area using ImageJ.

- After measuring the area at each time point, wound closure percentage can be calculated as follows:

Wound Closure% = $(A_{(0)}-A_{(t)})/A_{(0)})*100$

$A_{(0)}$ - is the area at time 0; $A_{(t)}$ is the area after incubation time

Anti-oxidant Assay

Materials

TMSC exosomes, TM cells, DMEM low glucose medium, ascorbic acid (positive control), 96 well flat bottom plates, 100µl and 20µl tips, pipettes, hydrogen peroxide (H_2O_2), Thiazolyl blue tetrazolium bromide (MTT), PBS, Inverted phase contrast microscope, CO_2 incubator, Plate reader with 560 and 670 nm filters.

Note: H_2O_2 concentration has to be standardized previously by treating cells with different concentrations of H_2O_2 (25µM to 200 µM) followed by MTT assay to measure the functional viability. The concentration required will vary for each cell type, which must be optimized prior to the anti-oxidant assay.

Procedure

- Seed 1 x 10^3 TM cells/well in 96 well plates
- At 60-70% confluency, treat the cells with 100µM H_2O_2 (along with medium) twice a day for four days to create a chronic oxidative stress model.
- After four days, add TMSC exosomes, positive control, or sham along with the medium and allow it to recover for 72 hours.
- Measure the viability of TM cells using MTT assay to identify the effect of exosome treatment under oxidative stress.

MTT Assay to Identify the Effect of Exosome Treatment

MTT (3-(4,5-Dimethylthiazol-2-yl)-2,5-diphenyltetrazolium bromide) assay is a colorimetric method for measuring the activity of enzymes in living cells that reduce MTT (yellow) to formazan crystals, giving a purple color. It is commonly used to determine the cytotoxicity of potential medicinal agents and toxic materials. Here, the protocol is described to carry out an MTT assay on TM cells exposed to chronic oxidative stress followed by exosome treatment.

Procedure

- After the removal of medium from the wells, add medium (serum-free, phenol red-free medium) with MTT reagent (0.5mg/ml) and incubate for 4 hours at 37°C in a CO_2 incubator.

  Note: The optimal working concentration of MTT is 0.2-0.5mg/ml for one to four hours. Generally, serum free media is recommended to reconstitute MTT to minimize the effect of serum components in MTT metabolization.

  The usage of phenol red indicator-free serum-free medium improves the experimental accuracy as there is no need for background correction.

  If it is not available, a normal phenol red-containing medium can be used, which needs to be measured at 670nm additionally for background correction.
- Use the wells treated with the cytotoxic chemical (1% Triton X-100) before MTT addition as a positive control for cytotoxicity.
- Carefully remove media and add 100µl of DMSO for 10 minutes.

  Note: As an alternative to DMSO, formazan crystal can be solubilized with 100µl of 0.01N SDS-HCl solution by keeping it in a humidified chamber in the dark under rocking conditions at room temperature for 4 to 18 hours.
- Read optical density at 560 nm and subtract background at 670nm (only for

phenol red-containing medium).

- Optical density should be directly correlated with cell quantity.
- Calculate the cell viability under different treatment conditions using the following formula:

Cell Viability (%) = $A_{Test} - A_{Blank} / A_{Control} - A_{Blank}$ X 100

A Test - Absorbance of wells treated with Test / Drug Compound

A Blank - Absorbance of blank

A Control – Absorbance of wells treated with sham

As an example, the calculations for TM cell viability with and without exosome treatment under chronic oxidative stress are given below in Table **1**:

Table 1. Anti-oxidant effect of TMSC exosomes on TM cell survival under chronic oxidative stress evaluated by MTT assay (phenol red-free serum-free method). TMSC exosomes enhanced TM cell survival under chronic oxidative stress compared to sham.

Condition	OD at 570nm	Cell viability %
Control (untreated)	0.29	Not applicable
Blank (MTT assay done in well without cells)	0.001	Not applicable
Sham (media alone after H_2O_2 *treatment)*	0.08	(0.08-0.001)/ (0.29-0.001) x100= **27.3%**
Positive control (ascorbic acid-containing media after H_2O_2 *treatment)*	0.21	(0.21-0.001)/ (0.29-0.001) x100= **72.3%**
Test (TMSC exosomes containing media after H_2O_2 *treatment)*	0.15	(0.15-0.001)/ (0.29-0.001) x100= **51.6%**

CONCLUSION

The protocols described above provides complete guidelines to isolate and characterize exosomes from stem cell-derived conditioned medium based on our standardized procedures using human TM cells. However, readers are encouraged to consult the original publications where the procedures have been used. For each user, minor modifications might be required based on their cell source and isolation and culturing procedures.

ACKNOWLEDGEMENTS

Rotary Aravind International Eye Bank, Madurai, and Rotary Aravind Eye Bank, Tirunelveli, are acknowledged for providing tissues. SunPharma is acknowledged for funding and Proteintech, Illinois, USA, is acknowledged for providing primary antibodies.

REFERENCES

Ammar, DA, Hamweyah, KM & Kahook, MY (2012) Antioxidants protect trabecular meshwork cells from hydrogen peroxide-induced cell death. *Transl Vis Sci Technol,* 1, 4-4. [http://dx.doi.org/10.1167/tvst.1.1.4] [PMID: 24049700]

Du, Y, Roh, DS, Mann, MM, Funderburgh, ML, Funderburgh, JL & Schuman, JS (2012) Multipotent stem cells from trabecular meshwork become phagocytic TM cells. *Invest Ophthalmol Vis Sci,* 53, 1566-75. [http://dx.doi.org/10.1167/iovs.11-9134] [PMID: 22297497]

Li, G, Luna, C, Liton, PB, Navarro, I, Epstein, DL & Gonzalez, P (2007) Sustained stress response after oxidative stress in trabecular meshwork cells. *Mol Vis,* 13, 2282-8. [PMID: 18199969]

Li, K, Wong, DK, Hong, KY & Raffai, RL (2018) Cushioned–Density Gradient Ultracentrifugation (C-DGUC): A Refined and High Performance Method for the Isolation, Characterization, and Use of Exosomes. *Methods Mol Biol,* 1740, 69-83. [http://dx.doi.org/10.1007/978-1-4939-7652-2_7] [PMID: 29388137]

Li, Y, Zheng, J, Wang, X, Wang, X, Liu, W & Gao, J (2021) Mesenchymal stem cell-derived exosomes protect trabecular meshwork from oxidative stress. *Sci Rep,* 11, 14863. [http://dx.doi.org/10.1038/s41598-021-94365-4] [PMID: 34290351]

Shabbir, A, Cox, A, Rodriguez-Menocal, L, Salgado, M & Badiavas, EV (2015) Mesenchymal Stem Cell Exosomes Induce Proliferation and Migration of Normal and Chronic Wound Fibroblasts, and Enhance Angiogenesis *In Vitro*. *Stem Cells Dev,* 24, 1635-47. [http://dx.doi.org/10.1089/scd.2014.0316] [PMID: 25867197]

Stamer, WD, Hoffman, EA, Luther, JM, Hachey, DL & Schey, KL (2011) Protein profile of exosomes from trabecular meshwork cells. *J Proteomics,* 74, 796-804. [http://dx.doi.org/10.1016/j.jprot.2011.02.024] [PMID: 21362503]

Stamer, WD, Seftor, REB, Williams, SK, Samaha, HAM & Snyder, RW (1995) Isolation and culture of human trabecular meshwork cells by extracellular matrix digestion. *Curr Eye Res,* 14, 611-7. [http://dx.doi.org/10.3109/02713689508998409] [PMID: 7587308]

Sundaresan, Y, Veerappan, M, Ramasamy, KS & Chidambaranathan, GP (2019) Identification, quantification and age-related changes of human trabecular meshwork stem cells. *Eye Vis (Lond),* 6, 31. [http://dx.doi.org/10.1186/s40662-019-0156-z] [PMID: 31641682]

Sundaresan, Y, Manivannan, LP, Radhakrishnan, S, Ramasamy, KS, Veerappan, M & Chidambaranathan, GP (2021) Reduction in trabecular meshwork stem cell content in donor eyes with primary open angle glaucoma. *Sci Rep,* 11, 24518. [http://dx.doi.org/10.1038/s41598-021-03345-1] [PMID: 34972817]

Théry, C, Witwer, KW, Aikawa, E, Alcaraz, MJ, Anderson, JD, Andriantsitohaina, R, Antoniou, A, Arab, T, Archer, F, Atkin-Smith, GK, Ayre, DC, Bach, JM, Bachurski, D, Baharvand, H, Balaj, L, Baldacchino, S, Bauer, NN, Baxter, AA, Bebawy, M, Beckham, C, Bedina Zavec, A, Benmoussa, A, Berardi, AC, Bergese, P, Bielska, E, Blenkiron, C, Bobis-Wozowicz, S, Boilard, E, Boireau, W, Bongiovanni, A, Borràs, FE, Bosch, S, Boulanger, CM, Breakefield, X, Breglio, AM, Brennan, MÁ, Brigstock, DR, Brisson, A, Broekman, MLD, Bromberg, JF, Bryl-Górecka, P, Buch, S, Buck, AH, Burger, D, Busatto, S, Buschmann, D, Bussolati, B, Buzás, EI, Byrd, JB, Camussi, G, Carter, DRF, Caruso, S, Chamley, LW, Chang, YT, Chen, C, Chen, S, Cheng, L, Chin, AR, Clayton, A, Clerici, SP, Cocks, A, Cocucci, E, Coffey, RJ, Cordeiro-da-Silva, A, Couch, Y, Coumans, FAW, Coyle, B, Crescitelli, R, Criado, MF, D'Souza-Schorey, C, Das, S, Datta Chaudhuri, A, de Candia, P, De Santana, EF, De Wever, O, del Portillo, HA, Demaret, T, Deville, S, Devitt, A, Dhondt, B, Di Vizio, D, Dieterich, LC, Dolo, V, Dominguez Rubio, AP, Dominici, M, Dourado, MR, Driedonks, TAP, Duarte, FV, Duncan, HM, Eichenberger, RM, Ekström, K, EL Andaloussi, S, Elie-Caille, C, Erdbrügger, U,

Falcón-Pérez, JM, Fatima, F, Fish, JE, Flores-Bellver, M, Försönits, A, Frelet-Barrand, A, Fricke, F, Fuhrmann, G, Gabrielsson, S, Gámez-Valero, A, Gardiner, C, Gärtner, K, Gaudin, R, Gho, YS, Giebel, B, Gilbert, C, Gimona, M, Giusti, I, Goberdhan, DCI, Görgens, A, Gorski, SM, Greening, DW, Gross, JC, Gualerzi, A, Gupta, GN, Gustafson, D, Handberg, A, Haraszti, RA, Harrison, P, Hegyesi, H, Hendrix, A, Hill, AF, Hochberg, FH, Hoffmann, KF, Holder, B, Holthofer, H, Hosseinkhani, B, Hu, G, Huang, Y, Huber, V, Hunt, S, Ibrahim, AGE, Ikezu, T, Inal, JM, Isin, M, Ivanova, A, Jackson, HK, Jacobsen, S, Jay, SM, Jayachandran, M, Jenster, G, Jiang, L, Johnson, SM, Jones, JC, Jong, A, Jovanovic-Talisman, T, Jung, S, Kalluri, R, Kano, S, Kaur, S, Kawamura, Y, Keller, ET, Khamari, D, Khomyakova, E, Khvorova, A, Kierulf, P, Kim, KP, Kislinger, T, Klingeborn, M, Klinke, DJ, II, Kornek, M, Kosanović, MM, Kovács, ÁF, Krämer-Albers, EM, Krasemann, S, Krause, M, Kurochkin, IV, Kusuma, GD, Kuypers, S, Laitinen, S, Langevin, SM, Languino, LR, Lannigan, J, Lässer, C, Laurent, LC, Lavieu, G, Lázaro-Ibáñez, E, Le Lay, S, Lee, MS, Lee, YXF, Lemos, DS, Lenassi, M, Leszczynska, A, Li, ITS, Liao, K, Libregts, SF, Ligeti, E, Lim, R, Lim, SK, Linē, A, Linnemannstöns, K, Llorente, A, Lombard, CA, Lorenowicz, MJ, Lörincz, ÁM, Lötvall, J, Lovett, J, Lowry, MC, Loyer, X, Lu, Q, Lukomska, B, Lunavat, TR, Maas, SLN, Malhi, H, Marcilla, A, Mariani, J, Mariscal, J, Martens-Uzunova, ES, Martin-Jaular, L, Martinez, MC, Martins, VR, Mathieu, M, Mathivanan, S, Maugeri, M, McGinnis, LK, McVey, MJ, Meckes, DG, Jr, Meehan, KL, Mertens, I, Minciacchi, VR, Möller, A, Møller Jørgensen, M, Morales-Kastresana, A, Morhayim, J, Mullier, F, Muraca, M, Musante, L, Mussack, V, Muth, DC, Myburgh, KH, Najrana, T, Nawaz, M, Nazarenko, I, Nejsum, P, Neri, C, Neri, T, Nieuwland, R, Nimrichter, L, Nolan, JP, Nolte-'t Hoen, ENM, Noren Hooten, N, O'Driscoll, L, O'Grady, T, O'Loghlen, A, Ochiya, T, Olivier, M, Ortiz, A, Ortiz, LA, Osteikoetxea, X, Østergaard, O, Ostrowski, M, Park, J, Pegtel, DM, Peinado, H, Perut, F, Pfaffl, MW, Phinney, DG, Pieters, BCH, Pink, RC, Pisetsky, DS, Pogge von Strandmann, E, Polakovicova, I, Poon, IKH, Powell, BH, Prada, I, Pulliam, L, Quesenberry, P, Radeghieri, A, Raffai, RL, Raimondo, S, Rak, J, Ramirez, MI, Raposo, G, Rayyan, MS, Regev-Rudzki, N, Ricklefs, FL, Robbins, PD, Roberts, DD, Rodrigues, SC, Rohde, E, Rome, S, Rouschop, KMA, Rughetti, A, Russell, AE, Saá, P, Sahoo, S, Salas-Huenuleo, E, Sánchez, C, Saugstad, JA, Saul, MJ, Schiffelers, RM, Schneider, R, Schøyen, TH, Scott, A, Shahaj, E, Sharma, S, Shatnyeva, O, Shekari, F, Shelke, GV, Shetty, AK, Shiba, K, Siljander, PRM, Silva, AM, Skowronek, A, Snyder, OL, II, Soares, RP, Sódar, BW, Soekmadji, C, Sotillo, J, Stahl, PD, Stoorvogel, W, Stott, SL, Strasser, EF, Swift, S, Tahara, H, Tewari, M, Timms, K, Tiwari, S, Tixeira, R, Tkach, M, Toh, WS, Tomasini, R, Torrecilhas, AC, Tosar, JP, Toxavidis, V, Urbanelli, L, Vader, P, van Balkom, BWM, van der Grein, SG, Van Deun, J, van Herwijnen, MJC, Van Keuren-Jensen, K, van Niel, G, van Royen, ME, van Wijnen, AJ, Vasconcelos, MH, Vechetti, IJ, Jr, Veit, TD, Vella, LJ, Velot, É, Verweij, FJ, Vestad, B, Viñas, JL, Visnovitz, T, Vukman, KV, Wahlgren, J, Watson, DC, Wauben, MHM, Weaver, A, Webber, JP, Weber, V, Wehman, AM, Weiss, DJ, Welsh, JA, Wendt, S, Wheelock, AM, Wiener, Z, Witte, L, Wolfram, J, Xagorari, A, Xander, P, Xu, J, Yan, X, Yáñez-Mó, M, Yin, H, Yuana, Y, Zappulli, V, Zarubova, J, Žėkas, V, Zhang, J, Zhao, Z, Zheng, L, Zheutlin, AR, Zickler, AM, Zimmermann, P, Zivkovic, AM, Zocco, D & Zuba-Surma, EK (2018) Minimal information for studies of extracellular vesicles 2018 (MISEV2018): a position statement of the International Society for Extracellular Vesicles and update of the MISEV2014 guidelines. *J Extracell Vesicles,* 7, 1535750.
[http://dx.doi.org/10.1080/20013078.2018.1535750] [PMID: 30637094]

Wang, M & Zheng, Y (2019) Oxidative stress and antioxidants in the trabecular meshwork. *PeerJ,* 7, e8121.
[http://dx.doi.org/10.7717/peerj.8121] [PMID: 31788363]

Yun, H, Zhou, Y, Wills, A & Du, Y (2016) Stem cells in the trabecular meshwork for regulating intraocular pressure. *J Ocul Pharmacol Ther,* 32, 253-60.
[http://dx.doi.org/10.1089/jop.2016.0005] [PMID: 27183473]

CHAPTER 46

Protocol for Single-Cell RNA-Sequence Analysis of Genetic Models of Glaucoma

Jack Hopkins[1], **Alex Leung**[1], **Youichi Shinozaki**[2,3], **Schuichi Koizumi**[2] and **Shin-ichi Ohnuma**[1,*]

[1] *UCL Institute of Ophthalmology, University College London, London, United Kingdom*

[2] *Department of Neuropharmacology, Interdisciplinary Graduate School of Medicine & GLIA Center, University of Yamanashi, Yamanashi, Japan*

[3] *Visual Research Project, Tokyo Metropolitan Institute of Medical Science, Tokyo, Japan*

Abstract: We used two genetically modified mouse models to elucidate the role of different cell types in the initiation and progression of glaucoma. Retinal ganglion cell death has been strongly associated with glaucoma development, and several key genes expressed in certain cell types have been identified. This includes the astrocyte-specific *ABCA1* gene and the *P2RY6* gene, which are found in non-pigmented epithelial cells of the ciliary body. This section describes the protocols for performing scRNA-sequencing to elucidate crucial mechanisms in cell populations and data analysis of sequencing data using the 10X Genomics platform and Seurat package in R.

Keywords: ABCA1, Astrocytes, Eye, Glaucoma, Glia, Intraocular pressure, Mouse models, Normal tension glaucoma, P2Y6 receptors, Protocol, Retina, Retinal ganglion cell, Single-cell RNA-sequencing.

INTRODUCTION

The purpose of this chapter is to describe the process of dissecting the murine retina and isolating cells for use in single cell-RNA sequencing to examine the progression of glaucoma from specific cell populations (Shinozaki *et al*., 2022). These procedures allow us to identify the molecular pathways and biological events in cell-line-specific mouse models of glaucoma and their effects on surrounding cell populations that contribute to the glaucoma-like phenotype observed in these mice. The use of these mice models can be combined with existing treatments for glaucoma to elucidate novel therapeutic strategies or prognostic markers to diagnose glaucoma early.

* **Corresponding author Shin-ichi Ohnuma:** UCL Institute of Ophthalmology, University College London, London, United Kingdom; E-mail: s.ohnuma@ucl.ac.uk

Najam A. Sharif and Sunny E. Ohia (Eds.)

Glaucoma is an age-related disease that affects over 70 million people worldwide, with approximately 10% presenting with full blindness (Quigley & Broman, 2006). Blindness in the most common forms of glaucoma arises due to increased intraocular pressure (IOP) in the anterior chamber of the reduced drainage of the aqueous humor through the trabecular meshwork, resulting in progressive damage to retinal neurons. The focal point of mechanical IOP-associated stress is the optic nerve head, which is enriched with retinal ganglion cell (RGC) axons (Burgoyne *et al.*, 2005). The subsequent loss of this population leads to irreversible injury to axons in the optic nerve head and at the lamina cribrosa (Fig. **1**). This is followed by the loss of RGC soma. Rarer forms of the disease, such as normal tension glaucoma (NTG), are also caused by the progressive loss of RGCs due to ischemia, glutamate neurotoxicity, inflammation, and hypoxia, but without high IOP in patients (Shen *et al.*, 2023).

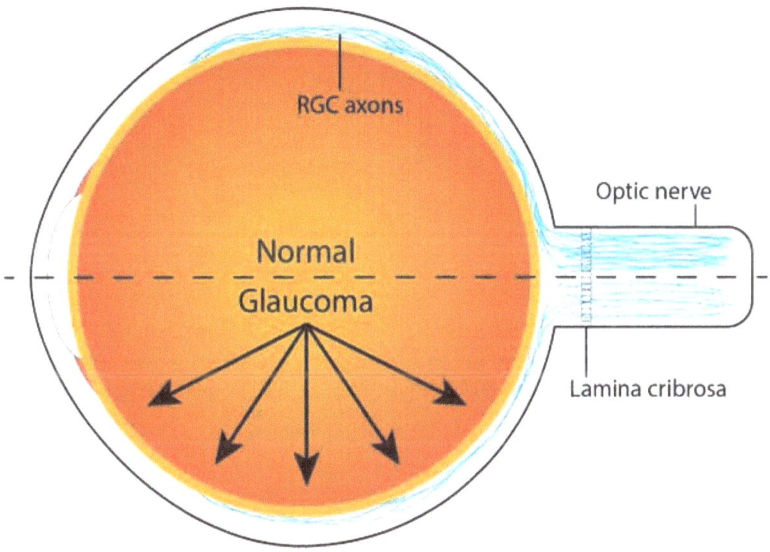

Fig. (1). Schematic representation of the eye depicting loss of RGCs. In the normal eye, RGC function and status is maintained. With the development of glaucoma and increased intraocular pressure (arrows), RGC function is destroyed and cells undergo apoptosis, leading to thinning of the nerve fibre layer.

Most *in vivo* glaucoma models induce IOP or other symptoms of glaucoma in an attempt to replicate the disease, while few genetic knockout models exist. This is, in part, due to the complexity of the disease progression. However, genetic mouse models are still crucial in elucidating specific mechanisms that may initiate or play a role in glaucoma development.

Several candidate driver genes of glaucoma have been described in genome-wide association studies (GWAS). At least four large-scale GWAS from independent, international cohorts have identified single nucleotide polymorphisms clustered by the ATP-binding cassette transporter 1 (*ABCA1*) gene on chromosome nine (Chen *et al*., 2014; Gharahkhani *et al*., 2014, 2021; Hysi *et al*., 2014). The *ABCA1* gene encodes a membrane-associated cholesterol and phospholipid efflux pump and has already been implicated in other age-related retinal diseases such as AMD and Alzheimer's disease (Lewandowski *et al*., 2022; Lupton *et al*., 2014). Indeed, patients with Alzheimer's disease present with a two- to three-fold increased risk of developing glaucoma. Furthermore, other studies have suggested a link between cholesterol levels and glaucoma (Kang *et al*., 2019; Posch-Pertl *et al*., 2022).

An *Abca1*$^{-/-}$ mouse model was constructed from a DBA1/lacJ mouse strain using homologous recombination to excise 910 base pairs from exon 17-22 using methods from the study by Hamon (2000). A reduction of the retinal ganglion marker, *Brn3a,* and elevation of apoptotic cells in the absence of IOP elevation in 12-month-old mice suggested that *Abca1*$^{-/-}$ mice are a suitable model for normal tension glaucoma.

These promising observations warranted further refining of the model. ABCA1 was found to co-localize in cells expressing GFAP, indicating specific expression in astrocytes. Additional studies have since confirmed *Abca1* expression in astrocytes (Y. Zhang *et al*., 2014; Y. Zhang & Wallace, 2015). Thus, astrocyte-specific, conditional *Abca1*$^{-/-}$ mice were generated by crossing *ABCA1* floxed mice with GFAP-Cre mice (Timmins *et al*., 2005). Similar phenotypes to non-specific *ABCA1*$^{-/-}$ mice were observed, along with reduced visual response to multifocal electroretinograms. These findings confirmed the importance of *ABCA1* expression in retinal astrocytes and how their dysregulation can contribute to the apoptosis and degeneration of RGCs.

While *Abca1*$^{-/-}$ mice appear to be useful models for normal-tension glaucoma, a model for the most common variant of the disease, primary angle-closure glaucoma, is yet to be identified. A candidate for primary angle-closure glaucoma became apparent with the discovery of elevated nucleotide levels in the aqueous humor of human patients with glaucoma (Li *et al*., 2011; Markovskaya *et al*., 2008; X. Zhang *et al*., 2007). These molecules bind to P2 receptors, which are divided into P2X and P2Y subfamilies, and they are found to be expressed in tissues within the eye such as the cornea, ciliary processes, trabecular meshwork, photoreceptors, and ganglion cells (Pintor *et al*., 2004; Shinozaki *et al*., 2023).

Extensive studies on the P2X and P2Y receptor families highlighted P2Y6 as a strong nominee for glaucoma-like phenotypes *in vivo* (Shinozaki *et al*., 2017). Administration of UDP in wild-type C57BL/6J mice reduced IOP by suppressing aqueous humor production in a manner analogous to that of the beta-blocker timolol, which is currently used to relieve IOP in the treatment of glaucoma (Shinozaki *et al.*, 2017). In *P2ry6*$^{-/-}$ mice, UDP did not alter aqueous humor production, and the mice demonstrated age-associated chronic IOP and retinal thinning. These contributed to retinal ganglion cell damage and impairment of visual acuity. As such, the *P2ry6*$^{-/-}$ mouse is considered an appropriate vector to model IOP-related glaucoma, including primary angle-closure glaucoma.

Both the *Abca1*$^{-/-}$ and *P2ry6*$^{-/-}$ mouse models demonstrate that cell-specific alterations can elicit a detrimental impact on RGC in the development of glaucoma. Thus, a deeper analysis of the pathways and genes regulated by *Abca1* and *P2y6* in astrocytes and ocular cells, respectively, and the mechanism of RGC degeneration is essential to elucidate the progression of glaucoma. scRNA sequencing of the mouse retina can solve this issue.

EXPERIMENTAL PROTOCOLS

The following procedures were used following the guidelines published by the Physiological Society of Japan and with the approval of the Animal Care Committee of Yamanashi University and the University College London.

Mouse Eye Dissection

Note: Upon culling of animals, eyes should be dissected and the retinal cells should be extracted immediately to prevent cell death that would interfere with the quality of scRNA-sequencing.

Enucleation of Mouse Eye

- Melt 10 mL of paraffin wax in an oven at 65 °C and pour into a 60 mm dish.
- Allow paraffin wax to solidify over two hours.
- Prepare a 1X phosphate-buffered saline (PBS) solution (137 mM NaCl, 2.7 mM KCl, 10 mM Na_2HPO_4, 1.8 mM KH_2PO_4, pH 7.6) and add 6 mL to a 60 mm dish containing paraffin wax base.
- Euthanize adult C57BL/6 mice by CO_2 overdose.

Note: CO_2 overdose should be used over cervical dislocation to avoid placing mechanical pressure or strain on the eye.

- Immediately transfer the mouse to a working environment and sever the neck using scissors.
- Holding the head still with two fingers on each side of the eye, exert slight pressure on the cranium to expose the eye and slide 45° forceps underneath.

- Ensure forceps have passed to the eye towards the sagittal plane, and firmly grip the optic nerve.
- Twist and pull the eye to enucleate.
- Submerge the eye immediately in a 60 mm dish containing PBS.

Retinal Dissection

Note: See Fig. (**2**) for a diagram of retinal dissection.

- Pin the eye in place by using a microdissection needle to fix the optic nerve to paraffin wax.
- Using forceps to stabilize the eye and a dissection microscope for precision, locate the iris and pierce with a second microdissection needle.
- Insert the tip of spring scissors into the pierced iris and make a small incision just above the iris.
- Make a second incision just below the iris using the spring scissors.
- Rotate the spring scissors 90° and make another two incisions to the boundary between the cornea and sclera.
- Using 45° forceps, gently pinch at the boundary to dislodge and remove the lens.
- Insert spring scissors parallel to the corneal-scleral boundary and cut 180° around the eye, rotating as you do so.
- Using a P1000 pipette tip at the optic nerve and facing the base of the eye, gently blow 1X PBS solution to dislodge the retina from RPE.
- Continue gently pumping water at the back of the eye until retina is fully removed and floating in solution. If performed correctly, the entire retina should be removed as a whole. In some cases, 45° forceps can be used to help extract the retina from the optic cup.

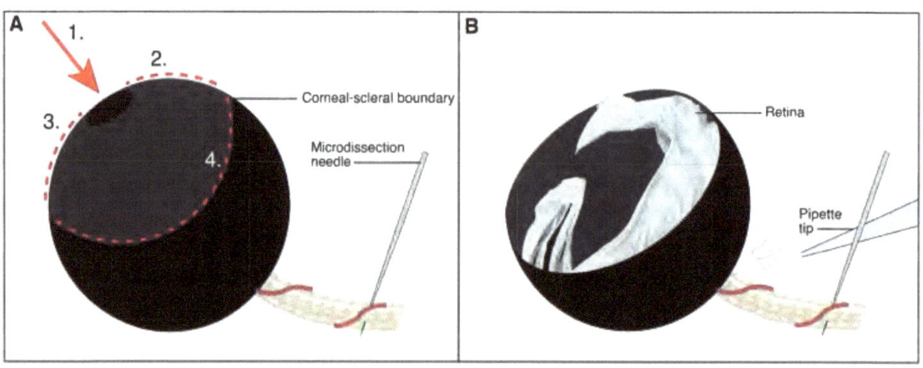

Fig. (2). Mouse retinal dissection. (A) The eye is first pinned in place by a microdissection needle and the iris is pierced. Incisions are then made from the iris to the corneal-scleral boundary. The eye is then cut at this boundary and the lens is carefully extracted. (B) A P1000 pipette is used to blow 1X PBS solution at the base of the eye, dislodging the retina, which can then be removed for dissociation.

Retinal Dissociation and Single-Cell Isolation

Note: In preparation for our chapter, we optimized dissociation with a number of kits and proteases before selecting the Worthington Papain Dissociation System to dissociate retinal tissues. To dissociate tissues of up to 0.4 cm^3, the following steps were taken:

- Place all solutions in vials 1-4 in a 37 °C incubator for 30 mins prior to use.
- Dissolve albumin ovomucoid inhibitor in 32 mL Earle's Balanced Salt Solution (EBSS) and equilibrate at 95% O_2:5% CO_2, pH 7.4.
- Reconstitute papain to 20 units/mL in 5 mL equilibrated EBSS containing 1 mM L-cysteine, 0.5 mM EDTA, and place it in a 37 °C water bath for 10 mins.
- Add 100 μL papain solution and 5 μL 2,000 units/mL DNase solution to each dissected retina.
- Displace air with sterile O_2:CO_s and cap tube.
- Triturate gently and incubate on a rocker for 15 mins at 37 °C.
- Dilute dissociated retina in 900 μL 1X PBS and pass through 35 μm cell filter to obtain single cell solution.

Preparation for 10X Genomics Sequencing

Note: scRNA-seq was performed using the 10X Genomics system. For a detailed step-by-step protocol of scRNA-seq using this platform, refer to the manufacturer's instructions.

- 9 μL retinal cell solution was added to 1 μL propidium iodide/acridine orange solution and mixed with a wide-bore pipette tip.
- A 10 μL cell solution was added to the Luna FL Count Slide.
- Calculate cell concentration using a LUNA-FL™ Dual Fluorescence Cell Counter.

Note: Cell clumping and viability were measured using propidium iodide/acridine orange. Only solutions with fully dissociated single cells and a viability of at least 80% were processed further.

- Adjust cell concentration to 3X the total number of cells to be sequenced and load 43.2 μL into 10X chips for scRNA-sequencing.

scRNA-seq Analysis Pipeline

Note: Our analysis was completed with 10X Genomics' CellRanger software (v3.0.2) and R package Seurat (v3.1.4) developed by Satija lab.

- Upload raw base-calling sequencing files from the 10X Genomics system to Cell Ranger software.
- Use the cellranger *mkfastq* command to demultiplex sequences and generate FASTQ files.
- Use the cellranger *count* command to perform splice-aware alignment to the GRCm38 mouse genome, basic quality control filtering, cell barcode counting, and calculating UMI counts.
- CellRanger employs *emptyDrops* to determine if each droplet contains cell materials or background contamination. Both raw and filtered cell count matrices are then generated.
- Download the filtered feature count matrix (barcodes, features, and matrix) and load it into RStudio as Seurat objects.
- Perform quality control filtering based on the number of UMIs, number of genes detected, and percentage of mitochondrial genes in each cell. *SoupX* can also be employed to estimate the profile of background contamination and remove it from the rest of the dataset.
- Employ *Normalize Data* to perform global-scaling log-normalization.
- Execute *Find Variable Features* to identify a subset of genes that exhibit high cell-to-cell variation.
- Perform linear transformation *Scale Data*to scale gene expression across cells.
- Integrate samples using *Find Integration Anchors* and *Integrate Data* functions.
- Employ linear dimensional reduction Principal Component Analysis (PCA) to reduce the dimension of data while preserving data variation, and UMAP or tSNE can be generated using non-linear dimensional reduction to project data into 2D plots
- Execute *Find Neighbors* and *Find Clusters* to perform KNN graph-based clustering, creating clusters of cells based on gene expression.
- Use *Find All Markers* to perform the Wilcox Rank test between different clusters to identify highly differentially expressed genes. Cell cluster markers can then be used to label cell types based on well-known cell type markers (Table **1**).
- Perform sub-clustering to further separate similar cell clusters to identify cellular subtypes
- Use differentially expressed gene lists created from a comparison between cell clusters (*e.g.*, Neurons *vs.* Microglia) or sample conditions (WT *vs.* ABCA1 KO) for ontological analysis using GO enrichment analysis or Ingenuity Pathway Analysis (IPA).

Table 1. Retinal cell-type biomarkers.

Cell type	Biomarker
Amacrine cells	*Tfap2b, Gad1, Lrrn3, Gad2*
Astrocyte	*Ndrg2, Aqp4, Slc6a11, Aldoc, Apoe*
Bipolar cells	*Gng13, Vsx2, Prkca, Isl1, Sebox, Scgn*
Cone bipolar cells	*Tac3, Vsx1, Gja7*
Rod bipolar cells	*Glrb, Grm6, Pcp2, Prkca*
Cone cells	*Arr3, Gngt2, Opn1sw, Cngb3, Gnat2*
Endothelial cells	*Cldn5, Itgb1, Cxcl12, Pecam1*
Horizontal cells	*Calb1, Onecut1, Onecut2*
Lens	*Cryga, Crygf, Lenep*
Microglia/Macrophage	*P2ry12, C1qa*
Muller glia	*Clu, Dkk3, Glul, Vim, Abca8a*
Microglia	*Hla-dpa1, Hla-dpb1, Hladra*
Photoreceptor progenitor	*Arrb1, Prdm1*
Progenitors	*Hes1, Hes5, Pax6, Vsx2*
Retinal ganglion cells	*Nefl, Stmn2, Vsnl1, Thy1, Resp18, Pou4f1, Opn4*
Rod cells	*Rho, Sag, Gnat1, Pde6a, Cnga1, Nrl*
Retinal pigment epithelium	*Rgr, Rpe65, Rrh, Ttr*

CONCLUSION

The protocols described above have endeavored to provide sufficient experimental details. However, readers are encouraged to look into original publications where such methods have been described. Additional literature searches may also be beneficial in order to find suitable modifications or refinements to the procedures described herein.

REFERENCES

Bar, I, Guns, PJ, Metallo, J, Cammarata, D, Wilkin, F, Boeynams, JM, Bult, H & Robaye, B (2008) Knockout mice reveal a role for P2Y6 receptor in macrophages, endothelial cells, and vascular smooth muscle cells. *Mol Pharmacol,* 74, 777-84.
[http://dx.doi.org/10.1124/mol.108.046904] [PMID: 18523137]

Burgoyne, CF, Crawford Downs, J, Bellezza, AJ, Francis Suh, JK & Hart, RT (2005) The optic nerve head as a biomechanical structure: A new paradigm for understanding the role of IOP-related stress and strain in the pathophysiology of glaucomatous optic nerve head damage. In Progress in Retinal and Eye Research (Vol. 24, Issue 1, pp. 39–73). *Prog Retin Eye Res*
[http://dx.doi.org/10.1016/j.preteyeres.2004.06.001] [PMID: 15555526]

Chen, Y, Lin, Y, Vithana, EN, Jia, L, Zuo, X, Wong, TY, Chen, LJ, Zhu, X, Tam, POS, Gong, B, Qian, S, Li,

Z, Liu, X, Mani, B, Luo, Q, Guzman, C, Leung, CKS, Li, X, Cao, W, Yang, Q, Tham, CCY, Cheng, Y, Zhang, X, Wang, N, Aung, T, Khor, CC, Pang, CP, Sun, X & Yang, Z (2014) Common variants near ABCA1 and in PMM2 are associated with primary open-angle glaucoma. *Nat Genet,* 46, 1115-9. [http://dx.doi.org/10.1038/ng.3078] [PMID: 25173107]

Gharahkhani, P, Burdon, KP, Fogarty, R, Sharma, S, Hewitt, AW, Martin, S, Law, MH, Cremin, K, Bailey, JNC, Loomis, SJ, Pasquale, LR, Haines, JL, Hauser, MA, Viswanathan, AC, McGuffin, P, Topouzis, F, Foster, PJ, Graham, SL, Casson, RJ, Chehade, M, White, AJ, Zhou, T, Souzeau, E, Landers, J, Fitzgerald, JT, Klebe, S, Ruddle, JB, Goldberg, I, Healey, PR, Mills, RA, Wang, JJ, Montgomery, GW, Martin, NG, Radford-Smith, G, Whiteman, DC, Brown, MA, Wiggs, JL, Mackey, DA, Mitchell, P, MacGregor, S & Craig, JE (2014) Common variants near ABCA1, AFAP1 and GMDS confer risk of primary open-angle glaucoma. *Nat Genet,* 46, 1120-5. [http://dx.doi.org/10.1038/ng.3079] [PMID: 25173105]

Gharahkhani, P, Jorgenson, E, Hysi, P, Khawaja, A P, Pendergrass, S, Han, X, Ong, J S, Hewitt, A W, Segrè, A v, Rouhana, J M, Hamel, A R, Igo, R P, Choquet, H, Qassim, A, Josyula, N S, Cooke Bailey, J N, Bonnemaijer, P W M, Iglesias, A, Siggs, O M & Wiggs, J L (2021) Genome-wide meta-analysis identifies 127 open-angle glaucoma loci with consistent effect across ancestries. *Nature Communications,* 12, 1-16. [http://dx.doi.org/10.1038/s41467-020-20851-4]

Hysi, PG, Cheng, CY, Springelkamp, H, Macgregor, S, Bailey, JNC, Wojciechowski, R, Vitart, V, Nag, A, Hewitt, AW, Höhn, R, Venturini, C, Mirshahi, A, Ramdas, WD, Thorleifsson, G, Vithana, E, Khor, CC, Stefansson, AB, Liao, J, Haines, JL, Amin, N, Wang, YX, Wild, PS, Ozel, AB, Li, JZ, Fleck, BW, Zeller, T, Staffieri, SE, Teo, YY, Cuellar-Partida, G, Luo, X, Allingham, RR, Richards, JE, Senft, A, Karssen, LC, Zheng, Y, Bellenguez, C, Xu, L, Iglesias, AI, Wilson, JF, Kang, JH, van Leeuwen, EM, Jonsson, V, Thorsteinsdottir, U, Despriet, DDG, Ennis, S, Moroi, SE, Martin, NG, Jansonius, NM, Yazar, S, Tai, ES, Amouyel, P, Kirwan, J, van Koolwijk, LME, Hauser, MA, Jonasson, F, Leo, P, Loomis, SJ, Fogarty, R, Rivadeneira, F, Kearns, L, Lackner, KJ, de Jong, PTVM, Simpson, CL, Pennell, CE, Oostra, BA, Uitterlinden, AG, Saw, SM, Lotery, AJ, Bailey-Wilson, JE, Hofman, A, Vingerling, JR, Maubaret, C, Pfeiffer, N, Wolfs, RCW, Lemij, HG, Young, TL, Pasquale, LR, Delcourt, C, Spector, TD, Klaver, CCW, Small, KS, Burdon, KP, Stefansson, K, Wong, TY, Viswanathan, A, Mackey, DA, Craig, JE, Wiggs, JL, van Duijn, CM, Hammond, CJ & Aung, T (2014) Genome-wide analysis of multi-ancestry cohorts identifies new loci influencing intraocular pressure and susceptibility to glaucoma. *Nat Genet,* 46, 1126-30. [http://dx.doi.org/10.1038/ng.3087] [PMID: 25173106]

Kang, JH, Boumenna, T, Stein, JD, Khawaja, A, Rosner, BA, Wiggs, JL & Pasquale, LR (2019) Association of Statin Use and High Serum Cholesterol Levels With Risk of Primary Open-Angle Glaucoma. *JAMA Ophthalmol,* 137, 756-65. [http://dx.doi.org/10.1001/jamaophthalmol.2019.0900] [PMID: 31046067]

Lewandowski, CT, Laham, MS & Thatcher, GRJ (2022) Remembering your A, B, C's: Alzheimer's disease and ABCA1. *Acta Pharm Sin B,* 12, 995-1018. [http://dx.doi.org/10.1016/j.apsb.2022.01.011] [PMID: 35530134]

Li, A, Zhang, X, Zheng, D, Ge, J, Laties, AM & Mitchell, CH (2011) Sustained elevation of extracellular ATP in aqueous humor from humans with primary chronic angle-closure glaucoma. *Exp Eye Res,* 93, 528-33. [http://dx.doi.org/10.1016/j.exer.2011.06.020] [PMID: 21745471]

Lupton, MK, Proitsi, P, Lin, K, Hamilton, G, Daniilidou, M, Tsolaki, M & Powell, JF (2013) The role of ABCA1 gene sequence variants on risk of Alzheimer's disease. *J Alzheimers Dis,* 38, 897-906. [http://dx.doi.org/10.3233/JAD-131121] [PMID: 24081377]

Markovskaya, A, Crooke, A, Guzmán-Aranguez, AI, Peral, A, Ziganshin, AU & Pintor, J (2008) Hypotensive effect of UDP on intraocular pressure in rabbits. *Eur J Pharmacol,* 579, 93-7. [http://dx.doi.org/10.1016/j.ejphar.2007.10.040] [PMID: 18031728]

Pintor, J, Sánchez-Nogueiro, J, Irazu, M, Mediero, A, Peláez, T & Peral, A (2004) Immunolocalisation of P2Y receptors in the rat eye. *Purinergic Signal,* 1, 83-90. [http://dx.doi.org/10.1007/s11302-004-5072-5] [PMID: 18404404]

Posch-Pertl, L, Michelitsch, M, Wagner, G, Wildner, B, Silbernagel, G, Pregartner, G & Wedrich, A (2022) Cholesterol and glaucoma: a systematic review and meta-analysis. *Acta Ophthalmol,* 100, 148-58. [http://dx.doi.org/10.1111/aos.14769] [PMID: 33506616]

Huang, B-Q, Yang, J & Shen, W-C (2023) Regulatory mechanisms of retinal ganglion cell death in normal tension glaucoma and potential therapies. *Neural Regen Res,* 18, 87-93. [http://dx.doi.org/10.4103/1673-5374.344831] [PMID: 35799514]

Shinozaki, Y, Kashiwagi, K, Namekata, K, Takeda, A, Ohno, N, Robaye, B, Harada, T, Iwata, T & Koizumi, S (2017) Purinergic dysregulation causes hypertensive glaucoma–like optic neuropathy. *JCI Insight,* 2, e93456. [http://dx.doi.org/10.1172/jci.insight.93456] [PMID: 28978804]

Shinozaki, Y, Leung, A, Namekata, K, Saitoh, S, Nguyen, HB, Takeda, A, Danjo, Y, Morizawa, YM, Shigetomi, E, Sano, F, Yoshioka, N, Takebayashi, H, Ohno, N, Segawa, T, Miyake, K, Kashiwagi, K, Harada, T, Ohnuma, S & Koizumi, S (2022) Astrocytic dysfunction induced by ABCA1 deficiency causes optic neuropathy. *Sci Adv,* 8, eabq1081. [http://dx.doi.org/10.1126/sciadv.abq1081] [PMID: 36332025]

Shinozaki, Y, Saito, K, Kashiwagi, K & Koizumi, S (2023) Ocular P2 receptors and glaucoma. *Neuropharmacology,* 222, 109302. [http://dx.doi.org/10.1016/j.neuropharm.2022.109302] [PMID: 36341810]

Timmins, JM, Lee, JY, Boudyguina, E, Kluckman, KD, Brunham, LR, Mulya, A, Gebre, AK, Coutinho, JM, Colvin, PL, Smith, TL, Hayden, MR, Maeda, N & Parks, JS (2005) Targeted inactivation of hepatic Abca1 causes profound hypoalphalipoproteinemia and kidney hypercatabolism of apoA-I. *J Clin Invest,* 115, 1333-42. [http://dx.doi.org/10.1172/JCI200523915] [PMID: 15841208]

Quigley, H & Broman, AT (2006) [http://dx.doi.org/10.1136/bjo.2005.081224]

Zhang, Y, Chen, K, Sloan, SA, Bennett, ML, Scholze, AR, O'Keeffe, S, Phatnani, HP, Guarnieri, P, Caneda, C, Ruderisch, N, Deng, S, Liddelow, SA, Zhang, C, Daneman, R, Maniatis, T, Barres, BA & Wu, JQ (2014) An RNA-sequencing transcriptome and splicing database of glia, neurons, and vascular cells of the cerebral cortex. *J Neurosci,* 34, 11929-47. [http://dx.doi.org/10.1523/JNEUROSCI.1860-14.2014] [PMID: 25186741]

Zhang, Y & Wallace, BC (2015) A Sensitivity Analysis of (and Practitioners' Guide to) Convolutional Neural Networks for Sentence Classification.

Zhang, X, Li, A, Ge, J, Reigada, D, Laties, AM & Mitchell, CH (2007) Acute increase of intraocular pressure releases ATP into the anterior chamber. *Exp Eye Res,* 85, 637-43. [http://dx.doi.org/10.1016/j.exer.2007.07.016] [PMID: 17822699]

CHAPTER 47

Protocols for Studying Nanotubes and their Role in Human Ocular Cell Communication in the Anterior Chamber of the Eye

Saima Chaudhry[1,*]

[1] *University of Texas at Arlington, 701 S Nedderman Dr, Arlington, TX-76019, USA*

Abstract: Communication between cells can be accomplished through the release and receipt of soluble chemical messenger molecules *via* endocrine and/or paracrine mechanisms. Additional connections can be made *via* the transmission of signals across gap junctions amongst neighboring cells. In recent years, however, a novel means of cellular communication, tunneling nanotubes (TNTs), has been identified that involves physical contact between cells such as trabecular meshwork (TM) cells in the anterior chamber of the eye aqueous humor drainage system that regulates intraocular pressure (IOP). The current chapter describes such TNTs in human TM cells to study them and to gain a better understanding of their role in the physiology and pathophysiology of human IOP regulation. Comparisons of TNTs in glaucomatous and normal TM cells can shed light on how TM cell communication or dysfunctions in TNTs may negatively impact IOP regulation and cause ocular hypertension.

Keywords: Actin cytoskeleton, Cellular communication, Filopodia, Glaucoma, Myosin-X, Trabecular meshwork, Tunneling nanotube.

INTRODUCTION

A heterogeneous population of trabecular meshwork (TM) cells possessing smooth muscle cells, endothelial cells, and structural features are present in the aqueous humor (AQH) drainage system in the anterior chamber of the eye (Abu-Hassan *et al.*, 2014; Acott *et al.*, 2020). The TM is inexorably connected to the Schlemm's canal (SC), which is an extension of the veinous micro-vessels through which the AQH finally drains as it exits the anterior chamber. This TM/SC pathway is a pressure-dependent system that regulates the intraocular pressure (IOP) by controlling the AQH drainage. When this outflow route of AQH egress is blocked due to the accumulation of unwanted proteins, lipids, and

* **Corresponding author Saima Chaudhry:** University of Texas at Arlington, 701 S Nedderman Dr, Arlington, TX-76019, USA; E-mail: saimachaudhry095@gmail.com

cellular debris, the IOP rises and damages the retinal-optic nerve-brain structures and reduces axonal connectivity, thereby starting the process of glaucomatous damage and inducing visual impairment. If this elevated IOP (ocular hypertension [OHT]) is not reduced by drugs or surgery and is allowed to keep rising, more and more damage is exerted to the optic nerve and retinal ganglion cells. After decades of slow but progressive vision loss, the patient can become blind unless the OHT is diagnosed and timely treated.

Under normal circumstances, cells within the TM and SC monitor their environment and the IOP and somehow regulate the efflux of AQH to maintain a steady IOP. How these cells achieve IOP homeostasis has been a mystery until the recent discovery of nanometer-sized tunneling nanotubes (TNTs) through which cells transfer signaling chemicals and organelles (mitochondria, hormones, transmitters, micro-RNAs, neurotrophins, enzymes, endosomes, lysosomes, *etc.*). Such a communication system has evolved in the eye, presumably since the traditional means of diffusional delivery of extracellularly secreted signaling molecules in the anterior chamber is not optimally possible. Here, the unidirectional AQH fluid flow from the ciliary body, where it is produced through the anterior chamber and out the TM/SC outflow system in the eye, would otherwise be constantly diluting the compounds and the resident time on the various cells and their receptors/ion-channels/transporters would be severely limited. Hence, communication through the TNTs should largely be unaffected by the fluid flow. Indeed, TNTs connect different TM/SC cells to permit intercellular communication and permit transfer of agents directly between the cells. These nano-scaled membranous tubes are 50-200 nm in diameter (Gerdes *et al.*, 2013), and they play a prominent role in intercellular trafficking between TM cells and to and from SC cells (Marzo *et al.*, 2012; Keller *et al.*, 2017, 2019). TNTs are a unique form of filopodia that advance from cell to cell, which, upon fusion, create a hollow connectome through which proteins and other molecules can travel between the cells by an "actin-myosin driven" system. In the second format of the cellular information transfer mechanism, cells can combine, and then a nanotube forms when the cells migrate away in different directions (Sun *et al.*, 2019a). Myosin-10 (Myo-X) is important and intimately involved in filopodia and TNT formation and cargo transfer. The myosin head binds to actin filaments, and the tail, which contains a special protein, helps transport cargo to the filopodia tips (Sun *et al.*, 2019a,b). In this manner, sensing of elevated IOP by TM cells probably triggers intra- and inter-cellular communication *via* such nanotubes to promote protease release to help digest excess ECM within the TM/SC and thus keep the outflow pathway open for AQH to egress and hence regulate IOP. These coordinated activities help lower IOP and maintain it at a desired and optimal level. Using the protocols described herein, the research scientists can observe the existing and newly formed TNTs and compare and contrast the dimensions, the number, and potentially the functions of the TNT in normal and glaucomatous TM and SC cells *via* live-cell imaging techniques (Fig. **1**). Protocols to permit the isolation, study, and quantification of various TM cell functions, including TNTs, are provided below.

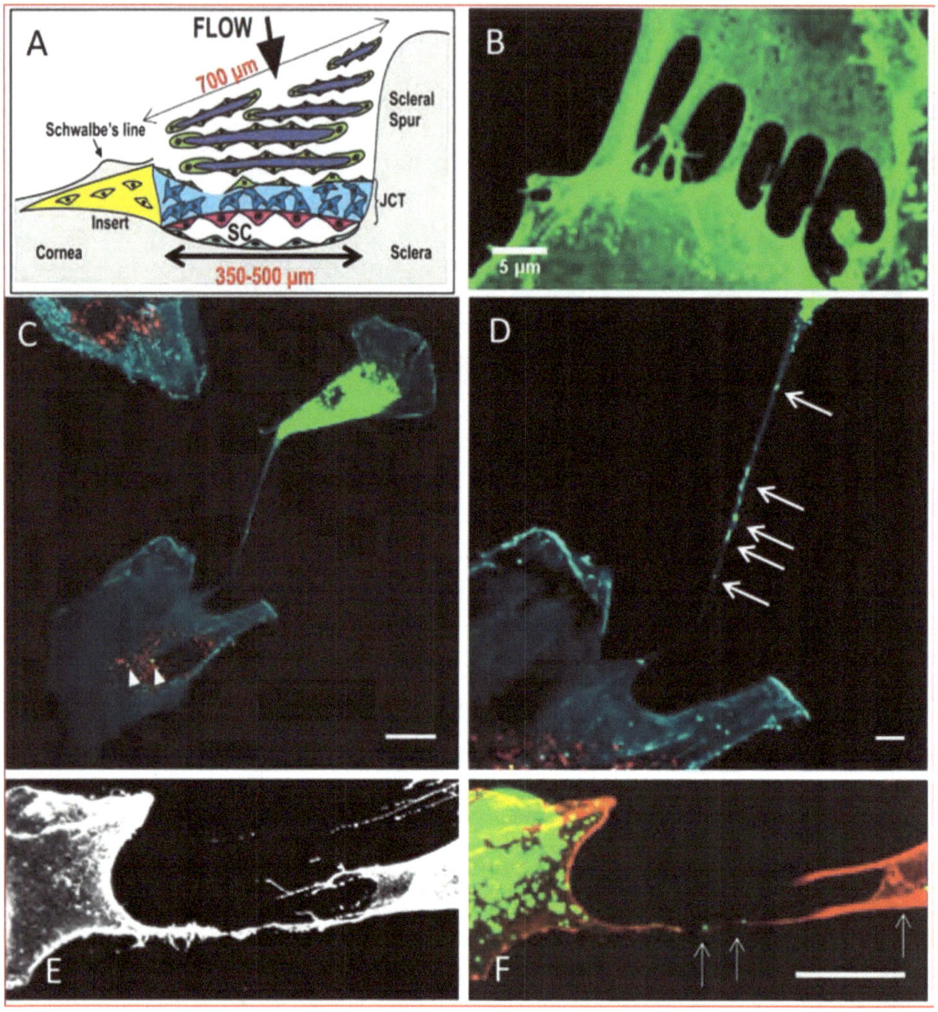

Fig. (1). (A) Schematic of a cross-section of the TM, with the regions and approximate dimensions of the tissue indicated. TM cells (green); corneoscleral beams (purple), the JCT region (blue); the inner wall cells of Schlemm's canal (pink); the putative stem cell insert region (yellow); and Schlemm's canal. (B) TM cells immunostained with CD-44 to label the cell membrane. Filopodia from neighboring cells appear to touch and fuse to form a tube. Scale bar: 5 um. (C) In coculture experiments, Dio-labeled vesicles (green) were present in a DiD-labeled (red) cell (arrowbeads). Cyan: CD44; scale bar: 20 µm. (D) At higher magnification, DiO-labeled vesicles are clearly visible (arrows) within a long cell process connecting the two cells. Scale bar: 5 µm. (E) CD44 immunostaining (gray) of a TNT connecting two TM cells. (F) DiO-labeled vesicles (green; arrows) are clearly visible within the SiR-actin-labeled cell process (red). Scale bar. 20 µm. Keller *et al.*, (2017).

EXPERIMENTAL PROTOCOLS

Isolating and Establishing Primary Human TM Cells

- Obtain whole human eyes postmortem from donors <60 years of age and sterilize them with 70% alcohol in a laminar flow hood.
- Bisect whole globes near the equator with a pair of sharp scissors or a scalpel.
- Under a dissecting microscope, gently remove various intraocular tissues (*e.g.*, lens, iris). Then, remove the TM from the anterior segment.
- Dissect 2-5mm strips of the TM tissue.
- Place 4-6 strips into one well of a 35 mm^2 six-well culture plate.
- Carefully add culture media to minimize tissue disturbance. TM cell culture medium should be composed of Dulbecco's Modified Eagle's Medium (DMEM), with 10% fetal bovine serum (FBS), 2 mM L-glutamine, low glucose (1 mg/L), and antibiotics (0.5% gentamicin or penicillin (100 units/ml) and streptomycin (100 µg/ml)).
- Maintain the cultures in a humidified incubator with 5% CO_2 at 37°C.
- Allow the TM cells to move out from the TM strips during 1-2 weeks in culture and begin to attach to the bottom of the wells.
- The TM strips can now be removed and placed into new plate wells to allow more TM cells to populate the new wells. Carefully change the culture medium every 3-5 days.
- TM cells can then be passaged/split to increase the number of isolated cells.
- Another procedure to obtain TM cells is to allow either dispase (10 mg/ml) or collagenase (10 mg/ml) to gently dissociate the TM tissue following incubation at 37 °C for 30 minutes in a rotary shaker. The enzymes should be inactivated either by adding 2% BSA or by diluting the samples with fresh medium lacking any other ingredients. More detailed information about the TM cell isolation and characterization procedures is available in Keller *et al.*'s paper (2017).

Immunostaining Protocol

- Using a viability-cytotoxicity kit for mammalian cells, take a sample of the anterior segment for live-dead cell staining.
- Take the remaining piece and place it in 10% neutral-buffered formalin for 24 hours.
- Using a decalcifying solution allows easier sectioning through the sclera.
- Cut approximately 8 to 10 wedges and embed each in a single paraffin block.
- Proceed by cutting 5-micrometer serial radial sections perpendicular to the Schlemm's canal and collecting them on microscope slides.
- Use hematoxylin and eosin to stain slides with several quadrants from each eye.

- Examine the presence of cells and evaluate the structural organization of the tissues.
- After deparaffinization and hydration, immunostaining can be performed.
- Using chondroitin's ABC 0.2 U/mL in PBS (Sigma-Aldrich) for 30 minutes at room temperature allows reactivity of CS GAG chain antibodies.
- Block all slides with 2% normal goat serum in PBS. Next, add primary antibodies to the tissue section. The antibodies include the following: mouse anti-heparan sulfate (1:100); mouse anti-C4S (1:100); rabbit anti-fibronectin (1:500, mouse anti-C6S (1:100); biotinylated HA-binding protein (1:100).
- Perform a negative control using no primary antibody.
- Begin washing with PBS after 3-5 minutes, and then add secondary antibodies diluted 1:500 in PBS. The secondary antibodies used are AlexaFluor 594–conjugated goat anti-rabbit, AlexaFluor 488–conjugated streptavidin, and AlexaFluor 488–conjugated goat anti-mouse.
- Following a 1hr incubation at room temperature, the slides should be washed in excess PBS for 5 minutes 3 times.
- Now, mount the coverslips over the sections and examine each slide by confocal and immunofluorescence microscopy (Keller *et al.*, 2008).

Phagocytosis Assay

The papers by Sun *et al.* (2019a,b) should be consulted. However, a brief overview of the procedures is presented below.

- Suspend pHrodo *Staphylococcus aureus* fluorescent bioparticles (1 mg/ml; from ThermoFisher) in PBS and gently disperse by shaking or using a vortex machine.
- To the above, add 50 µl of an opsonizing reagent, mix gently, and allow the mixture to sit for 1hr at 37°C.
- Centrifuge the mixture, decant the liquid, and wash the pellet by resuspension in PBS.
- Seed batches of TM cells in 6-well plates containing shMyo10 silencing lentivirus for three days and then change the medium.
- When TM cells attain about 80% confluency, treat them with 100 µM CK-666 prepared in DMSO for 2 hours.
- Control wells should include shCtrl silencing lentivirus and 0.04% DMSO vehicle control and should be pretreated for 30 minutes with 0.78 µM cytochalasin D to disrupt the actin cytoskeleton.
- Opsonized pHrodo BioParticles (100 µl) should now be added to each well.
- Place the plate in the Incucyte ZOOM instrument (Essen Bioscience, Ann Arbor, MI, USA) for imaging the cells.

- Allow the instrument to capture images of each well at 9 points every 15 min for up to 16 hours using the phase and fluorescence channels when imaging at 20x Objective.
- The phagocytosis assay should be repeated 3 times using three biological replicates. Fluorescence intensity at each point should be measured using FIJI software.
- For more information, readers can consult the papers by Sun *et al.* (2019a,b).

Cell Senescence Assay

- First, obtain TM cells derived from normal (NTM) and/or glaucomatous (GTM) donor TM tissues.
- Use a specific β-galactosidase enzyme staining kit (Cell Signaling Technologies, Danvers, MA, USA) and proceed according to the manufacturer's guidelines.
- Take images (at least 3 for each strain) of the cells *via* a suitable microscope equipped with a DC500 digital camera (*e.g.*, BX51 (Olympus, Waltham, MA USA; Leica, Deerfield, IL, USA).
- Calculate the average and determine any statistical significance using a 1-way ANOVA for every 2 minutes over a 2hr period.
- Create a timelapse movie by taking 3 frames per second and exporting them as MP4 files.
- Export any individual frames as TIFF files.
- Additional information can be found in the papers by Sun *et al.* (2019a,b).

Live-Cell Imaging of GTM in Culture

- Begin by growing GTM or NTM (1 x 10^5 cell/mL) overnight on 4-well micrometer slides.
- The next day, add 0.1 lM SiR-actin and 10 μM verapamil to the media for 1 hour.
- Be sure to wash cells with phosphate-buffered saline.
- Next, add serum-free Dulbecco's modified Eagle's medium.
- Image the cells using a TiE inverted microscope (Nikon, Melville, NY, USA) with a CSU- W1 spinning disk confocal attachment (Yokogawa, Sugar Land, TX, USA)
- House the slides in an enclosed environment and make sure humidity and CO_2 are controlled.
- Every 2 minutes for 2 hours, acquire images using NIS software (Nikon) on the 647 nm channel.
- For time-lapse movies, you need 3 frames per second, exported as MP4 files. All individual frames should be exported as TIFFs (Sun *et al.*, 2019a,b).

Immunostaining of Human TM Cells and Tissue

- Obtain NTG and GTM cells and allow them to grow overnight or at least when they are 70-90% confluent.
- Now, using SiR-actin, stain and visualize the cellular actin cytoskeleton.
- Be sure to fix cells for immunostaining using rabbit polyclonal Myo10 (PA5-55029; ThermoFisher) and 488-conjugated goat anti-rabbit secondary antibodies.
- For tissues, dissect the front of the eye segments from human cadaver eyes and place them in 4% paraformaldehyde to fix the tissues.
- Cut thin sections (1–1.5 mm thick) perpendicular to the other surface and capture them on microscope slides.
- Following tissue section permeabilization with 0.02% Tween-20, incubate with Myo-10 primary antibodies overnight. After this, perform 594-conjugation of goat anti-rabbit secondary antibodies.
- After the above procedures, dip the slides in the mounting medium (ProLong gold) containing 4',6-diamindino-2-phenylindole (DAPI).
- Then, image the labeled sections on a confocal microscope and digitally capture the required images.
- Further details are available in the following publications: Lu *et al.* (2008); Sun *et al.* (2019a,b).

Immunostaining and Measurement of Cell Size and Cellular Protrusions

- Begin with NTM and GTM cell strains (2x3 105 cells/mL)
- Culture on collagen I-coated BioFlex plates for 16 hours.
- After fixing the cells in 4% paraformaldehyde, expose them to a CD44 primary antibody solution (*e.g.*, rat, monoclonal anti-CD44; clone IM-7) (Stem Cell Technologies, Vancouver BC, Canada), followed by the Alexa-fluor 594-conjugated donkey anti-rat secondary antibody.
- Be sure to mount using coverslips in ProlongGold mounting medium, which contains DAPI. Now, visualize the TNT on a confocal microscope.
- In order to capture the whole depth of the cells, set Z-stacks 0.5 μm above and 0.5 μm below the fluorescent signal.
- Calculation of the area and volume of the cells based on the Z-stacks can be accomplished using the "surfaces" module Imaris software.
- Ensure the cells are not touching; they must be manually separated on the software, and if you cannot separate them easily, those images are to be discarded.
- To measure filopodia's number and length, use the module "filaments."
- Manually assign the beginning of the protrusion on the cell surface and the end of the filaments using the software.

- Measure colocalization of myosin-10 (Myo-10) and cortactin using the module "coloc". This will produce Pearson's value.
- Assignment of the colocalization is somewhat arbitrary but can be as follows: extra strong (0.88-1.0), quite strong (0.61-0.87), fairly moderate (0.4-0.6), quite weak (0.13-0.39), and very weak (0-0.12).
- Use ImageJ software to determine the actin stress fiber diameters from the confocal images.
- Additional information can be obtained from Keller *et al.* (2017).

Vesicle Transfer Assay

- Obtain confluent cultures of TM cells and proceed to dissociate them with trypsin using procedures described above in earlier sections of this chapter. Dilute the enzyme at the conclusion of the incubation and harvest the cells by centrifugation and resuspension. Split the cells into two. Then, label one half with Vybrant DiO dye (488nm) and the other half with DiD dye (647nm) (from ThermoFisher).
- Following centrifugation/washing/resuspension in fresh culture medium, mix the fluorescently-labeled cells (1:1 basis) and seed into culture plates (at a density of $1x10^5$ cells/mL, allowing them to attach in a humified incubator with CO_2 at 37^0C overnight.
- Next, label the NTM cells (n=5 wells) cells with DiO and incubate with the DiD-labeled GTM cells (n=6 wells).
- Now, fix the cells and then immuno-stain them with a CD44 monoclonal antibody solution, and after the appropriate time, image them on a confocal microscope.
- Count the DiO (green) and DiD (red) positive transferred vesicles in cells in each of the images.
- Determine the number of TM cells containing at least 5 vesicles of the opposing color.
- Now calculate the percentage of green-NTM cells that contain red-GTM-derived vehicles. Then, also determine the percentage of red-NTM cells that contain green-GTM-derived vesicles.
- Additional information for performing all the aforementioned procedures can be found in the papers by Keller *et al.* (2017) and Sun *et al.* (2019a,b).

Images of the TNTs between TM cells, with and without vesicles in the process of transport/transfer, can be seen in Fig. (**1**).

CONCLUSION

To conclude, the experimental protocols described herein are based on the original publications cited throughout this chapter. They help demonstrate procedures for isolating, culturing, and visualizing primary GTM and NTM cells that are established from postmortem human cadaver eyes. By following the measurement of the transferred vibrant DiO and DiD-labeled vesicles *via* TNT connections, the process of molecular transfer of cargo from cell to cell can be captured (*e.g.*, Fig. **1**). For more in-depth information about the TNTs and their imaging, readers are encouraged to consult the original publications where such methods are described. Appropriate references are provided below.

REFERENCES

Abu-Hassan, DW, Acott, TS & Kelley, MJ (2014) The trabecular meshwork: a basic review of form and function. *J Ocul Biol,* 2, 9.
[PMID: 25356439]

Acott, TS, Vranka, JA, Keller, KE, Raghunathan, V & Kelley, MJ (2021) Normal and glaucomatous outflow regulation. *Prog Retin Eye Res,* 82, 100897.
[http://dx.doi.org/10.1016/j.preteyeres.2020.100897] [PMID: 32795516]

Gerdes, HH, Rustom, A & Wang, X (2013) Tunneling nanotubes, an emerging intercellular communication route in development. *Mech Dev,* 130, 381-7.
[http://dx.doi.org/10.1016/j.mod.2012.11.006] [PMID: 23246917]

Keller, KE, Bhattacharya, SK, Borrás, T, Brunner, TM, Chansangpetch, S, Clark, AF, Dismuke, WM, Du, Y, Elliott, MH, Ethier, CR, Faralli, JA, Freddo, TF, Fuchshofer, R, Giovingo, M, Gong, H, Gonzalez, P, Huang, A, Johnstone, MA, Kaufman, PL, Kelley, MJ, Knepper, PA, Kopczynski, CC, Kuchtey, JG, Kuchtey, RW, Kuehn, MH, Lieberman, RL, Lin, SC, Liton, P, Liu, Y, Lütjen-Drecoll, E, Mao, W, Masis-Solano, M, McDonnell, F, McDowell, CM, Overby, DR, Pattabiraman, PP, Raghunathan, VK, Rao, PV, Rhee, DJ, Chowdhury, UR, Russell, P, Samples, JR, Schwartz, D, Stubbs, EB, Tamm, ER, Tan, JC, Toris, CB, Torrejon, KY, Vranka, JA, Wirtz, MK, Yorio, T, Zhang, J, Zode, GS, Fautsch, MP, Peters, DM, Acott, TS & Stamer, WD (2018) Consensus recommendations for trabecular meshwork cell isolation, characterization and culture. *Exp Eye Res,* 171, 164-73.
[http://dx.doi.org/10.1016/j.exer.2018.03.001] [PMID: 29526795]

Keller, KE, Bradley, JM, Sun, YY, Yang, YF & Acott, TS (2017) Tunneling Nanotubes are Novel Cellular Structures That Communicate Signals Between Trabecular Meshwork Cells. *Invest Ophthalmol Vis Sci,* 58, 5298-307.
[http://dx.doi.org/10.1167/iovs.17-22732] [PMID: 29049733]

Keller, KE, Sun, YY, Yang, YF, Bradley, JM & Acott, TS (2012) Perturbation of hyaluronan synthesis in the trabecular meshwork and the effects on outflow facility. *Invest Ophthalmol Vis Sci,* 53, 4616-25.
[http://dx.doi.org/10.1167/iovs.12-9500] [PMID: 22695958]

Keller, KE, Bradley, JM, Kelley, MJ & Acott, TS (2008) Effects of modifiers of glycosaminoglycan biosynthesis on outflow facility in perfusion culture. *Invest Ophthalmol Vis Sci,* 49, 2495-505.
[http://dx.doi.org/10.1167/iovs.07-0903] [PMID: 18515587]

Marzo, L, Gousset, K & Zurzolo, C (2012) Multifaceted roles of tunneling nanotubes in intercellular communication. *Front Physiol,* 3, 72.
[http://dx.doi.org/10.3389/fphys.2012.00072] [PMID: 22514537]

Sun, YY, Bradley, JM & Keller, KE (2019) Phenotypic and Functional Alterations in Tunneling Nanotubes Formed by Glaucomatous Trabecular Meshwork Cells. *Invest Ophthalmol Vis Sci,* 60, 4583-95. a
[http://dx.doi.org/10.1167/iovs.19-28084] [PMID: 31675075]

Sun, YY, Yang, YF & Keller, KE (2019) Myosin-X Silencing in the Trabecular Meshwork Suggests a Role for Tunneling Nanotubes in Outflow Regulation. *Invest Ophthalmol Vis Sci,* 60, 843-51. b
[http://dx.doi.org/10.1167/iovs.18-26055] [PMID: 30807639]

CHAPTER 48

Protocol for Aqueous Humor Metabolite Measurements for Glaucoma Research

Anna Mueller[1], **Isabella Moceri**[2] and **Sanjoy K. Bhattacharya**[3,*]

[1] *Bascom Palmer Eye Institute, University of Miami Miller School of Medicine, Miami, FL 33136, USA*

[2] *Miami Integrative Metabolomics Research Center, Miami, FL, 33136, USA*

[3] *University of Miami Miller School of Medicine, Miami, 1638 NW 10th Avenue, Suite 707A, FL 33136, USA*

Abstract: Ultra-high-performance liquid chromatography-mass spectrometry is commonly used in the untargeted analysis of metabolites within mammalian aqueous humor samples. Aqueous humor is a transparent fluid that bathes the anterior segment of the eye to nourish the cornea and lens. Aqueous humor also assists in the maintenance of intraocular pressure. In glaucoma, aqueous humor flow is impeded, leading to ocular hypertension and optic nerve damage. The application of metabolomics to study aqueous humor allows for advancements in knowledge of the molecular mechanisms in glaucoma. In this chapter, we put forth a protocol using hydrophilic interaction liquid chromatography (HILIC) coupled with tandem mass spectrometry to accurately identify metabolomic data of the aqueous humor samples. The purpose of this chapter is to provide an extraction and identification method of mammalian aqueous humor metabolites using liquid chromatography-tandem mass spectrometry.

Keywords: Aqueous humor, Glaucoma, HILIC, LC-MS/MS, QC Samples, Untargeted metabolomics, Ultra-high-performance liquid chromatography-mass spectrometry (UHPLC-MS).

INTRODUCTION

Glaucoma is a group of progressive diseases that leads to optic nerve degeneration. It is the leading cause of irreversible blindness worldwide, with about 70 million people affected by primary open-angle glaucoma—the most common type (Zhang *et al.*, 2021). With life expectancy increasing globally, res-

* **Corresponding author Sanjoy K. Bhattacharya:** University of Miami Miller School of Medicine, Miami, 1638 NW 10th Avenue, Suite 707A, FL 33136, USA; Tel: +3054824103; E-mail: SBhattacharya@med.miami.edu

Najam A. Sharif and Sunny E. Ohia (Eds.)

earchers have estimated that by 2040, glaucoma will affect 111.8 million patients (Tham *et al*., 2014). Up to half of glaucoma cases remain undetected due to their symptomless nature, which has resulted in biomarker advancements to aid in early diagnosis and potential therapy treatments (Barbosa Breda *et al*., 2020).

Metabolomics is defined as the analytical measurement of all known and unknown metabolites within a fluid, tissue, or cell (Han *et al*., 2020). The recent emerging approach of metabolomics has allowed researchers to identify biomarkers within diseases, study the natural effects of drugs, and explore the metabolic pathways performed by a specific disease (Pietrowska *et al*., 2017). Mass spectrometry-based analysis is highly effective when identifying metabolites within biological samples. The analyses are typically performed by gas chromatography-mass spectrometry (GC-MS) or liquid chromatography-mass spectrometry (LC-MS/MS). When using LC-MS/MS, metabolites are subject to contamination and background noise. Therefore, it is essential that sample preparation and extraction are done efficiently, as well as to ensure the performance of the instrument through quality controls, internal standards, and extraction blanks (Jauregui *et al*., 2023). Pooled quality control samples (Pooled QCs) are a pool of all samples within the study used to monitor the instruments' stability and the quality of the data being produced. Blank samples like blank mobile phases and extraction blanks provide information on the origin of the metabolites being identified. Both of these data filtering techniques reduce the size of the dataset by limiting the inclusion of non-biological metabolites (Ivanisevic and Want, 2019). For optimal results in identification, two ion modes are applied when looking for results in metabolite identification. In positive mode, the ions analyte is charged *via* protonation, whereas in negative ion mode, the analyte is charged *via* deprotonation (Banerjee and Mazumdar, 2012). In complexes such as plasma, urine, or tissue, hundreds to thousands of metabolites can be identified within the database. It is important to acknowledge that polar compounds do not bind well on the reverse phase column compared to the HILIC column, which is specifically created for separating highly polar compounds (Jauregui *et al*., 2023). The data results are most efficient when using both HILIC and reversed phase methods to identify both water-soluble charged metabolites and semi-polar metabolites (Najdekr *et al*., 2019).

In this chapter, we present an untargeted mass spectrometry method utilizing HILIC to identify metabolites of interest in aqueous humor samples from mammalian species. We present here the example of UHPLC- MS/MS instruments. However, these protocols are useful across the board with any LC-MS/MS system with additional adjustments to the specific instruments used.

EXPERIMENTAL PROTOCOLS

The following procedures were performed in compliance with the guidelines of the American Association for Laboratory Animal Science for the use of animals and adhered to the Statement for the Use of Animals in Ophthalmic and Visual Research from the Association for Research in Vision and Ophthalmology (ARVO).

MATERIALS AND CHEMICALS

- Ammonium formate
- 200 Mm Ammonium acetate
- Acetonitrile (ACN)
- Formic Acid
- Methanol (MeOH)
- Extraction solvent (for extraction from plasma): 1 mL stock solution of MeOH: ACN (v/v, 1:1)

ULTRA-HIGH-PERFORMANCE LIQUID CHROMATOGRAPHY AND MASS SPECTROMETRY

Instruments

- Thermo Scientific™ Vanquish™ Horizon UHPLC.
- Thermo Scientific™ Q ExactiveTM Orbitrap™ Mass Spectrometer coupled to a heated electrospray ionization source (HESI).
- Thermo Scientific™ Xcalibur™
- Vacuum centrifuge
- Sonicator

ULTRA HIGH-PERFORMANCE LIQUID CHROMATOGRAPHY COLUMNS AND VIALS

- AccucoreTM 150 Amide HILIC Column (150 mm x 2.1 mm, 2.6 µm, Thermo Scientific™).
- HPLC vials (catalog number: 6PRV11-03FIVP) and caps (catalog number: 11PSN(B)-8RT1).

Methods

Sample Preparation

Aqueous Humor Sample Collection

- Obtain approximately 100 μL of aqueous humor sample *via* anterior chamber paracentesis [usually performed by a surgeon (or a person trained in paracentesis for animals)].
- Once collected, centrifuge each sample at 15,000 rcf for 5 minutes (**See note 1**).
- Transfer supernatant to sterile Eppendorf tubes.
- Store at −80°C until ready for extraction and analysis.

Metabolite Extraction

- When ready for analysis, thaw aqueous humor samples on ice.
- Vortex-mix 400 μL of cold (-20°C) methanol/acetonitrile (v/v, 1:1) into 100 μL of sample for 1 minute.
- After extraction, sonicate for 1 hour in an ice bath **(See note 2).**
- Incubate at -20°C for 1 hour and centrifuge at 14,000 rcf for 20 minutes at 4°C.
- Harvest supernatants into sterile Eppendorf tubes **(See note 3).**
- SpeedVac until dry **(See note 4).**
- Once dry, dissolve the remaining extracts in 50% ACN.
- Filter each sample through 0.22 μm cellulose acetate membrane (ThermoFisher Scientific, Waltham, Massachusetts, USA).
- Transfer samples into 2 mL HPLC vials and store at -80°C until ready for analysis (**See note 5**).

Extraction Blank Sample Preparation

- Control samples should be processed as above without a biological sample present.

Pooled Quality Control Sample Preparation

- Place into new Eppendorf tube 10 μL aliquots of ("Pooled QC") and mix on a vortex machine for 30 seconds (**See note 6).**
- Split the pooled QC into 10 μL aliquots and place them into individual HPLC vials.

Mobile Phases

Preparation of Ammonium Formate and Ammonium Acetate 200 mM stock Solution

- Into 200mL of water, add 2.52 g of ammonium formate, and allow it to dissolve (200 mM final concentration) and sonicate to aid dissolution.
- Into 200mL of water, add 3.08 g of ammonium acetate, and allow it to dissolve (200 mM solution) and sonicate to aid dissolution.
- Place these stock solutions at 4°C (up to 1 month is fine).

Preparation for Mobile Phases A and B for HILIC UPLC-MS/MS Positive Ion Mode

- Use water to rinse 1L mobile-phase bottles.
- Now, to 450 mL of acetonitrile, add 50 mL of 200 mM ammonium formate stock. This mobile phase A is used for positive ionization and has 10 mM ammonium formate in 95% acetonitrile: 5% water with 0.1% formic acid.
- Sonicate the above mixture until it becomes clear.
- Now, add 500mL of acetonitrile and 1 mL of formic acid to the above mixture, thus preparing 1L of the mobile-phase solution.
- Now, add 50 mL of the 200 mM ammonium formate stock solution and 1.0 mL of formic acid to 450mL of water to 500 mL of acetonitrile. This mobile-phase B is used for positive ionization, and it is composed of 10 mM ammonium formate in 50% acetonitrile: 50% water with 0.1% formic acid.
- At this stage, mobile-phase A and B need to be sonicated for 30 minutes and left to stabilize overnight at 24°C (Najdekr *et al.*, 2019).

Preparation for Mobile Phases A and B for HILIC UPLC-MS/MS Negative Ion Mode

- Mix 450mL of acetonitrile with 50mL of the 200 mM ammonium acetate stock. Mobile phase A is used for negative ionization and is composed of 10 mM ammonium formate in 95% acetonitrile/5% water with 0.1% acetic acid. This mixture should be sonicated for 15 minutes until it becomes clear.
- Once clear, add 500mL of acetonitrile with 1mL of acetic acid to create a 1L mobile phase solution.
- Mobile phase B is used for negative ionization, and it contains 10 mM ammonium formate in 50% acetonitrile: 50% water with 0.1% acetic acid. Mix 450mL of water with 500mL of acetonitrile. Add 50 mL of the 200 mM ammonium acetate stock solution and 1 mL of acetic acid to create a 1L stock solution.

- Mobile phases A and B should be sonicated for 30 minutes (Najdekr *et al.*, 2019).

UHPLC and MS Methods

HILIC UHPLC Gradient

- Gradient values, including flow rates, are presented in Table **1**.
- Set the column to 35°C.
- Set injection volume to 5μL

Table 1. Hydrophilic interaction liquid chromatography (HILIC) method gradient using an Accucore™ 150 Amide HILIC column.

Retention Time (min)	Flow (mL/min)	%B
0.000	0.500	1.0
1.000	0.500	1.0
9.000	0.500	95.0
10.000	0.500	95.0
10.500	0.500	1.0
15.000	0.500	1.0

Q Exactive and HESI ion Source Settings

- Set the mass range to 67 – 1000 m/z.
- Set the resolution to 140,000 for full scan and 35,000 for ddMS^2.
- The AGC target for full scan = 3e6 and ddMS^2 = 2e5.
- The max injection time (IT) is 200 seconds for full scan mode and 50 seconds for ddMS^2.
- The number of microscans is 2.
- The normalized collision energy (NCE) should be set to 20, 35, and 50.
- Details of the source parameters are presented in Table **2**.

Table 2. Q Exactive heated electrospray ionization source (HESI) ion source settings for the HILIC method for both positive and negative acquisition mode.

In-source CID (kV)	0.5
Sheath Gas Flow Rate *Both* Modes	55
Aux Gas Flow Rate *Both* Modes	14
Sweep Gas Flow Rate *Both* Modes	4

(Table 2) cont.....

Spray Voltage (kV) *Positive* Mode *Negative* Mode	3.5 2.5
Capillary Temperature (°C) *Positive* Mode *Negative* Mode	350 380
S-lens RF Level *Both* Modes	30
Aux Gas Heater Temperature (°C) *Both* Modes	438

Setting up the Instrument

- Evaluate and calibrate the mass spectrometer using calibration solutions. For the positive ionization method, use Pierce™ ESI positive ion calibration solution, and for negative ionization mode, use Pierce™ ESI negative ion calibration solution.
- Purge lines A and B on the UHPLC system for 5 minutes.

HPLC Column Cleaning

After the data analysis, the column should be cleaned using an LC method setting with 95% B mobile phase for 60 minutes.

NOTES

1. Centrifuging the samples separates the supernatant and the concentrated particles within the sample.
2. Sonication allows for effective dissolving and mixing of the chemicals while releasing air bubbles.
3. Eppendorf tubes and laboratory plastic pipettes should be used to allow for optimal extraction without contamination. Do not disturb the protein pellet, as this will contaminate the instrument.
4. To avoid over drying the sample, SpeedVac for 20 minutes. If there is still liquid in the tube, keep checking on the samples (every 5 minutes) to prevent sample loss.
5. For long-term storage, place samples at -80°C. Samples remain viable at -20°C for up to 1 week.
6. Pooled QCs are used for metabolite normalization and identification.

CONCLUSION

The protocol above provides experimental outcomes of polar metabolites in the aqueous humor of mammals. Coupling HILIC chromatographic fractionation with tandem mass spectrometry allows for a vast profile of metabolite species that may prove interesting in diagnosing and treating ocular diseases. Using high-resolution instruments such as the Q Exactive ensures the information is both accurate and reproducible. The raw spectral data should be further analyzed using metabolomic identification software, such as Compound Discoverer 3.3 from Thermo Fisher. Further statistical analysis can be done using open-source software such as MetaboAnalyst 5.0. These data can be used to draw conclusions on potential metabolomic biomarkers for glaucoma and other ocular diseases. It may also play a role in developing therapeutic avenues utilizing metabolites of interest (Table 3).

Table 3. Sample data table showing metabolite data from aqueous humor samples in µg/ml.

Metabolites identified in aqueous humor samples						
Metabolite	**Sample 1**	**Sample 2**	**Sample 3**	**Sample 4**	**Sample 5**	**Sample 6**
4-aminobutanoate	0.43	1.678	1.592	1.544	1.423	0.943
Isoleucylarginine	0	0.387	0.228	0.137	0.33	0.062
L-phenylalanine	0.4	0.525	0.895	0.87	0.797	0.871
L-lysine	0.161	0.222	0.229	0.358	0.405	0.79
5-isobutyl-1-nitrobiuret	4.067	3.002	3.115	3.793	2.564	2.728
Indoline	0.192	0.1	0.432	0.555	0.841	1.075
Calystegin B2	0	3.411	0	0	0	0
Diacetyl	2.597	2.296	2.244	2.672	2.785	2.749
Guanine	0	0.008	0.008	0.002	0.002	0.006
Hypoxanthine	0	0	0	0	0	0
Proparacaine	0	0	0	0	0	0
2-Methyl-N-Phenylmaleimide	0.293	0.305	0.617	0.855	1.072	1.033
L-Proline	12.039	19.817	41.313	14.843	52.436	27.855
L-Arginine	3.061	3.68	1.658	2.255	1.742	2.632
Libramycin A	8.234	3.863	0.543	4.981	0	0
Bis-D-Fructose 2',1:2,1'-Dianhydride	0	0	0	0	0	0
4-Oxoproline	160.983	64.532	26.552	328.592	10.172	77.788
Argpyrimidine	0	0	0	2.118	0	0
4-Chloroacetophenone	5.395	12.074	12.972	2.835	4.622	81.642
2-Naphthylamine	0	0	3.6	0	0	0.134
His-Leu	0	1.099	0.015	0.104	0	0
L-Histidine	98.402	0.155	25.119	0.441	11.393	7.799
L-Tryptophan	0	0	0	0	0	0
L-Glutamic Acid	0	0	0	0	0.322	0.572

ACKNOWLEDGEMENTS

The authors would like to acknowledge the assistance offered by Ms. Faith Harvey. The authors would also like to acknowledge partial support provided by an unrestricted grant from Research to Prevent Blindness to the University of Miami.

REFERENCES

Banerjee, S & Mazumdar, S (2012) Electrospray ionization mass spectrometry: a technique to access the information beyond the molecular weight of the analyte. *Int J Anal Chem,* 2012, 1-40. [http://dx.doi.org/10.1155/2012/282574] [PMID: 22611397]

Barbosa Breda, J, Croitor Sava, A, Himmelreich, U, Somers, A, Matthys, C, Rocha Sousa, A, Vandewalle, E & Stalmans, I (2020) Metabolomic profiling of aqueous humor from glaucoma patients - The metabolomics in surgical ophthalmological patients (MISO) study. *Exp Eye Res,* 201, 108268. [http://dx.doi.org/10.1016/j.exer.2020.108268] [PMID: 33011236]

Han, G, Wei, P, He, M, Teng, H & Chu, Y (2020) Metabolomic Profiling of the Aqueous Humor in Patients with Wet Age-Related Macular Degeneration Using UHPLC–MS/MS. *J Proteome Res,* 19, 2358-66. [http://dx.doi.org/10.1021/acs.jproteome.0c00036] [PMID: 32293180]

Ivanisevic, J & Want, EJ (2019) From Samples to Insights into Metabolism: Uncovering Biologically Relevant Information in LC-HRMS Metabolomics Data. *Metabolites,* 9, 308. [http://dx.doi.org/10.3390/metabo9120308] [PMID: 31861212]

Jauregui, AM, Parellada, SE, Neag, E & Bhattacharya, SK (2023) Analysis of Brain Metabolites Using Two Complementary Ultrahigh-Performance Liquid Chromatography–Mass Spectrometry Methods. *Methods Mol Biol,* 2571, 133-42. [http://dx.doi.org/10.1007/978-1-0716-2699-3_13] [PMID: 36152157]

Najdekr, L, Blanco, GR & Dunn, WB (2019) Collection of Untargeted Metabolomic Data for Mammalian Urine Applying HILIC and Reversed Phase Ultra Performance Liquid Chromatography Methods Coupled to a Q Exactive Mass Spectrometer. *Methods Mol Biol,* 1996, 1-15. [http://dx.doi.org/10.1007/978-1-4939-9488-5_1] [PMID: 31127542]

Pietrowska, K, Dmuchowska, DA, Samczuk, P, Kowalczyk, T, Krasnicki, P, Wojnar, M, Skowronska, A, Mariak, Z, Kretowski, A & Ciborowski, M (2017) LC-MS-Based Metabolic Fingerprinting of Aqueous Humor. *J Anal Methods Chem,* 2017, 1-13. [http://dx.doi.org/10.1155/2017/6745932] [PMID: 28154769]

Tham, YC, Li, X, Wong, TY, Quigley, HA, Aung, T & Cheng, CY (2014) Global prevalence of glaucoma and projections of glaucoma burden through 2040: a systematic review and meta-analysis. *Ophthalmology,* 121, 2081-90. [http://dx.doi.org/10.1016/j.ophtha.2014.05.013] [PMID: 24974815]

Zhang, N, Wang, J, Li, Y & Jiang, B (2021) Prevalence of primary open angle glaucoma in the last 20 years: a meta-analysis and systematic review. *Sci Rep,* 11, 13762. [http://dx.doi.org/10.1038/s41598-021-92971-w] [PMID: 34215769]

CHAPTER 49

Protocols for Performing CRISPR Gene Editing in Anterior Chamber Eye Cells

Sam Yacoub[1,*], **Charles E. Amankwa**[1] and **Gulab Zode**[1]

[1] *Department of Pharmacology and Neuroscience and The North Texas Eye Research Institute, University of North Texas Health Science Center, Fort Worth, TX 76107, USA*

Abstract: The Clustered Regularly Interspaced Short Palindromic Repeats (CRISPR) technology has revolutionized genetics and opened up new possibilities for research and therapy. The CRISPR system is composed of single guide RNA (sgRNA) and the endonuclease (Cas9), which can be combined into a ribonucleoprotein complex (RNP). RNP can be used to target and cut specific DNA regions. The introduction of foreign DNA at the cut's site allows for precise genome editing, such as insertion, deletion, or substitution of specific genes. This powerful technology has been widely adopted in many fields, including basic research, drug discovery, and biotechnology. Its ability to efficiently edit genes has made it an essential tool for studying gene function, developing new therapies for genetic diseases, and improving crops and livestock. This chapter will discuss the utility of CRISPR/Cas9 and sgRNA using trabecular meshwork Cells (GTM3 cells), highlighting the limitations and potential alternative methods. We will also describe the T7 endonuclease I (T7EI) assay, a protocol used to confirm gene editing.

Keywords: Clustered regularly interspaced short palindromic repeats, Delivery methods, Guide RNA, Gene modification.

INTRODUCTION

The Clustered Regularly Interspaced Short Palindromic Repeats (CRISPR) system is a revolutionary gene editing technology that has revolutionized the field of genetics and created many exciting possibilities for research and therapeutic development. (Doudna & Charpentier, 2014). The CRISPR/Cas system is a bacterial immune system composed of short repetitive sequences and DNA fragments from previously encountered foreign DNA that provides adaptive im-

* **Corresponding author Sam Yacoub:** Department of Pharmacology and Neuroscience and The North Texas Eye Research Institute, University of North Texas Health Science Center, Fort Worth, TX 76107, USA;
E-mail: Sam.Yacoub@unthsc.edu

Najam A. Sharif and Sunny E. Ohia (Eds.)

munity in most prokaryotic organisms (Barrangou *et al*., 2007; Jinek *et al*., 2012). Recently, this system has been adapted for use as a gene-editing tool and has transformed the field of genetic research and opened up the possibility of treating a wide range of genetic diseases (Doudna & Charpentier, 2014).

The CRISPR/Cas9 system is a highly versatile and efficient gene-editing tool that uses a guide RNA (gRNA) to direct the Cas9 endonuclease to specific target sequences in the genome. Upon binding to the target site, Cas9 cleaves the DNA, allowing for the insertion, deletion, or substitution of specific genetic sequences with high precision (Hsu *et al*., 2014; Doudna & Charpentier, 2014). This system has been widely adopted in various fields, including basic research, drug discovery, and biotechnology, and has facilitated significant advancements in these areas (Sander & Joung, 2014).

However, the delivery of CRISPR/Cas9 to target cells remains a challenge due to the large size of the system and the potential toxicity associated with some delivery methods (Wang *et al*., 2016). Several approaches have been developed to overcome this limitation, including viral, non-viral, and physical methods of delivery, which can be used to deliver plasmids, ribonucleoprotein complex (RNPs), or other components of the CRISPR system (Wang *et al*., 2016; Chen *et al*., 2019).

Here, we will review the various methods for delivery of CRISPR/Cas9 and gRNA to ocular cell lines (We will use the GTM3 cell line as an example) and ways to confirm gene editing, highlighting the limitations of each approach and suggesting possible alternative methods.

EXPERIMENTAL PROTOCOLS

The following procedures were approved by the University of North Texas Health Science Center Institutional Animal Care and Use Committee review board.

Cell Selection: GTM3

Transformed GTM3 cell line (Pang, I. H *et al*., 1994) were cultured in DMEM (Sigma) supplemented with 10% fetal bovine serum (Atlas Biologicals, Fort Collins, CO), 1% L-glutamine (Gibco, Life Technologies), and 1% penicillin-streptomycin (Gibco, Life Technologies).

Cell Seeding: Forward Versus Reverse Seeding

Forward seeding and reverse seeding are two methods used to introduce cells into a culture. In forward seeding, cells are added to the culture at a low density and allowed to grow and divide over time to reach confluence. This method is commonly used when growing cells for long-term experiments or cell-based assays (Freshney, 2010). In reverse seeding, cells are added to the culture at a high density, often close to confluence, and then allowed to attach and spread. This method is commonly used for short-term experiments or for cells that do not adhere well to the culture surface (Masters *et al.*, 2018). The choice between forward and reverse seeding depends on the specific research goals and the studied cells' characteristics. For example, forward seeding may be preferred for long-term studies or for cells that require time to adjust to the culture environment, while reverse seeding may be used for short-term studies or for cells that do not adhere well (Estrada *et al.*, 2017).

Selection of CRISPR System Components

Selection of gRNA

Single-guide RNA (sgRNA) is a crucial element of the CRISPR-Cas9 gene-editing system, and its design is essential for the efficiency and specificity of the system. The following guidelines are used for designing efficient and specific sgRNA for gene editing, and several online tools are available to help with this process:

a. **Choose the target site:** The target site should be conserved across different alleles, specific to the gene of interest, and located near a protospacer adjacent motif (PAM) sequence that is required for Cas9 binding and cleavage.
b. **Avoid off-target effects:** To avoid off-target effects, sgRNA should not target sites with homology to non-targeted genes. Various online tools such as CRISPOR (Haeussler *et al.*, 2016) and E-CRISP (Heigwer *et al.*, 2014) are available to predict off-target effects and assist with sgRNA design.
c. **Optimize sgRNA design:** The design of the sgRNA should be optimized for efficiency and specificity, with consideration of factors such as the length of the sgRNA, the GC content, and the location of the PAM sequence. Various online tools such as Benchling (https://benchling.com/crispr) and CHOPCHOP (https://chopchop.cbu.uib.no) are available to help with sgRNA design and optimization.

By following these guidelines and utilizing online tools, one can design efficient and specific sgRNA for gene editing, allowing for precise and targeted modifications to the genome.

Selection of Appropriate Cas9 Enzyme

The CRISPR-Cas system for gene editing requires the selection of the appropriate Cas9 enzyme, which is a critical step. Among various Cas enzymes, Cas9 from

Streptococcus pyogenes is commonly used in genome editing due to its high efficiency and specificity (Jinek *et al*., 2012). However, other Cas enzymes, such as Cpf1 and Cas12a, have been developed that offer certain advantages. For instance, Cas12a is useful in some applications as it requires a shorter guide RNA (gRNA) and is more efficient than Cas9 (Zetsche *et al*., 2015). On the other hand, Cpf1 is often used when a smaller delivery vehicle is required, such as for *in vivo* gene editing, and its staggered DNA cleavage pattern can be beneficial for certain types of edits (Zetsche *et al*., 2017).

The choice of the Cas enzyme depends on several factors, including the target sequence, delivery method, and desired outcome. However, one should consider the limitations of these enzymes, such as the limited availability of Cas12a orthologs, which can make gene editing more challenging (Chen *et al*., 2018). Furthermore, the potential for off-target effects and the need for precise delivery methods are some of the critical challenges to consider when choosing a Cas enzyme (Kleinstiver *et al*., 2016).

To address these limitations, scientists are currently researching ways to optimize the CRISPR-Cas system, including the development of new Cas enzymes and delivery methods (Gao *et al*., 2020).

Protocols Based on Selected Delivery Methods

The delivery method for the CRISPR Cas9 system should also be considered. There are several methods available for delivery, such as transfection, electroporation, or viral transduction (Wang *et al*., 2019).

Non-viral Delivery Methods

There are several non-viral delivery methods for CRISPR/Cas9 gene editing technology. These methods do not use viral vectors, which can pose safety concerns and have cell type and efficiency limitations. Some common non-viral delivery methods for CRISPR include:

Lipid-based delivery: This method involves the use of lipid nanoparticles, such as liposomes, to deliver the CRISPR components into cells. The lipid nanoparticles can be functionalized to target specific cell types, increasing the efficiency of delivery (Yin, H. *et al.* (2014)).

Electroporation: This method uses an electric field to create transient pores in the cell membrane, allowing for the introduction of the CRISPR components (Porteus, M. H. (2015)).

Microinjection: This method involves physically injecting the CRISPR components into individual cells using a micropipette. This method is relatively low-throughput but can be useful for studying rare or difficult-to-transfect cells (Wang, L., *et al.* (2017)).

Sonoporation: This method uses high-frequency ultrasound to create temporary pores in the cell membrane, allowing for the introduction of the CRISPR components (Chen, Y. C., *et al.* (2015)).

Nanoparticle delivery: This method involves the use of nanoparticles, such as gold nanoparticles or polymeric nanoparticles, to deliver the CRISPR components into cells. The nanoparticles can be functionalized to target specific cell types, increasing the efficiency of delivery (Jiang, W. *et al.* (2015)).

Each of these non-viral delivery methods has its own advantages and disadvantages, and the choice of delivery method will depend on the specific requirements of the study.

Protocol for Non-Viral Delivery Method (Lipofection)

Lipofection is a non-viral method of delivering cargo proteins or nucleic acid; in our case, we will deliver CRISPR components into cells. It involves the use of lipid-based carriers, called liposomes, to encapsulate and transport its cargo into the target cells (Felgner, P. L. (1997).). The liposomes are formed by mixing the lipid and cargo in an aqueous solution, creating small, spherical structures that can then be added to the cells. Once the cells take up the liposomes, the lipid bilayer fuses with the cell membrane, releasing the cargo into the cytoplasm to manifest its function. (Wu, J., Huang, C. Y., & Langer, R. 1999).

3.1.1) Begin by placing both the supplied sgRNA and Cas9 endonuclease enzyme on ice. Gently mix them by briefly centrifuging and spinning them.

3.1.2) To prepare the sgRNA, use a nuclease-free buffer to create a 1μM stock solution. This solution can be stored in a -20°C freezer for up to 6 months.

3.1.3) Dilute the original stock of Cas9 using OptiMEM media to create a 1μM concentration.

3.1.4) Prepare 250 μL ribonucleoprotein complex (RNP) as follows:

a. 15 μL sgRNA (1 μM stock solution)
b. 15 μL Cas9 (1μM stock solution)
c. 6 μL Cas9 Plus Reagent (comes with the lipofectamine kit)
d. Add 214 μL OptiMEM media.
e. Incubate at room temperature for 5 min to assemble the RNP complexes.

Note: The RNP complex can be stored for up to 4 weeks at 4°C or for up to 6 months at –80°C. Store at 4°C for two days.

3.1.5) To the RNP complex mix, add 12 µL of transfection reagent (Lipofectamine) and 238 µL of Opti-MEM media. Incubate the resulting 500 µL transfection complex at room temperature for 20 minutes (Fig. **1**).

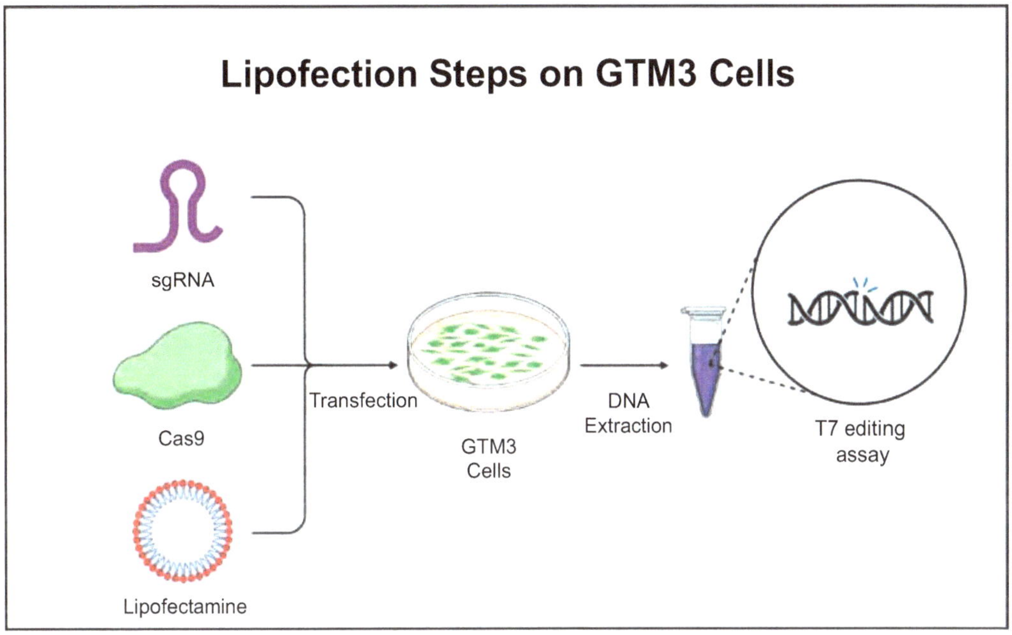

Fig. (1). Flow-chart illustrating non-viral transfection of GTM3 cells using lipofectamine..

3.1.6) Gently drop down the transfection mix on a 10 cm petri dish that has GTM3 cells with a confluency of 40% (volume of 1mL media without antibiotic; FBS can still be added at this stage); gently rock the plate back and forth till you have a homogenized media.

3.1.7) Incubate the plate containing the transfection complexes and cells in a tissue culture incubator (37ºC, 5% CO_2) for 24 hours.

3.1.8) After the incubation period, replace the media with fresh media and incubate for another 24 hours.

3.1.9) After the final incubation period, wash the cells with PBS twice and harvest the DNA using a DNA collection kit.

3.1.10) Store the DNA until you are ready to run the T7 assay, which will be explained in detail later in this chapter.

Viral Delivery Methods

The delivery of CRISPR components, including guide RNA (gRNA) and Cas9 or other endonucleases, into cells can be achieved using viral vectors. Common viral vectors used for CRISPR delivery include adenoviruses, lentiviruses, and adeno-associated viruses (AAVs).

Adenovirus-mediated delivery: The CRISPR components are packaged into the adenovirus, which is then used to infect target cells. Once the adenovirus enters the target cell, the CRISPR components are released and can initiate the gene editing process (Kim *et al.*, 2013).

Lentivirus-mediated delivery: Lentiviruses have also been widely used for CRISPR delivery due to their ability to infect a broad range of cell types, including non-dividing cells. Lentiviruses carrying CRISPR components are introduced into target cells, where the viral genome integrates into the cellular DNA and expresses the CRISPR components (Wang *et al.*, 2013).

Adeno-associated viruses (AAVs): AAVs are another popular viral vector for CRISPR delivery due to their low pathogenicity and ability to persist in target cells for long periods of time. AAVs carrying CRISPR components are introduced into target cells, where the viral genome integrates into a specific site on chromosome 19 and expresses the CRISPR components (Sudol *et al.*, 2019).

Protocol for Viral Delivery Method: AAV2

3.2.1) Select a viral vector: The first step in viral transduction is to select a suitable viral vector. The most commonly used viral vectors include retroviruses, lentiviruses, and adeno-associated viruses (AAVs).

3.2.2) Production of viral particles: Once a viral vector has been selected, the next step is to produce viral particles. The production of viral particles involves transfecting host cells with the viral vector plasmid and then collecting the viral particles that are secreted into the cell culture medium.

3.2.3) Purification of viral particles: The collected cell culture medium is then purified to isolate the viral particles. Common methods of viral particle purification include ultracentrifugation, column chromatography, or precipitation with polyethylene glycol.

3.2.4) Transduction of target cells: The purified viral particles are then used to transduce the target cells. This can be achieved by directly adding the viral particles to the cells or by incubating the cells with the viral particles.

3.2.5) Optimization of transduction efficiency: The efficiency of transduction can be influenced by various factors, such as the type of viral vector used, the amount of viral particles added, and the duration of incubation. Therefore, optimization of transduction efficiency is necessary to achieve the desired level of transduction.

3.2.6) Detection of transgene expression: Once the cells are transduced, the expression of the transgene can be detected by various methods, such as fluorescence microscopy, flow cytometry, or Western blotting.

Genome Editing Detection

The T7 Endonuclease I (T7EI) assay is a commonly used technique for verifying the results of gene editing experiments performed with the CRISPR-Cas9 system (Kleinstiver *et al.*, 2015). This assay is based on the ability of T7 endonuclease to cleave single-stranded DNA (ssDNA), producing a characteristic banding pattern that can be visualized on an agarose gel and used to confirm specific gene editing events (Sharma *et al.*, 2018).

The T7EI assay is a highly efficient method for gene editing confirmation and can be easily incorporated into high-throughput screening protocols (Kim *et al.*, 2016). Additionally, this assay is sensitive enough to detect even low levels of gene editing events (Perli *et al.*, 2017). It can be used to confirm a wide range of gene editing outcomes, including insertions, deletions, and substitutions (Szczepek *et al.*, 2016).

A T7 gene editing confirmation kit provides all necessary reagents and materials for performing the T7EI assay, making it a convenient solution for researchers who wish to quickly and accurately confirm their gene editing results. The kit typically includes T7 endonuclease, reaction buffer, and a detailed protocol, making it easy to set up the assay (Sharma *et al.*, 2018).

4.1) Extract genomic DNA: The first step in the assay is to extract genomic DNA from the edited cells. This can be done using a variety of methods, such as phenol-chloroform extraction or commercial DNA extraction kits.

4.2) The Polymerase Chain Reaction (PCR) amplification:

Subsequently, the specific genomic region of interest is amplified *via* PCR utilizing primers that flank the target site, as exemplified by MYOC gene primers presented in Table **1**. The technique necessitates several essential constituents, such as two oligonucleotide primers, a heat-resistant DNA polymerase, deoxynucleotide triphosphates (dNTPs), a reaction buffer, and magnesium, as described by Saiki *et al.*, (1988).

Table 1. Primers (MYOC gene) (Stock 100µM)

Forward Primer	**5'- GTT CTT CTG TGC ACG TTG C-3'**
Reverse Primer	**5'- GGG GAC ACT GGC CCC TTC TCA GC-3'**

4.2.1) To prepare the PCR reaction mix, add approximately 400 ng of DNA (2-4 µl) and adjust the total volume to 25µl using a variable amount of nuclease-free water according to Table **2**.

Table 2. Master mix.

Nuclease-Free Water	11.5 µL
5X Buffer (Promega Green GoTaq®)	5.0 µL
Taq Polymerase (Promega Green GoTaq®)	0.5 µL
dNTPs (10 mM)	1.0 µL
Forward Primer (10µM)	1.0 µL
Reverse Primer (10µM)	1.0 µL
$MgCl_2$ (25mM)	1.0 µL
DNA	4 µL
Total Volume	**25 µL**

4.2.2) To ensure accuracy, it is advised to conduct controls. Please prepare the controls as per Table **3**.

Table 3. PCR Protocol for Alt™ Control A & B Master mix.

Nuclease-Free Water	15.5 µL
5X Buffer (Promega Green GoTaq®)	5.0 µL
Taq Polymerase (Promega Green GoTaq®)	0.5 µL
dNTPs (10 mM)	1.0 µL
$MgCl_2$ (25mM)	1.0 µL
Alt™ Control A/ Alt™ Control B (template/primer mix)	2 µL
Total Volume	**25 µL**

4.3) After amplification, the PCR products are subjected to denaturation and reannealing to generate heteroduplex DNA molecules. This is achieved by heating the PCR products to 95°C for 5 minutes, followed by gradual cooling to 25°C. A thermal cycler is used to execute PCR, allowing for controlled temperature cycling through a series of repetitive steps that entail denaturation of the target

DNA template, annealing of primers to complementary sites on the template, and extension of primers by DNA polymerase, according to (McPherson *et al.*, 2002). This leads to the exponential amplification of the target DNA, enabling the production of millions or billions of copies of a particular DNA sequence in a single reaction. The PCR conditions must be optimized to ensure the specific amplification of the target sequence.

4.3.1) Amplify the 25µl of the final reaction mix in 38 thermal cycles (Table **4**), followed by the final chain extension step at 72°C for 7 minutes (Table **5**).

Table 4. Cycling conditions.

Step	Temperature (°C)	Time (min: sec)	Cycles
Denature	94	5:00	1
Denature	94	0:30	38
Anneal	56	0:45	
Extend	72	0:45	
Extend	72	7:00	1

Table 5. Cycling conditions.

Step	Temperature (°C)	Time (min: sec)	Cycles
Denature	95	5:00	1
Denature	98	0:20	38
Anneal	65	0:15	
Extend	72	0:30	
Extend	72	8:00	1

4.4) Treatment with T7 endonuclease I: Once the heteroduplex DNA molecules are formed, they are treated with T7 endonuclease I enzyme. This enzyme cleaves DNA at mismatched sites, which results in the generation of smaller DNA fragments.

4.4.1) Form heteroduplex for T7E1 Digestion Kit IDT (Alt-RTM Genome Editing Detection Kit) (Table **6**).

Table 6. Cycling conditions.

Component	Amount	Amount: Homoduplex control	Amount: Heteroduplex control
PCR product (From Step1)	10 µL	10 µL Control A	5 µL Control A 5 µL Control B

(Table 6) cont.....

T7E1 Reaction Buffer (10X)	2 µL	2 µL	2 µL
Nuclease-Free Water	6 µL	6 µL	6 µL
Total Volume	**18 µL**	**18 µL**	**18 µL**

4.4.2) Heat and cool PCR products in a thermal cycler according to Table **7**.

Table 7. Temperature cycling conditions to follow.

Step	Temperature (°C)	Time (min: sec)
Denature	95	10:00
Ramp1	95-85	Ramp rate -2°C/sec
Ramp 2	85-25	Ramp rate -0.3°C/sec

4.4.3) Combine the following in a microcentrifuge tube for the T7E1 Digestion (Table **8**).

Table 8. Combine the following in a microcentrifuge tube for the T7E1 Digestion.

Component	Amount
PCR Heteroduplexes (From step 4a)	18 µL
T7 endonuclease 1(1U/ µL)	2 µL
Total volume	**20 µL**

4.4.4) Incubate the T7E1 reaction at 37°C for 60 min.

4.5) Electrophoresis: The cleaved DNA fragments are then separated by gel electrophoresis on an agarose gel.

4.5.1) Prepare 2% agarose gel in 1X Tris Acetate EDTA (TAE) buffer (pH 8.3). Add 5µl of gel stain and cast the gel in the gel electrophoresis apparatus (Table **9**).

Table 9. Gel preparation for electrophoresis.

Component	Amount
0.5 gm agarose tablet	4 tablets
TAE Buffer	100 mL
Gel Stain	5.00 µL

4.5.2) Load the amplified products (~5 μL) and 5μl of 100bp DNA ladder into the wells.

4.5.3) Apply a voltage of 100 volts during electrophoresis and allow the process to continue for approximately 60-75 minutes.

4.5.4) The PCR products are visualized using the UV transilluminator.

4.5.4) The presence of cleaved DNA fragments indicates that the T7 endonuclease I has recognized and cleaved the mismatched sites in the heteroduplex DNA.

CONCLUSION

In the realm of genetics, CRISPR technology has had a profound impact on the way we approach gene editing and modification. The ability to precisely target and manipulate specific DNA sequences with high efficiency and specificity has opened up new avenues for research and treatment of genetic disorders. The CRISPR system, consisting of sgRNA and Cas9, has proven to be a powerful tool for scientists across different fields, enabling them to investigate gene function, develop new drugs, and enhance agricultural practices.

While CRISPR technology has significant potential, there are limitations and challenges that must be addressed. One such challenge is the delivery of CRISPR components to target cells. Researchers have developed various approaches to overcome this obstacle, including viral and non-viral methods, as well as physical delivery methods.

Another critical aspect of CRISPR technology is the verification of gene editing. The T7 Endonuclease I assay has become a widely used protocol to confirm the efficacy of gene modification.

Overall, CRISPR technology has ushered in a new era of genetic research, offering scientists an unprecedented ability to modify and manipulate genetic sequences with remarkable precision. As we continue to explore the potential of this technology, we must also remain mindful of its limitations and work to develop new and innovative approaches to overcome these obstacles. With continued progress and research, the possibilities of CRISPR technology are limitless, and we can expect to see many more exciting breakthroughs in the field of genetics in the years to come.

REFERENCES

Barrangou, R, Fremaux, C, Deveau, H, Richards, M, Boyaval, P, Moineau, S, Romero, DA & Horvath, P (2007) CRISPR provides acquired resistance against viruses in prokaryotes. *Science,* 315, 1709-12. [http://dx.doi.org/10.1126/science.1138140] [PMID: 17379808]

Chen, JS, Ma, E, Harrington, LB, Da Costa, M, Tian, X, Palefsky, JM & Doudna, JA (2018) CRISPR-Cas12a target binding unleashes indiscriminate single-stranded DNase activity. *Science,* 360, 436-9. [http://dx.doi.org/10.1126/science.aar6245] [PMID: 29449511]

Chen, YC (2015) *In vivo* CRISPR/Cas9-mediated gene editing in mice. *Methods Mol Biol,* 1259, 89-97.

Doudna, JA & Charpentier, E (2014) The new frontier of genome engineering with CRISPR-Cas9. *Science,* 346, 1258096.
[http://dx.doi.org/10.1126/science.1258096] [PMID: 25430774]

Estrada, Y & Garcia-Bates, BM (2017) Cell culture basics: Types of cell culture, cell growth, and assay methods. *In Vitro Cell Dev Biol Anim,* 53, 287-92.

Felgner, PL, Gaedigk, R, Tamir, H, Gref, R, Manthorpe, M & Liu, H (1997) Lipofection: a highly efficient, lipid-mediated DNA-transfection procedure. *Nature,* 387, 863-7.

Freshney, RI (2010) Culture of Animal Cells: A Manual of Basic Technique and Specialized Applications. *John Wiley & Sons, Inc*
[http://dx.doi.org/10.1002/9780470649367]

Gao, R (2020) Genome engineering *via* CRISPR-Cas systems: challenges and opportunities. *iScience,* 23, 100789.

Haeussler, M, Schönig, K, Eckert, H, Eschstruth, A, Mianné, J, Renaud, JB, Schneider-Maunoury, S, Shkumatava, A, Teboul, L, Kent, J, Joly, JS & Concordet, JP (2016) Evaluation of off-target and on-target scoring algorithms and integration into the guide RNA selection tool CRISPOR. *Genome Biol,* 17, 148.
[http://dx.doi.org/10.1186/s13059-016-1012-2] [PMID: 27380939]

Heigwer, F, Kerr, G & Boutros, M (2014) E-CRISP: fast CRISPR target site identification. *Nat Methods,* 11, 122-3.
[http://dx.doi.org/10.1038/nmeth.2812] [PMID: 24481216]

Hsu, PD, Scott, DA, Weinstein, JA, Ran, FA, Konermann, S, Agarwala, V, Li, Y, Fine, EJ, Wu, X, Shalem, O, Cradick, TJ, Marraffini, LA, Bao, G & Zhang, F (2013) DNA targeting specificity of RNA-guided Cas9 nucleases. *Nat Biotechnol,* 31, 827-32.
[http://dx.doi.org/10.1038/nbt.2647] [PMID: 23873081]

Jiang, W (2015) Multiplex genome engineering using CRISPR/Cas systems. *Nat Methods,* 11, 953-8.

Jinek, M, Chylinski, K, Fonfara, I, Hauer, M, Doudna, JA & Charpentier, E (2012) A programmable dual-RNA-guided DNA endonuclease in adaptive bacterial immunity. *Science,* 337, 816-21.
[http://dx.doi.org/10.1126/science.1225829] [PMID: 22745249]

Jinek, M, Chylinski, K, Fonfara, I, Hauer, M, Doudna, JA & Charpentier, E (2012) A programmable dual-RNA-guided DNA endonuclease in adaptive bacterial immunity. *Science,* 337, 816-21.
[http://dx.doi.org/10.1126/science.1225829] [PMID: 22745249]

Kim, D (2016) Efficient CRISPR/Cas9-mediated target mutagenesis in rice using the T7EI assay. *Plant Biotechnol J,* 14, 110-9.

Kim, D (2013) Efficient genome editing in human pluripotent stem cells using TALE-based transcription activator-like effector nucleases. *Nat Biotechnol,* 31, 681-3.
[http://dx.doi.org/10.1038/nbt.2646]

Kleinstiver, BP, Pattanayak, V, Prew, MS, Tsai, SQ, Nguyen, NT, Zheng, Z & Joung, JK (2016) High-fidelity CRISPR–Cas9 nucleases with no detectable genome-wide off-target effects. *Nature,* 529, 490-5.
[http://dx.doi.org/10.1038/nature16526] [PMID: 26735016]

Kleinstiver, BP (2015) High-fidelity CRISPR-Cas9 nucleases with no detectable genome-wide off-target effects. *Nature,* 523, 481-7.
[http://dx.doi.org/10.1038/nature14592] [PMID: 26098369]

Ladda, RL (1982) Resolution of DNA restriction fragments separated by agarose gel electrophoresis using a

non-denaturing system. *Anal Biochem,* 126, 206-13.
[PMID: 6285763]

Laemmli, UK (1970) Cleavage of structural proteins during the assembly of the head of bacteriophage T4. *Nature,* 227, 680-5.
[http://dx.doi.org/10.1038/227680a0] [PMID: 5432063]

Masters, JR & Huxley, TR (2018) Cells: A Laboratory Manual. *Cold Spring Harbor Laboratory Press.*

McPherson, M. J. *et al.* (1997) Principles and applications of PCR amplification. McPherson, M. J. and M. E. M. McPherson

McPherson, M. J. *et al.* (2002) Taq polymerase and PCR technology: Past, present, and future. McPherson, M. J. and M. E. M. McPherson

Pang, IH, Shade, DL, Clark, AF, Steely, HT & DeSantis, L (1994) Preliminary characterization of a transformed cell strain derived from human trabecular meshwork. *Curr Eye Res,* 13, 51-63.
[http://dx.doi.org/10.3109/02713689409042398] [PMID: 8156826]

Perli, SD (2017) Evaluation of T7 endonuclease I for assessment of CRISPR/Cas9-induced genomic deletions. *Biotechniques,* 63, 245-9.

Porteus, MH (2015) CRISPR-Cas9 gene editing in human stem cells. *Nat Biotechnol,* 33, 903-6.

Saiki, RK (1988) Enzymatic amplification of β-globin genomic sequences and restriction site analysis for diagnosis of sickle cell anemia. *Science,* 239, 487-91.
[http://dx.doi.org/10.1126/science.2448875] [PMID: 2448875]

Sander, JD & Joung, JK (2014) CRISPR-Cas systems for editing, regulating and targeting genomes. *Nat Biotechnol,* 32, 347-55.
[http://dx.doi.org/10.1038/nbt.2842] [PMID: 24584096]

Sharma, A (2018) A rapid and simple T7 Endonuclease I assay for gene editing confirmation. *J Vis Exp,* e56935-5.

Sudol, M (2019) The Gene Ontology Resource: 20 years and still GOing strong. *Nucleic Acids Res,* 47, D330-8.
[http://dx.doi.org/10.1093/nar/gky1055] [PMID: 30395331]

Szczepek, M (2016) T7 Endonuclease I-assisted generation and analysis of large genomic deletions. *Nat Commun,* 7, 13014-4.

Wang, H, Yang, H, Shivalila, CS, Dawlaty, MM, Cheng, AW, Zhang, F & Jaenisch, R (2013) One-step generation of mice carrying mutations in multiple genes by CRISPR/Cas-mediated genome engineering. *Cell,* 153, 910-8.
[http://dx.doi.org/10.1016/j.cell.2013.04.025] [PMID: 23643243]

Wang, L (2017) Microinjection of CRISPR/Cas9 components for targeted gene editing in mouse zygotes. *Nat Protoc,* 12, 851-62.

Wang, M (2016) Delivery of CRISPR/Cas9 by nonviral technology: bench to bedside. *Biotechnol J,* 11, 1558-69.
[http://dx.doi.org/10.1002/biot.201600]

Wang, M (2019) Efficient delivery of genome-editing proteins using bioreducible lipid nanoparticles. *Proc Natl Acad Sci USA,* 116, 10756-61.
[PMID: 26929348]

Wu, J, Huang, CY & Langer, R (1999) Preparation and characterization of liposome-entrapped plasmid DNA. *J Control Release,* 60, 27-40.

Yin, H (2014) Lipid-mediated delivery of RNA and protein for gene regulation and functional genomics. *Nat Protoc,* 9, 222-35.

Zetsche, B, Gootenberg, JS, Abudayyeh, OO, Slaymaker, IM, Makarova, KS, Essletzbichler, P, Volz, SE,

Joung, J, van der Oost, J, Regev, A, Koonin, EV & Zhang, F (2015) Cpf1 is a single RNA-guided endonuclease of a class 2 CRISPR-Cas system. *Cell,* 163, 759-71.
[http://dx.doi.org/10.1016/j.cell.2015.09.038] [PMID: 26422227]

Zetsche, B, Heidenreich, M, Mohanraju, P, Fedorova, I, Kneppers, J, DeGennaro, EM, Winblad, N, Choudhury, SR, Abudayyeh, OO, Gootenberg, JS, Wu, WY, Scott, DA, Severinov, K, van der Oost, J & Zhang, F (2017) Multiplex gene editing by CRISPR–Cpf1 using a single crRNA array. *Nat Biotechnol,* 35, 31-4.
[http://dx.doi.org/10.1038/nbt.3737] [PMID: 27918548]

SUBJECT INDEX

A

B

Najam A. Sharif and Sunny E. Ohia (Eds.)

C

D

E

F

G

H

I

J

K

L

M

N

O

P

Q

R

S

T

U

V

W

X

Y

Z

www.ingramcontent.com/pod-product-compliance
Lightning Source LLC
LaVergne TN
LVHW070942210926
848482LV00002B/73
* 9 7 8 9 8 1 5 3 2 4 3 5 8 *